IMMUNE NETWORKS

ANNALS OF THE NEW YORK ACADEMY OF SCIENCES
Volume 418

IMMUNE NETWORKS

Edited by Constantin A. Bona and Heinz Kohler

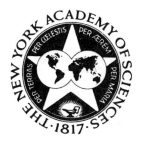

The New York Academy of Sciences
New York, New York
1983

Library of Congress Cataloging in Publication Data

Main entry under title:

Immune networks.

(Annals of the New York Academy of Sciences; v. 418)
"Result of a conference entitled International
Conference on Immune Networks, held on November 29–December 1, 1982, by the New York Academy of Sciences"—P.
   Bibliography: p.
   Includes index.
   1. Immunoglobulin idiotypes—Congresses.   2. Anti-antibodies—Congresses.   3. Immune response—Regulation—Congresses.   4. T cells—Congresses.   I. Bona, Constantin.
II. Kohler, Heinz, 1939–   .   III. International Conference on Immune Networks (1982: New York Academy of Sciences)   IV. Series.   [DNLM: 1. Immunoglobulin idiotypes —Immunology—Congresses.   W1 AN626YL v.418 / QW 601 I323 1982]
Q11.N5   vol. 418   [QR186.7]   500s [616.07'9]   83-26872
ISBN 0-89766-230-X
ISBN 0-89766-231-8 (pbk.)

SP
Printed in the United States of America
ISBN 0-89766-230-X (Cloth)
ISBN 0-89766-231-8 (Paper)
ISSN 0077-8923

ANNALS OF THE NEW YORK ACADEMY OF SCIENCES

VOLUME 418

December 29, 1983

IMMUNE NETWORKS[a]

Editors and Conference Organizers

CONSTANTIN A. BONA and HEINZ KOHLER

CONTENTS

Introductory Remarks. *By* CONSTANTIN A. BONA ix

Part I. Theoretical Aspects of the Immune Network

From Clonal Selection to Immune Networks: Induction of Silent Idiotypes. *By* J. URBAIN, M. FRANCOTTE, J. D. FRANSSEN, J. HIERNAUX, O. LEO, M. MOSER, M. SLAOUI, G. URBAIN-VENSANTEN, A. VAN ACKER, and M. WIKLER 1

Part II. Auto-Anti-Idiotypic Reactions

Studies of the Arsonate System Using Monoclonal Antibodies. *By* J. HIERNAUX, M. SLAOUI, O. LEO, M. MOSER, J. D. FRANSSEN, and J. URBAIN 9

Natural Regulation of Antibody Clones by Auto-Anti-Idiotypic Antibodies in Rabbits. *By* L. S. RODKEY, S. B. BINION, J. C. BROWN, and F. L. ADLER . 16

Regulation of the Anti-Trinitrophenyl Response by Anti-Idiotype Antibodies. *By* G. W. SISKIND, B. S. BHOGAL, J. J. GIBBONS, M. E. WEKSLER, G. J. THORBECKE, and E. A. GOIDL 26

An Independent Regulation of Distinct Idiotopes of the T15 Idiotype by Autologous T Cells. *By* J. CERNY and R. CRONKHITE.............................. 31

Part III. Classical Idiotypic Systems

Maternal-Fetal Transfer of a State of Idiotypic Suppression. *By* A. NISONOFF, M. F. GURISH, and T. F. KRESINA 40

Structural Correlates of Idiotypy in the Arsonate System. *By* M. N. MARGOLIES, E. C. JUSZCZAK, R. NEAR, A. MARSHAK-ROTHSTEIN, T. L. ROTHSTEIN, V. L. SATO, M. SIEKEVITZ, J. A. SMITH, L. J. WYSOCKI, and M. L. GEFTER... 48

Idiotype-Specific T-Helper Cells. *By* M. MCNAMARA, K. GLEASON, and H. KOHLER... 65

[a]This volume is the result of a conference entitled International Conference on Immune Networks, held on November 29–December 1, 1982, by The New York Academy of Sciences.

The Use of a Small Synthetic Antigen to Study Immune Regulation by Way
of Idiotypes. *By* C. J. BELLONE and S. JAYARAMAN 74

Auto-Anti-Allotype Antibody in Allotype-Suppressed Rabbits:
Immunoregulation of Immunoglobulin Synthesis by an Allotype-Idiotype
Network. *By* S. DRAY, A. GILMAN-SACHS, and W. J. HORNG 84

Part IV. Silent Repertoire

Idiotype-Anti-Idiotype Network. III. Genetic Control of Activation of A48Id
Silent Clones Subsequent to Manipulation of the Immune Network. *By*
L. J. RUBINSTEIN and C. A. BONA 97

The Role of Rabbit Immunoglobulin Allotypes in an Immune Network. *By*
J. A. SOGN, K. L. DREHER, L. J. EMORINE, E. E. MAX, S. JACKSON, and
T. J. KINDT 109

Part V. Idiotype Repertoire Analysis

Idiotypic Determinants Used in the Analysis of Antibody Diversification and
as Regulatory Targets. *By* K. BEYREUTHER, J. BOVENS, M.
BRÜGGEMANN, R. DILDROP, G. KELSOE, U. KRAWINKEL, C. MÜLLER, S.
NISHIKAWA, A. RADBRUCH, M. RETH, M. SIEKEVITZ, T. TAKEMORI, H.
TESCH, G. WILDNER, S. ZAISS, and K. RAJEWSKY 121

The Specificity Repertoire of Prereceptor and Mature B Cells. *By*
N. R. KLINMAN, R. L. RILEY, M. R. STONE, D. WYLIE, and D.
ZHARHARY 130

Detailed Analysis of the Public Idiotype of Anti-Hen Egg-White Lysozyme
Antibodies. *By* A. MILLER, L. K. CH'NG, C. BENJAMIN, E. SERCARZ, P.
BRODEUR, and R. RIBLET 140

Analysis of Idiotypic Heterogeneity in the Anti-α1-3 Dextran and
Anti-Phosphorylcholine Responses Using Monoclonal Anti-Idiotype
Antibodies. *By* J. F. KEARNEY, B. A. POLLOK, and R. STOHRER 151

The Effect of Somatic Mutation on Antibody Affinity. *By* P. J. GEARHART 171

Antibody-Specific Regulation of Primary and Secondary B-Cell Responses. *By*
S. K. PIERCE and N. A. SPECK 177

Part VI. Immune Circuits

Restricting Elements in the Immunological Circuitry: the Role of
I Region-Controlled Determinants. *By* T. TADA, K. OKUMURA, S.
MIYATANI, A. OCHI, H. NAKAUCHI, and H. KARASUYAMA 189

The Design of Regulatory Circuitry: Predominant Idiotypy and the Idea of
Regulatory Parsimony. *By* E. E. SERCARZ, B. ARANEO,
C. D. BENJAMIN, M. HARVEY, D. METZGER, A. MILLER, L. WICKER, and
R. YOWELL... 198

Similarities between Transplantation Antigens on
Methylcholanthrene-Induced Sarcomas and T-Cell Regulatory
Molecules. *By* P. M. FLOOD, A. B. DELEO, L. J. OLD, and R. K. GERSHON   206

Idiotype Determined Circuits in Maternally Suppressed Mice. *By* C. VICTOR,
C. BONA, and B. PERNIS 220

The Role of B-Cell I Region Encoded Antigens in T-Cell Dependent B-Cell Activation: I Region Encoded Antigen Density Correlates with Idiotype Expression. *By* K. BOTTOMLY and E. DUNN 230

Part VII. Internal Image and Parallel Sets in the Immune Network

The Internal Image of Catecholamines: Expression and Regulation of a Functional Network. *By* B.-Z. LÜ, P.-O. COURAUD, A. SCHMUTZ, and A. D. STROSBERG 240

Cross-Reactivity of Anti-Idiotypic Antibodies as a Tool to Study Nonimmunoglobulin Proteins. *By* K. SEGE 248

Induction of Anti-Arsonate CRI Positive Antibodies in BALB/c Mice. *By* O. LEO, M. MOSER, J. HIERNAUX, and J. URBAIN 257

Idiotypes of Anti-Major Histocompatibility Complex Antibodies. *By* D. H. SACHS, J. A. BLUESTONE, S. L. EPSTEIN, and R. RABINOWITZ 265

Internal Images of Major Histocompatibility Complex Antigens on T-Cell Receptors and Their Role in the Generation of the T-Helper Cell Repertoire. *By* G. K. SIM and A. A. AUGUSTIN 272

Idiotype Connection Between Anti-Arsonate and Anti-Dinitrophenyl Responses in BALB/c Mice. *By* G. K. LEWIS, Z. KAYMAKCALAN, J. YAO, and J. W. GOODMAN 282

The Level of Expression and the Molecular Distribution of ABPC 48 Idiotopes in Levan- or Anti-Idiotope-Primed BALB/c Mice. *By* P. LEGRAIN and G. BUTTIN 290

Regulation of the Response to $\alpha 1$–3 Dextran in $IghC^b$ Mice. *By* J. PÈNE, H. ZAGHOUANI, and M. STANISLAWSKI 296

Induction of Multi-Specific Antibodies to Bovine Serum Albumin after Production of Anti-Idiotype Antibodies to an Albumin-Specific Monoclonal Antibody. *By* N. J. KRIEGER, A. J. PESCE, and J. G. MICHAEL 305

Shared and Nonshared Idiotypes on Rabbit Anti-Allotype Antibodies. *By* D. W. METZGER 313

Bi-Directional Immune Responses within an Idiotype Network. *By* W. J. HORNG and D. S. KAZDIN 317

Part VIII. Immune Network and Diseases

Anti-Immunoglobulins and Their Idiotypes: Are They Part of the Immune Network? *By* H. G. KUNKEL, D. N. POSNETT, and B. PERNIS 324

Immune Networks in Immediate Type Allergic Diseases. *By* K. BLASER, A. WETTERWALD, E. WEBER, V. E. GERBER, and A. L. DEWECK 330

Cellular and Molecular Mechanisms That Regulate Idiotype Expression in Myeloma Cells. *By* R. G. LYNCH and G. L. MILBURN 346

Idiotypy of Clonal Responses of Mice to Influenza B Virus Hemagglutinin. *By* Y.-N. LIU, J. L. SCHULMAN, and C. A. BONA 356

Anti-Idiotypic Antibodies and Autoantibodies. *By* M. ZANETTI 363

A Monoclonal Antibody That Recognizes Anti-DNA Antibodies in Patients with Systemic Lupus. *By* B. DIAMOND and G. SOLOMON............................ 379

INDEX OF CONTRIBUTORS 387

SUBJECT INDEX 389

Financial assistance was received from:

- A. H. ROBINS COMPANY
- BOEHRINGER INGELHEIM LTD.
- E. I. DU PONT DE NEMOURS & COMPANY
- ELI LILLY & COMPANY
- FOGARTY INTERNATIONAL CENTER, NIH
- McNEIL PHARMACEUTICAL
- MERCK SHARP & DOHME RESEARCH LABORATORIES
- NATIONAL CANCER INSTITUTE, NIH
- NATIONAL SCIENCE FOUNDATION
- NEW ENGLAND NUCLEAR
- ORTHO PHARMACEUTICAL CORPORATION
- SCHERING-PLOUGH CORPORATION
- UNITED STATES AIR FORCE OFFICE OF SCIENTIFIC RESEARCH
- UNITED STATES OFFICE OF NAVAL RESEARCH
- THE UPJOHN COMPANY

Introductory Remarks

CONSTANTIN A. BONA

Department of Microbiology
Mt. Sinai School of Medicine
New York, New York 10029

The discovery of idiotypes in humans by Dr. Kunkel and the discovery of idiotypes in the rabbit by Dr. Oudin, as well as the formulation of the immune network concept by Dr. Jerne, has had a fundamental impact on the thinking of scientists interested in the areas of the structure of immunoglobulin, the generation of antibody diversity, and the regulation of immune responses. The program of this meeting covers various aspects of the immune network with particular emphasis on the new theoretical developments in this concept. We also discuss the idiotype-determined regulation in various antigenic systems, idiotype repertoire, T-cell circuitry, internal images of antigens, and parallel sets. The last session is devoted to the understanding of the mechanisms responsible for the alteration in the communication between clones bound by idiotype links in various diseases.

I hope that our discussions will cultivate new stimulating ideas that could provide impetus for directing future research and that could shed light on existing phenomena that are currently not fully understood.

But better than anticipating the results of our meeting, let us follow the advice of a Sanskrit proverb that says that it is better to wait until nightfall to reflect on the events of the day.

The Role of B-Cell I Region Encoded Antigens in T-Cell Dependent B-Cell Activation: I Region Encoded Antigen Density Correlates with Idiotype Expression. *By* K. BOTTOMLY and E. DUNN 230

Part VII. Internal Image and Parallel Sets in the Immune Network

The Internal Image of Catecholamines: Expression and Regulation of a Functional Network. *By* B.-Z. LÜ, P.-O. COURAUD, A. SCHMUTZ, and A. D. STROSBERG 240

Cross-Reactivity of Anti-Idiotypic Antibodies as a Tool to Study Nonimmunoglobulin Proteins. *By* K. SEGE 248

Induction of Anti-Arsonate CRI Positive Antibodies in BALB/c Mice. *By* O. LEO, M. MOSER, J. HIERNAUX, and J. URBAIN 257

Idiotypes of Anti-Major Histocompatibility Complex Antibodies. *By* D. H. SACHS, J. A. BLUESTONE, S. L. EPSTEIN, and R. RABINOWITZ 265

Internal Images of Major Histocompatibility Complex Antigens on T-Cell Receptors and Their Role in the Generation of the T-Helper Cell Repertoire. *By* G. K. SIM and A. A. AUGUSTIN 272

Idiotype Connection Between Anti-Arsonate and Anti-Dinitrophenyl Responses in BALB/c Mice. *By* G. K. LEWIS, Z. KAYMAKCALAN, J. YAO, and J. W. GOODMAN 282

The Level of Expression and the Molecular Distribution of ABPC 48 Idiotopes in Levan- or Anti-Idiotope-Primed BALB/c Mice. *By* P. LEGRAIN and G. BUTTIN 290

Regulation of the Response to $\alpha1-3$ Dextran in IghC^b Mice. *By* J. PÈNE, H. ZAGHOUANI, and M. STANISLAWSKI 296

Induction of Multi-Specific Antibodies to Bovine Serum Albumin after Production of Anti-Idiotype Antibodies to an Albumin-Specific Monoclonal Antibody. *By* N. J. KRIEGER, A. J. PESCE, and J. G. MICHAEL 305

Shared and Nonshared Idiotypes on Rabbit Anti-Allotype Antibodies. *By* D. W. METZGER 313

Bi-Directional Immune Responses within an Idiotype Network. *By* W. J. HORNG and D. S. KAZDIN 317

Part VIII. Immune Network and Diseases

Anti-Immunoglobulins and Their Idiotypes: Are They Part of the Immune Network? *By* H. G. KUNKEL, D. N. POSNETT, and B. PERNIS 324

Immune Networks in Immediate Type Allergic Diseases. *By* K. BLASER, A. WETTERWALD, E. WEBER, V. E. GERBER, and A. L. DEWECK 330

Cellular and Molecular Mechanisms That Regulate Idiotype Expression in Myeloma Cells. *By* R. G. LYNCH and G. L. MILBURN 346

Idiotypy of Clonal Responses of Mice to Influenza B Virus Hemagglutinin. *By* Y.-N. LIU, J. L. SCHULMAN, and C. A. BONA 356

Anti-Idiotypic Antibodies and Autoantibodies. *By* M. ZANETTI 363

A Monoclonal Antibody That Recognizes Anti-DNA Antibodies in Patients
with Systemic Lupus. *By* B. DIAMOND and G. SOLOMON 379

INDEX OF CONTRIBUTORS 387

SUBJECT INDEX 389

Financial assistance was received from:
- A. H. ROBINS COMPANY
- BOEHRINGER INGELHEIM LTD.
- E. I. DU PONT DE NEMOURS & COMPANY
- ELI LILLY & COMPANY
- FOGARTY INTERNATIONAL CENTER, NIH
- McNEIL PHARMACEUTICAL
- MERCK SHARP & DOHME RESEARCH LABORATORIES
- NATIONAL CANCER INSTITUTE, NIH
- NATIONAL SCIENCE FOUNDATION
- NEW ENGLAND NUCLEAR
- ORTHO PHARMACEUTICAL CORPORATION
- SCHERING-PLOUGH CORPORATION
- UNITED STATES AIR FORCE OFFICE OF SCIENTIFIC RESEARCH
- UNITED STATES OFFICE OF NAVAL RESEARCH
- THE UPJOHN COMPANY

Introductory Remarks

CONSTANTIN A. BONA

Department of Microbiology
Mt. Sinai School of Medicine
New York, New York 10029

The discovery of idiotypes in humans by Dr. Kunkel and the discovery of idiotypes in the rabbit by Dr. Oudin, as well as the formulation of the immune network concept by Dr. Jerne, has had a fundamental impact on the thinking of scientists interested in the areas of the structure of immunoglobulin, the generation of antibody diversity, and the regulation of immune responses. The program of this meeting covers various aspects of the immune network with particular emphasis on the new theoretical developments in this concept. We also discuss the idiotype-determined regulation in various antigenic systems, idiotype repertoire, T-cell circuitry, internal images of antigens, and parallel sets. The last session is devoted to the understanding of the mechanisms responsible for the alteration in the communication between clones bound by idiotype links in various diseases.

I hope that our discussions will cultivate new stimulating ideas that could provide impetus for directing future research and that could shed light on existing phenomena that are currently not fully understood.

But better than anticipating the results of our meeting, let us follow the advice of a Sanskrit proverb that says that it is better to wait until nightfall to reflect on the events of the day.

From Clonal Selection to Immune Networks: Induction of Silent Idiotypes[a]

J. URBAIN, M. FRANCOTTE, J. D. FRANSSEN,
J. HIERNAUX, O. LEO, M. MOSER, M. SLAOUI,
G. URBAIN-VANSANTEN, A. VAN ACKER,
AND M. WIKLER

Laboratory of Animal Physiology
Department of Molecular Biology
Free University of Brussels
Brussels, Belgium

This year is the 100th anniversary of Darwin's death, during which there has been a flood of papers, conferences, and debates. The basic idea of Darwinism is nicely illustrated by the title of the famous book by Jacques Monod: *le Hasard et la Nécessité*.[1] The chance corresponds to the randomness of mutations at the DNA level and necessity can be equated with selective pressure. This basic idea has played a significant role in immunology. The clonal selection theory[2-4] is an extension of the Darwinian concept at the lymphocyte level. It seems to some of us, however, that Darwin did not sufficiently explain the rate of evolution and the emergence of complex networks and regulatory mechanisms that require the simultaneous presence of interacting elements. Let us take a simple example. Imagine that one has two RNAs in a "prebiotic soup," each coding for one enzyme, its own replicate. E_1, the products of RNA_1 is the replicate of RNA_1; the same holds for the other couple. If we leave things as such, all that can happen is competition between the two. Eventually, the most stable, the most accurate, and the fastest replicator will win the game. Similarly, one can describe the immune system as a library of independent clones. If we admit that the beauty of imagination and the logics of complex regulatory mechanisms cannot stem from competition and selection alone, another basic principle should be added. This new principle could look like the emergence of a hypercycle.[5,6] Suppose simply that enzyme one becomes the replicase of RNA_2 and that enzyme two is the replicase of RNA_1 (see TABLE 1). Now instead of being put into competition, the two RNAs are forced to cooperate and to evolve together. In the words of Eigen "the first catalytic couplings must have been weak and complex and the number of genetic participants very large. The hypercycle principle is nonetheless simple: enforced cooperation among otherwise competing genes allowed their mutual survival and regulated their growth. It also made possible a more refined kind of evolution than that open to quasi species alone." If we apply the hypercycle principle to the immune system, we go immediately from the clonal selection theory (competition between quasi species of lymphocytes) to idiotypic networks.[7-12] Clones are no more independent, but they are coupled, connected by the products that distinguish them from each other, namely by their idiotypes.

[a]The laboratory of Animal Physiology is supported by grants from the Belgian State and from Euratom. M. Francotte, O. Leo, and M. Moser have a fellowship from The National Foundation for Scientific Research. M. Slaoui is supported by a grant from the Van Buuren Foundation.

The idiotypic receptor of one clone can deliver inductive or suppressive signals to another clone bearing a receptor able to interact specifically with the idiotype (i.e. an anti-idiotypic receptor). Now idiotypic and anti-idiotypic families are forced to evolve jointly, and this evolution can provide an internal selective pressure allowing the conservation of genes apparently useless. A maximum diversity is maintained, even in the absence of antigen.

To be clear, I would like to define the concept idiotypic network. The word network implies a set of interconnected elements. Idiotypic network means that idiotypes are involved directly in clonal interaction. A minimum network theory does not claim that idiotypic interactions are the only ways of lymphocyte interactions. Also, a minimum idiotypic network hypothesis does not assume that all idiotopes are targets of regulatory mechanisms. An idiotope is first operationally defined by the fact that a corresponding anti-idiotypic antibody can be obtained. It is quite plausible that some idiotopes do not play any role in regulatory mechanisms, or to use the terminology of W. Paul and C. Bona,[13] the world of idiotopes can be divided into regulatory idiotopes and nonregulatory idiotopes. A minimum network theory does not state that functional signals are delivered through idiotypic-anti-idiotypic interactions.

TABLE 1. The Immunization Cascade or the Immune Hypercycle

Sequential sets of anti-idiotypic antibodies are obtained in allotype matched rabbits or syngeneic mice.

Ab1: idiotype of rabbit X.
Ab2: anti-idiotypic antibodies raised against Ab1.
Ab3: anti (anti-)idiotypic antibodies raised against Ab2 in rabbit Y.
  α) Ab3 that just recognize idiotopes of Ab2 and nothing else;
  β) Ab3 that do not bind antigen, but share idiotopes with Ab1. This represents the nonspecific parallel set. It is formally equivalent to immunoglobulins devoid of antibody function that often accompanies the synthesis of Ab1. This set of Ab3 was first demonstrated, using Ab4 antibodies.
  γ) Ab3 that share idiotopes and bind antigen. This subset contains the precursors of Ab1' antibodies that appear in large amounts after antigen injection in Ab3 animals. A large part of Ab1' antibodies are strongly idiotypically cross-reactive with Ab1 antibodies.
Ab4: anti (anti-anti) idiotypic antibodies are raised against Ab3. In many cases, a large part of Ab4 does recognize Ab1 and Ab1' antibodies.

It is now clear that any immune response depends on a complex set of interactions in which several kinds of lymphocytes are brought in close proximity. These lymphocytes are connected by several kinds of molecular interactions including (1) idiotypic-anti-idiotypic interactions, and (2) interactions between the products of the major histocompatibility complex (H2K, K2D, IA, IE, etcetera) and the physiological receptors of T lymphocytes (R anti-H or R anti-I). Antigen can bridge idiotypic communities that normally ignore each other (associative recognition of different epitopes linked on the same backbone).

As a result of these interactions, nonspecific factors are released in the vicinity of interacting partners. These factors, while not recognizing antigens or idiotypes, act on specific targets. Either they are linked to another polypeptide that is itself specific or they can interact only with activated lymphocytes because the receptor of these factors is only present on activated lymphocytes. Regulation in the immune system operates at two levels. The first is the selection of available or expressed repertoires. Newborn lymphocytes are constantly released from bone marrow to periphery. We do not yet understand the rules of positive or negative selection that lead to the available repertoire. The second is the regulation of ongoing responses. This includes feedback mechanisms, increase and decrease in binding affinity, and class switching.

Several kinds of immunological repertoires should be defined. There is first the initial repertoire (R_o), which is germ line encoded and a result of the assortment between germ line pieces (V_H, D_H, J_H, V_L, J_L). This R_o cannot simply be evaluated by $n_1 V_H \times n_2 D_H$, etcetera, because fluctuations occur at the border of recombinational events. This initial repertoire is furthermore expanded by somatic mutations (random nucleotide substitutions or, much more interestingly, genic conversion events). A potential repertoire is therefore created—R_p.

We know from a variety of experimental data that the available or expressed repertoire (R_d) is smaller than the potential repertoire. Of course, natural tolerance restricts the potential repertoire, but also available idiotypic repertoires can be easily modified. Recurrent idiotypes can be suppressed (for example, by maternal or neonatal treatment). The idiotypically suppressed animal is still able to respond to antigen by the compensatory synthesis of other idiotypes.[14]

Alternatively, silent idiotypes that are never expressed after antigen injection only can be induced easily in a variety of systems.[15-18] In those cases, the immune system is manipulated in a predetermined goal, that is, a rabbit can learn to make a predefined idiotype. Therefore, by this kind of experiment, we can expect to learn something about the rules that select available repertoires. We shall first summarize the principle of the immunization cascade. We shall then describe briefly three new sets of data. Finally, we shall "hypercycle" back to one of our first experiments that have been largely ignored or dismissed.

When rabbits X and Y are injected with the same antigen, they respond by the synthesis of different non-cross-reactive idiotypes idx and idy. In the systems, we have used the frequency of idiotypic cross-reactions in the range of a few percents. The available repertoires (idx and idy) could be different, because genetically speaking, the potential repertoires are different. Simply, rabbit Y does not possess the potentiality to make idx. Alternatively, rabbit Y could have the potentiality to make idx but suppressive mechanisms could operate to inhibit the synthesis of idx. If this is the case, the suppressor should be highly specific and discriminate between idx and idy. In other words, the suppressor should be something like Ab2 (an anti-idiotypic antibody). Therefore, if we induce an immune response against Ab2 (an Ab3 antibody), perhaps we shall relieve idx from suppression in rabbit Y. It should be stressed that instead of thinking about suppression of suppression, we could reason in terms of positive selection: Ab2 (anti-idx) injected into rabbit Y could select an idx-like "variant."

Very recently, we extended this kind of experiment. Instead of asking the question, can a randomly chosen rabbit learn to make the idiotype of another rabbit, we asked whether one rabbit could simultaneously make a collection of n idiotypes, characteristics of n other rabbits, having no familial relationships. The experiment proceeded as follows. Several rabbits were injected with antigen (*Micrococcus luteus*). They make specific antibodies, some of which are called Ab1a, Ab1b, Ab1c, and Ab1d. Conventional Ab2 are then raised in allotype-matched rabbits, and they are called Ab2a (anti-Ab1a), Ab2b (anti-Ab1b), etcetera. All these Ab2 are strictly specific for their corresponding Ab1 (Ab2a does not recognize Ab1b). The different Ab2 are then mixed and injected into other naive rabbits. These rabbits respond by the synthesis of a collection of Ab3 antibodies (Ab3a, Ab3b, Ab3c, etcetera). The same rabbits are then injected with Micrococcus antigen. The results are clear-cut and reproducible. One rabbit is now making simultaneously a collection of Ab1' antibodies, Ab1'a, Ab1'b, Ab1'c, etcetera. These antibodies are separate entities, each strongly idiotypically cross-reactive with their corresponding Ab1. For example, we can remove Ab1'a (with a column of Ab2a), and this procedure does not remove Ab1'b, c, etcetera. This finding is a strong confirmation of our earlier data and shows clearly that the potential idiotypic repertoire is the same in all rabbits. An immune response does not rely only on antigenic selection, but depends on the previous idiotypic history of the animal.

We can guide the immune response towards a predetermined goal (idiotypic engineering), and it is important to recall that maternal immunoglobulins of the Ab3 type can strongly influence the immune response of progeny.[19] More generally, we could say that the response of a complex network does not depend only on the structure of the network but also on the previous history. Furthermore, there is an early imprinting period that is crucial.

What is the meaning of the immunization cascade? One possibility is that all genes are there, but many clones are silent because of the presence of idiotype-specific T-suppressor cells. This has been demonstrated in the MOPC 460 system by W. Paul and C. Bona[20] and later confirmed by Dominique Juy et al.[21]

We shall now proceed to a description of three systems (two that are new and unpublished and one old) in which we can induce a silent idiotype. But in these three cases, we can state that the germ line genes responsible for the appearance of Ab1' antibodies are not identical with the genes governing the synthesis of Ab1. (1) BALB/c mice can be manipulated to express the major CRI_A idiotype of A/J mice (see the paper by Leo in this volume and reference 22). (2) BALB/c mice can be induced to make a rabbit idiotype. (3) Newborn lymphocytes from one rabbit, let us say rabbit X, when developing in the presence of "memory cells" from rabbit B, are selected to make the idiotype of rabbit B.

THE ARSONATE SYSTEM

Because the data will be presented in detail in another paper in this volume, we shall limit ourselves to a very brief description of the results. In A/J mice, immunized with arsonate-keyhole limpet hemocyanin (Ars-KLH), there is a major CRI_A that is not expressed in BALB/c mice. DNA data suggest that there is no compelling evidence for the presence of the A/J germ line genes in BALB/c DNA. Nevertheless, BALB mice can be induced to make CRI_A after suitable manipulations. We shall return to this, but we would now like to emphasize a few points. When BALB/c mice are immunized with Ab2, they make Ab3 antibodies. A part of Ab3 antibodies recognizes arsonate. In most of the systems that have been investigated previously, it has been difficult to detect in Ab3 sera the presence of antigen-binding immunoglobulins. Furthermore, BALB/c mice are poor responders to arsonate, but pretreatment with Ab2 leads to a significant amplification of the primary response to arsonate.

We can therefore distinguish at least three subsets of Ab3 antibodies. Subset one is made up of Ab3 antibodies that are just anti-idiotypic antibodies to Ab2 (we shall denote this as subset Ab3α). The second subset does not bind antigen, but is sharing the same idiotopes with Ab1. We shall call this subset Ab3 (id$^+$) or Ab3-1. A third subset not only shares idiotopes but also binds antigen. This subset is already Ab1'. This small subset is clonally amplified when Ab3 animals are primed with antigen. We shall come back to these results at the end.

INDUCTION OF RABBIT IDIOTYPES IN MICE

We and others have shown that the potential idiotypic repertoire is more or less similar in different individuals from one species (rabbits and mice). We would now like to ask the question: Is the idiotypic repertoire similar in different species? Some immunologists will think that the question is nearly trivial. They will argue that diversity is such that one can always find immunoglobulins that can perform the job of others. No special genetic relationships should exist between these immunoglobulins. We can return them the question and ask: If so, why do different individuals injected with the same antigen express different idiotypes? They will probably answer that it is just for stochastic reasons. Now, the answer to our question is yes. This answer has been demonstrated in several ways.

Rabbit anti-idiotypic antibodies (Ab2) were raised against rabbit Ab1 (anti-tobacco mosaic virus (TMV) and anti-Micrococcus). These anti-idiotypic antibodies will be called $Ab2_{TMV}$ and $Ab2_{Mi}$. These are conventional discriminatory Ab2 that do not behave like internal images. As expected, these rabbit anti-idiotypic antibodies do not recognize anti-TMV or anti-Micrococcus antibodies from mice. Each purified Ab2 was coupled to a polyclonal activator, lipopolysaccharide (LPS), and the purified conjugate Ab2-LPS was injected into groups of ten mice. All BALB/c mice injected with rabbit $Ab2_{TMV}$- LPS synthesize Ab3 antibodies that recognize the immunogen $Ab2_{TMV}$ but not $Ab2_{Mi}$ or other control rabbit immunoglobulins. At first sight, these Ab3 could just be anti-idiotypic antibodies that recognize idiotopes of Ab2. The sera of Ab3 mice, however, do bind specifically tobacco mosaic virus. (Remember that these mice have never seen TMV.) Mice injected with rabbit $Ab2_{Mi}$ − LPS do not have such TMV-binding activity.

The level of anti-TMV antibodies is comparable to what is observed during a primary response against tobacco mosaic virus. The sera of Ab3 mice were affinity purified on Ab2 columns. The antibodies that bind to Ab2 were found to be enriched in anti-TMV activity. Furthermore, the appearance of anti-TMV antibodies was found to be strongly T cell dependent. Similar results are obtained when mice are injected with rabbit Ab2 alone, but the level of anti-TMV antibodies is 50-fold lower. The anti-TMV antibodies in Ab3 mice are typically mouse immunoglobulins. They carry Fc markers of mouse immunoglobulin and do not react with rabbit anti-α anti-allotypic antibodies. It is therefore quite certain in this system that the genes coding for Ab1 (rabbits) and for Ab1' (mice) are not identical, although they give rise to antibodies that are strongly idiotypically cross-reactive.

THE OLD AND NEW TALE OF IRRADIATED RABBITS[23,24]

Irradiated recipient rabbits were grafted with lymphoid cells from a donor rabbit hyperimmunized with tobacco mosaic virus. Donor and recipient rabbits were characterized by different allotypes of the a group (the donor was a1/a1 and the recipient a2 or a3). Recipient rabbits then received antigen, and donor cells survived during one or two weeks. Afterwards, all antibody synthesized bore the allotypic a markers of the recipients. Antibodies were therefore produced by host cells that differentiated during radiation recovery. The three most striking findings were the following. (1.) Anti-TMV antibodies synthesized in the recipient were immediately of high affinity. (2.) Despite the fact that donor and recipient antibodies displayed different allotypic a markers, both were idiotypically very similar. It does seem clear that newborn host B lymphocytes that differentiated during radiation recovery, could have been strongly influenced by "the idiotypic network" of donor cells. Host B lymphocytes displaying cross-reactive lymphocytes have been positively selected or imprinted by the idiotypic environment. (3.) Because a1, a2, and a3 are V_H markers, associated with residues of FR1 and FR3, it seems clear that the genes responsible for the appearance of cross-reactive recipient idiotypes are not the same that govern the synthesis of donor antibodies.[25]

It seems clear from the three systems described above, that Ab1′ antibodies must be derived from germ line genes that are not identical to those responsible for the synthesis of starting Ab1.

We could say that every gene is submitted to somatic mutations, nucleotide substitutions giving rise to a quasi species of lymphocytes. (The master lymphocyte is the one still expressing the germ line.) The injection of Ab2 would then provide a selective pressure to favor the variants expressing cross-reactive idiotypes with Ab1. It seems to us, however, that the events leading to the appearance of a silent idiotype occur too frequently and too repeatedly to be accounted for by classical somatic mutations. In other words, these events look like programmed mutations. This proposal is based on the measure of the frequency of B cells able to make CRI$^+$ antibodies in BALB/c mice under conditions of polyclonal activation (in the total absence of antigenic or idiotypic selection). This frequency is something around 10^{-4}. Furthermore, this frequency is tenfold higher in manipulated BALB/c mice. A more plausible hypothesis would be that the nature of the event is genic conversion, by which one gene can interact with another and exchange part of the sequence. If we accept genic conversion as a frequent event in multigenic families and particularly between V_H genes, then we can say that from a logical point of view, the minigene hypothesis of Kabat is fundamentally correct, even for the V piece.[26]

What do we know about physiological networks? Is the immune system a functional idiotypic network? Can we now make a critical evaluation of the network hypothesis? A detailed answer to these questions is dependent upon a careful analysis of the dynamics of immune response in nonmanipulated animals.

Such studies are now at hand, given the present state of immunoengineering. Nonetheless, we would like to make three points. (1.) It is almost impossible to prove that a hypothesis is correct. All we can do is to prove that a crucial point is wrong (Karl Popper).[27] (2.) The idiotype network hypothesis has allowed fascinating manipulations of the immune response and has provided tools for exploring fields that otherwise would have been neglected. (3.) Without the network hypothesis, many data become obscure and are difficult to explain (e.g., the decrease in binding affinity, the sharing of idiotypic specificities between different antibody subpopulations present in the same serum, the occurrence of immunoglobulins devoid of antibody function, but sharing idiotypic specificities, T-helper or -suppressor cells bearing anti-idiotypic receptors, and the matching of idiotypes between T and B cells).

It is hard to escape the conclusion that the network hypothesis has been, is, and will be a useful one in the history of immunology.

We would like to make the following proposals. (1.) The germ line repertoire is very large, perhaps enough to cover the antigenic universe. (2.) The minigene hypothesis is one of the secrets of diversity. This hypothesis is formally proven for D and J pieces. If genic conversion is a frequent event in the set of V genes, then V genes behave as if they were made up of minigenes. (3.) The immune system is a functional idiotypic network. (4.) Self recognition (idiotype interactions and H2 restriction) is the secret of a system whose purpose is to recognize and eliminate nonself. (5.) The idiotypic network could furnish an internal selective pressure, allowing the conservation of genes apparently useless. As we have pointed out elsewhere, this idea does not imply that every V gene is frozen once and forever. All that is needed is the conservation of V genes coding for families of idiotypically interacting molecules.[28]

I would like to close with a few appreciative words. I am deeply grateful to J. Oudin and H. Kunkel who discovered idiotypy and many facets of this fascinating polymorphism. We should not forget N. K. Jerne, whose thoughts on the role and importance of idiotypes and the histocompatibility antigen are invaluable.

ACKNOWLEDGMENT

The authors thank Lea Neirinckx for editorial assistance.

REFERENCES

1. MONOND, J. 1970. Le Hasard et la Nécessité. Editions Le Seuil. Paris.
2. JERNE, N. K. 1955. The natural selection theory of antibody formation. Proc. Natl. Acad. Sci. USA **41**: 849–856.
3. LEDERBERG, J. 1959. Genes and Antibodies. Science **129**: 1649–1653.
4. BURNET, F. M. 1959. The clonal selection theory of acquired immunity. Cambridge University Press.
5. EIGEN, M., M. GARDINER, P. SCHUSTER & R. WINKLER. 1982. The origin of genetic informations. Sci. Am. **246**: 78–94.
6. EIGEN, M. & P. SCHUSTER. 1978. The hypercycle: A principle of natural self-organization. Die Naturwissenschaften **64**: 541–565.
7. JERNE, N. K. 1974. Towards a network theory of the immune system. Ann. Immunol. Inst. Pasteur (Paris) **125C**: 373–389.
8. LINDENMANN, J. 1973. Speculations on idiotypes and homobodies. Ann. Immunol. Inst. Pasteur (Paris) **124C**: 171–184.
9. URBAIN, J. 1976. Idiotypes, expression of antibody diversity and network concepts. Ann. Immunol. Inst. Pasteur (Paris) **127C**: 357–374.
10. BONA, C. & H. HIERNAUX. 1980. Immune response: idiotype-antiidiotypic network. Crit. Rev. Immunol. **2**: 33.
11. ROWLEY, D., H. KOHLER & J. D. COWAN. 1980. An immunological network. Contemp. Top. Immunobiol. **9**: 205–223.
12. URBAIN, J., C. WUILMART & P. A. CAZENAVE. 1981. Idiotypic regulation in immune networks. Contemp. Top. Mol. Immunol. **8**: 113–148.
13. PAUL, W. & C. BONA. 1982. Regulatory idiotypes and immune networks: a hypothesis. Immunology Today **3**: 230–235.
14. WEILER, I. I. 1981. Neonatal and maternally induced idiotypic suppression in Lymphocytic Regulation. C. Bona and P. A. Cazenave, Eds: 245–267. Wiley Press. London.
15. URBAIN, J., M. WIKLER, J.-D. FRANSSEN & C. COLLIGNON. 1977. Idiotypic regulation of the immune system by the induction of antibodies against antiidiotypic antibodies. Proc. Natl. Acad. Sci. USA **74**: 5126–5130.
16. CAZENAVE, P. A. 1977. Idiotypic-antiidiotypic regulation of antibody synthesis in rabbits. Proc. Natl. Acad. Sci. USA **74**: 5122–5125.
17. BONA, C., H. HEBER-KATZ & W. PAUL. 1981. Immunization with a levan-binding myeloma protein leads to the appearance of auto-anti (anti-id) antibodies and to activation of silent clone. J. Exp. Med. **153**: 951–967.
18. WIKLER, M., J.-D. FRANSSEN, C. COLLIGNON, O. LEO, B. MARIAME, P. VAN DE WALLE, D. DEGROOTE & J. URBAIN. 1981. Idiotypic regulation of the immune system. J. Exp. Med. **150**: 184–195.
19. WIKLER, M., C. DEMEUR, G. DEWASME & J. URBAIN. 1980. Immunoregulatory role of maternal idiotypes. Ontogeny of immune networks. J. Exp. Med. **152**: 1024–1035.
20. BONA, C. & W. E. PAUL. 1979. Cellular basis of expression of idiotypes. J. Exp. Med. **149**: 532–539.
21. JUY, D., D. PRIMI & P. A. CAZENAVE. 1982. Idiotype regulation: evidence for the involvement of Igh-C restricted T cells in the M 460 idiotype suppressive pathway. Eur. J. Immunol. **12**: 24–30.
22. MOSER, M., O. LEO, J. HIERNAUX & J. URBAIN. 1983. Induction of silent idiotypes in BALB/c mice. Submitted for publication.
23. VAN ACKER, A., G. URBAIN-VANSANTEN, C. DEVOS-CLOETENS, N. TASIAUX & J. URBAIN. 1979. Synthesis of high affinity antibodies in irradiated rabbits grafted with allogeneic cells from hyperimmune donors. Ann. Immunol. Inst. Pasteur (Paris) **130C**: 385–396.

24. URBAIN-VANSANTEN, G., A. VAN ACKER, B. MARIAME, N. TASIAUX, C. DE VOS-CLOETENS & J. URBAIN. 1979. Synthesis of antibodies and immunoglobulins bearing recipient allotypic markers and donor idiotypic specificities in irradiated rabbits grafted with allogeneic cells from hyperimmune donors. Ann. Immunol. Inst. Pasteur (Paris) **130C:** 397–406.
25. BERNSTEIN, K. E., E. P. REDDY, C. B. ALEXANDER & R. G. MAGE. 1982. A cDNA sequence encoding a rabbit heavy chain variable region of the V_H a2 allotype showing homologies with human heavy chain sequences. Nature (London) **300:** 74–76.
26. KABAT, E. A., T. T. WU & H. BILOFSKY. 1978. Variable region genes for immunoglobulin framework are assembled from small segments of DNA. Proc. Natl. Acad. Sci. USA **75:** 2429–2433.
27. POPPER, K. 1972. The logics of scientific discovery. Hutchinson of London.
28. URBAIN, J. & C. WUILMART. 1982. Some thoughts on idiotypic networks and immunoregulation. Immunology Today **3:** 88–92, 125–127.

DISCUSSION OF THE PAPER

B. PERNIS (*Columbia University, New York*): I think you have shown how many elegant manipulations you can perform on the network, which begins to remind us of the manipulations the neurophysiologists do with the nervous system.

C. A. BONA (*Mt. Sinai School of Medicine, New York*): I have two remarks. First of all, we have just started to learn how heterogeneous the AB2 population is. With respect to the affinity to the specificity for the combined-site-associated or framework-associated idiotypes for the recognition of some paratypic idiotopes (and also with respect to the internal image), I think that if you take several hundred anti-idiotype antibodies specific for a particular idiotope, you will find very few, perhaps just one, that behaves as internal image that mimics the antigen. This is the first point.

J. URBAIN: May I comment about the internal image problem? There is no doubt that, let's say, Ab2 is a heterogeneous population, and, for example, Jerne is distinguishing between Ab2-α and Ab2-β.

BONA: I think you can go over the entire Greek alphabet, because from a functional point of view, the Ab2 are very heterogeneous. I find Ab2-α and β terminology confusing, and it certainly does not cover all functions of Ab2s.

URBAIN: Now, as we look at the internal image, I think one of the most important questions is, Are they just experimental curiosities or do they play a role in the regulation of the immune system? I think that the answer to this question should come from a measurement of the frequency of occurrence of these internal images, and I also think that anti-idiotypic antibodies that behave like antigen and that can be called internal image are always present in very small frequencies.

BONA: I agree. My second point is that we do not know anything about the molecular basis of the idiotype network. And I think that a lot of speculation about the V genes looking as antigens are very "versatile." For example, all of these silent genes that are activated, can actually just be interactions between genes that belong to the same family of gene. I do not rule out so easily random mutation events that are directed or driven by anti-idiotype antibodies or by idiotype that can lead to the expansion of some clones that generally belong to the silent fraction of the repertoire.

Studies of the Arsonate System Using Monoclonal Antibodies[a]

J. HIERNAUX,[b] M. SLAOUI, O. LEO, M. MOSER, J.D. FRANSSEN, AND J. URBAIN

[b]Department of Chemistry and Physics II
and
Laboratory of Animal Physiology
Department of Molecular Biology
Free University of Brussels
Brussels, Belgium

INTRODUCTION

The immune response of A/J mice to arsonate keyhole limpet hemocyanin (Ars-KLH) is characterized by the production of antibodies expressing a cross-reactive idiotype (CRI_A).[1,2] It has been shown that the expression of this CRI_A is linked to Ig C_H d and e haplotype and to the VK-1 locus.[2,3] A more detailed study, using CRI_A^+ hybridoma proteins (HP), has revealed a microheterogeneity within this family of antibodies. Indeed, the amino acid sequences analysis of various CRI_A^+ Ars-binding HP show that they present a few differences within the framework as well as the hypervariable region.[2,4,5] Capra and his collaborators have shown that all CRI_A^+ HP belong to a single family that includes a few CRI^- molecules.[6] Moreover, studies at the DNA level suggest that a very limited number of V genes code for the variable region of the heavy chain of CRI_A^+ antibodies.[7] Therefore, a process involving somatic mutations must be invoked to explain the generation of this heterogenous family of CRI_A^+ hybridoma proteins. Moreover, it has been shown that the serum from A/J mice immunized with Ars-KLH can inhibit the binding of any CRI^+ HP with its autologous rabbit anti-idiotypic antibody, whereas no other CRI^+ HP can inhibit this reaction.[8,9] This phenomenon suggests that any restricted idiotypic specificity of the CRI_A^+ HP can be expressed on the A/J anti-Ars antibodies. The surprising recurrence of those restricted idiotypic specificities seems to argue that similar somatic events occur in any A/J mouse. The complex character of the CRI_A stimulates the interest of its dissection with monoclonal antibodies recognizing distinct idiotopes. We succeeded in preparing several monoclonal anti-idiotypic antibodies. Various properties of one of them (2D3) are discussed here.

CHARACTERIZATION OF THE HYBRIDOMA PROTEIN 2D3

2D3 was obtained by the fusion of the spleen cells of a BALB/c mouse hyperimmunized with A/J anti-Ars antibodies coupled to KLH with the SP2/0 plasmacytoma.

[a]The Laboratory of Animal Physiology is supported by grants from the Belgian State and from Euratom. O. Leo and M. Moser have a fellowship from the National Foundation for Scientific Research. M. Slaoui is supported by a grant from the Van Buuren Foundation.

9

TABLE 1. Inhibition of the Binding of ^{125}I-Labeled 36.65 on 2D3[a]

Unlabeled Inhibitor	Nanograms Required for 50% Inhibition
36.65 (CRI$^+$)	31
36.60 (CRI$^-$)	>2000
R16.7 (CRI$^+$)	28
93G7 (CRI$^+$)	>2000
serum A/J anti-Ars I	218
serum A/J anti-Ars II	170
serum BALB/c anti-Ars	>2000

[a]Polyvinyl plates were coated with 200 ng of affinity purified 2D3.

2D3 is a γ_{2b} κ immunoglobulin that recognizes a cross-reactive idiotope expressed in all individual A/J anti-Ars sera. This idiotope is absent from preimmune A/J serum and has not been detected in the sera from 25 individual BALB/c mice immunized with arsonate keyhole limpet hemocyanin. Interestingly, 2D3 binds the HP 36.65 and R 16.7, but not the HP 93G7 (see TABLE 1). All three are CRI$_A$$^+$ HP[4,5] that have very similar amino acid sequences. Moreover, 2D3 does not recognize 36.60, a CRI$_A$$^-$ hybridoma protein.[4] The HP 36.60 and 36.65 were the kind gift of Dr. M. Gefter; 93G7 and R 16.7 were respectively the kind gift of Dr. J. D. Capra and Dr. A. Nisonoff. A conventional rabbit anti-CRI$_A$ antibody prepared in our laboratory[10] recognizes equally well the three CRI$_A$$^+$ HP 93G7, R 16.7, and 36.65, because each of these HP completely inhibits the binding of any other one to this anti-idiotypic antibody. It seems thus that 2D3 recognizes a cross-reactive idiotype distinct from the idiotypic specificities recognized by our rabbit anti-CRI$_A$ antibody. A binding assay has indicated that the 2D3 idiotope is expressed on 15% of A/J anti-Ars antibodies (see TABLE 2). This percentage is higher than the one found by Marshak-Rothstein et al. for private determinants associated with CRI$_A$$^+$ hybridoma proteins.[9] This finding and the fact that we are dealing with a monoclonal anti-idiotypic reagent having a unique specificity pattern argues against the notion that 2D3 recognizes a private specificity.

SUPPRESSION OF THE EXPRESSION OF THE 2D3 IDIOTOPE IN A/J MICE

Nisonoff and his collaborators have shown that the pretreatment of A/J mice with rabbit anti-CRI$_A$ antibodies results in the suppression of the production of CRI$_A$$^+$ anti-Ars antibodies.[11,12] Nevertheless, those hyperimmunized suppressed mice produce a CRI$^-$ anti-Ars antibody response quite comparable to a normal response. Similar observations have been made when two different BALB/c anti-CRI$_A$ HP were used to

TABLE 2. Binding of Radiolabeled Specifically Purified A/J Anti-Ars Antibodies to Anti-idiotypic Antibodies

^{125}I-labeled Ligand	Unsolubilized Anti-idiotypic Reagent	
	Rabbit Anti-CRI	2D3
Serum A/J anti-Ars I	85%[a]	14%
Serum A/J anti-Ars II	77%	13%

[a]Percentage of total radioactivity bound to the anti-idiotypic reagent

TABLE 3. Anti-Arsonate Response of Mice Pretreated with 2D3[a]

Number of Mice	Dose of 2D3	Amount of Serum Required for 50% Binding[b]
	μg	μl
4	—	0.00032 ± 0.00015
5	10	0.056 ± 0.018
5	150	0.034 ± 0.013
5	250	0.025 ± 0.010

[a]Adult A/J mice were inoculated intraperitoneally with 2D3 (in saline) on days 0 and 3, immunized on days 14 and 28 with 100 μg Ars-KLH emulsified in CFA, and bled on day 46.

[b]500 ng of Ars-bovine serum albumin were unsolubilized on polyvinyl plates. Various dilutions of A/J anti-Ars antisera were incubated overnight at 4° C. The anti-Ars antibody bound to the plate was revealed with a ^{125}I-labeled goat anti-mouse reagent.

pretreat the mice.[13] We performed similar experiments with 2D3, that is, we pretreated A/J mice with various doses of 2D3 before immunization with arsonate keyhole limpet hemocyanin.

By contrast with the experiments of Nisonoff *et al.*,[11,13] we observed that pretreated mice produce 100 times less anti-Ars antibodies that control mice (see TABLE 3). It appears that mice pretreated with large doses of 2D3 (150 μg and 250 μg) do not produce anti-Ars antibodies expressing the 2D3 idiotope, because their sera cannot inhibit the binding of radiolabeled 36.65 on unsolubilized 2D3 (see FIGURE 1). Nevertheless, the sera of those mice can still inhibit the binding of A/J anti-Ars antibodies to the rabbit anti-CRI$_A$ antibody. Mice pretreated with a small dose of 2D3 (10 μg) can still produce anti-Ars antibodies expressing the 2D3 idiotope (see FIGURE 1), although their overall response to Ars-KLH is suppressed.

EXPRESSION OF THE 2D3 IDIOTOPE IN BALB/c MICE

Various experiments performed in our laboratory have shown that silent clones can be activated by an immunization cascade process.[14,15] The presentation of Dr. Leo at this meeting clearly shows that BALB/c mice hyperimmunized with a polyclonal rabbit anti-CRI$_A$ antibody (Ab3 mice) produces CRI$_A$[+] antibodies after injection of

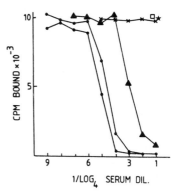

FIGURE 1. Inhibition of the binding of ^{125}I-labeled 36-65 on unsolubilized 2D3. Polyvinyl microtiter plates were coated with 200 ng of 2D3. □: Total binding, ★: Normal A/J serum, ●: A/J mice immunized twice with Ars-KLH, ×: A/J mice pretreated with 150 or 250μg of 2D3 before immunization with Ars-KLH, ▲: A/J mice pretreated with 10μg of 2D3 before immunization with Ars-KLH.

Ars-KLH (Abl' mice). It was obviously interesting to discover whether we could induce a silent idiotope by using a monoclonal instead of a polyclonal antibody. Therefore, we performed similar experiments by immunizing BALB/c mice with 2D3-KLH. Those mice clearly produced Ab3 antibodies as shown by a solid phase radioimmunoassay. Nevertheless, we could not detect Abl' antibodies (i.e. anti-Ars antibodies expressing the 2D3 idiotope) after immunization with arsonate keyhole limpet hemocyanin. Obviously, it can be argued that the lack of detection of anti-Ars antibodies expressing the 2D3 idiotope in Ab3 mice immunized against Ars-KLH does not constitute a final proof that such antibodies cannot be induced. In order to study further the expression of the 2D3 idiotope in BALB/c mice, we measured the frequency of mitogen-reactive BALB/c B cells secreting 2D3 positive immunoglobulins after lipopolysaccharide (LPS) activation. Indeed, polyclonal activation of B cells constitutes another way to reveal the silent repertoire.[16] Under our conditions, one B cell out of twenty is stimulated to proliferation and maturation into antibody secreting cells by LPS, as measured in a protein A plaque-forming cell assay.[17] The data presented in TABLE 4 indicate that it is possible to detect 2D3 positive LPS-reactive B cells in normal BALB/C mice. It is rather unlikely that the observed frequency can be explained by a simple somatic mutation process triggered by lipopolysaccharide. Moreover, our results show that this frequency is significantly enhanced in Ab3 BALB/c mice (i.e.

TABLE 4. Frequency of 2D3 Positive B Cells in BALB/c Mice[a]

Treatment of the Mice	Frequency Among LPS-Reactive B Cells
—	$1/1.7 \times 10^4$
Ab3	$1/2.9 \times 10^3$
Abl'	$1/1.2 \times 10^3$
Abl' control[b]	$1/1.6 \times 10^4$

[a]The number of positive wells was determined by hemagglutination of 2D3 coated sheep erythrocytes.
[b]BALB/c mice immunized with an unrelated antibody and then with Ars-KLH

mice hyperimmunized with 2D3-KLH). Among the 2D3 positive BALB/c B cells detected in our assay, 50% were Ars-binding molecules as determined by an inhibition of hemagglutination assay. Interestingly, the frequency of Ars-reactive B cells is increased in Ab3 mice when compared to normal mice. (Ab3 individuals have never seen the antigen.) The frequency increases from 1 cell out of 250 LPS reactive B cells in the naive BALB/c mice to 1 cell out of 60 LPS reactive B cells in Ab3 mice.

DISCUSSION

This paper deals with some properties of a monoclonal anti-CRI_A antibody that recognizes an idiotope expressed on the CRI_A^+ HP 36.65 and R 16.7, but nonexpressed on another CRI_A^+ HP 93G7. Injection of large doses of 2D3 (150 to 250 μg) into A/J mice prevents the occurrence of $2D3^+$ anti-Ars antibodies after immunization with Ars-KLH, although CRI_A^+ anti-Ars antibodies are still detected in the sera of those suppressed mice.

We investigated this idiotope to see if it was part of the silent repertoire of BALB/c mice that never express it after immunization with arsonate keyhole limpet hemocyanin. First, we tried to reveal it by using the immunization cascade process.[14,15] We assumed that in Ab3 mice (i.e. BALB/c mice hyperimmunized with 2D3), the mechanisms suppressing the expression of 2D3 might be released, as it has been suggested in other systems.[18,19] Nevertheless, we could not detect 2D3[+] anti-Ars Ab1' antibodies after immunization of Ab3 mice with arsonate keyhole limpet hemocyanin. BALB/c mice hyperimmunized with a rabbit anti-CRI$_A$ antibody, however, could produce CRI$_A{}^+$ antibodies.[10] So far, we have been unsuccessful in inducing a silent idiotope with monoclonal anti-idiotypic antibody in our laboratory. Obviously, it should be emphasized that 2D3 only recognizes one idiotope, whereas the rabbit anti-CRI$_A$ antibody recognizes a broader spectrum of determinants. Therefore, it can be expected that the nature of the regulatory events induced by 2D3 or by a rabbit anti-CRI$_A$ antibody are different. The latter seems to be able to induce a total release of the suppression of the expression of the CRI$_A$. On the contrary, it appears that 2D3 can only induce a partial release of suppression and its expression can still be prevented by cross-suppressive mechanisms. Obviously, it can also be argued that the 2D3 idiotope is absent from the repertoire of BALB/c mice. To further test this hypothesis, we studied the expression of the 2D3 idiotope on LPS-reactive B cells. The presence of the 2D3 idiotope could be detected on anti-Ars antibodies secreted by naive BALB/c spleen cells stimulated with LPS *in vitro*. Moreover, the frequency of 2D3 positive B cells was enhanced in Ab3 mice, indicating that hyperimmunization with 2D3-KLH could trigger some idiotypic regulatory mechanisms. The existence of the 2D3 idiotope in the repertoire of BALB/c mice is compatible with the immune network hypothesis of Jerne.[20] Indeed, this hypothesis assumes that the immune network is complete, that is, it should contain any potential antigenic specificity. Therefore, one would expect to find the image of any idiotope in any immune network. It should also be pointed out that CRI$_A{}^+$ plaque-forming cells have been detected in BALB/c mice immunized with Ars-*Brucella*.[21] It seems thus that polyclonal activators can bypass some regulatory signals and induce the production of CRI$_A{}^+$ antibodies in BALB/c mice. CRI$_A{}^+$ clones have also been detected in BALB/c mice by using a splenic fragment culture assay system.[22]

The regulatory mechanisms controlling the expression of certain idiotypes selected among the potential repertoire are not well known. Clearly, a part of the repertoire is silent.[15,19] It seems that the expression of an idiotype depends on a balance between positive and negative signals. Indeed, it has been shown that Id-specific T-suppressor cells could prevent the expression of a given idiotype.[23] No CRI$_A$-specific T-suppressor cells, however, have been evidenced in naive BALB/c mice.[24] It has also been suggested that Id-specific T-helper cells are required for the expression of a given idiotype.[25,26] Such cells might be induced in manipulated mice (Ab3 mice). In this case, it could be argued that there is a hole in the repertoire of Id-specific T-helper cells for the 2D3 idiotope.

ACKNOWLEDGMENT

The authors thank Mrs.L. Neirinckx for editorial assistance.

REFERENCES

1. KUETTNER, M. G., A. L. WANG & A. NISONOFF. 1972. Quantitative investigation of idiotypic antibodies. VI. Idiotypic specificity as a potential genetic marker for the variable regions of mouse immunoglobulin polypeptide chains. J. Exp. Med. **135:** 579.

2. GREENE, M. I., M. I. NELLES, M. S. SY & A. NISONOFF. 1982. Regulation of immunity to the azobenzenearsonate hapten. Adv. Immunol. **32**: 253.
3. LASKIN, J. A., A. GRAY, A. NISONOFF, N. R. KLINMAN & P. D. GOTTLIEB. 1977. Segregation of a locus determining an immunoglobulin genetic marker for the light chain variable region affects inheritence of expression of an idiotype. Proc. Natl. Acad. Sci. USA **74**: 4600.
4. MARSHAK-ROTHSTEIN, A., M. SIEKEVITZ, M. N. MARGOLIES, M. MUDGETT-HUNTER & M. L. GEFTER. 1980. Hybridoma proteins expressing the predominant idiotype of the antiazophenylarsonate response of A/J mice. Proc. Natl. Acad. Sci. USA **77**: 1120.
5. ESTESS, P., E. LAMOYI, A. NISONOFF & J. D. CAPRA. 1980. Structural studies on induced antibodies with defined idiotypic specificities. IX. Framework differences in the heavy- and light-chain-variable regions of monoclonal anti-p-azophenylarsonate antibodies from A/J mice differing with respect to a crossreactive idiotype. J. Exp. Med. **151**: 864.
6. MILNER, E. C. B. & J. D. CAPRA. 1982. V_H families in the antibody response to p-azophenylarsonate: correlation between serology and amino acid sequence. J. Immunol. **129**: 193.
7. SIMS, J., T. H. RABBITS, P. ESTESS, C. SLAUGHTER, P. W. TUCKER & J. D. CAPRA. 1982. Somatic mutation in genes for the variable portion of the immunoglobulin heavy chain. Science. **216**: 309.
8. LAMOYI, E., P. ESTESS, J. D. CAPRA & A. NISONOFF. 1980. Heterogeneity of an intrastrain crossreactive idiotype associated with anti-p-azophenylarsonate antibodies of A/J mice. J. Immunol. **124**: 2834.
9. MARSHAK-ROTHSTEIN, A., J. D. BENEDETTO, R. L. KIRSCH & M. L. GEFTER. 1980. Unique determinants associated with hybridoma proteins expressing a crossreactive idiotype: frequency among individual immune sera. J. Immunol. **125**: 1987.
10. MOSER, M., O. LEO, J. HIERNAUX & J. URBAIN. 1983. Idiotypic manipulations in mice: BALB/c mice can express the crossreactive idiotype of A/J mice. Proc. Natl. Acad. Sci. USA **80**: 4474.
11. HART, D. A., A. L. WANG, L. L. PAWLAK & A. NISONOFF. 1972. Suppression of idiotypic specificities in adult mice by administration of antiidotypic antibody. J. Exp. Med. **135**: 1293.
12. PAWLAK, L. L., D. A. HART & A. NISONOFF. 1973. Requirements for prolonged suppression of an idiotypic specificity in adult mice. J. Exp. Med. **137**: 1442.
13. NELLES, M. J., L. A. GILL-PAZARIS & A. NISONOFF. 1981. Monoclonal antiidiotypic antibodies reactive with a highly conserved determinant on A/J serum anti-p-azopheny-larsonate antibodies. J. Exp. Med. **154**: 1752.
14. URBAIN, J., M. WIKLER, J.-D. FRANSSEN & C. COLLIGNON. 1977. Idiotypic regulation of the immune system by the induction of antibodies against antiidiotypic antibodies. Proc. Natl. Acad. Sci. USA **74**: 5126.
15. URBAIN, J., C. WUILMART & P. A. CAZENAVE. 1981. Idiotypic regulation in immune networks. Contemp. Top. Mol. Immunol. **8**: 113.
16. ANDERSSON, J., A. COUTINHO, W. LERNHARDT & F. MELCHERS. 1977. Clonal growth and maturation to immunoglobulin secretion *in vitro* of every growth-inducible B lymphocyte. Cell **10**: 27.
17. GRONOWICZ, E., A. COUTINHO, F. MELCHERS. 1976. A plaque assay for all cells secreting Ig of a given type or class. Eur. J. Immunol. **6**: 588.
18. BONA, C., R. HOOGHE, P. A. CAZENAVE, C. LEGUERN & W. E. PAUL. 1979. Cellular basis of the regulation of expression of idiotype II. Immunity to anti-MOPC 460 idiotype antibodies increases the level of anti-trinitrophenyl antibodies bearing 460 idiotypes. J. Exp. Med. **149**: 815.
19. BONA, C., J. HIERNAUX. 1981. Immune response: idiotype antiidiotype network. CRC Crit. Rev. Immunol. **2**: 35.
20. JERNE, N. K. 1974. Towards a network theory of the immune system. Ann. Immunol. Inst. Pasteur (Paris) **125C**: 373.
21. LUCAS, A. & C. HENRY. 1982. Expression of the major crossreactive idiotype in a primary anti-azobenzenearsonate response. J. Immunol. **128**: 802.
22. SIGAL, N. H. 1982. Regulation of azophenylarsonate-specific repertoire expression. I. Frequency of crossreactive idiotype-positive B cells in A/J and BALB/c mice. J. Exp. Med. **156**: 1352.

23. BONA, C., W. E. PAUL. 1979. Cellular basis of regulation of expression of idiotype. I. T suppressor cells specific for MOPC 460 idiotype regulate the expression of cells secreting anti-TNP antibodies bearing 460 idiotype. J. Exp. Med. **149:** 592.
24. HIRAI, Y., Y. DOHI, M. S. SY, M. I. GREENE & A. NISONOFF. 1981. Suppressor T cells induced by idiotype-coupled cells function across an allotype barrier. J. Immunol. **126:** 2064.
25. WOODLAND, R. & H. CANTOR. 1978. Idiotype-specific T helper cells are required to induce idiotype-positive B memory cells to secrete antibody. Eur. J. Immunol. **8:** 600.
26. BOTTOMLY, K. & E. D. MOSIER. 1979. Mice whose B cells cannot produce the T15 idiotype also lack an antigen-specific helper T cell required for T15 expression. J. Exp. Med. **150:** 1399.

DISCUSSION OF THE PAPER

C. A. BONA (*Mt. Sinai School of Medicine, New York*): If I were to try to characterize anti-Id antibody in the old way by hemagglutinin inhibition, (if one gets inhibition with immunizing antibody protein, and not with the other protein that carries a cross-reactive idiotype, defined by other antibody), I would say that it is possible that your anti-Id antibody recognizes individual idiotype.

J. HIERNAUX: I know that you could make the argument that 2D3 recognizes a private idiotope. Our argument is that 2D3 recognizes an idiotope that is expressed on two monoclonals. One is R16.7 and the other is 36-65.

BONA: Is this expressed from the same fusion?

HIERNAUX: No, it is not. R16.7 was provided to us by Dr. Nisonoff and 36-65 is from another fusion obtained in a different laboratory. Moreover, this idiotope is expressed in any A/J mouse. It also depends on how you define a private idiotope.

T. MARION (*Yale University School of Medicine, New Haven, Conn.*): Can you find this idiotope, the 2D3, in normal mouse serum? Second, do you know to what antigen the non-Ars binding idiotope molecules bind?

HIERNAUX: To answer your first question, we cannot find this idiotope in normal mouse serum. For the second question, I do not know. I think there might be another talk this morning that addresses that type of question.

MARION: In Janeway's lab, a similar observation has been made in the MOPC 460 idiotype system. One can immunize mice with lipopolysaccharide (LPS) or simulate B cells with LPS, and one finds idiotype-positive, but non-dinitrophenylated (DNP)-binding hybridoma products. Among those non-DNP binding products are antibodies that bind to opportunistic pathogens in mice, for example, *Pasteurella pneumotropica*. Furthermore, these same antibodies can be generated, or hybridomas that make these antibodies can be generated by immunizing mice with anti-MOPC 460 idiotype antibody. In this case, one can find the idiotype-positive antibodies in normal mouse serum, and one can find that those antibodies in normal mouse serum do not bind to dinitrophenol. So we think that what these data may represent, at least, in the MOPC 460 system is that idiotype-positive antibodies that bind to *Pasteurella pneumotropica* may represent a nonspecific parallel set, whereas those that are generated against the DNP epitope may represent the specific parallel set of part of the Ab_3 repertoire.

BONA: Do you know if these antibodies bind to Menadion, because MOPC 315 that binds DNP, also binds to Vitamin K.

MARION: No, we do not know.

Natural Regulation of Antibody Clones by Auto-Anti-Idiotypic Antibodies in Rabbits[a]

L. SCOTT RODKEY,[b] STEVEN B. BINION,[c] JOHN C.
BROWN,[d] AND FRANK L. ADLER[e]

[b]Department of Pathology and Laboratory Medicine
University of Texas Medical School
Houston, Texas 77025

[c]Department of Pathology
University of Iowa Medical School
Iowa City, Iowa 52242

[d]Department of Microbiology
University of Kansas
Lawrence, Kansas 66045

[e]Division of Immunology
St. Jude Children's Research Hospital
Memphis, Tennessee 38101

INTRODUCTION

The purpose of this paper is to review and summarize data accumulated in our laboratories that relate to the ability of normal outbred rabbits to produce auto-anti-idiotypic (AAI) antibodies specific for their own previously synthesized antibody idiotopes. Data collected during the last seven to eight years by numerous laboratories suggest that the immune system can recognize and respond to both foreign and self epitopes. Recent data suggests that a variety of strategies may be employed by the immune system to regulate different elements and compartments within the immune system using the idiotope as the element of recognition.

The outbred rabbit has been used in these studies as a model more similar to the human than the inbred strains of mice, and the rationale behind many of the experimental approaches is to determine what strategies of specific immunoregulation predominate under specified conditions in an outbred species. Further, the well-characterized immunoglobulin (Ig) allotypic markers in rabbits provide convenient markers for controlling purity of reagents and for use as antigens. The *a* locus markers *a*1, *a*2, and *a*3 are particularly useful because they are known to be V-region markers and are heterogenous, with each set possessing several subsets of molecules that share some epitopes and also express unique epitopes.

ARTIFICALLY INDUCED AUTO-ANTI-IDIOTYPIC ANTIBODIES

The initial studies in this series were designed to determine whether it was possible for a normal outbred animal to mount an antibody response specific for its own

[a]This work was supported in part by National Science Foundation Grant PCM79-21110, and National Institutes of Health Grants AI16220 and CA23709.

TABLE 1. Characteristics of Artifically Induced Auto-Anti-Idiotypic Antibodies

- AAI antibodies are specific for autologous antibodies. No cross-reactivity was detected for antibodies of the same specificity from other littermates.
- Idiotype-AAI reactions were hapten inhibitable.
- Maximal proportion of antibodies recognized as bearing an idiotype was 40 percent.

previously synthesized antibody idiotypes.[1] Rabbits were immunized for a period of 189 days with the hapten trimethylammonium (TMA) coupled by diazotization to keyhole limpet hemocyanin, and the anti-TMA antiserum was collected. The immunizations were stopped, and the rabbits were rested for a period of 432 days. Anti-TMA antibodies from each rabbit were purified by affinity chromatography, and the Fab'$_2$ fragments were prepared by pepsin digestion at pH 4.3. Each rabbit was then immunized on day 621 with its own anti-TMA Fab'$_2$ fragments that were polymerized with glutaraldehyde, and sera were collected for the next 39 days. A radioimmunoassay (RIA) was used to assay for auto-anti-idiotypic antibodies in the late sera. The results of this study are summarized in TABLE 1.

This study confirmed the concept that normal outbred animals possess the genetic and biosynthetic capacity to mount auto-anti-idiotypic antibody responses specific for the individual's own, previously synthesized antibody idiotypes. This work verified a fundamental prerequisite in the network concept, namely, that AAI antibodies can be synthesized by normal outbred animals under the appropriate conditions.

The demonstration that AAI antibodies could be regularly elicited under the appropriate conditions led us to question whether the groups of molecules that were recognized as idiotypic by the AAI antibodies were the same or a different set of antibodies as those that were recognized using isologous anti-idiotypic (IAI) antisera.[2] In this paper, IAI antisera are anti-idiotypic antisera elicited in another rabbit that was matched for allotype. Outbred rabbits were immunized with TMA coupled to keyhole limpet hemocyanin, and the anti-TMA antibodies were purified. These antibodies were treated with pepsin to produce the Fab'$_2$ fragments. These fragments were reinjected into the animal that synthesized the antibodies to make the AAI antibodies, and other aliquots of the same antibodies were injected into an allotype-matched recipient to make the IAI reagent. These reagents were used in an RIA in which percentages of molecules bearing idiotypic markers were measured. In further assays, antisera were used in sequential binding assays to determine if the set of molecules recognized by the AAI antisera was contained within the larger set of molecules recognized by the IAI antisera. Hapten inhibition assays were also done to determine if the differences in the sets of molecules recognized by the AAI and the IAI antisera were attributable to any inherent differences in antibody affinity. The results of these studies are summarized in TABLE 2.

TABLE 2. Comparison of Auto-Anti-Idiotypic and Isologous Anti-Idiotypic Reagents

- AAI reagents consistently recognize smaller subsets of idiotypes than do IAI reagents.
- The smaller subset of idiotypes recognized by AAI reagents is included within the set of idiotypes recognized by IAI reagents.
- The differences in the sets of idiotypes recognized by IAI and AAI reagents are not related to affinity of different subsets of antibodies for hapten.

The results of these studies leave little doubt that outbred normal animals have the genetic machinery and synthetic capacity to mount AAI responses under the right conditions. There still remain some interesting unanswered questions related to the possible differences in populations of molecules that were recognized by the AAI as compared to IAI antisera. It is quite possible that the rabbits were tolerant to certain of the idiotopes at the time of reimmunization and that the recipient rabbits that made the IAI antisera were not tolerant. Another possibility that should be considered is whether or not T-helper cells are available for all idiotopes within the individual, as a deficit of T-helper cells for one or more sets of idiotopes could explain the apparent inability of the individual to make AAI antibody for all of its own idiotopes.

NATURALLY OCCURRING AUTO-ANTI-IDIOTYPIC ANTIBODIES

A fundamental requirement of the idiotype network concept of Jerne[3] is that the network be idiotope driven. The network is assumed to work naturally in immunocompetent individuals. The data confirming the existence of the genetic and biosynthetic machinery for making AAI responses are consistent with the network concept, but do not reveal whether or not the system functions naturally to limit immune responses. During a period of approximately three years, work in this laboratory was devoted exclusively to the design of experiments that could detect the presence of naturally occurring AAI antibodies. The general experimental design was to induce immune responses, purify the resulting antibodies, rest the animals, and look for the presence of immunoregulatory AAI antibodies during the rest period. This was done with numerous variations on the general experimental design, and we were consistently unable to detect the presence of AAI antibodies. During these experiments we began using the gram positive bacterium *Micrococcus lysodeikticus* as an antigen for a number of reasons. Work by Wilker, Strosberg, and Urbain with rabbits had demonstrated the extremely immunogenic nature of the micrococcal carbohydrate (CHO) in eliciting antibody responses in rabbits. We reasoned that the AAI response might be similar to other antibody responses in that it might be dose dependent. We felt that limiting the number of clonotypes in the response to a smaller number with higher concentration of each clonotype might favor the triggering of AAI antibodies.

One group of rabbits was immunized with micrococcus vaccine three times weekly for a three-week period followed by a rest period. A second round of injections was followed by another rest period. A total of four rounds of immunizations occurred over a period of one year. In this group of rabbits, one was found that exhibited a strong AAI response, and this response was shown to modify the subsequent immune response to the micrococcal vaccine.[4]

The characteristics of the anti-micrococcal CHO antibody response and the subsequent AAI response are shown in TABLE 3. The AAI response was initially

TABLE 3. Summary of Natural Auto-Anti-Idiotypic Response in Rabbit 102

- AAI antibodies were detected in alternate rounds of the response (second and fourth rounds).
- The idiotype-AAI reaction was hapten inhibitable.
- Circulating complexes were seen in whole serum during AAI synthesis.
- The quantity of AAI cycled during the time it was detectable.
- The presence of AAI was initially detected by dilution precipitation.
- New sets of anti-micrococcal clonotypes were synthesized in response to challenge by vaccine when previous clonotypes were suppressed by AAI antibodies.

TABLE 4. Summary of Idiotope Destruction by Low Concentrations of Reducing Agents

---

- Idiotopes were destroyed by reducing agents and not by oxidizing agents. Allotype epitopes were unaffected by reducing agents.
- Molar ratios as low as 0.025:1 of sulfite:Fab′$_2$ destroyed as much as 50% of idiotopes in some samples.
- Reducing agents have no detectable effect on the antigen-binding capacity of the molecules.
- Mercaptoethanol at concentrations of $1-5 \times 10^{-5}$ M destroyed 10–60% of idiotopes detectable with natural AAI antisera.
- Reducing agents have been shown to destroy idiotopes both in anti-micrococcal and anti-allotype antibody preparations when natural AAI antisera are used for detecting the reactions.

---

detected in this rabbit (number 102) because of an unusual precipitation that occurred whenever second round antiserum from this rabbit was diluted 1:10 to 1:30 in buffered saline. The studies on this animal showed that this precipitation was due to a reaction of idiotype:AAI:rheumatoid factor. Numerous inhibition assays verified the presence of each component of this triplex reaction. The mechanism of this reaction has not been clear until just recently. Nichol *et al.*[5] have recently established a theoretical basis for the dilution-induced precipitation of a three-member interacting system such as we identified. It should be mentioned that a similar dilution-induced precipitation system was noted earlier by Christian[6] in some human sera.

Although the studies of rabbit 102 were clearcut, showing the AAI antibodies had been induced naturally and that the presence of these antibodies had a profound effect on the clonality of the subsequent antibody response, the fact that this animal was one out of a group of fourteen suggested that this characteristic may not have been a common feature of immune responses. Several other groups of animals were immunized in an attempt to detect the natural synthesis of AAI antibodies.

During studies with one group of rabbits, we altered our method of radiolabeling and changed from using the Chloramine-T method[7] to the iodine monochloride (ICl) method.[8] In these studies[9] purified anti-micrococcal Fab′$_2$ fragments were labeled with the Chloramine-T method, and a second aliquot was labeled with the ICl method. Late sera from several animals were assayed for the presence of AAI antibodies using both labeled preparations. The results of these studies are shown in TABLE 4. It was evident from these studies that some of the idiotypic structures that induced the natural AAI antibodies were extremely sensitive to the action of reducing agents, suggesting that these structures were stabilized by a disulfide bond. This bond was sensitive to the action of several reducing agents at concentrations much lower than those needed for intra- or interchain disulfide cleavage in rabbit antibodies. It was found that the concentrations of 2-mercaptoethanol needed for significant destruction of some of the idiotopes was in the range of $1-5 \times 10^{-5}$ M. It is intriguing that this concentration range was the one originally described by Click[10,11] and by Chen and Hirsch[12,13] to dramatically enhance the production of antibodies *in vitro*. Because the addition of such levels of reducing agents has been shown to enhance secondary responses *in vitro*, but not primary responses,[14,15] it is possible that the destruction of the idiotopes that are recognized by natural AAI antibodies could have prevented the recognition of these idiotopes by either idiotype-specific T-suppressor cells or by AAI antibodies. In either case, an enhanced immune respone to the antigen should occur.

Once the extreme reduction sensitivity of the idiotopes was understood, we changed to the use of ICl-labeled Fab′$_2$ fragments of antibodies in our RIA and surveyed a group of nineteen rabbits that had been immunized through several rounds of immunizations with micrococcus.[16] The results of these studies are summarized in TABLE 5. The group of rabbits was surveyed for the presence of AAI antibodies in each individual by RIA, and 42% of those studied showed the presence of AAI antibodies following micrococcal immunizations. The sera were assayed for individual reactivity, and the results showed that there was substantial cross-reactivity in this group of sera. Some degree of cross-reactivity was noted in all but one combination of seven different antibody preparations and seven AAI antisera. Many of the cross-reactions were equal to or greater in quantity of labeled idiotypes recognized than were the homologous reactions. These cross-reactions were shown to be due to identical idiotopes on the antibodies of the different rabbits and not due to the presence of structurally similar, yet nonidentical, idiotope structures. These data are in direct contrast to the data usually obtained in studies of outbred animals even using artifically induced AAI sera from the same individual in that these latter sera recognize individually unique idiotopes.[1] These studies have suggested that the idiotopes that are normally recognized through network-mediated AAI antibodies may be a special group of molecules.

Although we felt that the preceeding study had substantially verified that AAI responses seemed to be an integral part of many immune responses, questions remained about the practical significance of these studies because all animals studied had undergone hyperimmunization and the antibody levels of all these animals were significantly above those usually encountered in most natural immunological responses. For this reason, we sought to find a system for inducing immune responses that was a much more natural system and that did not involve hyperimmunization or any undue amount of experimental manipulation.

In 1963, Steinberg and Wilson[17] described an immunological response in humans that resulted when a child was born of a mother that was heterozygous for two Ig allotypes and the father was homozygous for a different allotype coded at the same locus. This child would then be exposed *in utero,* and by colostral Ig transfer, to Ig of an allotype that was foreign to the child. Their work showed that these offspring made immune responses to these allotypic markers that could be detected as early as seven months and for as long as thirty-five years. This was an immunological system in which the antigenic exposure was a normal developmental event. This system required no external manipulation and thus seemed useful for studies of natural AAI antibody responses.

TABLE 5. Summary of Characteristics of Naturally Induced Auto-Anti-Idiotypic Antibodies

- Naturally induced AAI antibodies were detected in a large fraction (42%) of the animals studied.
- Unlike artifically induced AAI antibodies, naturally induced AAI antibodies showed substantial cross-reactivity with idiotypic antibodies from other AAI-positive rabbits.
- The cross-reactivity was shown by quantitative inhibition assays to be due to the presence of identical idiotopes on anti-micrococcal antibodies from different rabbits.
- These idiotopes were highly reduction sensitive.
- The cross-reactive idiotopes were shown to be the same as idiotopes expressed on antibodies of the same specificity from the father of all of the AAI-positive rabbits.

TABLE 6. Summary of Auto-Anti-Idiotypic Regulation of Natural Anti-Allotype Responses in Rabbits

---

- All offspring studied mounted anti-allotype responses with the day of onset of the responses varying from day 78 to day 176 and with some responses detectable for over 300 days.
- Anti-b5 responses varied in antibody concentration, but variations in specificity were not detected.
- Anti-a1 responses were shown to vary with respect to specificity for different a1 subgroup epitopes.
- AAI antibodies were detected when specificity changes in anti-a1 populations occurred.
- Deliberate immunization re-elicited the anti-a1 specificities that were deleted by AAI responses.
- Idiotopes eliciting natural AAI responses were cross-reactive.

Several studies have shown that a similar type of response can be expected in rabbits in which heterozygous females are crossed with homozygous males. Adler and Noelle,[18] Hagen *et al.*,[19] and Adler and Adler[20] have shown that this type of experimental design frequently induced natural production of anti-allotype antibodies in the offspring to the maternal allotype that was not inherited by the offspring.

This system seemed to be a good one for studying the potential production of a naturally induced antibody, and then following this response, for determining if there was any modification of the response by naturally induced AAI antibodies. A doubly heterozygous female rabbit of allotype a1a2b4b5 was mated with a homozygous male rabbit of allotype a3b4. Seven offspring resulted from this mating, with four of the offspring being a2a3b4, two being a2a3b4b5, and one being a1a3b4. These rabbits were first bled on day 78, and small serum samples were taken at approximately fourteen-day intervals for over a year. These sera were all tested in sensitive RIA protocols for the presence of antibodies specific for the allotype missing from each of the individuals. For example, the a2a3b4 offspring were assayed for anti-a1 antibodies and also for anti-b5 antibodies. The a2a3b4b5 offspring were tested for anti-a1 and the a1a3b4 were tested for the presence of anti-a2 and anti-b5. The results of these RIA experiments[21] showed that all seven of the offspring made antibodies to at least one of the noninherited allotypes, and one of the offspring made antibodies to both a1 and b5 determinants, neither of which were inherited. The time of onset of these responses was found to be highly variable, with some responses detected as early as day 78 and some as late as day 176, indicating that this property is highly variable from individual to individual. Experiments were set up to study the anti-b5 and the anti-a1 responses that were detected in these rabbits. The summary of these experiments is shown in TABLE 6. As indicated in the summary, responses of several rabbits to the noninherited b5 markers showed that all sera bound all b5 molecules in the radioimmunoassay. The only difference in the various anti-b5 antisera was a difference in the quantity of anti-b5 antibodies from different bleedings of each individual. On the other hand, the anti-a1 antisera were shown to be highly variable in their capacity to bind a1 molecules within different bleedings of the same individual. This difference, which was reflected in the RIA results as an apparent cycling of the response, was shown to be due to differences in the specificities of the antibodies that were present at different times and not due to changes in the concentration of anti-a1 antibodies in the consecutive bleedings. The data showed that each succeeding wave of antibody cycle appeared to be specific for a smaller subset of a1 molecules than was the cycle just preceeding it.

Anti-a1 antibodies were purified from the first wave of anti-a1 antibodies from each of two individual's sera. These were pepsin digested and labeled with the ICl method. These antibodies were used in an RIA to attempt to detect anti-idiotypic antibodies specific for the anti-a1 antibodies. These assays showed that AAI antibodies specific for the anti-a1 antibodies were present following each anti-a1 cycle of antibodies. The AAI antibodies showed peaks during the valleys of anti-a1 responses, and the AAI antibodies dropped to minimal levels during peaks of anti-a1 responses. The experimental design used immunization with a1 molecules after the natural anti-a1 had been lowered by AAI action in an attempt to determine if this AAI modulation of the response was permanent or temporary. After injection, sera were taken and titrated against labeled a1 molecules in an RIA to determine if all anti-a1 specificities had been recovered by immunization. The results showed that anti-a1 antibodies specific for all a1 subgroups had been elicited by the deliberate immunization, which suggested that the natural AAI modulating effect was reversible. Other results showed cross-reactivity of the idiotopes that elicited the natural AAI responses. This is in agreement with the data on the characteristics of the natural AAI responses to anti-micrococcal antibodies.[16]

CONCLUDING REMARKS

Evidence has been presented that strongly suggests that normal outbred rabbits possess the genetic and biosynthetic machinery to mount AAI antibody responses. Further evidence was described in which AAI antibodies were found to be synthesized naturally following antibody responses. The antibodies were shown to exert strong influences on the subsequent response to antigen with substantial clonotype shifts occurring in one case and demonstrable shifts in specificity occurring in the second case. It is not yet clear whether these observed shifts are due to the direct action of AAI antibodies, to mechanisms that involve T-suppressor cells, or to the action of AAI antibody on accessory cells such as T-helper cells. Further studies are necessary to clarify the mechanism(s) affected. Studies that have been done in individual idiotype systems in inbred mice suggest that any or all of the mechanisms mentioned above might be functional in a natural outbred animal's immune response.

Results have been presented drawn from two systems in outbred rabbit experiments that suggest that the natural AAI-mediated suppression, regardless of the mechanism, is a transient and reversible suppression. Data from one system[4] show that deleted clonotypes reappeared spontaneously in the absence of AAI antibodies, and those from another system[21] showed that injection of antigen restimulated suppressed clones to synthesize antibodies with specificities that were earlier suppressed by the appearance of AAI antibodies. These data are in agreement with studies done by Strayer et al.[22,23] in which anti-idiotype suppression of T15 responses in adults is a transient type of suppression. Thus, the accumulated evidence suggests that AAI-mediated suppression in the adult outbred animal appears to be a transient rather than permanent type of suppression.

One of the areas we have attempted to clarify to some extent is related to the question of whether all inducible antibodies have idiotopes that can elicit natural AAI responses. Early quantitative studies[1] could not detect more than 40% of antibody molecules capable of eliciting AAI antibodies even after treating the antibody with glutaraldehyde and giving multiple injections of it in complete Freund's adjuvant. The acknowledged general heterogeneity of anti-hapten antibody responses makes these data difficult to interpret, however. Recent work[9] leads us to suggest that the question of possible unique subsets of antibodies with idiotopes that are unusually immunogenic for eliciting AAI production may be valid. The extreme reduction sensitivity of the identical idiotope made in eight of nineteen rabbits studied suggests that a specific disulfide bond may position idiotopes such that they are unusually immunogenic. O'Donnell *et al.*[24] have shown that many variant Ig molecules exist in rabbits with variations in the number and location of cysteine residues in the N-terminal portion of the molecules. These sequence variants were present in low concentrations in normal IgG pools isolated from the serum of nonimmunized rabbits, but they certainly could be dramatically increased in concentration by immunization.

Numerous studies in the past have dealt with the immunological interrelation of mother and fetus. Studies described here show that maternal Ig allotypes are among the first foreign antigens encountered by the developing immune system. This potentially tolerizing stimulus frequently serves as an excellent stimulant for antibody production. This has been documented in humans,[17] rabbits,[18] and mice.[25] Adler and Adler[20] have shown that a complex tolerance-immune state seems to exist in this system. Maternal-fetal effects of placental transfer of idiotypes have been documented as well as have effects of passive transfer of anti-idiotype to neonates. Transfer of anti-idiotype to neonates in the T15 system rendered the offspring unresponsive to antigen challenge.[22,23] Olson and Leslie[26] have shown that antigen-induced maternal immune responsiveness exerts a permanent regulatory influence on idiotype expression by progeny. Kindred and Roelants[27] have shown that adult offspring of immunized mothers exhibit a more restricted clonal response to the antigen to which the mother was immunized. These data lend strong support to the idea that allotypic and idiotypic relationships between mother and offspring can provide early and lasting effects on the immune potential of the offspring.

REFERENCES

1. RODKEY, L. S. 1974. Studies of idiotypic antibodies. Production and characterization of autoantiidiotypic antisera. J. Exp. Med. **139:** 712–720.
2. RODKEY, L. S. 1976. Studies of idiotypic antibodies: reactions of isologous and autologous anti-idiotypic antibodies with the same antibody preparations. J. Immunol. **117:** 986–989.
3. JERNE, N. K. 1974. Towards a network theory of the immune system. Ann. Immunol. Inst. Pasteur (Paris) **125C:** 373–389.
4. BROWN, J. C. & L. S. RODKEY. 1979. Autoregulation of an antibody response via network-induced auto-anti-idiotype. J. Exp. Med. **150:** 67–85.
5. NICHOL, L. W., M. J. SCULLEY & D. J. WINZOR. 1982. The composition-dependence of the extent of reaction between a multivalent acceptor and a bivalent ligand: Implications of self-interaction of the ligand in precipitin effects. J. Theor. Biol. **96:** 723–740.
6. CHRISTIAN, C. L. 1959. A study of rheumatoid arthritis sera: Comparison of spontaneous precipitates and gamma globulin-induced precipitates. Arthritis Rheum. **2:** 289–298.
7. HUNTER, W. M. & F. C. GREENWOOD. 1962. Preparation of iodine-131 labeled human growth hormone of high specific activity. Nature (London). **194:** 495–496.
8. MCFARLANE, A. S. 1958. Efficient trace labeling of proteins with iodine. Nature (London) **182:** 53.
9. BINION, S. B. & L. S. RODKEY. 1983. Destruction of antibody idiotopes with ultra-low concentrations of reducing agents. Mol. Immunol. **20:** 475–483.
10. CLICK, R. E., L. BENCK & B. J. ALTER. 1972. Enhancement of antibody synthesis *in vitro* by Mercaptoethanol. Cell. Immunol. **3:** 156–160.
11. CLICK, R. E., L. BENCK & B. J. ADLER. 1972. Immune responses *in vitro*. I. Culture conditions for antibody synthesis. Cell. Immunol. **3:** 264–276.

12. CHEN, C. & J. G. HIRSCH. 1972. Restoration of antibody forming capacity in cultures of nonadherent spleen cells by Mercaptoethanol. Science **176:** 60–61.
13. CHEN, C. & J. G. HIRSCH. 1972. The effects of mercaptoethanol and of peritonealmacrophages on the antibody forming capacity of nonadherent mouse spleen cells *in vitro.* J. Exp. Med. **136:** 604–617.
14. LUZZATI, A. L. & C. RAMONI. 1981. Primary antibody response of rabbit blood lymphocytes *in vitro.* J. Immunol. Methods. **47:** 201–208.
15. READ, S. E. & D. G. BRAUN. 1974. *In vitro* antibody response of primed rabbit peripheral blood lymphocytes to group A variant streptococcal polysaccharide. Eur. J. Immunol. **4:** 422–426.
16. BINION, S. B. & L. S. RODKEY. 1982. Naturally induced auto-anti-idiotypic antibodies. Induction by identical idiotopes in some members of an outbred rabbit family. J. Exp. Med. **156:** 860–872.
17. STEINBERG, A. G. & J. A. WILSON. 1963. Hereditary globulin factors and immune tolerance in man. Science **140:** 303–304.
18. ADLER, F. L. & R. J. NOELLE. 1975. Enduring antibody responses in "normal" rabbits to maternal immunoglobulin allotypes. J. Immunol. **115:** 620–625.
19. HAGEN, K. L., L. E. YOUNG, R. G. TISSOT & C. COHEN. 1978. Factors affecting natural antiallotype antibody production in rabbits. Immunogenetics **6:** 355–366.
20. ADLER, F. L. & L. T. ADLER. 1982. Consequences of prenatal exposure to maternal alloantigens. Ann. N.Y. Acad. Sci. **392:** 266–275.
21. RODKEY, L. S. & F. L. ADLER. 1983. Regulation of natural anti-allotype antibody responses by idiotype network-induced auto-anti-idiotypic antibodies. J. Exp. Med. **157:** 1920–1931.
22. STRAYER, D. S., H. COSENZA, W. M. F. LEE, D. A. ROWLEY & H. KOHLER. 1974. Neonatal tolerance induced by antibody against antigen-specific receptor. Science **186:** 640–643.
23. STRAYER, D. S., W. M. F. LEE, D. A. ROWLEY & H. KOHLER. 1975. Anti-receptor antibody. II. Induction of long-term unresponsiveness in neonatal mice. J. Immunol. **114:** 728–733.
24. O'DONNELL, I. J., B. FRANGIONE & R. R. PORTER. 1970. The disulphide bonds of the heavy chain of rabbit immunoglobulin G. Biochem. J. **116:** 261–268.
25. WARNER, N. L. & L. A. HERZENBERG. 1970. Tolerance and immunity to maternally derived incompatible IgG_2a-globulin in mice. J. Exp. Med. **132:** 440–447.
26. OLSON, J. C. & G. A. LESLIE. 1981. Inheritance patterns of idiotype expression: Maternal-fetal immune regulatory networks. Immunogenetics **13:** 39–56.
27. KINDRED, B. & G. E. ROELANTS. 1974. Restricted clonal response to DNP in adult offspring of immunized mice: A maternal effect. J. Immunol. **113:** 445–448.

DISCUSSION OF THE PAPER

D. W. SCOTT (*Duke Medical Center, Durham, N.C.*): Do you have any evidence for how restrictive that auto-anti-idiotypic response is?

L. S. RODKEY: We have started working on this problem and that is difficult in the system, but we are looking at this problem by isoelectric focusing. Our preliminary results seem to indicate that the response is substantially smaller than the initial idiotypic response but how much smaller, we cannot yet say. The AAI response does seem to narrow the idiotypic antibody response at different steps.

UNIDENTIFIED SPEAKER: Do you know if these idiotopes require the interaction of both heavy and light chain idiotypes?

RODKEY: Not so far. We have not successfully performed that experiment. We have tried, but we have the problem in this spontaneous auto-anti-idiotype system of incredibly small amounts of material to work with. That particular experiment is difficult to do.

A. GILMAN-SACHS (*University of Illinois Medical School, Chicago, Ill.*): Dr. Rodkey, you said that in the system with the auto-anti-idiotype, antigen is not inhibitable; what were you using for the hapten?

RODKEY: All we could use were Fab fragments, pooled Fab fragments.

GILMAN-SACHS: And that did not inhibit the binding of antigen?

RODKEY: Not at all.

GILMAN-SACHS: Very surprising.

RODKEY: Yes, it is. It was surprising to us.

H. KÖHLER (*Roswell Park Memorial Institute, Buffalo, N.Y.*): Have you observed any quenching of idiotype complexes in your assays?

RODKEY: I am not quite sure what you mean.

KÖHLER: If you have idiotype and anti-idiotype present in the same serum and you measure it, have you observed any quenching of complexes?

RODKEY: Occasionally, yes.

KÖHLER: Could that account for your cycling pattern?

RODKEY: No, I do not think so, not in these particular cases. We looked very hard for complexes in those patterns, looking for the free idiotype when we were looking for auto-anti-idiotype. It appears that the idiotype from the first round seems to be gone. We cannot detect it by trying an inhibition type experiment. It just does not seem to be there in detectable quantities.

Regulation of the Anti-Trinitrophenyl Response by Anti-Idiotype Antibodies[a]

GREGORY W. SISKIND,[b] BALBIR S. BHOGAL,[d]
JAMES J. GIBBONS,[b] MARC E. WEKSLER,[c]
G. JEANETTE THORBECKE,[d] AND EDMOND A. GOIDL[e]

[b]Division of Allergy and Immunology
[c]Division of Geriatrics and Gerontology
Department of Medicine
Cornell University Medical College
New York, New York 10021
[d]Department of Pathology
New York University Medical School
New York, New York 10016
[e]Department of Microbiology
University of Maryland
Baltimore, Maryland 21201

It has been suggested by Jerne[1] that the immune system is self regulated as a consequence of a network of interactions between idiotypes (ids) and anti-idiotypes (anti-id). One of the key predictions from such a hypothesis is that anti-id should be spontaneously produced during the immune response to traditional foreign antigens. Such spontaneous production of auto-anti-id has been observed by several groups[2–5] including our own.[6–10]

We have employed the observation that in some cases the presence of a low concentration of hapten in the assay medium results in an increase in the number of plaque-forming cells (PFC) observed in a Jerne[11] assay, as the basis for the detection of auto-anti-idiotype antibody.[6,7] We suggested that auto-anti-id can bind to Ig on the surface of potential antibody secreting cells, thereby causing a reversible inhibition of antibody secretion. Hapten competes with anti-id for cell-surface antigen receptors (id). Therefore, in the presence of hapten, bound auto-anti-id is displaced, the inhibition of secretion is reversed, and an increase in the number of PFC is observed. Thus, hapten-augmentable PFC represent B cells whose secretion of antibody has been blocked as a consequence of the binding of auto-anti-id to cell surface idiotype. Evidence justifying the use of this assay has been previously published[6,10] and includes (a) the ability to elute with hapten a factor from spleen cells that can cause a specific hapten-reversible inhibition of plaque formation and that has binding and antigenic properties consistent with its being an IgG auto-anti-id; (b) the fact that under certain experimental conditions the number of hapten-augmentable PFC detected in the spleen correlates with the results obtained using a conventional enzyme-linked immunosorbent assay (ELISA) for anti-id in the serum.

With this approach we have demonstrated that auto-anti-id is produced spontaneously during the primary and secondary responses to both T-dependent and T-independent antigens;[5,8] auto-anti-id is produced spontaneously by mice,[5,8,10] rabbits

[a]This work was supported in part by research grants from the National Institutes of Health, U.S.P.H.S. numbers: AG-02347, AG-00541, AG-00239, AI-11694, and AI-03076.

26

TABLE 1. Hapten-Augmentable Plaque-Forming Cells in the Spleens of Rabbits Four Days after the Intravenous Injection of Antigen[a]

Antigen	Direct Anti-TNP PFC/Spleen	Percentage Hapten-Augmentable PFC
	(Geom. Mean $\overset{\times}{\div}$ S.E.) (n)[b]	(Mean ± S.E.)
TNP-BA	26,700 $\overset{\times}{\div}$ 1.3 (4)	33 ± 8
TNP-F	10,600 $\overset{\times}{\div}$ 1.3 (7)	59 ± 16

[a]Rabbits were injected intravenously with 500 µg TNP-F or 3×10^9 TNP conjugated *Brucella abortus* organisms. Hapten-augmentable PFC were detected in the presence of 10^{-9} M TNP-ε-amino-n-caproic acid (TNP-EACA).

[b]N = number of animals

(TABLE 1), and chickens (TABLE 2) after the injection of foreign antigen; auto-anti-id production is T-cell dependent in the mouse[7] and chicken (TABLE 2); there is an age-associated shift in idiotype expression;[7] there is an age-associated increase in auto-anti-id production.[9] The age-related increase in auto-anti-id production has been confirmed serologically using an ELISA assay. Binding of enzyme-labeled anti-2,4,6-trinitrophenyl (TNP) ids, obtained from mice immunized with TNP-Ficoll (F), to anti-TNP-F antiserum, averaged 48 ± 6 optical density (O.D.) units (405 nm) with antiserum from 1½ to 2 month-old mice and 108 ± 13 O.D. units with antiserum from 12 to 15 month-old animals. Binding to normal mouse serum averaged 22 ± 3 O.D. units. That aged mice produce high auto-anti-id responses is also suggested by studies of Klinman.[13]

We have carried out a series of cell transfer experiments to determine the cellular basis for the increased incidence of hapten-augmentable PFC following immunization of old mice with trinitrophenyl-lysyl-Ficoll. Normal young C57BL/6 mice were lethally irradiated (950R), were reconstituted with spleen cells from either young or old normal syngeneic mice, were immunized with 10 µg TNP-F one day after cell transfer, and were sacrificed seven days later. As indicated in TABLE 3, mice reconstituted with spleen cells from aged donors have a high incidence of hapten-augmentable PFC, whereas mice reconstituted with spleen cells from young donors have relatively few. Transfer of thymus cells from young donors together with the spleen cells from old mice does not eliminate the production of a marked hapten-augmentable PFC response (data not shown). Thus the tendency of aged mice to produce a marked auto-anti-id response appears to be an intrinsic property of their spleen-cell population. Treating the spleen cells from aged donor with anti-Thy-1 and complement prior to transfer does not eliminate this ability to generate a marked auto-anti-id response (data not shown), suggesting that the auto-anti-id response of

TABLE 2. Hapten-Augmentable Plaque-Forming Cells in the Spleen of Normal and Neonatally Thymectomized Chickens Four Days after the Intravenous Injection of Trinitrophenyl-lysyl-Ficoll[a]

Treatment	Direct Anti-TNP PFC/Spleen	Percentage Hapten-Augmentable PFC
	(Geom. Mean $\overset{\times}{\div}$ S.E. (n))	Mean ± S.E.)
Normal	31,700 $\overset{\times}{\div}$ 1.2 (6)	38 ± 6
Thymectomized	21,500 $\overset{\times}{\div}$ 1.1 (4)	5 ± 2

[a]Eight month-old chickens were injected with 100 µg TNP-F. Hapten-augmentable PFC were detected in the presence of 10^{-7} M TNP-EACA.

TABLE 3. Irradiated Mice Reconstituted with Spleen Cells from Normal Aged C57BL/6 Donors Have a High Incidence of Hapten-Augmentable Plaque-Forming Cells after Immunization with Trinitrophenyl-lysyl-Ficoll[a]

Donor Age	Anti-TNP PFC/Spleen	Percentage Hapten-Augmentable PFC
(Months)	(Mean ± S.E.)	(Mean ± S.E.)
4	17,000 ± 3,000	6 ± 5
18	10,000 ± 1,200	109 ± 25

[a]Assayed seven days after antigen injection. Assays were performed in the presence of concentrations of TNP-EACA ranging from 10^{-9} to 10^{-7} M in half-log increments. The maximum hapten-augmentation of plaque formation observed is reported. Results presented are based upon groups of four or five mice.

aged mice is less T-cell dependent than is that of young mice. Similar cell transfer experiments were performed reconstituting mice with bone marrow cells from young or old donors. As indicated in TABLE 4, recipients of bone marrow from young and from old donors both have a low incidence of hapten-augmentable plaque-forming cells.

Thus the bone marrows of old and young mice behave similarly, whereas the peripheral spleen cell populations of old and young mice are clearly different. It would appear that the bone marrow of aged mice is capable of producing a distribution of B-cell clones (ids) indistinguishable from that of young mice, but that the populations of B-cells resident in the spleens of old and young mice are different in this respect. It was hypothesized that id-anti-id interactions between B cells arising from the bone marrow and long-lived T cells in the periphery could result in a difference in id distribution in the peripheral B-cell system as compared with that generated from the bone marrow. This hypothesis was tested by mixed cell transfer experiments in which lethally irradiated, thymectomized, young mice were reconstituted with bone marrow from young or old donors together with splenic T cells from young or old donors. The recipients were immunized with TNP-F five days after cell transfer. It can be seen from the data presented in TABLE 5 that if the peripheral T-cell population comes from young donors, the recipients produce relatively few hapten-augmentable PFC regardless of whether the bone marrow is from old or young mice. Conversely, if the peripheral T cells are obtained from old donors, the recipients produce relatively more hapten-augmentable PFC regardless of the source of the bone marrow. Thus the results are consistent with the hypothesis developed above.

In conclusion, it appears that the bone marrow of aged mice is capable of producing

TABLE 4. Irradiated Mice Reconstituted with Bone Marrow from Normal Aged C57BL/6 Mice Have a Low Incidence of Hapten-Augmentable Plaque-Forming Cells after Immunization with Trinitrophenyl-lysyl-Ficoll[a]

Donor Age	Direct Anti-TNP PFC/Spleen	Percentage Hapten-Augmentable PFC
(months)	(Mean ± S.E.)	(Mean ± S.E.)
2–3	4,000 ± 600	13 ± 3
18	1,380 ± 220	7 ± 5

[a]Assayed seven days after antigen injection. Assays were performed in the presence of concentrations of TNP-EACA ranging from 10^{-9} to 10^{-7} M in half-log increments. The maximum hapten-augmentation of plaque formation observed is reported. The results presented are based upon groups of four mice.

TABLE 5. Influence of Splenic T Cells on the Incidence of Hapten-Augmentable Plaque-Forming Cells Produced by Transferred Bone Marrow[a]

Bone Marrow Donor	Splenic T-Cell Donor	Percentage Hapten-Augmentable PFC
(months)	(months)	(Mean ± S.E. (n))
2–3	2–3	12 ± 4 (6)
2–3	18	55 ± 12 (9)
18	2–3	16 ± 5 (10)
18	18	38 ± 12 (7)

[a]Assayed seven days after injection of 10 μg TNP-F. Assays were performed in the presence of concentration of TNP-EACA ranging from 10^{-9} to 10^{-7} in half-log increments. The maximum hapten-augmentation of plaque formation observed is reported. Splenic T cells (95% or greater Thy-1 positive) were prepared by passing spleen-cell suspensions through an anti-Ig-mouse Ig column (Wigzell column).

a distribution of B cells comparable to that produced by bone marrow of young mice. Idiotype anti-idiotype antibody interactions between B cells arising from the bone marrow and peripheral T cells result in a shift in the distribution of clones in the B-cell population and lead to the high auto-anti-id response typical of aged mice. It is suggested that the long-lived peripheral T-cell population serves as repository for information on shifts in ids resulting from life-long intereactions with environmental and self antigens. Unpublished observations (Bhogal *et al.*) on antigen-fed rabbits suggest that ingested antigens might be important in this respect.

REFERENCES

1. JERNE, N. K. 1974. Towards a network theory of the immune system. Ann. Immunol. Inst. Pasteur (Paris) **125**(C): 373.
2. KLUSKENS, L. & H. KOHLER. 1974. Regulation of the Immune Response by autogenous antibody against receptor. Proc. Nat'l Acad. Sci. USA **71**: 5083.
3. COSENZA, H. 1976. Detection of anti-idiotype reactive cells in the response to phosphorylcholine. Eur. J. Immunol. **6**: 114.
4. BANKERT, R. B. & D. PRESSMAN. 1976. Receptor-blocking factor present in immune serum resembling auto-anti-idiotype antibody. J. Immunol. **117**: 457.
5. MCKEAN, T. J., F. P. STUART & F. W. FITCH. 1974. Anti-idiotypic antibody in rat transplantation immunity. I. Production of antibody in animals repeatedly immunized with alloantigens. J. Immunol. **113**: 1876.
6. SCHRATER, A. F., E. A. GOIDL, G. J. THORBECKE & G. W. SISKIND. 1979. Production of auto-anti-idiotypic antibody during the normal immune response to TNP-Ficoll. I. Occurrence in AKR/J and BALB/c mice of hapten-augmentable anti-TNP plaque forming cells and their accelerated appearance in recipients of immune spleen cells. J. Exp. Med. **150**: 138–153.
7. GOIDL, E. A., A. F. SCHRATER, G. W. SISKIND & G. J. THORBECKE. 1979. Production of auto-anti-idiotypic antibody during the normal immune response to TNP-Ficoll. II. Hapten-reversible inhibition of anti-TNP plaque forming cells by immune serum as an assay for auto anti-idiotype antibody. J. Exp. Med. **150**: 154–165.
8. SCHRATER, A. F., E. A. GOIDL, G. J. THORBECKE & G. W. SISKIND. 1979. Production of auto-anti-idiotypic antibody during the normal immune response to TNP-Ficoll. III. Absence in nu/m mice: evidence for T cell dependence of the anti-idiotypic antibody response. J. Exp. Med. **150**: 808–817.
9. GOIDL, E. A., A. F. SCHRATER, G. J. THORBECKE & G. W. SISKIND. 1980. Production of auto-anti-idiotypic antibody during the normal immune response. IV. Studies of the

primary and secondary responses to thymic-dependent and independent antigens. Eur. J. Immunol. **10:** 810–814.

10. GOIDL, E. A., G. J. THORBECKE, M. E. WESKLER & G. W. SISKIND. 1980. Production of auto-anti-idiotypic antibody during the normal immune response. V. Changes in the auto-anti-idiotypic antibody response and the idiotype repertoire associated with aging. Proced. Natl. Acad. Sci. USA **77:** 6788–6792.

11. GOIDL, E. A., T. HAYAMA, G. M. SHEPHERD, G. W. SISKIND & G. J. THORBECKE. 1983. Production of auto-anti-idiotypic antibody during the normal immune response. VI. Hapten augmentation of plaque formation and hapten-reversible inhibition of plaque formation as assays for anti-idiotypic antibody. J. Immunol. Methods **58:** 1–17.

12. JERNE, N. K. & A. A. NORDIN. 1963. Plaque formation in agar by single antibody-producing cells. Science **140:** 405.

13. KLINMAN, N. 1981. Antibody-specific immunoregulation and the immunodeficiency of aging. J. Exp. Med. **154:** 547.

DISCUSSION OF THE PAPER

C. A. BONA (*Mt. Sinai School of Medicine, New York*): Dr. Siskind, is it possible that in your anti-idiotype antibodies you have a fraction displaying rheumatoid activity?

G. W. SISKIND: This is all, of course, hapten reversible, so certainly there may be rheumatoid factor there. It would not be the material, however, that we are particularly measuring here, because this particular auto-anti-id is site specific, in the sense that it is hapten reversible.

An Independent Regulation of Distinct Idiotopes of the T15 Idiotype by Autologous T Cells[a]

JAN CERNY AND RICHARD CRONKHITE

Department of Microbiology
University of Texas Medical Branch
Galveston, Texas 77550

INTRODUCTION

The immune response to phosphorylcholine (PC) in BALB/c mice is one of several experimental models in which the existence of autochthonous anti-idiotypic reactivity has been demonstrated, both at humoral[1,2] and cellular[3] levels. Furthermore, there is evidence that the self-recognition of the T15 idiotype on PC-reactive immunocytes contributes to the regulation of the anti-PC response.[4,5]

The anti-idiotypic response, which has been measured using the whole T15 idiotype represented by PC-reactive myeloma proteins, TEPC-15 and HOPC-8, may be a sum of different responses. It appears that an immunoglobulin bearing the T15 idiotype is an extremely complex antigen consisting, perhaps, of a dozen or more distinct determinants, called idiotopes. If these idiotopes were recognized independently by non-cross-reacting autoimmune anti-idiotopic clones, measurements of the response against the whole antigen complex (the idiotype) might obscure the specific response involved in the immune regulation. The image of the network could be further confounded by a possible idiotopic heterogeneity of PC-reactive lymphocytes.

In this article, we will summarize the evidence for the antigenic complexity of the T15 idiotype and for the idiotopic heterogeneity of PC-reactive, T15-bearing lymphocyte populations of inbred mouse strains, including BALB/c. Data will be presented suggesting that the individual idiotope(s) constituting T15 are recognized by sets of specific T cells and that various idiotope positive lymphocyte clones are regulated independently of one another, in a genetically determined fashion, by the autochthonous T-cell responses.

ANTIGENIC COMPLEXITY OF THE T15 IDIOTYPE AND THE IDIOTOPIC HETEROGENEITY OF T15-POSITIVE, PHOSPHORYLCHOLINE-REACTIVE LYMPHOCYTES

An important tool for the analysis of the T15 idiotype has been the monoclonal antibody generated against TEPC-15 or HOPC-8 myeloma proteins in several laboratories. The list in TABLE 1 includes the hybridomas selected for their private specificity towards TEPC-15/HOPC-8 and no other PC-reactive myeloma protein.[6-8]

Does each monoclonal antibody recognize a different, non-cross-reactive idiotope

[a]This work was supported in part from United States Public Health Service Grant R01 AI 19072.

TABLE 1. Monoclonal Antibodies against Individual Epitopes (=Idiotopes) of the T15 Idiotype (TEPC-15/HOPC-8)

Antibody		Hapten-inhibition		Expression on IgM Anti-PC
Clone	Ig Class	PC-chloride (mol)	PC-KLH (μg)	Antibody-forming Cells from BALB/c
AB1-2[a]	γ^1	−	+ ⎫	Frequent ($\geq$80% PFC
MaId 5-4[b]	γ^1	−	+ ⎬	all mice)
B36-82[c]	μ	−	30 ⎭	
B39-38[c]	γ^1	−	− ⎫	
B36-39[c]	γ^1	−	− ⎬	(Frequent?)[d]
B36-69[c]	γ^1	10^{-5}	10 ⎭	
B36-75	γ^1	10^{-3}	20 ⎫	
B24-50[c]	γ^{2b}	−	− ⎬	Rare (40% PFC
B24-44[c]	γ^1	10^{-5}	1 ⎭	$\leq$1/2 of the mice)

[a] John Kearny, University Alabama in Birmingham (reference 7).
[b] Christoph Heusser, CIBA, Basel (reference 8).
[c] G. Hammerling, DFKZ, Heidelberg (reference 6).
[d] Only a small number of BALB/c mice have been tested.

on the T15 molecule (which would be designated by the name of the hybridoma, i.e., the antibody AB1-2 binds to the AB1-2 idiotope, etcetera)? The answer seems to be yes, but the evidence is circumstantial.

First, the inhibition of binding of the antibodies to TEPC-15 by the PC hapten reveals significant differences among anti-idiotopes (TABLE 1). Some idiotopes, like B36-69, B36-75, and B24-44, are displaced by PC-chloride, suggesting that the antibodies bind to a paratopic idiotope. Other idiotopes, AB1-2, MaId5-4, and B36-82 are displaced only by PC coupled to a large protein, which implies that the target idiotope is "near paratopic." The remaining two, B39-38 and B24-50, appear to react

TABLE 2. T15 Idiograms of Individual C57BL/6 Mice[a]

		PFC Inhibitable With:					
Experiment	Animal No.	AB1-2	MaId5-4	B36-82	B36-75	B24-50	B24-44
A	1	+	−	+	−	−	−
	2	+	+	+	−	−	−
	3	−	+	+	−	−	−
	4	+	+	+	+	−	−
B	5	+	−	+	−	−	−
	6	+	+	+	+	−	+
	7	+	+	+	−	−	+
	8	+	+	+	−	+	+
C	9	+	nt	nt	−	nt	+
	10	+	nt	nt	−	nt	−
	11	−	nt	nt	−	nt	−
	12	−	nt	nt	−	nt	−

[a] PC-specific plaque-forming cells (PFC, day 4 after immunization of spleen cells *in vitro*) from individual donors were analyzed by inhibition with various monoclonal anti-idiotopic Ab described in TABLE 1 and in the text. + = inhibition by 30% to >80%; − = lack of idiotopic expression (inhibition <15%); nt = not tested.

with nonparatopic determinants. Second, the pattern of reactivity of the monoclonal anti-idiotope(s) with PC-immune sera and with PC-reactive cells indicates that idiotope determinants recognized by individual antibodies can be independently expressed. Hammerling and Wallich tested pooled PC-immune sera from various inbred mouse strains for reactivity with the monoclonal anti-T15 antibodies using a radioimmunoassay. They found that a given antiserum reacted, for example, with AB1-2, but not with B24-50. When antisera collected from six different mouse strains were assayed against the panel of anti-T15 antibodies, a pattern of independent expression of each putative idiotope emerged.[6] This pattern has been confirmed and extended in our studies on PC-specific IgM antibody-forming cells from individual mice.[9] We have added monoclonal anti-idiotopic antibodies into the plaque assay, and have taken the proportion of inhibitable plaques (direct, IgM plaques) as a measure of cells expressing a given idiotope. As indicated in TABLE 1, some anti-idiotopic antibodies ("frequent") inhibited a majority of plaque-forming cells from every BALB/c mouse, whereas others ("rare") inhibited only a portion (varying from 20% to 60%) of PFC in no more than half of the animals tested. A similar analysis of immunocytes from C57BL/6 mice revealed an even more diverse pattern. An example is given in TABLE 2. By comparing the reactivity among twelve individual mice, we find that every anti-idiotope tested can inhibit the PFC in the absence of inhibition by any other antibody in the panel, in other words, that individual idiotopes of the T15 idiotype are expressed in the PFC population independently of one another.

Collectively, the preceding data suggest two things: the TEPC-15 molecule carries several distinct idiotopic determinants distinguished by individual monoclonal anti-idiotopic antibodies that differ in their relative position to the paratope; the PC-reactive lymphocyte population is idiotopically heterogenous in that a given clone may produce IgM antibody expressing some, but not other, idiotopic determinants of the prototype T15 idiotype.

It should be stressed that an accurate determination of the number of distinct idiotopic determinants in TEPC-15 and in its somatic variants awaits a molecular, immunochemical analysis. By the same token, an indisputable evidence for the distinct specificity of every monoclonal anti-idiotopic antibody listed in TABLE 1 remains tentative.

AUTOLOGOUS T CELLS REGULATE AN INDEPENDENT EXPRESSION OF DISTINCT IDIOTOPE WITHIN THE T15 COMPLEX IN A GENETICALLY DETERMINED MANNER

The existence of natural idiotope-specific T-cell regulation becomes apparent when the idiotypic profiles of anti-PC responses in cultures of splenocytes and B cells stimulated with *Streptococcus pneumoniae* R36a (Pn) are compared. In BALB/c mice (TABLE 3), the elimination of T cells did not change the expression of AB1-2, MaId 5-4, or B36-82 by Pn-stimulated B cells *in vitro* even though the magnitude of the response was significantly reduced compared to the cultures of spleen cells. The B-cell response was restored by addition of either a T-cell-replacing helper factor (TRF, a supernatant from concanavalin A-stimulated spleen cells) or syngeneic T cells; however, the idiotopic profile of the response remained the same.

Quite different results were obtained with lymphocytes from other inbred mice. In DBA/2 (TABLE 4), Pn-stimulated splenocytes produced PFC, expressing all three idiotopes. Two of them, AB1-2 and MaId 5-4, disappeared from the response following depletion of T cells, whereas the B36-82 remained as dominantly in the B cell cultures

TABLE 3. T-Cell Independent Expression of T15 by B Cells from BALB/c

Pn-stimulated Responder Cells (10^6/well)	Added to Culture	PC-specific PFC			
		Total[c]	Proportion Expressing[d]		
			AB1-2	MaId5-4	B36-82
Spleen	—	162	68%	80%	>85%
B cells[a]	—	51	72%	70%	>85%
	TRF[b]	184	61%	75%	83%
	T cells[e] (2×10^5)	150	75%	74%	>85%

[a] B cells were prepared by repeated treatment of splenocytes with a monoclonal anti-Thy-1.2 antibody and complement.
[b] Con A-induced spleen-cell supernatant (25% v/v).
[c] PFC/well, mean from quadruplicate cultures. Standard error was ≤20% of the means.
[d] Percent plaques inhibitable by a given anti-idiotopic antibody.
[e] Nonadherent cell fraction from plates coated with a goat anti-mouse Ig antiserum. Prepared from the same splenotype pool as the B cells.

as it was in the splenocyte cultures. Addition of TRF again increased the anti-PC response to the control level, but it did not stimulate the expression of either AB1-2 or MaId 5-4. Syngeneic T cells, on the other hand, restored the idiotopic profile of the response. Thus it appears that B cells expressing AB1-2 or MaId 5-4 idiotopes of T15, but not those bearing B36-82, are absolutely T-helper dependent in DBA/2 mice, although they are helper independent in BALB/c mice. The result with TRF and T cells shows that these B cells require idiotope-specific help that cannot be replaced merely by a nonspecific activating signal. We speculate that the apparent difference in requirement for activation between B cells expressing distinct idiotope has resulted from a network selection process, as discussed in the concluding chapter.

Results obtained with C57BL/6 lymphocytes (TABLE 5) are opposite of those in DBA/2; the expression of AB1-2 and MaId 5-4 appears to be under a T-suppressor cell (T_S) regulation in these mice, because the removal and addition of T cells respectively enhanced and inhibited the expression of B cells bearing those idiotopes. Again, the third T15 idiotope, B36-82, was expressed equally well in all types of Pn-stimulated cultures.

Another piece of evidence suggesting that autologous T cells can be activated to

TABLE 4. T-Cell Depletion Abolishes the Expression of Some T15 Idiotopes by B Cells from DBA/2[a]

Pn-stimulated Responder Cells (10^6/well)	Added to Culture	PC-specific PFC			
		Total	Proportion Expression		
			AB-12	MaId5-4	B36-82
Spleen	—	190	38%	58%	75%
B cells	—	84	<15%[b]	<15%	>85%
	TRF	205	<15%	<15%	80%
	T cells (2×10^5)	168	47%	51%	>85%

[a] See TABLE 3 for legend.
[b] Inhibition by <15% is considered not significant (=Id not expressed).

TABLE 5. Effect of T Cells on T15 Profile of the Anti-Phosphorylcholine Response of Lymphocytes from C57BL/6[a]

Pn-stimulated Responder Cells (10^6/well)	Added to Cultures	PC-specific PFC			
			Proportion Expressing:		
		Total	AB-12	MaId5-4	B36-82
Spleen	—	122	27%	32%	84%
B cells	—	80	>85%	75%	83%
	T cells (2×10^5)	116	42%	28%	>85%

[a]See TABLES 3 and 4 for legend.

regulate the function of B cells bearing different idiotopic determinants of the T15 idiotype independently of one another came from an experiment on neonatally suppressed mice (carried out in collaboration with Christoph Heusser, CIBA-Geigy, Basel).[10] BALB/c mice were injected with the monoclonal anti-T15 antibody, MaId 5-4 (20 μg/mouse) within twenty-four hours after birth. The response of the splenic lymphocytes from these mice to Pn *in vitro* was studied when the animals reached the age of two to five months. As seen in TABLE 6, the spleen cells from adult, neonatally treated mice responded to Pn immunization as well as cells from control littermates, except that the PFC did not express T15 idiotope. Neonatal treatment with MaId 5-4 antibody suppressed the expression of the corresponding idiotope as well as two other idiotopes, AB1-2 and B36-82. When we eliminated T cells from the lymphocyte suspension of MaId 5-4-suppressed donors and stimulated the remaining B cells with Pn (FIGURE 1), the PFC generated in these cultures expressed no MaId 5-4 idiotope, but they occasionally did express near normal levels of either B36-82 or both B36-82 and AB1-2 (FIGURE 1, B cells $_S$). This result prompted us to set up cultures containing reciprocal mixtures of T and B cells from normal (N) and MaId 5-4-suppressed mice (S). Results of several experiments are shown in FIGURE 2. T cells from idiotope-suppressed donors (T_S) inhibited the expression of the target determinant, MaId 5-4, in all cultures of Pn stimulant, normal B cells (B_N). Occasionally, the T_S also inhibited the expression of either AB1-2 or B36-82, or both; this pattern has varied from one experiment to another. In other words, there were distinct suppressor cells for the three T15 idiotopes, and a given T_S pool might contain a subset specific for one idiotope but not for another. B cells from suppressed mice cocultured with normal T cells were never able to express the MaId 5-4, but did occasionally express the other idiotope (FIGURE 2). This supports the notion that the neonatal administration of MaId 5-4 antibody induced central tolerance (functional B-cell paralysis) and active T_S specific

TABLE 6. Phosphorylcholine-Specific Response and T15 Expression in Cultures of Spleen Cells from MaId5-4-Suppressed Mice[a]

Source of Cells	PFC			
	Total/Well	Percent Expressing Idiotope:		
		MaId5-4	AB1-2	B36-82
Normal	642	74	82	>85
Suppressed	598	<15	<15	<15

[a]See TABLES 3 and 4 for legend.

T15 profile of P anti-PC response in
Mald 5.4 - suppressed (S) BALB/c

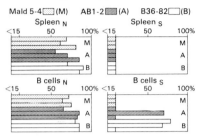

FIGURE 1. Each column represents an independent experiment carried out with spleen cells pooled from two to four mice, either normal (N) or neonatally suppressed with MaId5-4 (S). Columns in corresponding positions show data from the same experiment, such that the first column in each category (M, A, and B) in each panel shows experiment No. 1, etcetera. Cultures containing 10^6 lymphocytes per well were stimulated with an optimal dose of *S. pneumoniae* R36a vaccine. The number of PC-specific PFC per well varied from 160 to 400 for spleen cells and from 80 to 150 for B cells. Data are expressed as percent of PFC expressing a given T15 idiotope-MaId5-4 (M), AB1-2 (A), or B36-82(B) as determined by a specific plaque-inhibition assay (reference 9) with the corresponding monoclonal anti-idiotope.

for MaId 5-4 idiotope, as well as cosuppression of at least two other idiotopic determinants of T15 family that appeared to involve either an active suppression by idiotope-specific T cells or, less frequently, a central tolerance. The relative contribution of the mechanisms of cosuppression may vary from one animal to another.

DISCUSSION AND CONCLUSIONS

Evidence has been presented that TEPC-15, the prototype of T15 idiotypic molecules, carries several distinct idiotopes that may be distinguished by different monoclonal antibodies. The position of different idiotopes on the immunoglobulin molecule is not precisely known, and proof that any two monoclonal anti-idiotopic

T15 profile of anti-PC response in mixed
cultures of cells from normal (N) and
Mald 5.4 - suppressed (S) BALB/c

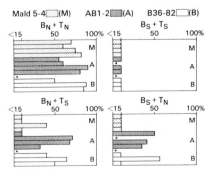

FIGURE 2. The assay system and data presentation are the same as in FIGURE 1. B and T cells were isolated from the same pool of splenocytes (as described in TABLE 3) for each experiment. Each well contained 10^6 B cells and 3×10^5 T cells. * = not tested.

antibodies react with different Ig structures awaits more precise, competitive binding studies using monoclonal anti-PC antibodies as target molecules. The emerging pattern, however, of antigenic complexity of T15 is compatible with results of a similar analysis of idiotypes on antibodies to p-azophenylarsonate,[11-13] dextran,[14] and, in particular, nitrophenyl.[15,16]

More important is the notion that the T15-positive IgM antibodies to PC in BALB/c mice are highly heterogenous. The data from TABLE 1 (details in reference 9) and FIGURES 1 and 2 can be explained only if we assume that there are lymphocyte clones producing IgM expressing some (e.g., MaId 5-4), but not all (e.g., AB1-2), idiotopes of T15. These data and their interpretation are consistent with previous studies at the level of lymphocyte populations by Kearney et al.[7] and Owen et al.[17] They appear to contradict the molecular analysis of selected anti-PC IgM antibodies that revealed uniform amino acid sequences in both V_H and V_L regions.[18] Owen et al. estimated that an inbred murine strain can synthesize more than 10^7 different IgM antibodies, and suggested[17] that the apparent restriction in the IgM repertoire based on sequencing may be an artifact of the sampling technique. Since there appears to be a single V_H-coding sequence for anti-PC antibodies,[19] the idiotopic heterogeneity of IgM would likely arise through a process of somatic diversification.

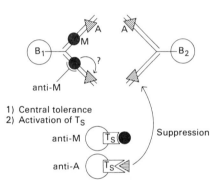

FIGURE 3. A possible mechanism of idiotopic cosuppression in BALB/c mice injected neonatally with monoclonal antibody against MaId5-4 idiotope (M, ●). The cosuppressed idiotope is AB1-2 (A, △). The T15 idiotype of clone B_1 is M^+, A^+, that of clone B_2 is M^-, A^+. The allosteric change in the A region following the anti-M-M interaction is shown by the arrow and question mark. See text for details.

The main point of this paper is the demonstration that different idiotopic determinants of T15 idiotype are recognized by specific sets of distinct, autologous T cells. Because the T15 lymphocytes are idiotopically heterogenous, the clones bearing distinct idiotopes may be regulated independently of each other by the corresponding anti-idiotopic T cells.

The experiments with neonatally suppressed mice show that administration of monoclonal antibody against one determinant, MaId 5-4 may activate T_S specific for other, presumably non-cross-reacting, determinants—AB1-2 and B36-82. The situation is schematically depicted in Figure 3. We speculate that when the anti-MaId5-4 antibody reacts with the corresponding idiotope on the B-cell receptor (B_1), a conformational change occurs (allosteric mechanism?) in the adjacent region of the molecule bearing another idiotope, AB1-2. The change is recognized by T cells and leads to triggering of AB1-2-specific T_S that can, once activated, react with "unchanged" AB1-2 expressed on other lymphocyte clones (B_2) that do not share the target determinant, MaId 5-4. The target clone (M^+, A^+) is suppressed (functionally paralyzed) by the direct action of anti-M, and the M-specific T_S are activated, but not required for the suppression of M^+ cells. On the other hand, the suppression of M^-, A^+ clones will depend on active T-suppressor cells.

Data shown in TABLES 3–5 suggest that the genetic control of idiotopic expression operates through anti-idiotopic T cells and that it is independent for various determinants of T15. Lymphocytes bearing a given idiotope may be helped in DBA/2, suppressed in C57BL/6, or left to be autonomous in BALB/c. Preliminary studies (not shown) on congeneic mice indicate that genes in both H-2 and Ig loci participate in the process. It appears that the recognition of idiotopes develops in context of the self environment and that the network influences the balance of the naturally occurring anti-idiotopic T-helper and -suppressor cells. It is tempting to speculate that the anti-idiotopic help and suppression represent a mechanism for selection of appropriate somatic variants of immunoglobulins. B cells expressing those variants will multiply and differentiate at different rates under the selective pressure from anti-idiotopic clones. In an adult mouse, clones with different idiotopes will be more or less functionally mature, thereby having different requirements for activation. This hypothesis predicts that idiotopically distinct T15 clones will differ not only in their dependence on T-cell help, as already indicated by the present data, but also in respect to the optimal immunizing dose of the antigen, the macrophage dependence, and the Lyb phenotype.

ACKNOWLEDGMENT

The authors are indebted to Dr. Garnett Kelsoe for critical evaluation of the manuscript.

REFERENCES

1. KLUSKENS, L. & H. KOHLER. 1974. Regulation of immune response by autogenous antibody against receptor. Proc. Nat. Acad. Sci. USA 71: 5083–5087.
2. COSENZA, H. 1976. Detection of anti-idiotype reactive cells in the response to phosphorylcholine. Eur. J. Immunol. 6: 114–116.
3. KELSOE, G. & J. CERNY. 1979. Reciprocal expansion of idiotype and anti-idiotypic clones following antigen stimulation. Nature (London) 279: 333–334.
4. KELSOE, G., D. ISAAK & J. CERNY. 1980. Thymic requirement for cyclical idiotypic and reciprocal anti-idiotypic immune responses to a T-independent antigen. J. Exp. Med. 151: 289–300.
5. CERNY, J. & M. J. CAULFIELD. 1981. Stimulation of specific antibody-forming cells in antigen-primed nude mice by the adoptive transfer of syngeneic anti-idiotypic T cells. J. Immunol. 126: 2262–2266.
6. HAMMERLING, G. J. & R. WALLICH. 1980. Monoclonal anti-idiotypes as a probe for the analysis of the diversity of anti-phosphorylcholine antibodies. In Protides of Biological Fluids. H. Peeters, Ed.: Vol. 28: 569–574. Pergamon Press. Oxford.
7. KEARNEY, J. I., R. BARLETTA, Z. A. QUARE & J. QUINTANS. 1981. Monoclonal versus heterogeneous anti-H8 antibodies in the analysis of the anti-phosphorylcholine response in BALB/c mice. Eur. J. Immunol. 11: 877–882.
8. HEUSSER, C. H., S. POSKOCIL & M. H. JULIUS. 1980. A major idiotype (T15-MI-1) on T15-positive B and T cells. Immunobiology 157: 227.
9. CERNY, J., R. WALLICH & G. J. HAMMERLING. 1982. Analysis of T15 idiotopes by monoclonal antibodies: Variability of idiotopic expression on phosphorylcholine-specific lymphocytes from individual inbred mice. J. Immunol. 128: 1885–1891.
10. CERNY, J., R. CRONKHITE & C. H. HEUSSER. 1983. Antibody response of mice following neonatal treatment with a monoclonal anti-receptor antibody. Evidence for B cell tolerance and T suppressor cells specific for different idiotopic determinants. Eur. J. Immunol. 13: 244.

11. ESTESS, P., E. LAMOYI, A. NISONOFF & J. D. CAPRA. 1980. Structural studies on induced antibodies with defined idiotypic specificities. IV. Framework differences in the heavy- and light-chain variable regions of monoclonal anti-p-azophenyl-arsonate antibodies from A/J mice differing with respect to a cross-reactve idiotype. J. Exp. Med. **151:** 863–875.

12. MARSHAK-ROTHSTEIN, A., M. SIEKEVITZ, M. N. MAERGOLIES, M. MUDGETT-HUNTER & M. L. GEFTER. 1980. Hybridoma proteins expressing the predominant idiotype of the anti-azophenyl-arsonate response of A/J mice. Proc. Natl. Acad. Sci. USA **77:** 1120–1124.

13. LAMOYI, E., P. ESTESS, J. D. CAPRA & A. NISONOFF. 1980. Heterogeneity of an intrastrain cross-reactive idiotype associated with anti-p-azophenylarsonate antibodies of A/J mice. J. Immunol. **124:** 2834–2840.

14. CLEVINGER, B., J. SCHILLING, R. GRIFFITH, D. HANSBURG, L. HOOD & J. DAVIE. 1980. Antibody diversity patterns and structure of idiotypic determinants on murine anti-α(1-3) dextran antibodies. *In* Monoclonal Antibodies. R. H. Kennett, T. J. McKearn & K. B. Bechtol, Eds.: 37–48. Plenum Press. New York.

15. RETH, M., T. IMANISHI-KARI & K. RAJEWSKY. 1979. Analysis of the repertoire of anti-NP antibodies in C57BL/6 mice by cell fusion. II. Characterization of idiotypes by monoclonal anti-idiotype antibodies. Eur. J. Immunol. **9:** 1004–1013.

16. KELSOE, G., M. RETH & K. RAJEWSKY. 1980. Control of idiotype expression by monoclonal anti-idiotype antibody. Immunol. Rev. **52:** 75–88.

17. OWEN, J. A., N. H. SIGAL & N. R. KLINMAN. 1982. Heterogeneity of the BALB/c IgM anti-phosphorylcholine antibody response. Nature (London) **295:** 347–348.

18. GEARHART, P. J., N. D. JOHNSON, R. DOUGLAS & L. HOOD. 1981. IgG antibodies to phosphorylcholine exhibit more diversity than their IgM counterparts. Nature (London) **291:** 29–34.

19. CREWS, S., J. GRIFFIN, H. HUANG, K. CALAME & L. HOOD. 1981. A single V_H gene segment encodes the immune response to phosphorylcholine: Somatic mutation is correlated with the class of antibody. Cell **25:** 59–66.

DISCUSSION OF THE PAPER

H. KOHLER: *(Roswell Park Memorial Institute, Buffalo, N.Y.):* Dr. Cerny, in one of your slides I could see that the addition of normal cells did rescue a suppressed idiotype. Is that correct?

J. CERNY: That is correct. I did not want to dwell on this topic too much because I am not quite sure how it compares statistically with the response of B cells alone from suppressed mice. They also sometimes express some of those idiotopes. I agree with you. I think that addition of normal cells does rescue a suppressed idiotype. We tried to interpret this finding as lack of suppression, but since I do not know what that will really mean, I did not want to go into that point.

KOHLER: Dr. Cerny, could you block the T-suppressor cells from your culture by antigen or by anti-idiotopes?

CERNY: You are looking for a control of specificity.

KOHLER: I am looking into whether one can block the T-suppressor cells with anti-id, antigen, or something in the culture.

CERNY: I have no evidence either way.

Maternal-Fetal Transfer of a State of Idiotypic Suppression[a]

ALFRED NISONOFF AND MICHAEL F. GURISH

Rosenstiel Basic Medical Sciences Research Center
Department of Biology
Brandeis University
Waltham, Massachusetts 02254

THOMAS F. KRESINA

Division of Rheumatology
Case Western Reserve School of Medicine
Cleveland, Ohio 44906

INTRODUCTION

In this paper we will review recent data indicating that a state of idiotypic suppression is transferred from a female mouse to its offspring when the mother is given T cells or serum from a syngeneic donor that has been suppressed with respect to that idiotype and hyperimmunized. The serum factor (or factors) can also induce idiotype suppression when inoculated directly into a neonatal mouse. The component of serum that initially induces suppression appears not to be an immunoglobulin; however, the nature of the suppressive substance that is transferred from mother to fetus is not yet known. Before presenting these data some of our earlier work on suppression of idiotype will be reviewed briefly.

PROPERTIES OF THE IDIOTYPIC SYSTEM

The idiotype investigated is associated with the anti-*p*-azophenylarsonate (anti-Ar) antibodies of the A/J strain of mice. An average of about one-half of the antibodies carries a major idiotype,[1] which we have designated CRI_A, to distinguish it from an apparently unrelated minor idiotype, or group of idiotypes, CRI_m,[2-4] associated with a small proportion of the anti-Ar antibodies of the same strain. About one-third of the CRI_m population is closely related serologically to an idiotype, CRI_C, present in a substantial proportion of the anti-Ar antibodies of BALB/c mice.[5,6]

The molecules constituting the CRI_A population exhibit microheterogeneity, as evidenced by serological and amino acid sequence analyses of the products of hybridomas secreting CRI_A-positive anti-Ar antibodies.[7-17] The molecules of this family, however, have in common one or more idiotopes. This was shown by experiments in which anti-idiotypic antibodies specific for one monoclonal $CRI_A{}^+$ antibody was allowed to react with a different, ^{125}I-labeled $CRI_A{}^+$ monoclonal antibody. Each of a large number of $CRI_A{}^+$ hybridoma products proved to be equally strong inhibitors of this interaction. This "criss-cross" experiment was carried out in

[a]This work was supported by Grants AI-17751 and AI-12895 from the National Institutes of Health.

order to eliminate effects due to private idiotopes that are present on individual monoclonal $CRI_A{}^+$ antibodies.[7,15]

IDIOTYPE SUPPRESSION

When adult A/J mice are treated with idiotype-specific rabbit or monoclonal mouse antibodies[9,18] and then immunized with keyhole limpet hemocyanin (KLH)-Ar, they produce normal concentrations of anti-Ar antibodies. These antibodies, however, are devoid of CRI_A. Such suppressed mice, when hyperimmunized with KLH-Ar and then allowed to rest for eight to twelve weeks, develop substantial concentrations of T-suppressor cells with anti-idiotypic receptors[19,20] that can adoptively transfer the idiotypically suppressed state to syngeneic recipients. The presence of anti-idiotypic receptors on T cells was demonstrated by rosette formation, using A/J red blood cells conjugated with CRI^+ Fab fragments. Selective removal from the T-cell population of those cells with anti-idiotypic receptors depleted the suppressor activity, whereas the rosettes themselves proved to be much more suppressive, on a numerical basis, than the unfractionated lymphocytes.

We have also identified T-cell derived factors that are capable of inducing idiotype suppression in native mice. When mice were suppressed with respect to CRI_A, hyperimmunized, and allowed to rest for three weeks, their T cells, when placed in culture, elaborated suppressive factors with both idiotypic and anti-idiotypic receptors.[21] The specificity of the receptors was demonstrated by adsorption experiments using Sepharose 4B to which idiotype-positive or anti-idiotypic immunoglobulins were conjugated.

Adoptive transfer of idiotype suppression is possible with B cells as well as with T cells from hyperimmunized, idiotype-suppressed (HIS) donors.[22] Here, the mechanism is thought to be clonal dominance. The primed, CRI^- B cells from the HIS donor dominate in the anti-Ar antibody response and prevent the appearance of normal levels of the idiotype.

TRANSFER OF THE SUPPRESSED STATE
FROM MOTHERS TO OFFSPRING

The experiments next described demonstrated that a state of idiotype suppression, induced by T cells, can be transferred from the mother to a fetus.[23] Following adoptive transfer of enriched T cells or B cells from HIS A/J donors to female recipients, the latter were mated. Mice that became pregnant within seven days were studied further. Such mice were immunized intraperitoneally with 100 μg KLH-Ar on the first day after parturition (day 0) and again 14 days later; they were bled on day 28. The offspring were immunized and bled on the same days, but only 25 μg KLH-Ar was used for immunization.

The results of these experiments, shown in TABLE 1, lead to the following conclusions. (1) The mothers that received HIS T cells by adoptive transfer produced normal quantities of anti-Ar antibodies upon immunization, but these antibodies lacked CRI_A. The state of idiotype suppression was induced by as few as 2.5×10^6 HIS T cells, but 5×10^5 T cells were ineffective. (2) Offspring of mothers that had received HIS T cells also produced substantial amounts of anti-Ar antibodies; these were CRI_A negative. In addition, the dose response was similar to that observed in the mothers of

TABLE 1. Expression of CRI in Litters from Dams Given Cells from Hyperimmune or Idiotypically Suppressed Hyperimmune Mice

Group	Cells Transferred[a]	Number of Litters	Mothers (M) or Litters (L)	Day 28 Sera	
				Anti-Ar Titer mg/ml	Anti-Ar Antibody Required for 50 Percent Inhibition[b] ng
1	none	1	M	1.7	44
			L	[0.18, 0.14, 0.27, 0.55]	[62, <10, <10, <10]
2	2.5×10^6 hyperimmune T cells	2	M	2.1, 2.7	71, <10
			L	[0.68, 0.13] [0.21, 0.23, 0.13]	[77, 73] [<10, <10, 26]
3	2.5×10^6 hyperimmune suppressed T cells	3	M	1.1, 2.2, 2.2	>5,000(0), <5,000(9), <5,000(0)
			L	[0.29, 0.20, 0.23] [0.67, 0.12, 0.97] [0.99, 0.72, 0.22]	[>5,000(5), 2600, >5,000(48)] [2600, 2800, 2900] [3300, 3900, 2600]
4	1×10^7 hyperimmune suppressed T cells	2	M	2.5, 1.9	>5,000(6), >5,000(3)
			L	[0.63, 0.25] [0.29, 0.13, 0.98]	[>5,000(3), >5,000(0)] [>5,000(1), >5,000(0), >5,000(0)]
5	5×10^5 hyperimmune suppressed T cells	2	M	1.5, 0.60	<10, <10
			L	[0.82, 0.31] [0.20, 0.33, 0.12, 0.10]	[<10, <10] [<10, <10, <10, <10]
6	2.5×10^6 hyperimmune B cells	2	M	2.0, 5.4	33, <10
			L	[0.26, 0.13, 0.27] [0.26, 0.22, 0.53, 0.22, 0.37]	[<10, <10, <10] [<10, <10, <10, <10, <10]
7	2.5×10^6 hyperimmune suppressed B cells	4	M	3.2, 1.7, 0.16, 0.27	18, 440, 310, <10
			L	[0.021, 0.18, 0.033] [0.93, 0.047, 0.061] [0.61, 0.13, 0.24] [0.30, 0.34, 0.023]	[44, 21, 67] [170, 50, 79] [220, <10, 370] [<10, <10, 27]
8	1×10^7 hyperimmune suppressed B cells	3	M	0.57, 0.32, 1.3	400, 370, >5,000(30)
			L	[0.056, 0.011, 0.017, 0.20] [0.31, 0.37, 0.34, 0.32, 0.44] [0.49, 0.59, 0.24]	[29, 21, 80, 21] [320, 53, 10, 690, 2,600] [490, 730, 650]

[a] Recipients became pregnant within 7 days after cell transfer. Cell donors were A/J mice hyperimmunized or idiotypically suppressed and hyperimmunized with KLH-Ar.

[b] ... equal to 5,000 ng of anti-Ar antibody

these litters. Offspring were suppressed when their mothers had received 2.5×10^6 or 1×10^7 HIS T cells, but 5×10^5 cells were ineffective.

The results obtained with groups 7 and 8 indicate that some suppression of CRI_A occurred in both mothers and offspring, when mothers had received 2.5×10^6 or 1×10^7 HIS B cells (rather than T cells). The degree of suppression, however, was much weaker than that observed with the corresponding numbers of HIS T cells, and a substantial percentage of the mothers and offspring were not suppressed when the dosage of HIS B cells was 2.5×10^6. We cannot decide from these data whether B cells actually have some suppressive activity or whether the activity noted was due to contamination by T cells.

Groups 1, 2, and 6 served as the controls for the experiments of TABLE 1. Results obtained with these groups indicate that no suppression of idiotype occurred in either mothers or offspring when the mothers had received no cells by adoptive transfer or had received T cells or B cells from hyperimmunized but nonsuppressed donors.

SUPPRESSIVE FACTOR(S) IN THE SERA OF HYPERIMMUNIZED, IDIOTYPE-SUPPRESSED MICE

The data in TABLE 2 indicate the presence, in HIS serum, of a soluble factor or factors that when inoculated into pregnant female mice, caused a suppression of CRI_A production in some of the mothers and in their offspring.[23] In these experiments the mothers received HIS serum five to seven days before parturition. Mothers and neonates were then immunized according to the protocol described above.

As shown by group 2, TABLE 2, one of the four mothers that received HIS serum was very strongly suppressed and two of the others were partially suppressed with respect to idiotype production. Suppression was also observed in three of the four litters of this group; all of the mice in one litter and one half of the mice in two other litters were idiotypically suppressed. In examining these data it should be noted that we have never observed the absence of CRI_A in the anti-Ar antibodies of an adult immunized mouse, and only on very rare occasions in a neonatal mouse. Hence, any suppression of CRI_A in these experiments is significant. Controls for this experiment (group one) received serum from hyperimmunized but nonsuppressed mice. Both the mothers and their offspring, when immunized, produced normal amounts of CRI_A upon immunization.

A question that arises is whether the suppressive agent in these experiments is an immunoglobulin. Candidates for the suppressive agent include the rabbit anti-idiotype used initially to suppress the donors, or mouse anti-idiotype that might somehow have been stimulated in the donors. Both of these possibilities seemed unlikely. With respect to the rabbit anti-idiotype, it should be noted that the anti-idiotype had been administered to donors at least three months before the passive transfer of serum and that the half life of rabbit IgG in mice was about six days.[24] Radioimmunoassays for mouse anti-idiotype showed that it was present at a level below 50 ng/ml (the lower limit of sensitivity of this assay) in the donor mice.

To examine this question directly, adsorption experiments were carried out using columns of Sepharose 4B conjugated with rabbit anti-mouse Fab (specifically purified antibody) or with an IgG fraction of goat anti-rabbit IgG. The effectiveness of the columns was monitored in each case by adding to the serum to be adsorbed trace amounts of the appropriate, ^{125}I-labeled mouse or rabbit immunoglobulin. It was observed that at least 95%, and probably more than 99%, of the immunoglobulin was removed by the columns. (A small amount of radioactivity may be associated with

TABLE 2. Suppressive Effects in Female Parents and Their Litters of Serum from Idiotypically Suppressed Mice

Group	Serum Transferred[a]	Volume of Serum ml	Treatment of Serum	Number of Litters	Mothers (M) or Litters (L)	Day 28 Anti-Ar titer mg/ml	Day 28 Anti-Ar Antibody Required for 50 Percent Inhibition[b] ng
1	Hyperimmune	0.2	none	2	M	0.021, 0.70	61, 58
					L	[0.024, 0.071] [0.31, 0.022]	[10, 10] [21, 43]
2	Hyperimmune Suppressed	0.2	none	4	M	0.084, 0.92, 0.28, 1.2	250, 360, 10, >5,000(36)
					L	[0.051, 0.034] [0.18, 0.20, 0.22, 0.24, 0.21] [0.10, 0.13, 0.26, 0.09] [0.027, 0.055, 0.12, 1.1]	[29, 175] [200, >5000(43), >5000(46), 22, 750] [10, 380, >1300(0), 2900] [1000, >1000(17), 52, 50]
3	Hyperimmune Suppressed	0.2	adsorbed with anti-mouse Fab	2	M	0.020, D^c	>5000(8), D
					L	[0.57, 0.39, 0.26 0.40] [0.78, 0.13, 0.18]	[>5000(14), >5000(48), 2500, >5000(14)] [440, >5000(4), >5000(9)]
4	Hyperimmune Suppressed	0.2	adsorbed with anti-rabbit IgG	2	M	0.011, 0.062	>5000(8), >5000(9)
					L	[0.021, 1.5] [0.14, 0.27, 0.63, 0.26, 0.73]	[>5000(0), >5000(5)] [>5000(14), >5000(4), >5000(12), 3300, >5000(17)]
5	Hyperimmune Suppressed	0.02	none	2	M	0.44, 0.75	1400, 31
					L	[0.2, 0.14] [0.06, 0.033, 0.035]	[1000, 42] [31, 36, 22]

molecules other than immunoglobulin.) It is evident from TABLE 2 that the adsorption of immunoglobulins from the serum had no effect on the suppressive activity of HIS serum, either in mothers or their offspring. Furthermore, when 0.02 ml, rather than 0.2 ml, of unadsorbed serum was administered, very little suppression of idiotype was noted. The latter result indicated that the suppressive activity of the adsorbed HIS serum was not due to traces of an immunoglobulin that might have remained after adsorption.

SUPPRESSIVE EFFECTS OF SERUM FROM HYPERIMMUNIZED, IDIOTYPE-SUPPRESSED MICE ADMINISTERED DIRECTLY TO NEONATES[23]

The results in TABLE 3 demonstrate that HIS serum is also suppressive when administered to neonates (rather than to mothers prior to parturition). A/J mice were given 0.2 ml of HIS serum on the day of birth, then immunized with 25 μg KLH-Ar

TABLE 3. Suppression of Expression of the CRI in Neonatal Mice Given Serum from Idiotypically Suppressed Hyperimmune Mice

		Day 28	
Serum Administered[a]	Number of Litters	Anti-Ar Titer mg/ml	Anti-Ar Antibody Required for 50 Percent Inhibition[b] ng
Hyperimmune	1	0.22, 0.25, 0.14	10, 10, 50
Hyperimmune	2	0.21, 0.11, .09	1700, 230, 280
Suppressed		0.14, 0.07, 0.06	2200, 900, 340
		0.24	1800

[a] A/J mice were given 0.2 ml of serum on the day of birth, immunized with 25 μg KLH-Ar intraperitoneally on days 5 and 19, and bled on day 28.
[b] In the radioimmunoassay for CRI_A

intraperitoneally on days 5 and 19; the mice were bled on day 28. In three of the seven neonates the degree of suppression of CRI_A exceeded 90%; partial suppression was observed in the other three mice as well.

CRI_A PRODUCTION IN NEONATAL MICE NURTURED BY HYPERIMMUNIZED SUPPRESSED FOSTER MOTHERS[23]

The results obtained by Weiler[25] suggested the possibility that the suppression induced in neonatal mice might be attributable to factors transmitted in milk. To test this possibility four normal litters were transferred within 24 hours after birth to four foster mothers that had been idiotypically suppressed by the adoptive transfer of 2.5 × 10^6 T cells from HIS donor mice three to four weeks earlier. Each of these surrogate mothers was proven to be idiotypically suppressed after immunization, and each was lactating because it had recently given birth to its own litter. It was found that the neonatal mice raised by foster mothers produced anti-Ar antibodies containing normal amounts of CRI_A (data not shown). Thus, the maternal-fetal transfer of idiotype suppression is not due solely to factors found in the milk. We cannot as yet rule out the possibility that factors in milk may contribute to the transfer of suppression from mother to offspring.

DISCUSSION

The results presented here suggest a novel mechanism of regulation of antibody production in the neonatal mouse, apparently mediated without the participation of immunoglobulin. Idiotype suppression was observed in offspring of mothers that had received either T cells or serum from HIS donors. Our data do not indicate the nature of the active moiety that is transferred from mother to fetus. It seems somewhat more probable that a soluble suppressive factor, rather than cells, is transferred, because there is little evidence for cell transfer across the placenta or by way of the yolk sac.[25,26]

The nature of the suppressive factor or factors in HIS serum also remains to be elucidated. An obvious possibility is that the factor is elaborated by T cells, because the supernatants of cultured HIS T cells are known to contain idiotype-suppressor factors.[21] One might further speculate that a T-cell derived factor is transferred from mother to fetus. The mechanism of suppression might further require stimulation of T-suppressor cells by such a factor.[17] Further experiments are needed to answer these questions.

The experiments with HIS foster mothers indicate that a state of suppression is not transferred from such mice to neonates by way of the milk. We have not ruled out, however, the possibility that substances in milk may contribute to suppression in mice that are delivered by HIS mothers.

It should be of interest to ascertain whether other types of suppressive factors, for example antigen-specific T-cell derived factors, can be similarly transmitted from mother to fetus. Also the importance of this regulatory mechanism in normal neonatal mice remains to be determined.

REFERENCES

1. KUETTNER, M. G., A. L. WANG & A. NISONOFF. 1972. J. Exp. Med. 135: 579–595.
2. GILL-PAZARIS, L. A., A. R. BROWN & A. NISONOFF. 1979. Ann. Immunol. Inst. Pasteur (Paris) 130 C: 199–213.
3. GILL-PAZARIS, L. A., E. LAMOYI, A. R. BROWN & A. NISONOFF. 1981. J. Immunol. 126: 75–79.
4. NELLES, M. J. & A. NISONOFF. 1982. J. Immunol. 128: 2773–2778.
5. BROWN, A. R. & A. NISONOFF. 1981. J. Immunol. 126: 1263–1267.
6. BROWN, A. R., E. LAMOYI & A. NISONOFF. 1981. J. Immunol. 126: 1268–1273.
7. LAMOYI, E. L., P. ESTESS, J. D. CAPRA & A. NISONOFF. 1980. J. Immunol. 124: 2834–2840.
8. LAMOYI, E. L., P. ESTESS, J. D. CAPRA & A. NISONOFF. 1980. J. Exp. Med. 152: 703–711.
9. NELLES, M. N., L. A. GILL-PAZARIS & A. NISONOFF. 1981. J. Exp. Med. 154: 1752–1763.
10. ESTESS, P., A. NISONOFF & J. D. CAPRA. 1979. Mol. Immunol. 16: 1111–1118.
11. ESTESS, P., E. LAMOYI, A. NISONOFF & J. D. CAPRA. 1980. J. Exp. Med. 151: 863–875.
12. SIEGELMAN, M., C. SLAUGHTER, L. MCCUMBER, P. ESTESS & J. D. CAPRA. 1981. In Symposium on Immunoglobulin Idiotypes and Their Expression. C. Janeway, E. Sercarz and H. Wigzell, Eds.: 135. Academic Press. New York.
13. SIEGELMAN, M. & J. D. CAPRA. 1981. Proc. Natl. Acad. Sci. USA 78: 7679–7683.

14. ALKAN, S. S., R. KNECHT & D. G. BRAUN. 1980. Hoppe-Seyler's Z. Physiol. Chem. **361:** 191–195.
15. MARSHAK-ROTHSTEIN, A., A. M. SIEKEVITZ, M. N. MARGOLIES, M. MUDGETT-HUNTER & M. L. GEFTER. 1980. Proc. Natl. Acad. Sci. USA **77:** 1120–1124.
16. MARGOLIES, M. N., A. MARSHAK-ROTHSTEIN & M. L. GEFTER. 1981. Mol. Immunol. **18:** 1065–1077.
17. GREENE, M. I., M. J. NELLES, M-S. SY & A. NISONOFF. 1982. Adv. Immunol. **32:** 253–300.
18. HART, D. A., A. L. WANG, L. L. PAWLAK & A. NISONOFF. 1972. J. Exp. Med. **135:** 1293–1300.
19. OWEN, F. L. & A. NISONOFF. 1978. Cell. Immunol. **37:** 243–253.
20. OWEN, F. L. & A. NISONOFF. 1978. J. Exp. Med. **148:** 182–194.
21. HIRAI, Y. & A. NISONOFF. 1980. J. Exp. Med. **151:** 1213–1231.
22. EIG, B. M., S-T. JU & A. NISONOFF. 1977. J. Exp. Med. **146:** 1574–1584.
23. KRESINA, T. F. & A. NISONOFF. 1983. J. Exp. Med. **157:** 15–23.
24. SPIEGELBERG, H. C. & W. O. WEIGLE. 1965. J. Exp. Med. **121:** 323–338.
25. WEILER, E. 1981. *In* Lymphocytic Regulation by Antibodies. C. Bona & P-A Cazenave, Eds.: 245. John Wiley and Sons. New York.
26. MILLER, J. F. A. P. 1966. Immunity in the Fetus and the New Born. Br. Med. Bull. **22:** 21.

DISCUSSION OF THE PAPER

UNIDENTIFIED SPEAKER: Have you studied at all the factor in terms of id cell-type linkage—the ability to transfer factors from animals of different allotype?

A. NISONOFF: We could only study idiotype suppression in strains that produce the idiotype, so there would be no way to study this effect in strains other than the allotype A strains.

UNIDENTIFIED SPEAKER: Does that include the suppressor factors?

NISONOFF: Yes, because the suppressor factor is suppressing the idiotype. If you go to a strain other than one that is Igh-1e, it does not produce the idiotype, so there is no way to measure suppression.

UNIDENTIFIED SPEAKER: You could, however, take a factor from C.AL-20 or something similar and transfer it into the A/J.

NISONOFF: That would be a feasible experiment. We could use C.AL-20 which differs with respect to the H-2, and determine whether its suppressor factor works in A/J. We have not done that yet. These are tedious experiments, because each donor mouse requires roughly 14 weeks of preparation, and you can suppress one or at most two mice with one donor.

UNIDENTIFIED SPEAKER: With respect to the experiments with the fostering mother, do you know whether T cells can be transferred from breast milk of animals that are hypersuppressed?

NISONOFF: There is no really good evidence that cells travel from the mother to the fetus. A paper was published ten years ago that suggested, by chromosome analysis, that some transfer of cells was occurring. This notion is controversial, however, and has not been pursued.

UNIDENTIFIED SPEAKER: Actually, my point was not that an intact cell might do it, but rather that the population of cells that are represented within the breast may not be capable of suppressing or releasing a factor that can suppress, as opposed to spleen cells, lymph node cells.

NISONOFF: Do you mean from the suppressed foster mother?

UNIDENTIFIED SPEAKER: Right.

NISONOFF: That would be the implication.

Structural Correlates of Idiotypy in the Arsonate System[a]

MICHAEL N. MARGOLIES,[b] ELIZABETH C. JUSZCZAK,[c]
RICHARD NEAR,[d] ANN MARSHAK-ROTHSTEIN,[e]
THOMAS L. ROTHSTEIN,[f]
VICKI L. SATO,[g]
MIRIAM SIEKEVITZ,[d] JOHN A. SMITH,[h]
LAWRENCE J. WYSOCKI,[d] AND MALCOLM L. GEFTER[d]

*Departments of [b]Surgery, [c]Medicine, and [h]Pathology
Massachusetts General Hospital and Harvard Medical School
Boston, Massachusetts 02114*

*Departments of [f]Medicine and [e]Microbiology
Boston University Medical Center
Boston Massachusetts 02118*

*[g]Department of Cellular and Developmental Biology
Harvard University
Cambridge, Massachusetts 02138*

*[d]Department of Biology
Massachusetts Institute of Technology
Cambridge, Massachusetts 02138*

INTRODUCTION

Predominant idiotypes inherited in certain strains of mice represent phenotypic markers thought to be directly related to germ line genes encoding antibody variable regions. Nisonoff and coworkers[1] described and extensively characterized a heritable idiotype (here denoted Id^{CR}) represented in a large proportion of anti-para-azophenylarsonate (Ars) antibodies in all strain A mice immunized with arsonate-protein conjugates. Because it has been postulated that immune regulation is mediated through a network of idiotypes and anti-idiotypes,[2] it is important to determine whether the structural data is consistent with this model. We have analyzed the degree of diversity in the Ars-associated idiotype(s) and the origin of this diverse repertoire through structural analyses of antibody variable regions and the genes from which they are derived. The use of monoclonal antibodies of defined idiotype obtained following somatic cell fusion makes such characterization possible. In this report, for purposes of discussion the results of structural studies on hybridoma products are divided into four groups: a family of arsonate-binding monoclonal antibodies bearing the predominant cross-reacting idiotype (Id^{CR}); arsonate-binding monoclonal antibodies that lack Id^{CR}; arsonate-binding monoclonal antibodies that constitute a second idiotype family

[a]This work was supported by National Institutes of Health Grants CA24432, HL19259, AI13357, CA28900, and CA24368, and a grant from the American Cancer Society (NP-6L).

(Id^{36-60}) distinct from Id^{CR}; and an unusual group of monoclonal antibodies that bear Id^{CR}, but fail to bind arsonate.

ORIGIN OF DIVERSITY IN ANTI-PARA-AZOPHENYLARSONATE MONOCLONAL ANTIBODIES BEARING THE PREDOMINANT CROSS-REACTIVE IDIOTYPE

Amino acid sequence analyses of pooled serum anti-arsonate antibodies bearing the predominant idiotype (Id^{CR})[3,4] revealed a single sequence in the heavy chain variable region and in the light chain complementarity-determining regions (CDR) as well. These results were in accordance with the prediction that the reproducible appearance of a dominant idiotype of restricted heterogeneity in immune sera could be accounted for by that idiotype arising as the product of a single or limited number of germ line V genes.[1] Subsequently, however, a variety of analyses on monoclonal anti-arsonate antibodies indicated that Id^{CR} was diverse, analogous to the serologic heterogeneity reported among monoclonal antibodies in other systems.[5,6] A set of anti-arsonate Id^{CR+} hybridoma proteins proved to be serologically heterogeneous in reactions with conventional rabbit anti-idiotypic sera (raised against pooled Id^{CR+} antibodies) as well as antisera of more restricted specificity.[7] Hybridoma proteins bearing Id^{CR} may also be distinguished serologically by monoclonal anti-idiotypic reagents.[8,9] Isotypically identical hybridoma proteins varied in their isoelectric point.[7] Individual Id^{CR+} hybridoma products bear distinct private idiotypes, each of which are present in small quantities in Ars-immune sera, suggesting that the family of molecules expressing Id^{CR} is large.[10] Suppression induced by monoclonal anti-idiotopes may be idiotope specific, corresponding to the fine specificity of the anti-idiotope employed.[9] Although individual antibodies could be distinguished serologically, this family of monoclonal antibodies, nonetheless, possesses shared determinants.[7,11]

The serologic and functional diversity among Id^{CR+} monoclonal antibodies described above was proved by the results of amino acid sequence analysis that identified sequence differences among monoclonal Id^{CR+} variable regions in both framework and complementarity-determining regions.[7,12–14] Partial amino acid sequences of a set of Id^{CR+} hybridoma protein heavy chains,[7,14,15] are illustrated in FIGURE 1, where each sequence is compared to the hybridoma protein 36-65 that is identical to the V_H germ line sequence (see below). All of the Ars-binding Id^{CR+} sequences depicted resulted from independently derived hybridomas. Three of these Id^{CR+} hybridoma proteins (3A4, 3D10, and 1F6) do not bind arsonate. All of the heavy chains but one (44-10) exhibit scattered amino acid substitutions in both the framework region and complementarity-determining regions. In addition, they all share several linked substitutions[14] that differ from the reported sequence of pooled serum Id^{CR+} heavy chains. Similar results were found for the kappa light chains (FIGURE 2); scattered differences occur in both framework regions and complementarity-determining regions. These sequence results indicate that Id^{CR} constitutes a family of closely related but nonidentical V regions. It was thus necessary to address the question of whether these families of sequences for heavy and light chain V regions reflected the presence of multiple germ line genes for each, or was due to somatic diversification of a single germ line gene. In order to resolve this issue for the V_H region, Siekevitz and coworkers cloned the expressed V_H gene from the Id^{CR+} hybridoma cell line 36-65.[16] DNA hybridization studies using this probe under stringent hybridization conditions revealed only a single 6.4 kb band in Eco R-1 digested A strain DNA. In an analysis of strains of mice carrying recombinant IgH haplotypes, the presence or absence of the 6.4 kb band was directly correlated with the ability of each strain to

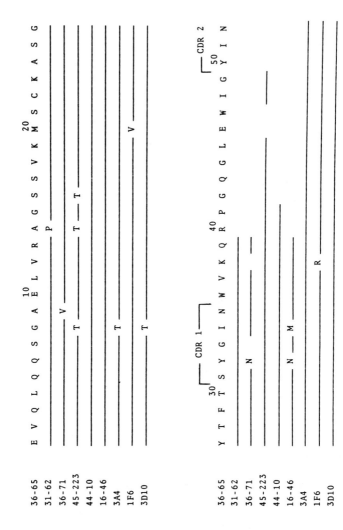

FIGURE 1. Amino acid sequences of murine A/J hybridoma protein heavy chains bearing Id^{CR}[7,14,15] compared to the V_H germ line sequence (hybridoma 36-65).[16,17] Amino acids are indicated in the one-letter code.[39] A line indicates identity with the topmost sequence. Numbering of residues and designation of CDR is according to Kabat et al.[40]

MARGOLIES *et al.*: STRUCTURAL CORRELATES OF IDIOTYPY

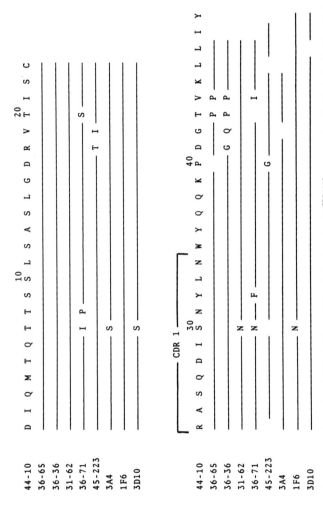

FIGURE 2. Amino acid sequences of murine A/J hybridoma light chains bearing $Id^{CR7,14,15}$ compared to light chain 44-10, which represents the most common sequence. See legend to FIGURE 1 for further details.

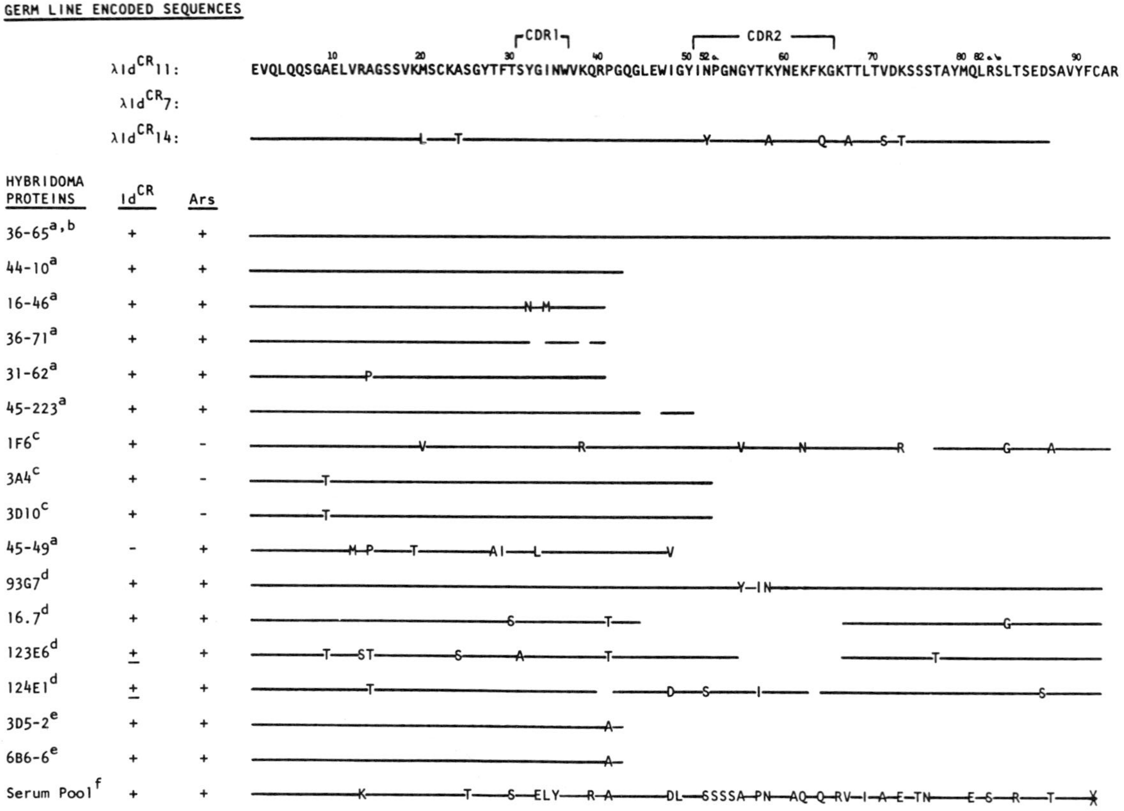
GERM LINE ENCODED SEQUENCES
CDR1
CDR2
λId[CR]11:
EVQLQQSGAELVRAGSSVKMSCKASGYTFTSYGINWVKQRPGQGLEWIGYINPGNGYTKYNEKFKGKTTLTVDKSSSTAYMQLRSLTSEDSAVYFCAR
λId[CR]7:
λId[CR]14:
HYBRIDOMA PROTEINS
Id[CR]
Ars
36-65[a,b]
44-10[a]
16-46[a]
36-71[a]
31-62[a]
45-223[a]
1F6[c]
3A4[c]
3D10[c]
45-49[a]
93G7[d]
16.7[d]
123E6[d]
124E1[d]
3D5-2[e]
6B6-6[e]
Serum Pool[f]

produce cross-reacting idiotype.[16] Strains of mice phenotypically negative for idiotype lacked the structural gene. Thus, there was no evidence for genes other than the structural gene controlling the expression of the Ars-associated predominant idiotype.

The detection of a single 6.4 kb band in Eco R-1-digested A/J embryonic DNA and a single rearranged band in all Id^{CR+} hybridoma DNA after hybridization with the 36-65 V_H probe was consistent with a single gene encoding the Id^{CR} V_H family. In all Ars-binding Id^{CR+} cell lines, the same germ line V_H gene was rearranged to the J_{H2} segment. Although three Id^{CR}-like genes were later cloned from the single 6.4 kb band, only one of these appeared to produce the Id^{CR+} family.[17] The protein sequence encoded by this gene is shown at the top of FIGURE 3 (λ phage $Id^{CR}11$) and is identical to the V_H-encoded portion of the rearranged hybridoma 36-65 for which the DNA sequence has also been determined.[16,17] Two other genes (λ phage $Id^{CR}7$ and λ phage $Id^{CR}14$) encoded heavy chain V regions that differ from 36-65 by at least eight amino acids (FIGURE 3). Because none of the sixteen hybridoma protein sequences tabulated in FIGURE 3 contain these substitutions, it is likely that all of the heavy chains are encoded by this single λ $Id^{CR}11$ gene corresponding to the 36-65 sequence. The serum V_H sequence of pooled serum Id^{CR+} antibodies previously reported[3] differs from this germ line gene-encoded sequence at 32 positions in V_H, some of which would require multiple nucleotide base changes. Only a minority of the amino acid substitutions are found in any of the hybridoma proteins. Because numerous linked nucleotide base changes would be necessary to produce the serum sequence from the germ line gene sequence, the V_H serum sequence could not have arisen from the Id^{CR} gene that gave rise to the hybridoma protein sequences.

The DNA and protein structural studies summarized above indicate that with respect to the heavy chain V regions, a large diverse collection of antibodies arises by somatic mutation from a single germ line gene, analogous to results for the T15 idiotype family[18] and for part of the predominant idiotype in the NP((4-hydroxy-3-nitrophenyl)acetyl) system.[19] Thus, the dominance of the idiotype associated with the response to para-azophenylarsonate cannot be accounted for on the basis of a large number of Id^{CR} V_H genes.

FIGURE 3 Comparison of the amino acid sequences encoded by A/J embryonic Id^{CR} V_H genes[16,17] sequences determined for Id^{CR}-derived hybridoma proteins and the serum pool. The amino acid sequence encoded by λ the $Id^{CR}11$ gene is shown at the top for reference. Horizontal lines indicate identity with this sequence. The DNA sequences of λ $Id^{CR}7$ and λ $Id^{CR}14$ are identical to each other, but differ from λ $Id^{CR}11$ at eight amino acids in V_H. Numbering of residues and designation of CDR is according to Kabat *et al.*[40] The Id^{CR+} hybridoma heavy chain sequences appear to be derived from the germ line gene λ $Id^{CR}11$. The substitutions found in the λ $Id^{CR}7$ and λ $Id^{CR}14$ sequences have not been found in any hybridoma heavy chains.

[a]Protein sequences reported by Marshak-Rothstein *et al.*[7] and Margolies *et al.*[14] All of these monoclonal antibodies bind to arsonate and all inhibit an anti-idiotype serum idiotype binding assay to an extent of 75–90%, except for 45-49, which lacks Id^{CR}. DNA hybridization studies[16] demonstrate that 45-49 is derived from the Id^{CR+} gene.

[b]The sequence of 36-65 is derived from the sequence of the rearranged DNA[16] and the protein sequence[14] (M.N. Margolies, unpublished).

[c]These arsonate-nonbinding Id^{CR+} monoclonal antibodies were produced following immunization with monoclonal anti-idiotype.[29] These sequences are from Margolies *et al.*,[15] except for the results for 1F6 (J.A. Smith and M.N. Margolies, unpublished).

[d]Protein sequences reported by Siegelman *et al.*[41] and Sims *et al.*[42] Proteins 123E6 and 124E1 are partially Id^{CR+} in that two micrograms of 123E6 are required to inhibit in an idiotype assay by 58%, and 2.9 micrograms of 124E1 are required to inhibit to an extent of 48 percent.

[e]Sequences were reported by Alkan *et al.*[23]

[f]Sequences of heavy chains from pooled Id^{CR+} A/J anti-Ars sera or ascites.[3]

ANTI-PARA-AZOPHENYLARSONATE HYBRIDOMA PROTEINS LACKING
THE PREDOMINANT CROSS-REACTIVE IDIOTYPE

Structural studies on anti-Ars monoclonal antibodies lacking the predominant Id^{CR} revealed significantly greater diversity in V region sequence than that contained within the set of Id^{CR+} proteins described above. This study suggested that multiple germ line genes encode anti-arsonate Id^{CR-} regions. The amino terminal sequences of nine randomly selected Id^{CR-} hybridoma proteins are displayed in FIGURE 4.[14,20] Four of these were blocked to Edman degradation, but could be sequenced following cleavage with pyroglutamyl aminopeptidase. By comparison to the germ line sequence for Id^{CR+}, the Id^{CR-} heavy chains contain multiple difference in both framework regions and complementarity-determining regions. All of the Id^{CR-} heavy chains with the exception of 45-49 belong to V region subgroups different from that of the Id^{CR+} heavy chains. The V_H sequence of 45-49 is closely related to the Id^{CR+} sequence. Although there is extensive sequence diversity in the Id^{CR-} heavy chains shown in FIGURE 4, three of these eight randomly selected proteins (36-60, 31-64, and 36-54) were highly homologous to each other, yet entirely distinct from the set of Id^{CR-} sequences. The striking structural similarity among these three Id^{CR-} antibodies pertains also for the light chains (see below, FIGURE 5) and is in accordance with the observation that they constitute a second idiotype family that is serologically cross-reactive, the member of which may be suppressed concordantly[20] (see next section).

The findings for Id^{CR-} light chains are similar to those for the corresponding heavy chains (FIGURE 5). There is marked diversity in both framework regions and CDR, including different chain lengths in CDR, suggesting that multiple light chain genes are utilized in the anti-Ars response in addition to those associated with cross-reacting idiotype. Analogous to the results for their Id^{CR-} heavy chains, the sequences of the Id^{CR-} light chains 36-60, 31-64, and 36-54 constitute a highly homologous set entirely distinct from the structure of the Id^{CR+} light chain family (FIGURE 5). Compared with the Id^{CR+} V_L sequences, these three light chains all contain a five residue insertion in CDR1 and belong to a different subgroup, V_k2. Thus, the structural data suggests for both light and heavy chains that different genes encode the predominant Id^{CR} and the minor idiotype[36-60].

The light chain of the Id^{CR-} hybridoma protein 45-49, unlike the other Id^{CR-} sequences, is indistinguishable from the Id^{CR+} associated sequence. As noted above, the 45-49 V_H sequence is also highly homologous to the Id^{CR} V_H sequence. By Northern and Southern blotting hybridization analyses, Siekevitz and coworkers[16] showed that the 45-49 V_H gene is derived from the same germ line gene that encodes the Id^{CR+} antibodies. In the same analyses, none of the other Id^{CR-} cell lines proved related to the Id^{CR+} V probe. Thus, the 45-49 V_H appears to be derived from the same gene as the Id^{CR+} family, but somatic mutation (or alternatively, changes in the D gene) has resulted in the loss of the cross-reacting idiotype. This conclusion is supported by the results of Milner and Capra[21] who raised an antiserum to an Id^{CR-} antibody 91A3. Like 45-49, 91A3 is similar in sequence to that of the Id^{CR+} family. The anti-91A3 antiserum reacts also with all Id^{CR+} hybridomas and the Id^{CR-} hybridoma protein 45-49.[21] The occurrence of Id^{CR-} proteins that are derived from the Id^{CR+} V_H gene indicates the possibility that somatic mutation can result in antibodies that, if one were to accept the tenets of the network hypothesis, could no longer be regulated by anti-cross-reacting idiotype. Thus, analysis of monoclonal antibodies has revealed that molecules lose idiotypic determinants despite preservation of the antigen binding site. The converse has been detected also, that is, molecules bear Id^{CR}, but do not bind to the Ars hapten (see below).

IDIOTYPE NEGATIVE ANTI-p-AZOPHENYLARSONATE
HYBRIDOMA HEAVY CHAINS

```
                         10                      20
Germ Line  IdCR+   E V Q L Q Q S G A E L V R A G S S V K M S C K A
36-60      IdCR-   — — — — — E P S — K P S Q T L S L T — S V
31-64      IdCR-   — — — — — E P S — K P S Q T L S L T — S V
36-54      IdCR-   — — — — — E P S — K P S Q T L S L T — S V
45-49      IdCR-   —
44-1-3     IdCR-     M   P           K P A       R I   T
31-41      IdCR-   < V   D           K P A         I
45-112     IdCR-   < — — D           K P A         I
45-165     IdCR-   < I V   P       K K P E T       I

                      |_____ CDR 1 _____|
                   30                      40
Germ Line  IdCR+   S G Y T F T S Y G I N W V K Q R P G Q G L E W I
36-60      IdCR-   T — D S I — D Y W     I R K F   N K     H M
31-64      IdCR-   T — D S I — N Y W     I R K F   N K     F M
36-54      IdCR-   T — D S I — N Y W     I R K F   N K
45-49      IdCR-   A I         L
44-1-3     IdCR-             T   Y V H
31-41      IdCR-             D H T   H — A       (T) E
45-112     IdCR-             D H T   H
45-165     IdCR-             D   R M                       V
```

FIGURE 4. Amino acid sequences of murine A/J anti-Ars Id[CR−] monoclonal antibody heavy chains [14,20] (E. Juszczak and M.N. Margolies, unpublished). They are compared to the Id[CR+] germ line V_H sequence of 36-65 (see FIGURES 1 and 9). The < indicates an amino terminal pyrrolidone carboxylic acid residue; the sequences of these chains were obtained following digestion with pyroglutamyl aminopeptidase. Hybridoma proteins 36-60, 31-64, and 36-54 constitute a highly homologous set bearing a minor idiotype (Id[36-60])[20] distinct from Id[CR] (see FIGURES 6 and 7).

IDIOTYPE NEGATIVE ANTI-p-AZOPHENYLARSONATE
HYBRIDOMA LIGHT CHAINS

										10									20					
Consensus	IdCR+	D	I	Q	M	T	Q	T	T	S	S	L	S	A	S	L	G	D	R	V	T	I	S	C R
36-60	IdCR-	-	V	V	-	-	-	-	-	P	L	T	-	-	V	T	I	-	-	Q	P	A	S	— K
31-64	IdCR-	-	V	V	-	-	-	-	-	P	L	T	-	-	V	I	I	-	-	Q	P	A	S	— K
36-54	IdCR-	-	V	V	-	-	-	-	-	P	L	T	-	-	V	T	I	-	-	Q	P	A	S	— K
31-41	IdCR-	E	N	V	L	-	-	-	S	P	A	I	M	-	-	-	-	P	-	E	K	-	-	M T — K
45-112	IdCR-								S	P										E			S	L T
45-165	IdCR-			V		S			S	P				A	V			A		E	K		-	M — K
45-49	IdCR-																							
44-1-3	IdCR-	Blocked																						

					30							CDR 1 34 a	b	c	d	e	f		W	Y	Q	Q	K	40 P	D	G
Consensus	IdCR+	A	S	Q	D	I	S	N	Y	L	N	-	-	-	-	-	-	-	W	Y	Q	Q	K	P	D	G
36-60	IdCR-	S	-	-	R	L	L	D	S	D	G	K	T	Y	L	N	-	-	-	-	L	L	-	R	—	G Q
31-64	IdCR-	S	-	-	S	L	L	D	S	D	G	K	T	Y	L	S	-	-	-	-	L	L	-	R	—	G Q
36-54	IdCR-	S	-	-	S	L	L	D	S	D	G	K	T	Y	L	N	-	-	-	-	L	-	-		—	G Q
31-41	IdCR-	-	S	-	S	S	V	S	Y	F	-	-	-	-	-	-	-	-	-	-	L					
45-112	IdCR-	-	-	-	E	-	G	-	S	-	-	-	-	-	-	-	-	-	-	-	L					
45-165	IdCR-	S	-	-	S	L	L	-	S	R	T	R	K	N	Y	L	T	-	-	-						
45-49	IdCR-	-	-	-	-	-	-	-	-	-	-	-	-	-	-	-	-	-	-	-					G	Q

FIGURE 5. Amino acid sequences of murine A/J anti-Ars IdCR- monoclonal antibody light chains [14,20] (E. Juszczak and M.N. Margolies, unpublished). They are compared to a reference IdCR+ light chain sequence (represented by light chain 44-10 in FIGURE 2). Among the IdCR- sequences, hybridoma protein 36-60, 31-64, and 36-54 represent a highly homologous set bearing a minor idiotype (Id36-60)[20] distinct from IdCR (see FIGURES 6 and 7).

A SECOND IDIOTYPE FAMILY IN THE A/J RESPONSE TO
PARA-AZOPHENYLARSONATE THAT IS SHARED BY BALB/c MICE

In addition to the predominant Id^{CR}, Nisonoff and collaborators[22] identified a heterogeneous population of minor idiotypes. As noted above, examination of several randomly selected Id^{CR-} hybridoma proteins by amino acid sequence analysis identified a set of closely related molecules that constituted a second idiotype family (FIGURES 4–7). Marshak-Rothstein and coworkers[20] prepared a rabbit antiserum against the Id^{CR-} hybridoma protein 36-60. This antiserum reacted only with the hybridoma proteins 36-60, 31-64, and 36-54 (see FIGURES 4 and 5), but not with any other Id^{CR-} nor Id^{CR+} hybridoma protein. This second idiotype family (Id^{36-60}) was present in virtually all A/J sera at a level of approximately 10 to 20% in comparison to cross-reacting idiotype. By means of appropriate adsorption experiments,[20] Id^{CR}, and Id^{36-60} were also shown to be nonoverlapping sets in immune sera. Unlike Id^{CR}, Id^{36-60} was present in BALB/c sera as a major component. The neonatal injection of anti-Id^{36-60} antisera prior to Ars-keyhole limpet hemocyanin immunization resulted in suppression of Id^{36-60} and was independent of the suppression of cross-reacting idiotype. Thus, Id^{CR} and Id^{36-60} provide two independent markers for monitoring network regulation of the anti-Ars antibody response in A/J mice.

Partial sequences similar to those of the Id^{36-60} group have been reported[13,23] and presumably represent other examples of this family of hybridoma proteins. The frequency of occurrence of sequences resembling 36-60 among randomly selected groups of Id^{CR-} proteins correlates with the amount of Id^{36-60} found in Ars-immune serum.

Nisonoff and his collaborators defined an idiotype, CRI_c, associated with the anti-Ars response in BALB/c mice.[24] They demonstrated that it is related to some of the heterogeneous minor idiotypes in the A/J strain[25] and is independently regulated. Idiotype[36-60] and Id-CRI_c may be very similar. Idiotype[36-60], however, was defined by antisera raised against monoclonal antibodies of known sequence. CRI_c was defined by an antisera raised against serum antibodies and might include other minor idiotype families.

On the basis of the structural and serologic data, it was predicted that the second idiotype family (Id^{36-60}) present in both murine strains is derived from one or a few germ line genes shared by A/J and BALB/c mice.[20] The slopes of the inhibition curves in a radioimmunoassay for Id^{36-60} in A/J and BALB/c sera suggested that the gene family for Id^{36-60} was shared by A/J and BALB/c strains despite the findings that Id^{36-60} consists of a closely related set of molecules, analogous to the findings for the predominant cross-reacting idiotype.

Recently, an anti-Ars hybridoma protein bearing Id^{36-60} has been derived from a BALB/c mouse following fusion with the Sp2/0 Ag-14 cell line (R. Near and M. Gefter, unpublished). The partial amino acid sequence of the light chain of hybridoma protein 1210.7 is exhibited in FIGURE 6, where it is compared to the set of Id^{36-60} sequences from A/J hybridomas. The 1210.7 light chain sequence is indistinguishable from the A/J Id^{36-60} associated light chain sequences, indicating that they likely arise from equivalent gene(s) in BALB/c and A/J mice, respectively.

The complete heavy chain variable region sequences of the hybridoma protein 36-60 (A/J) as well as for hybridoma protein 1210.7 (BALB/c) are displayed in FIGURE 7 (E. Juszczak and M.N. Margolies, unpublished), along with the partial sequences of the A/J heavy chains 31-64 and 36-54.[20] The 36-60 and 1210.7 heavy chains differ at only four positions in the V_H-encoded portions, suggesting that they arise from the same or very similar germ line genes. Both heavy chains use an identical D gene that corresponds to a core sequence of the BALB/c D gene FL16.2, reported by

STRUCTURAL CORRELATES OF THE ANTI-ARSONATE IDIOTYPE 36-60

HYBRIDOMA LIGHT CHAINS

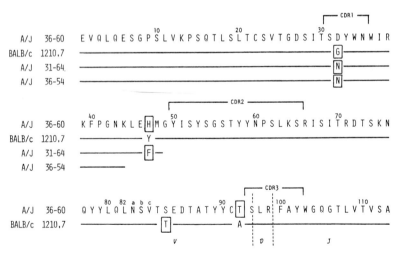

```
                              10                    20
A/J      36-60    D V V M T Q T P L T L S V T I G Q P A S I S C
A/J      31-64    ──────────────────────── I ────────────────
A/J      36-54    ──────────────────────────────────────────
BALB/c   1210.7   ──────────────────────────────────────────


                         ┌──────────── CDR1 ────────────┐
                              30        34  a  b  c  d  e            40
A/J      36-60    K S S Q R L L D S D G K T Y L N W L L Q R P G Q
A/J      31-64    ────── S ──────────────────── S ──────────
A/J      36-54    ────── S ─────────────────────────
BALB/c   1210.7   ────── S ──────────────────────────────────
```

FIGURE 6. Amino acid sequences of anti-Ars hybridoma light chains bearing the minor idiotype 36-60.[20] All of these hybridoma proteins reacted with a rabbit antiserum directed against hybridoma 36-60. Portions of the sequences of the A/J hybridomas 36-60, 31-64, and 36-54 have been reported previously.[20] The sequence of the BALB/c 1210.7 light chain bearing the same idiotype is from R. Near and M.N. Margolies (unpublished).

ID^{36-60} HYBRIDOMA HEAVY CHAINS

```
                                                          ┌─── CDR1 ───┐
                              10               20           30
A/J      36-60    E V Q L Q E S G P S L V K P S Q T L S L T C S V T G D S I T S D Y W N W I R
BALB/c   1210.7   ──────────────────────────────────────────── G ──────
A/J      31-64    ──────────────────────────────────────────── N ──────
A/J      36-54    ──────────────────────────────────────────── N ──────


                                   ┌──────────── CDR2 ────────────┐
                  40              50                  60                70
A/J      36-60    K F P G N K L E H M G Y I S Y S G S T Y Y N P S L K S R I S I T R D T S K N
BALB/c   1210.7   ──────────── Y ──────────────────────────────────
A/J      31-64    ──────────── F ──
A/J      36-54    ──────────


                                              ┌─── CDR3 ───┐
                  80  82 a b c            90            100              110
A/J      36-60    Q Y Y L Q L N S V T S E D T A T Y Y C T │ S L R │ F A Y W G Q G T L V T V S A
BALB/c   1210.7   ──────────────── T ──────────────── A │ ──────────
                                  v                      │  D  │        J
```

FIGURE 7. Amino acid sequences of anti-Ars hybridoma heavy chains bearing the minor idiotype (Id^{36-60})[20] shared by the A/J and BALB/c strains.[20] The complete V_H region sequences of 36-60 and 1210.7 are the results of E. Juszczak and M.N. Margolies (unpublished). The residues enclosed in the blocks are those that differ from the sequence encoded by an A/J germ line V_H gene sequence (R. Near and M. Gefter, unpublished). Portions of the sequence encoded by the V_H, D, and J_H genes (italics) are divided by vertical broken lines. Numbering of residues and designation of CDR are according to Kabat et al.[40]

Kurosawa and Tonegawa.[26] In addition, both hybridomas use the J_H3 gene sequence.[27] Whether the expression of Id^{36-60} requires sequences encoded in all three gene segments (V_H, D, and J_H) remains to be determined. In DNA hybridization studies, R. Near and M. Gefter (unpublished) have shown that all Id^{36-60} hybridomas use J_H3. In addition, their initial results indicate that all Id^{36-60} hybridoma protein V_H arise from a single germ line gene. The DNA sequence of the rearranged heavy chain V region of hybridoma protein 36-60 has been determined, and is indistinguishable from the independently derived amino acid sequence displayed in FIGURE 7. In addition, the A/J germ line gene DNA sequence for Id^{36-60} V_H has been established (R. Near and M. Gefter, unpublished). The heavy chain hybridomas 36-60 (A/J) and 1210.7 (BALB/c) each differ from this germ line sequence at only two positions in V_H, indicated by the boxes in FIGURE 7. Each of these substitutions may be accounted for by a single nucleotide base change from the germ line gene sequence. The data is thus consistent with the entire Id^{36-60} family arising by somatic mutation from a single germ line gene, analogous to the results for Id^{CR} summarized above. It is likely that the BALB/c germ line gene is identical or nearly identical in primary structure to that determined for the A/J germ line gene.

The frequent appearance of the Id^{CR} and Id^{36-60} idiotype families among anti-Ars antibodies suggested that both groups resulted from the direct expression of germ line genes.[20] Because Id^{CR} was predominant in A/J mice, as compared to Id^{36-60}, the possibility was entertained that Id^{CR} existed as multiple gene copies. A difference in gene number is not responsible for Id^{CR} being the predominant idiotype in A/J mice, because the Id^{CR} family has now been demonstrated to be derived from a single germ line V_H gene.[16,17] Whether other control mechanisms are used in regulating the level of gene expression,[20,25] or whether differences in affinity for antigen in the two families accounts for their disproportionate expression, remains to be determined. In this regard, the affinity for hapten of the Id^{CR+} hybridoma protein 36-65, which is identical in sequence to the germ line gene V_H sequence, is lower than all Id^{CR+} hybridoma proteins derived by somatic diversification from this germ line gene. In addition, the affinity of the Id^{CR+} hybridoma protein 36-65 is lower than the three representative hybridoma proteins bearing idiotype$^{36-60}$.[28]

MONOCLONAL ANTIBODIES BEARING THE PREDOMINANT Ars-ASSOCIATED IDIOTYPE THAT DO NOT BIND ARSONATE

In an examination of A/J nonimmune sera, Id^{CR+} Ars-nonbinding immunoglobulin was detected.[29] Following immunization with Ars-protein conjugates, although substantial Ars-binding Id^{CR} appeared, the level of Ars-nonbinding Id^{CR} remained low. Following immunization with a hapten-inhibitable rat monoclonal anti-Id^{CR}, however, large amounts of Ars-binding as well as Ars-nonbinding Id^{CR+} immunoglobulin resulted. As the Ars− component of the Id^{CR+} family in this experiment represents a substantial proportion of total Id^{CR}, any postulated regulatory mechanism that operated to expand Id^{CR} exclusively on the basis of idiotype would be expected to produce large amounts of Id^{CR+} Ars− immunoglobulin. These results are consistent with the postulated coordinate expression of related idiotypes proposed by Jerne.[2]

The finding of Ars-nonbinding Id^{CR+} antibodies recalls earlier reports of such molecules among heterogeneous antibodies elicited in rabbits[30,31] and in mice.[32,33] The structural relationship, however, between these antigen binding and antigen nonbinding forms of idiotype was unclear because of ambiguities in the serological identification of V regions. In addition, the structural differences between idiotype-bearing immunoglobulin elicited by antigen and that elicited by anti-idiotype could not be determined previously because of the heterogeneity of the antibodies produced in such immune responses. The molecular basis of idiotype-anti-idiotype interactions is best revealed through the analysis of (homogeneous) monoclonal antibodies. In the Ars-associated Id^{CR} system, three unusual hybridoma proteins possessing the predominant cross-reactive idiotype were produced from an A/J mouse immunized with a monoclonal rat anti-cross-reacting idiotype. These hybridomas reacted with all available anti-idiotypic sera from several species but did not bind to arsonate.[29] The availability of such Ars-nonbinding hybridoma proteins bearing the predominant Ars-associated idiotype provides a unique approach for monitoring network effects.

The results of amino acid sequence analyses on the heavy and light chains of these three Id^{CR+} Ars− hybridoma proteins are displayed in FIGURE 8.[15] Each is compared to the Id^{CR+} Ars+ sequences that, in the case of the heavy chain, correspond to the V_H germ line gene sequence.[16,17] Positions at which amino acid substitutions were found in individual Id^{CR+} Ars+ hybridoma proteins are indicated by an asterisk in FIGURE 8. For both V_H and V_L, the Id^{CR+} Ars− molecules are nearly identical to the Id^{CR+} Ars+ sequences. The sequences of 3D10 and 3A4 are thus far indistinguishable for both heavy and light chains. This data, taken together with the results of DNA hybridization studies[16,17] (L. Wysocki, unpublished) demonstrate that Id^{CR+} Ars− and Id^{CR+} Ars+ hybridoma proteins are derived from the same germ line V_H gene. Moreover, the marked homology between the corresponding two sets of V_L sequences indicate that both are derived from similar or identical V_L germ line genes. These structural studies indicate that immunization employing monoclonal anti-idiotype can lead to the production of "anti-anti-idiotype" that is nearly indistinguishable in V_H and V_L encoded sequences from the original idiotype, a result that could not be appreciated using heterogeneous idiotype-anti-idiotype systems.

The finding that segments of V region sequences contributing to idiotype and segments used in antigen binding are not identical is not unexpected. In order to further examine the structural changes rendering Id^{CR+} hybridoma proteins Ars-nonbinding, we undertook more extensive sequence analysis on protein 1F6 (J.A. Smith and M.N. Margolies, unpublished). In FIGURE 9, the heavy chain V region sequence of the Id^{CR+} Ars− 1F6 antibody is compared to that of the Id^{CR+} Ars+ antibody 36-65, which represents the germ line V_H sequence (residues 1–94). The heavy chain of the Ars-nonbinding protein 1F6 differs from the V_H gene-encoded sequence at eight positions. Employing a nucleic acid probe specific for Id^{CR+} heavy chains, it was demonstrated that Id^{CR+} Ars− hybridomas also use the same V_H gene.[16] Thus, the 1F6 V_H-encoded segment appears to arise from the Id^{CR+} germ line V_H gene by somatic mutation resulting in eight amino acid substitutions. Each of these substitutions can be accounted for by a single nucleotide base change.

The Id^{CR+} Ars− 1F6 heavy chain employs the same D gene core sequence, as does the 36-65 H chain (Y-Y-G-G-S-Y), except for a single mutation at position 100a. This core sequence corresponds to a combination of the D genes FL16.2 and SP2.3 reported for BALB/c mice by Kurosawa and Tonegawa.[26] Whether the amino acid interchange at position 96 arises as a result of V-D-joining diversity is unknown. Although 36-65 and 1F6 appear to use the same V_H and D genes, the Id^{CR+} Ars+ 36-65 antibody J region sequence may be assigned to the J_H2 gene, whereas that of the Id^{CR+} Ars− antibody corresponds to the J_H4 gene.[27] The results of the amino acid sequences are in accordance with the observations of Siekevitz et al.[16] that one V_H germ line gene rearranges with the J_H2 segment in all Id^{CR+} Ars+ hybridoma cell lines, but in the case of Id^{CR+} Ars− hybridomas, rearrangement occurs instead to J_H4[16] (L. Wysocki, unpublished). In the T15 anti-phosphorylcholine system, a single J_H segment (J_H1) is also used exclusively.[34] The monoclonal antibodies, however, binding alpha-1,3 dextran may employ several J regions.[35] The finding that the Id^{CR+} Ars− hybridomas use the

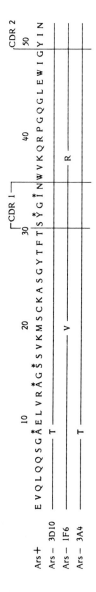

FIGURE 8. Amino acid sequences of heavy (top) and light (bottom) chains of murine A/J hybridoma proteins bearing a predominant cross-reacting idiotype.[15] Sequences of the heavy chains of the Ars-nonbinding hybridomas 3D10, 1F6, and 3A4 are compared to the V_H germ line sequence of the Ars-binding hybridoma 36-65.[16,17] The light chain sequences of the Ars-nonbinding hybridomas are compared to the most common V_L sequence of a set of CRI^+ Ars-binding hybridomas. Asterisks in the topmost sequences indicate positions where amino acid substitutions have been found in the Id^{CR+} Ars+ set of hybridomas. (M.N. Margolies, L.J. Wysocki & V.L. Sato.[15] With permission from *The Journal of Immunology*).

J_H4 rather than the J_H2 segment invites the conclusion that the loss of arsonate binding is due to the structural differences between the J_H2 and J_H4 segments or to D-J junctional changes in these proteins. This recalls the finding of Cook et al.[36] that a single amino acid difference in the J segment of the S107 heavy chain markedly alters binding to phosphorylcholine. Examination of the sequences in FIGURE 9, however, also raises the possibility that substitutions in CDR2 and/or those at the V-D joining site are instead responsible for the loss of antigen binding. This explanation requires that the other Id^{CR+} Ars− heavy chains each also possess changes in CDR other than those due to differences in D-J joining. Parenthetically, the partial sequence of the 1F6 light chain (J.A. Smith and M.N. Margolies, unpublished) is identical thus far to the Id^{CR+} Ars+ sequences.[37]

CRI⁺ HYBRIDOMA HEAVY CHAINS

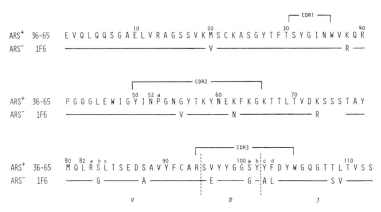

FIGURE 9. Amino acid sequences of Id^{CR+} A/J hybridoma heavy chains. The sequence of heavy chain 36-65 is identical to the germ line gene sequence for $Id^{CR16,17}$ in its V_H-encoded portion (residues 1-94). The Id^{CR+} hybridoma 1F6 does not bind arsonate and was produced following immunization with anti-idiotype.[29] The 1F6 heavy chain sequence is the work of J.A. Smith and M.N. Margolies (unpublished). Portions of the sequence encoded by the V_H, D, and J_H genes are divided by vertical broken lines. The precise limits of D gene-encoded residues with respect to those resulting from junctional diversity are unknown.

Because the Id^{CR+} Ars+ heavy chains and the Id^{CR+} Ars− heavy chains use different J_H segments, it is likely that the amino acid residues used in the predominant shared idiotype are not contributed by the J_H region. (It may, of course, be argued that the residues conserved between J_H2 and J_H4 (FIGURE 9) are used in the idiotypic determinants in concert with other portions of the heavy chain V region). In any case, the existence of antigen nonbinding molecules with preserved idiotype and of an Ars-binding molecule derived from the Id^{CR+}-associated V_H gene (hybridoma protein 45-49 discussed above) that has lost idiotype, are further reminders that "idiotopes" and "paratopes" are not necessarily synonymous.

The Id^{CR+} Ars− monoclonal antibodies were not selected on the basis of arsonate-binding, a property that may or may not be relevant to the evolution of genes controlling cross-reacting idiotype. The possibility was advanced that the Ars-associated idiotype might predominate, because Id^{CR+} antibodies have specificity for an antigen in the murine environment that is different from arsonate.[29] In this connection, the partial V_H sequence of an A/J hybridoma protein obtained following immunization with *Brucella abortus* is indistinguishable from that of the Id^{CR+} Ars+-associated V_H gene structure.[38]

ACKNOWLEDGMENTS

We thank Andrew Brauer and Christine Oman for their outstanding technical assistance.

REFERENCES

1. KUETTNER, M. G., A. L. WANG & A. NISONOFF. 1972. J. Exp. Med. **135:** 579–583.
2. JERNE, N. K. 1974. Ann. Immunol. Inst. Pasteur (Paris) **125C:** 373–389.
3. CAPRA, J. D. & A. NISONOFF. 1979. J. Immunol. **123:** 279–284.
4. CAPRA, J. D., A. S. TUNG & A. NISONOFF. 1977. J. Immunol. **119:** 993–999.
5. RETH, M., G. J. HAMMERLING & K. RAJEWSKY. 1978. Eur. J. Immunol. **8:** 393–400.
6. JU, S.-T., M. PIERRES, C. WALTENBAUGH, R. N. GERMAIN, B. BENACERRAF & M. E. DORF. 1979. Proc. Nat. Acad. Sci. USA **76:** 2942–2946.
7. MARSHAK-ROTHSTEIN, A., M. SIEKEVITZ, M. N. MARGOLIES, M. MUDGETT-HUNTER & M. L. GEFTER. 1980. Proc. Nat. Acad. Sci. USA **77:** 1120–1124.
8. MARSHAK-ROTHSTEIN, A., M. N. MARGOLIES, R. RIBLET & M. L. GEFTER. 1981. *In* Immunoglobulin Idiotypes. C. Janeway & E. Sercarz, Eds.: 739–749. Academic Press. New York.
9. ROTHSTEIN, T. L., M. N. MARGOLIES, M. L. GEFTER & A. MARSHAK-ROTHSTEIN. 1983. J. Exp. Med. **157:** 795–800.
10. MARSHAK-ROTHSTEIN, A., J. D. BENEDETTO, R. L. KIRSCH & M. L. GEFTER. 1980. J. Immunol. **125:** 1987–1992.
11. NELLES, M. J., L. A. GILL-PAZARIS & A. NISONOFF. 1981. J. Exp. Med. **154:** 1752–1763.
12. ESTESS, P., A. NISONOFF & J. D. CAPRA. 1979. Mol. Immunol. **16:** 1111–1116.
13. ESTESS, P., E. LAMOYI, A. NISONOFF & J. D. CAPRA. 1980. J. Exp. Med. **151:** 863–875.
14. MARGOLIES, M. N., A. MARSHAK-ROTHSTEIN & M. L. GEFTER. 1981. Mol. Immunol. **18:** 1065–1077.
15. MARGOLIES, M. N., L. J. WYSOCKI & V. L. SATO. 1983. J. Immunol. **130:** 515–517.
16. SIEKEVITZ, M., M. L. GEFTER, P. BRODEUR, R. RIBLET & A. MARSHAK-ROTHSTEIN. 1983. Eur. J. Immunol. **12:** 1023–1032.
17. SIEKEVITZ, M., S. Y. HUANG & M. L. GEFTER. 1983. Eur. J. Immunol. **13:** 123–132.
18. CREWS, S., J. GRIFFIN, H. HUANG, K. CALAME & L. HOOD. 1981. Cell **25:** 59–66.
19. BOTHWELL, A. L. M., M. PASKIND, M. RETH, T. IMANISHI-KARI, K. RAJEWSKY & D. BALTIMORE. 1981. Cell **24:** 625–637.
20. MARSHAK-ROTHSTEIN, A., M. N. MARGOLIES, J. D. BENEDETTO & M. L. GEFTER. 1981. Eur. J. Immunol. **11:** 565–572.
21. MILNER, E. C. B. & J. D. CAPRA. 1982. J. Immunol. **129:** 193–199.
22. GILL-PAZARIS, L. A., A. R. BROWN & A. NISONOFF. 1979. Ann. Immunol. Inst. Pasteur (Paris) **130C:** 199–213.
23. ALKAN, S. S., R. KNECHT & D. G. BRAUN. 1980. Hoppe-Seyler's Z. Physiol. Chem. **361:** 191–195.
24. BROWN, A. R. & A. NISONOFF. 1981. J. Immunol. **126:** 1263–1267.
25. BROWN, A. R., E. LAMOYI & A. NISONOFF. 1981. J. Immunol. **126:** 1268–1273.
26. KUROSAWA, Y. & S. TONEGAWA. 1982. J. Exp. Med. **155:** 201–218.
27. SAKANO, H., R. MAKI, Y. KUROSAWA, W. ROEDER & S. TONEGAWA. 1980. Nature (London) **286:** 676–683, 1980.
28. ROTHSTEIN, T. L. & M. L. GEFTER. 1983. Mol. Immunol. **20:** 161–168.

29. WYSOCKI, L. J. & V. L. SATO. 1981. Eur. J. Immunol. **11:** 832–839.
30. OUDIN, J. & P.-A. CAZENAVE. 1971. Proc. Nat. Acad. Sci. USA **68:** 2616–2620.
31. URBAIN, J., M. WIKLER, J. D. FRANSSEN & C. COLLIGNON. Proc. Natl. Acad. Sci. USA **74:** 5126–5130.
32. EICHMANN, K., A. COUTINHO & F. MELCHERS. 1977. J. Exp. Med. **146:** 1436–1449.
33. SEPPALA, I. J. T. & K. EICHMANN. 1979. Eur. J. Immunol. **9:** 243–250.
34. GEARHART, P. J., N. D. JOHNSON, R. DOUGLAS & L. HOOD. 1981. Nature (London) **291:** 29–34.
35. SCHILLING, J., B. CLEVINGER, J. M. DAVIE & L. HOOD. 1980. Nature (London) **283:** 35–40.
36. COOK, W. D., S. RUDIKOFF, A. GIUSTI & M. D. SCHARFF. 1982. Proc. Natl. Acad. Sci. USA. **79:** 1979–1983.
37. SIEGELMAN, M. & J. D. CAPRA. 1981. Proc. Natl. Acad. Sci. USA **78:** 7679–7683.
38. SATO, V. L., D. NEMAZEE & M. N. MARGOLIES. International Conference on Immune Networks. Dec., 1982.
39. IUPAC-IUB COMMISSION ON BIOCHEMICAL NOMENCLATURE. 1968. J. Biol. Chem. **243:** 3557–3559.
40. KABAT, E. A., T. T. WU & H. BILOFSKY. 1979. NIH Publ. **80-2008:** 865.
41. SIEGELMAN, M., C. SLAUGHTER, L. MCCUMBER, P. ESTESS & J. D. CAPRA. 1981. *In* Immunoglobulin Idiotypes. C. Janeway, E. E. Sercarz and H. Wigzell, Eds.: 135–158. Academic Press. New York.
42. SIMS, J., T. H. RABBITTS, P. ESTESS, C. SLAUGHTER, P. W. TUCKER & J. D. CAPRA. 1982. Science **216:** 309–310.

DISCUSSION OF THE PAPER

A. MILLER (*University of California, Los Angeles*): Could you clarify the situation with regard to the consensus sequence from serum and hybridoma antibodies; are they different or not?

M. N. MARGOLIES: They are different. My third slide showed the germ line sequence in the heavy chain. The hybridoma sequences all appear to be related to that heavy chain sequence from the germ line that is identical to the heavy chain sequence of the hybridoma 36-65. The pool sequence appears different at approximately thirty positions in the V region; a number of which would require two base changes.

C. A. BONA (*Mt. Sinai School of Medicine, New York*): Do you consider that this last group is really anti-anti-idiotype or is the group a parallel set?

MARGOLIES: I do not know. Operationally it was produced (I used the term in quotes) by immunization with anti-idiotype.

Idiotype-Specific T-Helper Cells

M. McNAMARA, K. GLEASON,[a] AND H. KOHLER

Department of Molecular Immunology
Roswell Park Memorial Institute
Buffalo, New York 14263

INTRODUCTION

The network hypothesis[1] describes the immune system as a web of interacting B and T cells. The specificity of these interactions is based on the complementarity of idiotypes.[2] For B cells, the idiotype repertoire consists of variable domains of immunoglobulins that are constructed by a pair of heavy and light chains. The nature of T-cell idiotypes is not clearly understood.[3] Despite this uncertainty on the chemistry of T-cell receptors and factors, idiotypic cross-reactions between B-cell idiotypes and so-called T-cell idiotypes have been documented in numerous reports.[4-6] The cross-reactivity of T cells does not necessarily indicate the presence of V_H-like structures on T cells, but could simply mean that T-cell receptors or factors mimic idiotypic structures.

Idiotype-specific suppressor cells and their factors have been studied extensively,[7-9] but very little is known about the role and specificity of idiotype-specific T-helper cells. The existence of such idiotype-recognizing T-helper cells can be easily demonstrated by priming T cells to become helper cells for a hapten-specific B-cell response where the carrier for the hapten is a well-defined B-cell idiotype, that is, a myeloma or hybridoma antibody. The physiological role of these idiotype-specific T-helper cells, however, is not clear and in one system is controversial.[10] The fact that these T cells exist,[11] however, and can be induced by priming with a defined antigen (hapten) attests to their biological significance. Therefore, the elucidation of specific network interactions between the B- and T-cell idiotype repertoires is an essential step towards a more complete understanding of the immune system.

In the present study, we have used the phosphorylcholine (PC) system[12] to generate idiotype-recognizing T-helper cells and compared the specificity of idiotype recognition by B cells with that by T cells. We find that T cells "see" idiotypes differently than B cells. T cells preferentially recognize a cross-reactive idiotope, whereas syngeneic or semiallogeneic anti-idiotypic antisera are specific for private idiotopes. Further, we demonstrate that the PC-hemocyanin (Hy) priming is inducing the idiotype-recognizing T cell by way of a T-cell intermediate.

MATERIALS AND METHODS

Mice and Immunizations

BALB/c male and female mice, 6 to 8 weeks old, were purchased from Cumberland View Farms, Clinton, Tennessee. A/He females, 6 to 8 weeks old, were purchased from Jackson Laboratory, Bar Harbor, Maine. (CBA/N × BALB/c)F1 (NBF1)

[a]Present address: Department of Microbiology, University of Illinois, Chicago, Ill. 60680.

males, 6 to 8 weeks old, were purchased from Lab Supply, Indianapolis, Indiana. Athymic, nu/nu BALB/c mice were purchased from Harlan Spraque-Dawley, Madison, Wisconsin and from our own breeding colony. Mice to be used as PC-Hy-primed donors received two intraperitoneal (i.p.) injections, the first with 100 μg Hy in complete Freund's adjuvant (CFA) 48 weeks before use, and the second with 100 μg PC-Hy in incomplete Freund's adjuvant (IFA) 4 weeks before use. Mice to be used as anti-T15-primed donors received .1 μg idiotype-binding capacity. A/He antiserum, intravenously (i.v.) was prepared as previously described.[13] Six to 10 weeks later, the mice sera were tested for T15 idiotype by radioimmunoassay (RIA). Serum levels of T15 were in the normal range (50–100 μg/ml) for BALB/c mice.

Myeloma Proteins

Plasmacytomas T15, M167, and MOPC-460 were obtained from Dr. M. Potter, National Cancer Institute, National Institutes of Health, Bethesda, Maryland, and were maintained by i.p. passage in BALB/c mice. T15, M167, and M460 were purified from the ascitic fluid by affinity-column chromatography.[14]

Antigens

Phosphorylcholine$_5$-hemocyanin was prepared by the reduction of p-aminophenyl-phosphorylcholine (Biosearch, San Rafael, Calif.) to diazophenylphosphorylcholine followed by reaction with hemocyanin.[15] Trinitrophenylated proteins were prepared by the reaction of 2,4,6-trinitrobenzene sulfonic acid (Sigma Chemical Co., St. Louis, Mo.), with purified T15, M167, or M460, which had their binding sites blocked by the appropriate hapten—either .1M PC chloride (Sigma Chemical Co.) or .1M dinitro-phenyl-glycine (Sigma Chemical Co.). After trinitrophenylation, the hapten was removed by dialysis against borate-buffered saline.

Splenic Fragment Cultures

The method for analyzing individual T-helper cells has been described in detail elsewhere.[13] Briefly, primed T-helper cells, obtained as previously described,[16] were transferred to athymic, nu/nu BALB/c recipient mice. Twenty-four to 48 hours later, the spleens were removed aseptically and diced into 1 mm cubes. Each fragment was cultured separately in sterile 96-well culture plates (Costar, Data Packaging, Cambridge, Mass.) in Dulbecco's modified Eagle's medium (DMEM) (Grand Island Biological Co., Grand Island, N.Y.) supplemented with 10% agammaglobulin horse serum (AHS) (Grand Island Biological Co.). The splenic fragment cultures were immunized with trinitrophenyl (TNP)-conjugated myeloma proteins at 5×10^{-7} to 5×10^{-8} M trinitrophenyl. Phosphorylcholine and PC-bovine serum albumin (BSA), used as in vitro inhibitors of T-cell function, were added at the time of immunization at 10^{-7} M phosphorylcholine. T15 and M167 were used also as inhibitors in vitro at 1.4, 7.0, and 14.0 $\times 10^{-9}$ M protein. Heavy and light chains, prepared as described previously,[16] were used similarly at 1.4×10^{-8} M protein. Three days after immunization, culture supernatants were removed and at 3-day intervals the supernatants were collected and assayed for the presence of anti-TNP antibody by enzyme-linked immunosorbent assay (ELISA) and RIA, as previously described.[13,16]

RESULTS

Generation of Idiotype Specific Help

Two methods of generating T15-idiotype-specific T cells have been used: low-dose priming of adult mice with anti-T15 or immunizing adult mice with phosphorylcholine-hemocyanin. The former method involves immunization of BALB/c mice with 10 μg idiotype binding equivalents of A/He anti-T15 antiserum and subsequent transfer, 8 to 10 weeks later, of the primed T cells to athymic, nu/nu, BALB/c recipients. Immunization of the splenic fragment cultures *in vitro* with TNP-T15 resulted in a TNP-specific B-cell response to the appropriate antigen, as seen in TABLE 1. No response was seen when the cultures were immunized with TNP-M460. Because M460 is an α, κ myeloma protein, as is T15, these results indicate that the T cells induced by priming are not specific for heavy or light chain class determinants.

TABLE 1. Anti-T15 Priming and Phosphorylcholine-Hemocyanin Priming Generates Idiotype-Specific Help for Trinitrophenyl-T15

BALB/c T Cell Donor Treatment[a]	T Cells Injected[b] ($\times 10^5$)	*In Vitro* Antigen[c]	Positive Wells[d]
—	0	TNP-T15	<1
Anti-T15-primed	5	TNP-T15	9
Anti-T15-primed	5	TNP-M460	1
Hy-primed	6	TNP-T15	3
Hy-primed	9	TNP-T15	2
PC-Hy-primed	3	TNP-T15	13
PC-Hy-primed	6	TNP-T15	22
PC-Hy-primed	9	TNP-T15	20

[a] Mice used as anti-T15-primed donors received 0.1μg A/He anti-T15 antisera intravenously 6–8 weeks before use. Mice used as Hy-primed donors received 100μg Hy in CFA 4 weeks before use; PC-Hy-primed donors received 100μg Hy in CFA 8 weeks before use and 100μg PC-Hy in IFA 4 weeks before use.

[b] T cells that had been nylon-wool purified were injected into BALB/c nu/nu recipients.

[c] The splenic fragment cultures were immunized *in vitro* with TNP$_7$-T15 at 5×10^{-7} to $5 \times 10^{-8} M$ TNP, or with TNP$_6$-M460 at $10^{-8} M$ TNP.

[d] Ninety-six to 288 cultures were assayed for anti-TNP activity on days 10 and 13 by radioimmunoassay.

Phosphorylcholine-hemocyanin priming of adult mice can also generate idiotype-specific help (TABLE 1). Graded doses of nylon wool-passaged T cells from either Hy-primed or PC-Hy-primed mice were transferred to nu/nu BALB/c recipients, and, as above, immunization of the splenic fragments with TNP-T15 resulted in an anti-TNP response. The antibody response was shown to be linearly dependent on the doses of donor T cells transferred up to 9×10^5 T cells. A decrease in the response to TNP-T15 is seen at the highest cell dose. Hemocyanin-primed donor cells were not able to help in the response to TNP-T15, demonstrating that PC-Hy priming is specifically generating T15-recognizing T help.

Specificity of the T-Helper Cells from Phosphorylcholine-Hemocyanin Immunized BALB/c Mice

T cells stimulated by PC-Hy priming were analyzed for their specificity. Previous data from our laboratory showed that these cells, which recognize T15, could also recognize M167, another anti-PC, non-T15 myeloma.[17] This lack of idiotype specificity in the recognition can be explained by either a single T-helper population that recognizes an idiotope shared by T15 and M167, or by two distinct T-helper populations, each of which recognizes a different idiotype on T15 and 167.

To further characterize the specificity of the T-helper cell induced by PC-Hy priming, we attempted to block *in vitro* the action of the idiotype-specific T-helper cell using various inhibitors. As can be seen from TABLE 2, free hapten PC or PC-BSA used as an inhibitor abrogated the response to TNP-T15 completely. This indicates that the binding site on the T15 protein, known to be a highly conserved determinant,[18] is a major portion of the determinant recognized by the T-helper cells. Next, unconjugated T15 and M167 were used as *in vitro* inhibitors at 1, 5, and 10 times molar excess over the antigen concentration. The results in TABLE 2 demonstrate that both idiotypes inhibit the response to TNP-T15 to the same extent.

In order to further localize the determinants recognized by idiotype-specific T-helper cells, isolated heavy and light chains from T15 and 167 were used as inhibitors *in vitro*. The results, seen in TABLE 2, show that the heavy chains of T15 and of M167 inhibit the response to the antigen 32% and 48% respectively, whereas neither light chain inhibited the response significantly. This fact indicates that the major part of the determinant recognized by the T-helper cells resides on the heavy chain. The complete expression of the determinant probably requires the intact structure of a complete immunoglobulin molecule. Collectively, these inhibition studies provide evidence that part of the idiotype recognized by these idiotype specific T cells is shared by T15 and M167. The helper cell that recognizes idiotype can be induced by priming with phosphorylcholine. An indirect method of T-help induction must be invoked to explain this induction. In the following experiments, we aimed to analyze the cellular circuits in this network interaction.

T-Helper Induction Circuit

To determine if the idiotype-recognizing T cell was being induced by another T cell, (CBA/N × BALB/c) (NBF1) male mice were primed with phosphorylcholine-

TABLE 2. Inhibition of the *In Vitro* Response to Trinitrophenyl-T15

BALB/c T Cell Donor Treatment[a]	*In Vitro* Antigen[b]	*In Vitro* Inhibitor[c]	Positive Wells[d]	Inhibition Percent
PC-Hy-primed	TNP-T15	—	29–40	—
PC-Hy-primed	TNP-T15	PC or PC-BSA	0	100
PC-Hy-primed	TNP-T15	T15	15	44
PC-Hy-primed	TNP-T15	M167	15	56
PC-Hy-primed	TNP-T15	T15 H chain	27	32
PC-Hy-primed	TNP-T15	T15 L chain	35	13
PC-Hy-primed	TNP-T15	167 H chain	24	40
PC-Hy-primed	TNP-T15	167 L chain	41	0

[a]PC-Hy-primed donor mice were prepared as in TABLE 1. Ly 2.2$^-$ nylon-wool purified T cells were prepared by treatment with anti-Ly 2.2 plus rabbit complement and then injected into BALB/c nu/nu recipients.
[b]Cultures were immunized with TNP$_7$-T15 at $10^{-8}M$ TNP.
[c]Cultures were inhibited with the hapten PC and PC-BSA at $10^{-7}M$ PC; T15, 167, and M460 at $1.4 \times 10^{-8}M$ protein; and T15, 167 H, and L chains at $1.4 \times 10^{-8}M$ protein.
[d]Culture supernatants were assayed for anti-TNP antibody by ELISA.

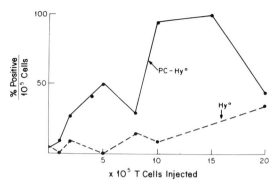

FIGURE 1. Titration of T-helper cells from PC-Hy primed NBF1 males for a response to TNP-T15. Percent positive cultures per 10^5 transferred cells are plotted against the number of transferred T-helper cells. One hundred percent is equivalent to 34 responding cultures per 1.5×10^6 transferred cells.

hemocyanin. These mice have an x-linked immune defect (xid gene) that renders their B cells unresponsive to PC in a primary response.[19] Graded doses of PC-Hy-primed Ly2⁻, nylon wool-passaged T cells were transferred to athymic, nu/nu, BALB/c recipients. Splenic fragment cultures were prepared and immunized with TNP-T15. The results in FIGURE 1 show that recipients that received no cells, or Hy-primed T-helper cells were not able to respond to the antigen. Those recipients, however, that received the PC-primed T-helper cells were able to mount a substantial response to TNP-T15. The number of positive responses to TNP-T15 is dependent on the number of transferred T cells (see FIGURE 1). The response increases linearly up to 5×10^5 transferred T cells. Then the response begins to decline, which is followed by a second increase. At the highest cell dose of 2×10^6 T cells, the response again decreases. This response pattern seems to be similar to that found by Eichmann.[20]

Because T15 recognizing T-helper cells can be induced by PC-Hy-priming in the immunodefective NBF1 male, anti-PC antibodies, in particular those of the T15 idiotype, are not involved in the induction circuit. Instead, PC-Hy stimulates a T cell, which in turn induces the idiotype-recognizing T-helper cells, demonstrating a T-T-cell induction network.

To further exclude the possibility that the induction of idiotype-recognizing T-helper cells occurs by way of a B-T circuit, B cells from PC-Hy-primed BALB/c B were cotransferred with normal T-helper cells from NBF1 mice. One, 2, or 3 weeks later, splenic fragment cultures were prepared and immunized with TNP-T15. The results in TABLE 3 indicate that the whole spleen population from PC-Hy primed donors exhibited a response to the antigen. By contrast, PC-primed B cells, cotransferred with normal NBF1 T cells, were not able to stimulate T15-specific help. Collectively, these adoptive transfer experiments provide evidence that T cells are able to induce idiotype-recognizing T-helper activity, whereas B cells are not able to induce the same.

DISCUSSION

Various manipulations of the network affecting B cells have been reported.[21–23] In the present study, we have investigated the T-cell compartment of the idiotypic network. Previous findings have shown that idiotype-specific T cells can be directly induced by priming with idiotype.[24,25] Here we show data on the generation of these cells through indirect routes. We provide evidence that the induction of helper cells specific for the T15-idiotype is possible in both T15 positive and T15 negative mice. In order to demonstrate idiotype-recognizing T-helper cells, priming with anti-idiotype antibody or with PC is necessary. The fact that anti-idiotype can be used to induce the idiotype-recognizing T cells is further evidence in support of regulation through complementary idiotypic interactions, and the fact that these cells can also be activated by exposure to antigen is evidence of their biological significance.

One point of interest is that T15-specific helper cells can be generated in a T15 negative mouse, the immunodefective NBF1 male. This finding contrasts with the claim of Bottomly et al.,[10,26] who reported that the NBF1 males are deficient in a T15-specific T-helper cell population. They suggest that because NBF1 males are incapable of responding to PC with T15 idiotype, the absence of idiotype-specific T cells may be due to the lack of cell-bound and circulating T15. Our data, however,

TABLE 3. B Cells from Phosphorylcholine-Hemocyanin Primed BALB/c Mice Do Not Induce Idiotype-Specific Help for Trinitrophenyl-T15

Cells Transferred from BALB/c PC-Hy-Primed[a]	T Cells Transferred from Normal NBF1 $(\times 10^6)$[b]	Anti-TNP Positive Wells[c]
—	—	0 ± 0
5×10^6 spleen cells	—	41.7
5×10^6 B cells	—	0 ± 0
5×10^6 B cells	10^6	1 ± 0

[a]Mice used as PC-Hy-primed donors were prepared as in TABLE 1. B cells were prepared by treating whole spleen cells with anti-Thy-1.2 plus complement. Cells were injected into normal NBF1 recipients that had not been x-irradiated 6–8 hours before cell transfer.

[b]The Ly 2.2⁻ T cells were prepared as in TABLE 2 and transferred into the x-irradiated recipients at the same time as the B cells. One, 2, or 3 weeks after cell transfer the mice were sacrificed.

[c]Splenic fragment cultures were immunized in vitro with TNP₇-T15 at $10^{-8}M$ TNP. Two hundred eighty-eight cultures were assayed for anti-TNP antibody at days 6, 12, and 15 by ELISA.

demonstrate that even in the absence of the T15 idiotype, a T-helper cell population can be induced in the F1 male that recognizes T15.

The PC system has been well studied at the B-cell idiotype level.[27,28] The present study on idiotype-specific T cells allows one to compare the idiotypic interaction sequence of both the T cell and the B cell compartment. An interesting parallelism emerges: as PC antigen induces a subsequent auto-anti-idiotypic antibody response,[29] so do T cells. Priming with PC-antigen induces a T cell that auto-recognizes a shared determinant on T15. By contrast to the auto-anti-idiotypic B-cell response that is not hapten inhibitable, the auto-anti-idiotypic T cells recognize a determinant that is intimately involved in the PC-binding site. Still, the biological significance of such auto-anti-idiotypic T cells remains an enigma. It is unlikely that its function is to promote the T15 dominance as proposed by Bottomly and colleagues.[26]

An interesting observation was made in the T-cell dose titration into nude BALB/c. The biphasic pattern (see FIGURE 1) is reminiscent of the data of Eichmann and colleagues.[20] These authors, however, used polyclonal activation to induce T-helper activity, whereas in our experiments T-helper cells were induced specifically with PC antigen. The finding can be interpreted by assuming that two different populations of T-helper cells exist with different frequencies. For each of these populations, T-suppressor cells are cotransferred. This process induces the decline of the response with increasing cell dose.

Viewed as a whole, these data suggest that T cells that recognize a shared determinant on anti-PC antibodies might be important for stimulating and maintaining a B-cell memory for anti-PC responsiveness. They might also indicate that the T-cell idiotype receptor repertoire is biochemically different from that of B-cell idiotypes. Its function might be, in general terms, to exert a regulatory control over B cells. In this task, T cells see B cells as families of idiotypes and not as individual members of a constantly changing and mutating B-cell repertoire.[28,30]

SUMMARY

In the present study we investigated the induction and fine specificity of T-helper cells that recognize idiotypes. The data presented show that both low-dose priming with anti-T15 antiserum and priming with PC-Hy are effective in stimulating T15-specific T help. Phosphorylcholine-hemocyanin priming can generate these T cells in either PC-responding or nonresponding strains of mice. Furthermore, the PC-primed T-helper cells can also recognize another anti-PC myeloma, M167, that is idiotypically different from T15. The fine specificity of the anti-PC-idiotype recognizing T-helper cells was examined by studying the effect of *in vitro* inhibitors on the T-cell help. Both PC and PC-BSA as well as T15 and M167 had an inhibitory effect on the T help. Free T15 and M167 heavy chains also blocked the helper activity for T15; T15 and M167 light chains had no effect, however. Viewed collectively, these results show that PC-Hy priming induces T-helper cells that recognize idiotypic determinants common to both T15 and M167, and that the proteins' H chain is the major structural component of the determinant. Finally, the generation of these idiotype-recognizing T cells was found to occur by way of a T-T interaction loop, based on the finding that T-helper cells are induced by PC-Hy priming in animals that lack PC-responding B cells.

REFERENCES

1. JERNE, N. K. 1974. Towards a network theory of the immune system. Ann. Immunol. Inst. Pasteur (Paris) **125C:** 373.
2. KOHLER, H., D. A. ROWLEY, T. DuClos & B. RICHARDSON. 1977. Complementary idiotypy in the regulation of the immune response. Fed. Proc. Fed. Am. Soc. Exp Biol. **36:** 221.
3. EICHMANN, K. 1978. Expression and functions of idiotype on lymphocytes. Adv. Immunol. **26:** 195.
4. BINZ, H. & H. WIGZELL. 1975. Shared idiotypic determinants on B and T lymphocytes reactive against the same antigenic determinants. I. Demonstration of similar or identical idiotypes on IgG molecules and T-cell receptors with specificity for the same alloantigen. J. Exp. Med. **142:** 197.
5. EICHMANN, K. & K. RAJEWSKY. 1975. Production of T and B cell immunity by anti-idiotypic antibodies. Eur. J. Immunol. **5:** 661.
6. JULIUS, M. H., H. COSENZA & A. A. AUGUSTIN. 1978. Evidence for autogenous production of T cell receptor bearing idiotypic determinants. Eur. J. Immunol. **8:** 484.
7. OWEN, F.L., S-T. JU & A. NISONOFF. 1977. Presence on idiotype-specific suppressor T cells of receptors that interact with molecules bearing the idiotype. J. Exp. Med. **145:** 1559.

8. KIM, B. S. 1979. Mechanisms of idiotype suppression. I. *In vitro* generation of idiotype-specific suppressor T cells by anti-idiotype antibodies and specific antigen. J. Exp. Med. **149:** 1371.
9. TAKEMORI, T. & T. TADA. 1974. Properties of antigen-specific suppressive T-cell factor in the regulation of antibody response of the mouse. I. *In vivo* activity and immunochemical characterizations. J. Exp. Med. **142:** 1241.
10. BOTTOMLY, K. & D. E. MOSIER. 1979. Mice whose B cells cannot produce the T15 idiotype also lack an antigen-specific helper T cell required for T15 expression. J. Exp. Med. **150:** 1399.
11. CANTOR, H. & E. A. BOYSE. 1976. Regulation of cellular and humoral immune response by T cell subclasses. Cold Spring Harbor Symp. Quant. Biol. **41:** 23.
12. LEE, W., H. COSENZA & H. KOHLER. 1974. Clonal restriction of the immune response to phosphorylcholine. Nature (London) **247:** 55.
13. GLEASON, K., S. PIERCE & H. KOHLER. 1981. Generation of idiotype-specific T cell help through network-perturbation. J. Exp. Med. **153:** 924.
14. CUATRECASAS, P. 1970. Protein purification by affinity chromatography: derivations of agarose and polyacrylamide beads. J. Biol. Chem. **245:** 3059.
15. GEARHART, P. J., N. H. SIGAL & N. R. KLINMAN. 1975. Heterogeneity of the BALB/c anti-phosphorylcholine antibody response at the precursor cell level. J. Exp. Med. **141:** 567.
16. GLEASON, K. & H. KOHLER. 1982. Regulatory Idiotypes. T helper cells recognize a shared V_H idiotype on phosphorylcholine-specific antibodies. J. Exp. Med. **156:** 539.
17. CREWS, S., J. GRIFFIN, H. HUANY, K. CALAME & L. HOOD. 1981. A single V_H gene segment encodes the immune response to phosphorylcholine. Somatic mutation is correlated with the class of the antibody. Cell **25:** 59.
18. CLAFLIN, J. L. & M. J. DAVID. 1974. Clonal nature of the immune response to phosphorylcholine. IV. Idiotypic uniformity of binding site associated antigenic determinants among mouse anti-phosphorylcholine antibodies. J. Exp. Med. **140:** 673.
19. MOND, J. J., R. LIEBERMAN, J. K. INMAN, D. G. MOSIER & W. G. PAUL. 1977. Inability of mice with a defect in B-lymphocyte maturation to respond to phosphorylcholine on immunogenic carriers. J. Exp. Med. **146:** 1138.
20. EICHMANN, K., I. FALK, I. MELCHERS & M. M. SIMON. 1980. Qualitative studies on T-cell diversity. I. Determination of the precursor frequency for two types of streptococcus A-specific helper cells in nonimmune polyclonally activated splenic T cells. J. Exp. Med. **152:** 477.
21. COSENZA, H. & H. KOHLER. 1972. Specific inhibition of plaque formation to PC by antibody against antibody. Science **176:** 1027.
22. KELSOE, G. & J. CERNY. 1979. Reciprocal expansions of idiotypic and anti-idiotypic clones following antigen stimulation. Nature (London) **279:** 333.
23. ROMBALL, C. G. & W. O. WEIGLE. 1976. Modulation of regulatory mechanisms operative in the cyclical production of antibody. J. Exp. Med. **143:** 497.
24. JANEWAY, C. A., Jr., N. SAKATO & N. H. EISEN. 1975. Recognition of immunoglobulin idiotypes by thymus-derived lymphocytes. Proc. Nat. Acad. Sci. USA **72:** 2357.
25. JULIUS, M. H., A. A. AUGUSTIN & H. COSENZA. 1977. Recognition of a naturally occurring idiotype by autologous T cells. Nature (London) **265:** 251.
26. BOTTOMLY, K. & F. JONES, III. 1981. Idiotypic dominance manifested during a T-dependent anti-phosphorylcholine response requires a distinct T helper cell. *In* B Lymphocytes in the Immune Response: Functional Development and Interactive Properties. 415. Elsevier/North Holland. Amsterdam, Holland.
27. KOHLER, H. 1975. The response to phosphorylcholine: dissecting an immune response. Transplant. Rev. **27:** 26.
28. GEARHART, P., N. D. JOHNSON, R. DOUGLAS & L. HOOD. 1981. IgG antibodies to phosphorylcholine exhibit more diversity than their IgM counterparts. Nature (London) **291:** 29.
29. KLUSKENS, L. & H. KOHLER. 1974. Regulation of immune response by autogenous antibody against receptor. Proc. Nat. Acad. Sci. USA. **71:** 5083.
30. BONA, C. A., E. HEBER-KATZ & W. PAUL. 1981. Idiotype-anti-idiotype regulation. I.

Immunization with a levan-binding myeloma protein leads to the appearance of auto-anti(anti-idiotype) antibodies and to the activation of silent clones. J. Exp. Med. **153**: 951.

DISCUSSION OF THE PAPER

T. TADA (*Tokyo University, Tokyo, Japan*): Would you say that these helper cells are not the ones that determine T15 dominance?

H. KOHLER: I really do not think these data address that question. I do not know.

TADA: If they have a broad cross-reactivity, what will be the result?

KOHLER: Then idiotype-recognizing T_H cells could not cross-react. We have not tested this function of the T cell that we are looking at.

D. E. MOSIER (*Institute for Cancer Research, Philadelphia, Pa.*): How do you imagine that this T cell would regulate an anti-PC response if its interaction with its target antigen idiotype is inhibited by PC. Would it be by antigen? It would seem that the function of this cell would be self limited.

KOHLER: I was careful not to say what the function of that T cell is, so I do not have to answer your question. But we can go on and speculate.

J. CERNY: Dr. Kohler, you made allusion to Eichmann's T-cell titration experiments in which I had participated. I have the following question for you. When you look at the wells that contain the positive fragments that mount response to TNP, would the same wells mount response to an unrelated antigen, or do you see a different distribution if you stimulate your fragments with a different antigen? Would you see a segregation or not?

KOHLER: We have, of course, used control antigens, like TNP coupled to a non-PC binding myeloma or monoclonal. These wells were negative.

CERNY: Do you mean that other wells are positive?

KOHLER: No, they are nothing. We could not detect anything above background if we used TNP coupled to a non-PC binding myeloma or monoclonal.

The Use of a Small Synthetic Antigen to Study Immune Regulation by Way of Idiotypes[a]

CLIFFORD J. BELLONE AND
SUNDARARAJAN JAYARAMAN

Department of Microbiology
Saint Louis University School of Medicine
Saint Louis, Missouri 63104

INTRODUCTION

There are many antigen-specific T-suppressor (T_S) systems described that study the regulation of antibody and delayed-type hypersensitivity (DTH) responses in mice.[1-7] Studies in various antigen systems have clearly revealed the heterogeneity of antigen-specific T_S that communicate by way of antigen, idiotype(s) (Id), and major histocompatibility complex (MHC) encoded gene products.[1-7] The induction of distinct waves of T_S has been demonstrated using antigen under tolerogenic conditions[8-11] or using factor(s) derived from one population to induce another T_S population.[12,13] Thus, it has not been demonstrated that different T_S subsets can be induced sequentially *in vivo* in the same experimental animals using an immunogenic form of antigen. Such an observation will contribute to the understanding of the proposed synergistic and antagonistic interaction between different T_S subsets under normal physiological conditions.

Our earlier studies indicated the possibility of using the synthetic monovalent antigen, L-tyrosine-*p*-azophenyltrimethylammonium (tyr(TMA)) as an agent to induce regulatory T-cell populations.[14,15] This report summarizes the data obtained in the TMA system using tyr(TMA) to induce T_S subpopulations. The data indicate that tyr(TMA) triggers the induction of two mechanistically distinct T_S in a temporal sequence in the same experimental animal after the induction of a T-helper population.[16,17] Moreover, the occurrence of anti-idiotypic second-order T_S (T_{S_2}) after a single injection of tyr(TMA) in A/J mice was accompanied by the loss of function of an idiotypic modulatory T cell (Tmod) that is critical for the function of T_{S_2}.[18] In addition, the preliminary data indicate that the "lesion" in the suppressor pathway might be due to an active suppressive mechanism that blocks Tmod function *in situ*. We also present results that provide information regarding mechanisms by which Tmod and T_{S_2} communicate in order to effect suppression.

MATERIALS AND METHODS

Mice

Male A/J (H-2^a, Igh-1^e) mice of 6 to 8 weeks old were obtained from the Jackson Laboratory, Bar Harbor, Maine.

[a]This work was aided by Basic Research Grant No. 1-665 from the March of Dimes Birth Defects Foundation and by the United States Public Health Service, National Institutes of Health Grant AI-13115.

Antigens

L-tyrosine-*p*-azophenyltrimethylammonium and trimethylaminoaniline were purchased from Biosearch, (San Raphael, Calif.) and Bachem, Inc. (Torrance, Calif.), respectively. Preparation of diazonium salt,[19] and TMA coupled syngeneic spleen cells (TMA-SC)[20] have already been described.

Immunization and Challenge

Mice were injected subcutaneously with freshly coupled 3×10^7 TMA-SC and 5 days later challenged in the footpad with 25 μl of 10mM diazotized TMA in saline.[20] The footpad swelling was recorded 24 hours later, and the response was expressed as the increment of footpad swelling between challenged and unchallenged footpads.

Suppressor Cells

To induce T_S cells mice were injected intraperitoneally (i.p.) with 0.2 ml containing 100 μg of tyr(TMA) and Freund's complete adjuvant (FCA). The T_S were purified either using nylon wool columns[16] or petri dishes coated with affinity purified rabbit anti-mouse immunoglobulin (RAMIg) as described previously.[17]

Monitoring Modulatory Cell Activity

Mice injected i.p. with tyr(TMA) 6 weeks before, served as the recipients. Modulatory T cells were obtained from lymph nodes of normal mice immunized 5 days earlier.[18] The immune lymph node cells were, in some cases, treated with several reagents, as previously described,[18] before intravenous (i.v.) transfer into recipients. The mice were challenged usually within 2 hours of cell transfer.

In vitro Arming of Modulatory T Cells

Either normal mice or tyr(TMA) injected mice (6 weeks before) were immunized with TMA-SC. Lymph nodes and spleens were collected and T cells were fractionated using RAMIg plates.[17] In some experiments, purified T cells were further fractionated on petri dishes coated with TMA coupled to bovine serum albumen (BSA).[16] Suppressor factors were extracted as described earlier.[16] Purified T cells were armed with suppressor factors *in vitro* following the procedure of Zembala *et al.*[21] In brief, T cells were suspended at 3×10^7 cells per ml in balanced salt solution containing 5% heat inactivated fetal calf serum and 3×10^7 cell equivalent suppressor factor. After 45 minutes of incubation at 37° C, the cells were spun and washed once in balanced salt solution before transfer.

Statistical Analysis

All data were analyzed for significance by using a two-tailed Student's *t*-test. Percent suppression was calculated using the formula:

$$\text{Percent suppression} = \left(\frac{\text{Positive control} - \text{experimental group}}{\text{Positive control} - \text{negative control}} \right) \times 100.$$

RESULTS

TABLE 1 summarizes the cellular sequence triggered by a single i.p. injection of tyr(TMA) in FCA in A/J mice. One week after the antigen injection, a TMA-specific helper population, bearing cross-reactive Id characteristic of anti-TMA antibodies in A/J mice, was detected.[14] A week later, the first-order T-suppressor cells (T_{S_1}) capable of suppressing both DTH and antibody responses specific to the TMA hapten were detected.[17] The Ly-1$^+$, 2$^-$, nylon wool adherent T_{S_1}, bearing idiotypic receptors, bind only to TMA coupled to protein carriers and not to Id associated with anti-TMA antibodies. Both the T_{S_1} and the suppressor factor(s) derived from them (T_SF_1) act at the induction, but not at the effector phase of the DTH response. T_SF_1 can suppress the DTH response across both H-2 and allotype barriers. T_{S_1}-bearing mice, when stimulated to anti-TMA antibody production, suppress both Id$^+$ and Id$^-$ plaque-forming cell (PFC) responses. This finding is in marked contrast to the T_{S_2}-bearing mice. Perhaps the most interesting observation is that the T_{S_1} are able to suppress the DTH response intrinsically in addition to their ability to suppress the response on adoptive transfer. This phenomenon is in marked contrast to the late appearing T_S population, T_{S_2}.

Six weeks after tyr(TMA) inoculation, the splenic suppressor activity is mediated by Ly-1$^-$, 2$^+$, I-J$^+$, nylon wool-nonadherent T_{S_2} cells.[16] These T_{S_2} do not bind antigen,

TABLE 1. Properties of tyr(TMA)-Induced Regulatory T Cells

Appearance	Designation	Properties
1 week	T_H	Idiotypic T helper specific for TMA hapten
2 weeks	First-order suppressors (T_{S_1})	*Cells:* Ly-1$^+$, 2$^-$, idiotypic, nylon wool adherent T cells that bind to TMA-BSA and not to idiotype(s); act at the induction phase of DTH only.
		Factor(s): Acts at the induction phase of DTH only; acts across H-2 and allotype barriers to suppress DTH; depends on Cy-sensitive cell type(s).
		Animals: Intrinsically suppress DTH responses; exhibit suppression of both Id$^+$ and Id$^-$ PFC responses.
6–7 weeks	Second-order suppressors (T_{S_2})	*Cells:* Ly-1$^-$, 2$^+$, nylon wool-nonadherent T cells that bind to idiotype(s) and not to TMA-BSA; act at both induction and effector phases of DTH; express function only on adoptive transfer into naive hosts; both H-2 and allotype restricted for action.
		Factor(s): Acts at induction and effector phases of DTH; restricted by both H-2 and allotype; depends on Cy-sensitive cell type(s).
		Animals: No intrinsic suppression of DTH responses; exhibit only Id$^+$ PFC suppression.

TABLE 2. Phenotype of Modulatory T Cells[a]

Cells Transferred	Response mm ± 1 SEM	Percent Suppression
Positive Controls	1.02 ± 0.03 (37)[b]	—
LNC + c	0.55 ± 0.03 (18)	70[c]
LNC + anti-Thy-1 + c	0.88 ± 0.09 (6)	21
LNC + anti-Id + c	0.85 ± 0.03 (10)	25
LNC + anti-Ly-2 + c	0.82 ± 0.05 (6)	30
LNC + anti-Ly-1 + c	0.64 ± 0.02 (5)	57[c]
Negative controls	0.35 ± 0.01 (30)	—

[a]T_{S_2}-bearing mice (A/J mice injected with tyr(TMA) plus FCA 6 weeks before) were immunized with 3×10^7 TMA-SC. Five days after immunization these mice were injected i.v. with 2×10^7 LNC derived from normal mice that were immunized with TMA-SC 5 days earlier. LNC were treated with indicated reagents and washed extensively before transfer. Positive controls represent T_{S_2}-bearing mice that received no cells, and negative controls represent naive mice challenged alone. All mice were challenged in the footpad within 1 hour of cell transfer, and the footpad response was monitored 24 hours later.
[b]Number of mice tested is given in parentheses.
[c]Significant suppression.

but do bind Id and act at the induction as well as the effector phases of delayed-type hypersensitivity. Unlike the T_SF_1, the suppressor factor(s) derived from T_{S_2} (T_SF_2) is both H-2 and allotype restricted for their function.[16] With regard to antibody suppression, unlike T_{S_1}, the T_{S_2}-bearing mice suppress only the Id^+ component of the PFC response.[15] One of the most interesting findings is that the T_{S_2} cells can readily suppress the DTH response on adoptive transfer into normal mice, but fail to function intrinsically.[18] Thus, T_{S_2}-bearing mice effectively suppress Id^+ antibody production,[15] but fail to alter the DTH response that is also mediated by Id^+ T cells mediating delayed-type hypersensitivity (T_{DTH}).[18]

A number of findings in our laboratory suggested that the inability of these mice to suppress DTH was due to a loss of a T_S subpopulation, termed the modulatory cells (Tmod).[18] We, as well as others, have found[18,22] that the function of T_{S_2} depends on a cyclophosphamide (Cy)-sensitive cell type in antigen-activated lymphoid cells derived from normal mice. Further, we found that the T_{DTH} from T_{S_2}-bearing mice were suppressible on adoptive transfer into naive mice when first mixed with antigen-activated lymph node cells (LNC) from normal mice.[18] This finding indicated that a normal constituent of the suppressor circuit was lacking in the T_{S_2}-bearing mice. Based on these findings, experiments were designed to make the T_{S_2} functional *in situ*. Antigen-activated LNC derived from normal mice were transferred i.v. into antigen-primed T_{S_2}-bearing mice just prior to challenge. As seen in TABLE 2, these cells provided the missing critical cellular function, because these recipients expressed suppression of delayed-type hypersensitivity. Treatment of the antigen-activated LNC from normal mice prior to the adoptive transfer with several reagents revealed that the missing cellular component was a $Thy-1^+$, $Ly-1^-$, 2^+, idiotype-bearing Tmod population. Thus, a single injection of tyr(TMA) in FCA in A/J mice triggers a sequence of cellular events that results in a loss of Tmod function.

There are several possible mechanisms by which this "lesion" could occur. Because normal immunization procedures induce Tmod activity in normal mice, but not in T_{S_2}-bearing mice, the possibility exists that these cells were either clonally deleted in the T_{S_2}-bearing mice or that they were quiescent due to some active suppressor mechanism. To test these possibilities, naive spleen cells were transferred into

TABLE 3. Inability of Normal Spleen Cells to Restore Tmod Activity[a]

Time of Cell Transfer	Response mm ± 1SEM	Percent Suppression
Positive controls	0.96 ± 0.05 (19)[b]	—
24 hours before immunization	0.78 ± 0.06 (13)	28[c]
24 hours before challenge	0.77 ± 0.07 (9)	30[c]
Negative controls	0.32 ± 0.08 (20)	—

[a] A/J mice injected i.p. with tyr(TMA) plus FCA 6 weeks before were immunized with 3×10^7 TMA-SC. Six $\times 10^7$ spleen cells from naive mice were transferred i.v. either before immunization with TMA-SC or before challenge in the footpad. The footpad swelling was measured 24 hours after challenge. Positive controls were not injected with cells. Negative controls represent naive mice challenged in the footpad.
[b] Number of mice tested per group is given in parentheses.
[c] Not significant.

T_{S_2}-bearing mice 24 hours before immunization for DTH or just prior to footpad challenge. As seen in TABLE 3, transfer at either time point did not result in DTH suppression, suggesting that the transferred precursor Tmod cells could not be triggered to function in the T_{S_2}-bearing hosts. These results suggest that the Tmod inactivity is due to some active mechanism that could result in a lesion at a number of levels. The experiments do not rule out the possibility that Tmod are activated to partially differentiate, but do not function *in situ* because of a defect in the communication between T_{S_2} and Tmod. Zembala *et al.*[21] have shown that effector-phase T_SF when "armed" on to the acceptor cells, trigger the release of inhibitor molecules that suppress the transfer of contact sensitivity. Minami *et al.*[23] have reported that the monoclonal T_SF_2, when incubated *in vitro* with T_{S_2} activates these cells to effect suppression. If the lesion in T_{S_2}-bearing mice were in fact at this level it might be possible to "arm" antigen-activated Tmod from these mice and reverse the lack of function. It was first necessary to determine whether arming of Tmod with T_SF_2 effects suppression of TMA-specific delayed-type hypersensitivity. To test this hypothesis, T cells from LNC and spleens obtained from normal mice, immunized 5 days earlier with TMA-SC were incubated *in vitro* with T_SF_2 after which these armed cells were transferred into recipients that had been previously immunized and treated with Cy to deplete the host of Tmod.[18] In some experiments, to better define the specificity and target of T_SF_2, these T cells were first incubated on antigen (TMA-BSA)-coated petri dishes, and the adherent and nonadherent populations were collected. These two populations were then incubated with T_SF_2 and transferred separately to monitor for suppression of delayed-type hypersensitivity. As seen in FIGURE 1, only the adherent or antigen-binding T population was suppressive after incubation with T_SF_2, indicating that Tmod bear antigen-specific receptors as well as acceptor sites for T_SF_2. To further test the specificity of arming of Tmod cells, antigen-activated T cells from normal mice were incubated *in vitro* with T_SF_1 rather than with T_SF_2. By contrast to the Tmod cells armed with T_SF_2, the Tmod armed with T_SF_1 could not suppress the DTH response (data not shown), indicating that the arming with T_SF_2 is a highly specific interaction.

The next experiment was performed to determine whether the lack of Tmod function in T_{S_2}-bearing mice might be overcome by *in vitro* arming of T cells from these mice. It is possible that T_SF_2 acceptor sites on Tmod are blocked or not expressed *in vivo* and could be reversed by the *in vitro* incubation period. As seen in FIGURE 2, T cells from normal mice, when armed with T_SF_2, suppress the DTH as observed earlier. When the T cells, however, from T_{S_2}-bearing mice were incubated with T_SF_2 and transferred back into T_{S_2}-bearing mice, no suppression was observed. It should be mentioned that the armed T cells from normal mice when transferred into T_{S_2}-bearing mice could effectively bring about suppression (data not shown).

DISCUSSION

This overview of the TMA system was intended primarily to show how the monovalent synthetic antigen tyr(TMA) can lend insight into regulatory networks that use restricted idiotypes. There are several points we wish to emphasize. We now have accumulated enough data to show that tyr(TMA) in FCA triggers a sequence of regulatory T cells beginning with a T_H population[14] followed in order by T_{S_1}[17] and T_{S_2}.[16] This sequential occurrence takes place over a period of several weeks and appears to be governed in part by Id-anti-Id interactions, because a single dose of a rabbit anti-Id antiserum will trigger essentially the same cellular pathway induced by tyr(TMA).[15] Further, the TMA-specific T_H and T_{S_1} populations bear Id, and precede the appearance of T_{S_2} that have receptors that recognize and bind to idiotype.[16] Unlike most systems, a nontolerogenic antigenic regimen is used to trigger the suppressor pathway. Further, no external manipulations are required to dissect out the various subpopulations, as they appear not to overlap at given points in time. As summarized in the RESULTS section (See TABLE 1), the early phase (2 week) and late phase (6 week) suppressor T_S are clearly different subpopulations, both with respect to surface antigenic markers, function, and most importantly, receptor specificity.[16,17] The

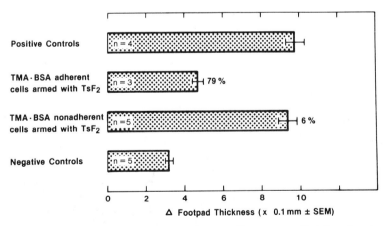

FIGURE 1. T_SF_2 arms the T cells bearing antigen-specific receptors. Both lymph nodes and spleens from normal mice immunized with TMA-SC were collected 5 days later. T cells enriched using RAMIg plates were incubated on dishes coated wth TMA-BSA. Both the adherent and nonadherent fractions were armed with T_SF_2 and washed before transfer into recipients. The recipients were normal mice immunized with TMA-SC and injected i.p. with 20 mg Cy/kg on day 1 to deplete Tmod cells. The armed cells (10×10^6 antigen adherent and 20×10^6 antigen nonadherent) were injected i.v., and the recipients were challenged within 2 hours of cell transfer. Positive controls are mice immunized and Cy treated but not transferred with cells. The figures show the percent suppression of DTH caused by the transfer of armed cells. n = number of mice tested.

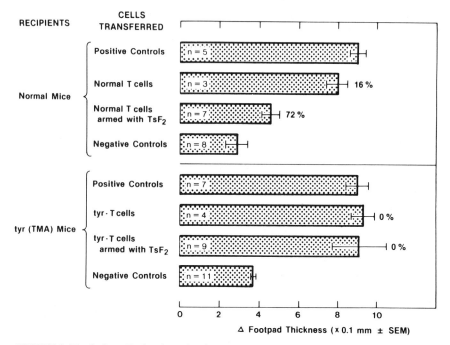

FIGURE 2. T cells from T_{S_2}-bearing mice do not mediate suppression after *in vitro* arming with T_SF_2. RAMIg plate-purified T cells obtained from normal and T_{S_2}-bearing mice 5 days after TMA-SC immunization were armed with T_SF_2. The armed cells ($30-40 \times 10^6$ per mouse) were injected i.v. into respective groups of mice immunized with TMA-SC 5 days earlier. The mice were challenged within 2 hours of cell transfer. The figures show the percent suppression of DTH caused by the transfer of armed cells. n = number of mice tested.

described T_{S_1}, and T_{S_2} plus their respective factors share many of the properties of previously described T_S in other Id-defined DTH systems.[7,8,10,24,25]

The T_SF_1 in the TMA system, however, is neither H-2 nor allotype restricted for its action on DTH responses, unlike the T_SF_1 that suppresses azobenzenearsonate (ABA)-specific DTH[26] and nitrophenylacetyl (NP)[24]-specific contact-sensitivity responses[27] that act across H-2 barriers, but are restricted by allotype. It should be noted that the ABA-T_SF_1[7] and NP-T_SF_1[24] were obtained from cells induced with a tolerizing dose of hapten-coupled syngeneic spleen cells, but the TMA-T_SF_1 was extracted from T_{S_1} cells induced after an immunogenic dose of the monovalent antigen tyr(TMA). In the synthetic polymer L-glutamic acid[50]-L-tyrosine[50] (GT)-induced suppressor pathway, the GT-T_{S_1} induced in the nonresponder strain of mice yield GT-T_SF_1 that suppresses the antibody response in an H-2 and allotype nonrestricted manner.[28]

In some systems, it has been shown that T_SF_1 serves to induce the genetically restricted T_{S_2} that are effector phase suppressors and restricted by both H-2 and allotype for their interaction with target cells.[7,9] The question remains whether T_{S_1} and T_SF_1 serve only to function as inducers, or whether they can act as suppressor effectors independent of T_{S_2}. Our data indicate that T_{S_1} and T_{S_2} might function in a mechanistically different fashion independent of each other. This is suggested by the observation that the suppression of antibody responses in the T_{S_1} and T_{S_2}-bearing mice is different. By contrast to the T_{S_2}-bearing mice wherein only the Id^+ PFC responses were suppressed, the T_{S_1}-bearing mice suppress both Id^+ and Id^- PFC responses.[15,17]

The unique observation in the TMA system is that the T_{S_2}-bearing mice, while suppressing the Id^+ PFC response, could not suppress the Id^+ DTH response.[18] The failure of T_{S_2} to suppress the DTH responses intrinsically was found to be due to the loss of function of another type of T_S called Tmod that is similar to T auxiliary,[29] or T_{S_3}.[7,22,30] Because antibody formation is suppressed in these mice, the possibility of whether the Tmod are required for the T_{S_2}-mediated suppression of antibody responses is raised. It has been shown that T_{S_3} are required for both the suppression of antibody responses[31] as well as contact sensitivity responses to nitrophenylacetyl.[22] On the other hand, there are data suggesting the direct action of anti-idiotypic T_{S_2} on idiotypic B cells in some systems.[32-34] It is still an open question, however, whether B cells can be regulated by the anti-idiotypic T_{S_2} directly without any intermediary cell type like the T_{S_3} or Tmod. If the idiotypic B cells producing anti-TMA antibodies can be regulated directly by anti-idiotypic T_{S_2} without the involvement of Tmod cells, unlike the DTH responses, this would represent a unique immune strategy regulating the idiotypic T and B cells in a different manner, which may be advantageous to the immune system under certain circumstances. On the other hand, if the idiotypic B cells also need Tmod for their regulation as in the NP system,[31] then the failure to demonstrate the function of Tmod in the T_{S_2}-bearing mice may only be temporary. This situation is possible because the time period affected in assaying for DTH is short (5 days) when compared to a 4 week period in assaying for antibody responses. Although this fact might explain the difference in the mode of action of anti-idiotypic T_{S_2} on idiotypic T and B cells, it remains to be proven. Regardless of the involvement of Tmod in B-cell suppression, the T_{S_2}-bearing mice are capable of a "split" suppression by inactivation of Tmod at least for a critical time period.

In order to understand this lesion in the suppressor pathway, it is essential to understand how the Tmod is triggered to function under normal conditions. Zembala et al.[21] have shown that T-acceptor cells, when incubated in vitro with effector phase T_SF, suppressed the transfer of contact sensitivity. Minami et al.[23] have reported that the incubation of monoclonal T_SF_2 with antigen-activated T_{S_3} in vitro results in an effector T_S population that suppresses the contact sensitivity responses specific to nitrophenylacetyl. Our data (FIGURE 1) show that the Tmod when armed with T_SF_2 in vitro can suppress the DTH responses in vivo. This fact is in line with the findings that the factors that act at the effector phases of immune responses have an acceptor site on T-acceptor cells.[21] In addition, we show that the Tmod cells have receptors that bind to the antigen, unlike T-acceptor cells in one system that apparently do not possess antigen-specific receptors.[35] In addition, the Tmod cells after arming with T_SF_2 in vitro can be activated to release suppressor substance(s) after a brief incubation with TMA-SC, which in turn can suppress the DTH response in Cy-treated mice (unpublished data). The data indicate that the suppression of DTH responses by armed Tmod cells is mediated by the release of soluble suppressor factor(s) as shown in other systems.[21,35]

Interestingly enough, the T cells from T_{S_2}-bearing mice could not be armed with T_SF_2 in order to effect suppression of DTH in T_{S_2}-bearing mice (FIGURE 2). This fact suggests that either the Tmod cells in these mice are clonally deleted, or alternatively, that the Tmod cells in these mice were not fully activated to be triggered by the binding of T_SF_2. In any case, it was not possible to reactivate the function of Tmod cells by incubating with T_SF_2 in vitro. It will be interesting to explore the possibility of activating the Tmod cells in T_{S_2}-bearing mice by some alternative manipulation, assuming that the Tmod are under active suppression. Whatever the reason for the lesion in the suppressor pathway, this model system appears to offer unique opportunities not only for exploring the mechanism by which Tmod control immune responses, but also the control of these critical T_S themselves.

ACKNOWLEDGMENTS

We wish to thank Mrs. Maria J. Weingartner for her expert secretarial assistance in the preparation of this manuscript.

REFERENCES

1. GERSHON, R. K. 1974. Contemp. Top. Immunobiol. 3: 1.
2. CANTOR, H. & E. A. BOYSE. 1977. Contemp. Top. Immunobiol. 7: 47.
3. TADA, T. & K. OKUMURA. 1979. Adv. Immunol. 28: 1.
4. MCKENZIE, I. F. C. & T. POTTER. 1979. Adv. Immunol. 27: 181.
5. BONA, C. A. 1981. Idiotypes and Lymphocytes. Academic Press. New York.
6. GERMAIN, R. N. & B. BENACERRAF. 1981. Scand. J. Immunol. 13: 1.
7. GREENE, M. I., M. J. NELLES, M.-S. SY & A. NISONOFF. 1982. Adv. Immunol. 32: 254.
8. WEINBERGER, J. Z., R. N. GERMAIN, S.-T. JU, M. I. GREENE, B. BENACERRAF & M. E. DORF. 1979. J. Exp. Med. 150: 761.
9. WEINBERGER, J. Z., B. BENACERRAF & M. E. DORF. 1980. J. Exp. Med. 151: 1413.
10. WEINBERGER, J. Z., R. N. GERMAIN, B. BENACERRAF & M. E. DORF. 1980. J. Exp. Med. 152: 161.
11. MILLER, S. D., L. D. BUTLER & H. N. CLAMAN. 1982. J. Immunol. 129: 461.
12. WALTENBAUGH, C., J. THEZE, J. A. KAPP & B. BENACERRAF. 1977. J. Exp. Med. 146: 970.
13. SY, M.-S., M. H. DIETZ, R. N. GERMAIN, B. BENACERRAF & M. I. GREENE. 1980. J. Exp. Med. 151: 1183.
14. ALEVY, Y. G., C. WITHERSPOON & C. J. BELLONE. 1981. J. Immunol. 126: 2390.
15. ALEVY, Y. G. & C. J. BELLONE. 1980. J. Exp. Med. 151: 528.
16. JAYARAMAN, S. & C. J. BELLONE. 1982. Eur. J. Immunol. 12: 278.
17. JAYARAMAN, S. & C. J. BELLONE. 1983. J. Immunol. 130: 2519.
18. JAYARAMAN, S. & C. J. BELLONE. 1982. J. Exp. Med. 155: 1810.
19. ALEVY, Y. G., C. D. WITHERSPOON, C. A. PRANGE & C. J. BELLONE. 1980. J. Immunol. 124: 215.
20. JAYARAMAN, S. & C. J. BELLONE. 1982. Eur. J. Immunol. 12: 272.
21. ZEMBALA, M., G. L. ASHERSON & V. COLIZZI. 1982. Nature (London) 297: 411.
22. SUNDAY, M. E., B. BENACERRAF & M. E. DORF. 1981. J. Exp. Med. 153: 811.
23. MINAMI, M., S. FURUSUWA & M. E. DORF. 1982. J. Exp. Med. 156: 465.
24. MINAMI, M., K. OKUDA, S. FURUSAWA, B. BENACERRAF & M. E. DORF. 1981. J. Exp. Med. 154: 1390.
25. OKUDA, K., M. MINAMI, S. FURUSAWA & M. E. DORF. 1981. J. Exp. Med. 154: 1838.
26. DEITZ, M. H., M.-S. SY, B. BENACERRAF, A. NISONOFF, M. I. GREENE & R. N. GERMAIN. 1981. J. Exp. Med. 153: 450.
27. OKUDA, K., M. MINAMI, D. H. SHERR & M. E. DORF. 1981. J. Exp. Med. 154: 468.
28. KAPP, J. A. & B. A. ARANEO. 1982. J. Immmunol. 128: 2447.
29. SY, M.-S., S. D. MILLER, J. W. MOORHEAD & H. N. CLAMAN. 1979. J. Exp. Med. 149: 1197.
30. SY, M.-S., A. NISONOFF, R. N. GERMAIN, B. BENACERRAF & M. I. GREENE. 1981. J. Exp. Med. 153: 1415.

31. SHERR, D. H. & M. E. DORF. 1982. J. Immunol. **128:** 1261.
32. BONA, C. & W. E. PAUL. 1979. J. Exp. Med. **149:** 592.
33. ABBAS, A. K., L. L. PERRY, B. A. BACH & M. I. GREENE. 1980. J. Immunol. **124:** 1160.
34. MILBURN, G. L. & R. G. LYNCH. 1982. J. Exp. Med. **155:** 852.
35. ZEMBALA, M. A., G. L. ASHERSON, B. M. B. JAMES, V. E. STEIN & M. C. WATKINS. 1982. J. Immunol. **129:** 1823.

Auto-Anti-Allotype Antibody in Allotype-Suppressed Rabbits: Immunoregulation of Immunoglobulin Synthesis by an Allotype-Idiotype Network[a]

SHELDON DRAY, ALICE GILMAN-SACHS, AND
WAYNE J. HORNG[b]

Department of Microbiology and Immunology
University of Illinois at Chicago
Health Sciences Center
Chicago, Illinois 60612

Since the initial characterization of rabbit immunoglobulin (Ig) allotypes,[1-4] the study of these genetic variants has greatly enhanced our basic understanding of the diversity, genetic control, structure, and functions of the Ig molecule.[5-8] The concept of allotype suppression,[9] the demonstration that lymphocytes have surface Ig,[10] and the characterization of idiotypes[11-13] were key elements in the development of the network theory of the immune system.[14] The subsequent demonstration of the induction of *auto*-anti-allotype antibodies (Ab)[15] and *auto*-anti-idiotype Ab[16] provided further experimental support for the theory. The recent characterization of common or similar idiotypic specificities of anti-allotype Ab has provided a system for testing some features of the immune network.[17-22] Here we present some concepts of how allotypes, idiotypes, and *auto*-antibodies may be affected in the immunoregulation of rabbit Ig synthesis.

When fetal or neonatal rabbits are given antibody directed to one of their inherited Ig allotypes, either by transfer *in utero* or by neonatal injections, a long-lasting inability to synthesize Ig molecules of that allotype develops. A compensatory increase, however, in other Ig gene products occurs, and serum levels are normal. These alternative gene products may be encoded either by an allelic gene product for rabbits heterozygous at the a V_H, $b\kappa$, or $nC\mu$ loci, by a linked gene product for rabbits homozygous at the a V_H locus, or by an unlinked gene product for rabbits homozygous at the $b\kappa$ locus (TABLE 1). This phenomenon, known as allotype suppression, reflects a basic mechanism that regulates the relative quantities of Ig allotypes and is the first example of an antibody-induced alteration in the expression of Ig genes[9] (reviewed in references 23–25).

The demonstration that anti-allotype antibodies induce blast transformation of lymphocytes from rabbits having the corresponding allotype[10] indicated that lymphocytes bear surface immunoglobulin. This finding suggested that allotype suppression was probably induced by the interaction of anti-allotype Ab with cell surface immunoglobulin. Allotype suppression has been demonstrated in rabbits heterozygous

[a]This work was supported by Research Grants PHS AI-07043 and PHS AI-15228 from the National Institutes of Health.

[b]Present address: Abbott Laboratories, North Chicago, Illinois 60064.

or homozygous with respect to allotypes encoded by the $b\kappa$ locus, which controls the synthesis of 80 to 90% of the light chains; the a V_H locus, which controls a subgroup of V_H regions present in 70 to 90% of the heavy chains; and the n $C\mu$ locus, which controls the constant region of the μ chain (reviewed in references 23–25). Thus far, however, attempts to induce suppression by anti-allotype Ab specific for the constant regions of the α or γ chain have not been successful.[23] Thus, the induction of allotype suppression *in vivo* appears to be mediated by the interaction of anti-allotype Ab with IgM molecules on the lymphocyte surface. This phenomenon is consistent with the finding that Ig-bearing lymphocytes of the spleen and lymph node have surface IgM, but not IgG or IgA (FIGURE 1).[26,27]

Recently, we and other investigators have shown that the *allo*-anti-allotype Ab used to induce allotype suppression of a designated allotype have a common or similar idiotype specificity.[17–22] In our laboratory, antibody to the a2 allotype (anti-a2 Ab) from an a^1a^1 homozygous rabbit was isolated and used as an immunogen in recipient rabbits of the same genotype. The resulting anti-idiotype Ab reacted not only with the immunogen anti-a2 Ab but also with anti-a2 Ab from fifteen other rabbits.[18] By immunodiffusion (FIGURE 2), direct binding radioimmunoassay (TABLE 2), or inhibi-

TABLE 1. Effects of Allotype Suppression in Rabbits Heterozygous or Homozygous for the b (κ light chain), a (V_H region subgroup), or n ($C\mu$ region) Locus[a]

Genotype	Suppressing Ab	Suppressed Ig Allotype	Compensated Ig Allotype	Gene That Compensates
b^4b^5	anti-b4	b4	b5	allelic
a^1a^3	anti-a1	a1	a3	allelic
$n^{81}n^{82}$	anti-n81	n81	n82	allelic
b^5b^5	anti-b5	b5	c7 & c21	unlinked (λ chains)
a^2a^2	anti-a2	a2	x32 & y33	linked (V_H subgroups)
$n^{81}n^{81}$	anti-n81	n81	new?	linked? ($C\mu$ subclass?)

[a] After Dray, 1979.

tion of binding (FIGURE 3), the idiotypic specificity of each of the anti-a2 Ab preparations was found to be very similar if not identical. Moreover, by direct binding radioimmunoassay (TABLE 2) and analysis by sequential radiobinding, virtually all of the anti-a2 Ab molecules that had the idiotypic specificity also reacted with the antigen, that is, the a2 allotype.[18] The expression of this common idiotypic specificity was not dependent on the expression of a V_H or light chain allotypic specificity, because the 15 anti-a2 Ab preparations were obtained from a1b4, a1b5, a3b4, and a3b5 noninbred rabbits. The idiotypic specificities of both anti-a1 and anti-a3 anti-allotype Ab were also characterized, and similar or cross-reacting idiotypic specificities were found for each set of eight nonimmunogen anti-a1 and eight nonimmunogen anti-a3 anti-allotype Ab preparations.[22] Recently, we induced anti-idiotype Ab to anti-y33 anti-allotype antibody. The y33 allotypic specificity is present among the minor V_H region allotypes (up to 5% of the Ig molecules are y33) and is greatly enhanced in the serum of a2-suppressed a^2a^2 rabbits (up to 50% of the Ig molecules are y33).[28] By immunodiffusion, radiobinding assay, and inhibition of binding radioimmunoassay, the idiotypic specificity detected on the immunogen anti-y33 Ab was found also on the anti-y33 Ab preparations from three other rabbits. Thus, as shown for anti-allotype Ab to the major a V_H locus allotypes, anti-allotype Ab induced in different rabbits to a minor y V_H locus allotype also bears a similar idiotypic specificity. The expression of a common idiotypic specificity on anti-allotype Ab molecules to a V_H allotype is in sharp contrast to the findings for other rabbit antibodies and suggests that the number of V region genes coding for an anti-allotype Ab is limited. With respect to an immune network, the finding of a common idiotype for anti-allotype Ab would facilitate regulation of these molecules by anti-idiotype antibody.

Although allotype suppression can be induced by administration of exogenous *allo*-anti-allotype Ab, this Ab is not required to maintain suppression because suppression is maintained for a very long time after anti-allotype Ab is no longer

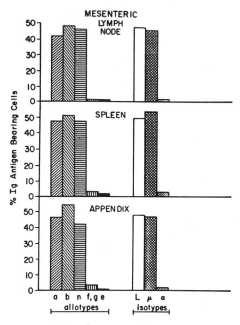

FIGURE 1. Lymphocytes from lymph node, spleen, and appendix cells have surface IgM, but not IgA or IgG. Lymphoid cells were mixed with sheep red blood cells conjugated to specifically isolated anti-allotype Ab to a V_H, $b\kappa$ light chain, $C\mu n$, $C\alpha$ f, g or $C\gamma e$ allotypes and with anti-isotype Ab to light chains (L), μ chains, or α chains. The rosetted Ig-bearing cells were counted microscopically.

detected in the serum. Eventually, however, the suppressed allotype escapes from suppression and gradually increases in quantity.[25] Indeed, allotype suppression in homozygous rabbits in comparison to that of heterozygous rabbits is not permanent or even very long lasting; the suppressed allotype generally escapes suppression more rapidly in homozygous than in heterozygous rabbits, suggesting that the compensation by a linked or nonlinked gene product in a homozygous rabbit is not as stable as that by an allelic gene product in a heterozygous rabbit (TABLE 1). To insure long lasting allotype suppression, however, a rabbit suppressed for the synthesis of an Ig allotype can be autoimmunized at two months of age with that allotype. In 1975, Lowe *et al.*[15] showed that complete allotype suppression can be continuously maintained by inducing *auto*-anti-allotype Ab in a suppressed rabbit; they induced Ab to the b6 allotype of

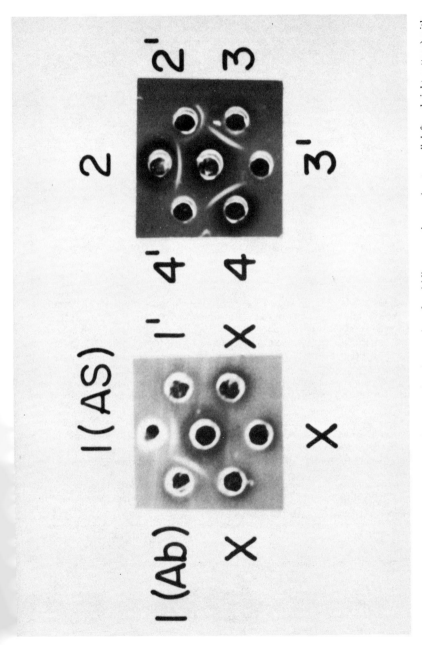

FIGURE 2. Immunodiffusion experiment demonstrating the reaction of anti-idiotype antiserum (center well, left and right pattern) with the pool of anti-a2 antiserum from which the immunogen was isolated, 1 (AS); the immunogen anti-a2 Ab isolated therefrom, 1(Ab); and the three anti-a2 antisera that constituted the pool, 2, 3, and 4. Note lack of reaction with the preimmune serum (1', 2', 3', and 4'). Twelve other anti-a2 antisera gave a similar precipitin reaction with anti-idiotype Ab (not shown).

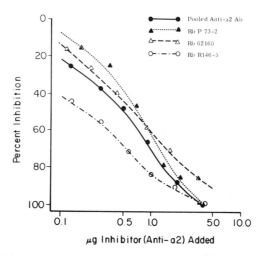

FIGURE 3. Inhibition curves obtained when the binding of ^{125}I-labeled pooled immunogen anti-a2 Ab to insolubilized anti-idiotype antiserum is inhibited by three nonimmunogen anti-a2 Ab preparations, P73-2, 62160, and R146-5. These inhibition curves were similar to that obtained with the immunogen.

κ-light chains in b^4b^6 or b^5b^6 heterozygous rabbits suppressed for the paternal b6 allotype. We extended these findings by inducing *auto*-Ab to the a1 V_H allotype in an a^1a^2 heterozygous rabbit suppressed for a1.[29] When *auto*-anti-a1 Ab was isolated from this rabbit, it reacted with the same percentage of a1 Fabγ molecules as did an *allo*-anti-a1 Ab (TABLE 3). When the IgG and IgM of this rabbit was analyzed by radioimmunoassay, essentially no a1 was detected. Indeed, virtually all of these Ig molecules were of the a2 allotype. The suppression was complete and apparently permanent, because the suppressed allotype was not detectable in serum after one year.

An additional development that resulted from the above procedures was the use of auto-immunized and suppressed heterozygous female rabbits as the mothers of homozygous suppressed and auto-immunized rabbits.[30] We used the following procedures to produce these rabbits (FIGURE 4). First, an a2-suppressed a^1a^2 heterozygous

TABLE 2. The Amount of Anti-a2 Allotype Antibody That Reacts with the Anti-Idiotype Antibody or with the a2 Allotype

	Percentage of [^{125}I]Anti-a2 Allotype Ab Bound to Insolubilized	
[^{125}I]Anti-a2 Ab from Rabbit:	Anti-Idiotype Antiserum	a2 Serum
Pool	52	52
62160	45	45
R146-5	50	52
P73-2	58	54
2L280-2	60	57
P28-7	43	35
H192-3	40	55

female was immunized to produce *auto* anti-a2 antibody. Next, the auto-immunized heterozygous female was mated to an a^2a^2 homozygous male to obtain a a2-suppressed offspring. The female progeny, while still suppressed for the a2 allotype at 2 months of age, were immunized to produce *auto*-anti-a2 Ab. This immunization resulted in complete and permanent suppression. An a2-suppressed and *auto*-anti-a2 Ab producing a^2a^2 homozygous female from this litter was mated with an a^2a^2 male to produce an entire litter of a^2a^2 homozygous rabbits, all suppressed for the a2 allotype. By the same procedure, we also induced *auto*-anti-b4 Ab and *auto*-b5 Ab in b4-suppressed b^4b^4 and b5-suppressed b^5b^5 homozygous rabbits, respectively. This procedure facilitates production of rabbits that are homozygous and suppressed for the synthesis of allotypes of the major V_H subgroup (encoded by the *a* V_H locus) or the dominant light chain type (encoded by the *b* κ locus). In these rabbits, the auto-antibody provides a self-regulating mechanism that permanently blocks the expression of a major Ig gene *in vivo*. Presumably this occurs by blocking the expansion of lymphocyte clones that might bear the suppressed allotype.

Auto-anti-a2 Ab was isolated and assayed for the common idiotypic specificity detected on *allo*-anti-a2 antibody. This *auto*-anti-Ab was isolated from the serum of

TABLE 3. Comparison of the Binding Capacity of *Auto*-Antibody and *Allo*-Antibody to the a1 Allotype[a]

		Percentage of a1 Fabγ Precipitated by	
Fabγ from Rabbit	Genotype of Rabbit	*Auto*-anti-a1	*Allo*-anti-a1
2P287-5	a^1a^1	76	79
2P287-6	a^1a^1	75	78
2L290-2	a^1a^1	72	75
N236-2	a^1a^1	74	76
2L93-1	a^1a^1	73	75
H151-1	a^1a^1	67	71

[a]In control experiments, less than 4% of Fabγ from an a^2a^2 or a^3a^3 rabbit was precipitated by *auto*-anti-a1 or *allo*-anti-a1 antibody.

either an a^1a^2 heterozygous or an a^2a^2 homozygous rabbit that had been autoimmunized after complete suppression for the synthesis of the a2 allotype.[22,31] These *auto*-anti-a2 Ab molecules not only reacted with the a2 allotype, but also had the common idiotypic specificity previously detected on *allo* anti-a2 Ab (TABLE 4). Thus, the *auto*-anti-a2 Ab that maintains allotype suppression permanently was found to have the same idiotypic specificity as the *allo*-anti-a2 Ab that induces allotype suppression. Similar findings have been reported for *auto*-anti-a1 Ab and *allo*-anti-a1 Ab by Metzger and Roux.[21] Because anti-allotype Ab can inhibit the expression of an allotype and because *auto*-anti-allotype Ab can be induced in suppressed rabbits, a rabbit must possess the genes coding for the allotype as well as for the anti-allotype antibody. In normal rabbits, however, only the allotype is ordinarily expressed at detectable levels, whereas in allotype-suppressed and auto-immunized rabbits, only the *auto*-anti-allotype Ab is expressed. Although the detection of naturally occurring *auto*-anti-allotype Ab has not been reported in unimmunized rabbits, it would be of great interest to demonstrate its existence either in the serum or on the surface of lymphocytes of normal or allotype-suppressed rabbits. The use of anti-idiotype Ab to anti-allotype Ab will greatly facilitate these studies and possibly provide information about the network that may regulate the expression of the allotype.

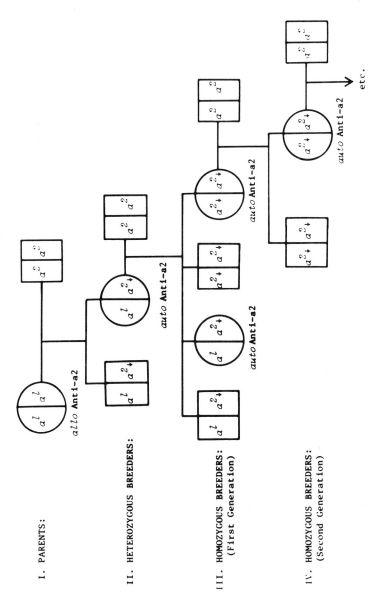

FIGURE 4. Rationale of inducing homozygous allotype suppression by means of an auto-immunized homozygous female breeder. The arrows indicate rabbits suppressed for the a2 allotype. The rabbits that were immunized to produce *allo-* or *auto-*Ab are indicated.

TABLE 4. The Presence of the Common Idiotypic Specificity of *Allo*-Anti-a2 Antibody on *Auto*-Anti-a2 Antibody Molecules

Rabbit No.[a]	Genotype	Percentage of [^{125}I] *Auto*-Anti-a2 Ab Molecules Bound to Insolubilized	
		Antiserum to the Common Idiotype of Anti-a2 Ab	Serum Containing the a2 Allotype
R12-3	$a^2 a^2$	34	34
T218-4	$a^1 a^2$	40	38

[a]For rabbit R12-3, essentially all of the V_H allotype was x32 or y33, whereas for rabbit T218-4, essentially all of the V_H allotype was a1.

Because perinatal exposure to *allo*-anti-allotype Ab suppresses the expression of Ig allotypes, the question arises whether *auto* anti-allotype Ab naturally appears and serves to regulate the synthesis of Ig allotypes. For example, the serum a2:a1 allotype ratio in heterozygous rabbits is relatively constant and is under genetic control, closely linked to the heavy chain chromosomal region.[32] If *auto*-anti-a2 Ab naturally occurs and depresses the level of the a2 allotype, it might be possible to suppress the anti-a2 Ab with anti-idiotype Ab, thereby allowing for an increase in the a2 allotype and an increase in the a2:a1 ratio. With this in mind, an $a^1 a^1$ homozygous dam immunized with anti-a2 Ab and producing anti-idiotype Ab was mated to an $a^2 a^2$ homozygous male. The serum Ig a2:a1 ratios for three offspring were then determined for the postnatal period of 3 to 15 weeks. For two of the progeny, the serum a2:a1 ratios increased from 0.6 or 0.8 at week 4 to 1.3 or 1.2 at week 9 and then decreased to 0.7 or 0.8 at week 12 (FIGURE 5).[31] The third rabbit already had a relatively high a2:a1 ratio of 1.1:1 when first tested at week 5; the ratio then decreased to 0.6 by week 12. Because the a2 allotype in the offspring is encoded by the paternally inherited gene, the a2 allotype level in the serum represents neonatal synthesis. On the other hand, the serum a1 allotype level includes not only neonatal synthesis, but also maternally transferred Ig that is essentially completely metabolized by the 7th or 8th week. The increase in the a2:a1 ratio seen at the 7th or 8th week is no longer affected by the passively transferred

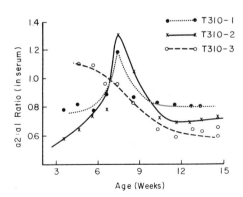

FIGURE 5. The serum a2:a1 ratio from 3 to 15 weeks of age for three $a^1 a^2$ heterozygous littermates, T310-1, -2, or -3, which were offspring of an $a^2 a^2$ male and an $a^1 a^1$ female producing anti-idiotype Ab to the common idiotype of anti-a2 antibody. Offspring from similar matings, but where the mother was not immunized have an a2:a1 ratio ranging from 0.3 to 0.7 at 8 weeks of age.

a1 allotype, but represents a ratio primarily of neonatally synthesized allotypes. An a2:a1 ratio > 1 at 7 to 8 weeks appears to be significant, because the a2:a1 ratio in the serum of 13 offspring from nonimmunized mothers ranged from 0.3 to 0.7 at 8 weeks of age.[32] Thus, the passive transfer of anti-idiotype Ab to the fetus apparently caused a transient increase in the a2:a1 ratio. Presumably, in the neonatal rabbit, the transient idiotype suppression is induced in a manner similar to allotype suppression, that is, by the interaction of anti-idiotype Ab with the idiotype (i.e., anti-a2 Ab) present as a lymphoid cell receptor.

In heterozygous rabbits, the relative amounts of serum allotypes are unequal and characteristic of a given genotype.[23,33] Thus, there is a preferential expression of one allotype over another. Nevertheless, the pre-B cells of heterozygous rabbits exhibit allelic exclusion and appear to be generated in equal allotype frequencies in the bone marrow.[34] Thus, during differentiation from pre-B cells to B cells, some mechanism must exist to induce this preferential increase of one allotype over another. Such a mechanism may be an allotype-idiotype network wherein naturally occurring anti-allotype Ab may inhibit or suppress synthesis of the corresponding allotype and regulate the relative amounts of allotypes in heterozygous rabbits. In addition, Ab to

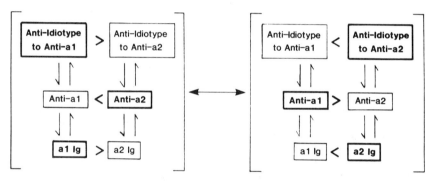

FIGURE 6. A proposed allotype-idiotype network that regulates the serum a1:a2 ratios in a^1a^2 rabbits. The left diagram shows the situation for an a1:a2 ratio >1, whereas the right diagram shows the situation for an a2:a1 ratio >1.

the common idiotypic specificity of anti-allotype Ab may also be generated and affect the level of the anti-allotype Ab (FIGURE 6).

According to concepts of the immune network,[14,35,36] the allotype-idiotype network would consist of a series of interacting auto-antibodies generated from an epitope of the allotype so as to have anti-allotype Ab (Ab1), anti-idiotype Ab (Ab2), anti-anti-idiotype (Ab3), etcetera. To test another aspect of this immune network, allotype-matched rabbits were immunized with anti-idiotype Ab to anti-a2 Ab (Ab2), and indeed the synthesis of anti-anti-idiotype Ab (Ab3) was induced.[37] These rabbits, however, produced primarily anti-a2 Ab (i.e., the idiotype, Ab1) in an Ab1:Ab3 ratio of approximately 4:1. Thus, immunization with anti-idiotype Ab apparently provided a bidirectional stimulus. The two populations of Ab could be isolated from the antiserum; one, the anti-a2 Ab (Ab1), reacted with a2 IgG and the anti-idiotype Ab (Ab2), whereas the other, anti-anti-idiotype Ab (Ab3), reacted only with the anti-idiotype antibody.[37] This finding indicates that Ab synthesis may be induced not only in response to antigen, but also in response to its anti-idiotype antibody. These results with the a2 allotype-idiotype immune network are in agreement with the findings of others who used either an immunoglobulin,[38] levan-binding myeloma,[39] or a microbial antigen.[40] The finding of an apparent stimulus by antibody to the common idiotype of anti-a2 Ab to evoke the synthesis of anti-a2 Ab can also be interpreted as resulting from the appearance of an epitope on the anti-idiotype Ab related to an epitope on the a2 allotype, that is, an internal image or related epitope.[14,41] On the one hand, the anti-idiotype Ab may act through its paratope to stimulate cells bearing anti-a2 Ab receptors expressing an idiotope (i.e., of the common idiotype). Whether a paratope acts to stimulate or suppress the synthesis of Ig by a cell bearing an interacting idiotope may be concentration dependent as shown by Roux *et al.* for primary antibody synthesis generated *in vitro* to sheep red blood cells in the presence of anti-allotype antibody.[42] In these experiments, high concentrations of anti-allotype Ab caused complete suppression, whereas low concentrations of anti-allotype Ab caused as much as a sixfold enhancement of the anti-sheep red blood cell plaque-forming cell (PFC) response. On the other hand, the anti-idiotype Ab may act through its epitope (i.e., an internal image related to the epitope of the a2 allotype) to stimulate cells bearing anti-a2 receptors with the interacting paratope. Whether the anti-idiotype Ab acts to stimulate cells through its paratope or idiotope may be difficult to distinguish.

When allotype suppression is induced perinatally by passive administration of anti-allotype Ab, the suppressed allotype sooner or later reappears. When, however, the allotype-suppressed rabbit is actively immunized to induce the production of *auto*-anti-allotype Ab, allotype suppression appears to be permanent. With this in mind, the question arises as to whether the active induction of *auto*-anti-idiotype Ab could prevent the appearance of *auto*-anti-allotype Ab in heterozygous a^1a^2 rabbits and thereby allow for a permanent increase in the a2:a1 ratio. In a preliminary experiment, however, the attempt to immunize an a^1a^2 heterozygous rabbit to produce antibody to the common idiotypic specificity of anti-a2 Ab resulted only in a transient increase of the a2:a1 ratio for about 10 to 15 weeks. Thus, it is not yet clear whether or not a permanent suppression of the idiotype can be induced.

We have shown that anti-allotype Ab or anti-idiotype Ab passively administered perinatally can alter the expression of immunoglobulin allotypes. We have also shown that the induction of *auto*-anti-allotype Ab provides a self-regulating mechanism for maintaining allotype suppression permanently. The induction of *auto*-anti-idiotype Ab to a common idiotype of anti-allotype Ab has provided tentative evidence that allotype expression is thereby altered. The ability to alter the expression of allotypes by anti-allotype Ab or anti-idiotype Ab, as well as the ability to simultaneously induce the synthesis of Ab1 and Ab3 by immunization with Ab2 are consistent with proposals of an immune network.

REFERENCES

1. OUDIN, J. 1956. C.R. Acad. Sci. **242:** 2489–2492.
2. DRAY, S. & G. O. YOUNG. 1958. J. Immunol. **81:** 142–149.
3. DUBISKI, S., Z. DUDZIAK, D. SKALBA & S. DUBISKA. 1959. Immunology **2:** 84–92.
4. DRAY, S., S. DUBISKI, A. KELUS, E. S. LENNOX & J. OUDIN. 1962. Nature (London) **195:** 785–786.
5. MAGE, R. G., R. LIEBERMAN, M. POTTER & W. D. TERRY. 1973. *In* The Antigens, M. Sela, Ed.: 299–376. Academic Press. New York.
6. KINDT, T. J. 1975. Adv. Immunol. **21:** 35–86.
7. KNIGHT, K. L. & W. C. HANLY. 1975. Contemp. Top Mol. Immunol. **4:** 55–88.
8. CAZENAVE, P. A. 1981. *In* Lymphocytic Regulation by Antibodies. C. Bona and P. A. Cazenave, Eds.: 109–138. John Wiley and Sons. New York.
9. DRAY, S. 1962. Nature (London) **195:** 677–679.
10. SELL, S. & P. H. GELL. 1965. J. Exp. Med. **122:** 423–440.

11. OUDIN, J. & M. MICHEL. 1963. C.R. Acad. Sci. (D). **257:** 805–808.
12. KUNKEL, H. G., M. MANNIK & R. C. WILLIAMS. 1963. Science **140:** 1218–1219.
13. GELL, P. G. H. & A. KELUS, 1964. Nature (London) **201:** 687–689.
14. JERNE, N. K. 1974. Ann. Immunol. Inst. Pasteur (Paris) **125:** 373–389.
15. LOWE, J. A., L. M. CROSS & D. CATTY. 1975. Immunology **28:** 469–484.
16. RODKEY, L. S. 1974. J. Exp. Med. **139:** 712–720.
17. ROLAND, J. & P. A. CAZENAVE. 1979. C.R. Acad. Sci. **388:** 571–574.
18. GILMAN-SACHS, A., S. DRAY & W. J. HORNG. 1980. J. Immunol. **125:** 96–101.
19. ROLAND, J. & P. A. CAZENAVE. 1981 Eur. J. Immunol. **11:** 469–474.
20. RODKEY, L. S. 1982. In The Immune System, 2. The present. G. Steinbury and I. Lefkovits, Eds.: 315–321. Karger Publishing. Basel.
21. METZGER, D. W. & K. H. ROUX. 1982. J. Immunol. **429:** 1138–1342.
22. GILMAN-SACHS, A., S. DRAY & W. J. HORNG. 1982. J. Immunol. **129:** 1194–1199.
23. MAGE, R. G. 1975. Transplant. Rev. **27:** 87–99.
24. DRAY, S. 1979. Ann Immunol. Inst. Pasteur (Paris) **130:** 481–494.
25. HORNG, W. J., A. GILMAN-SACHS & S. DRAY. 1980. In Lymphocytic Regulation by Antibodies. C. Bona and P.-A. Cazenave, Eds.: 139–155. John WIley and Sons. New York.
26. PERNIS, B., L. FORNI & L. AMANTE. 1970. J. Exp. Med. **132:** 1001–1018.
27. ESKINAZI, D. P., B. A. BESSINGER, G. MOLINARO & S. DRAY. 1980. Molec. Immunol. **17:** 403–411.
28. KIM, B. S. & S. DRAY. 1972 Eur. J. Immunol. **2:** 509–514.
29. HORNG, W. J., A. GILMAN-SACHS, K. H. ROUX, G. A. MOLINARO & S. DRAY. 1977. J. Immunol. **119:** 1560–1562.
30. HORNG, W. J., A. GILMAN-SACHS & S. DRAY. 1980. J. Immunol. **125:** 1250–1255.
31. HORNG, W. J., A. GILMAN-SACHS, D. KAZDIN & S. DRAY. 1980. Fourth Int. Congr. Immunol. Paris Abst. #2.5.07.
32. GILMAN-SACHS, A., S. DRAY & K. L. KNIGHT. 1981. Eur. J. Immunol. **11:** 1001–1005.
33. R. S. LOFTS, JR., L. S. RODKEY. 1981. Mol. Immunol. **18:** 433–438.
34. GAITHINGS, W. E., R. G. MAGE, M. D. COOPER, A. R. LAWTON & G. O. YOUNG-COOPER. 1981. Eur. J. Immunol. **11:** 200–206.
35. CAZENAVE, P. A. 1977. Proc. Natl. Acad. Sci. USA **74:** 5122–5125.
36. URBAIN, J., M. WIKLER, J. D. FRANSSEN & C. COLLIGNON. 1977. Proc. Natl. Acad. Sci. USA **74:** 5126–5130.
37. KAZDIN, D. & W. J. HORNG. 1981. Fed. Proc. Fed Am. Soc. Exp. Biol. Abst. **40:** 1063.
38. JERNE, N. K., J. ROLAND & P. A. CAZENAVE. 1982. Eur. Mol. Biol. Org. J. **1:** 243–247.
39. BONA, C. A., E. HEBER-KATZ & W. E. PAUL. 1981. J. Exp. Med. **153:** 951–967.
40. WIKLER, M., J. D. FRANSSEN, C. COLLIGNON, O. LEO, B. MARIAME, P. VAN DE WALLE & J. URBAIN. 1979. J. Exp. Med. **150:** 184–195.
41. NISONOFF, A. & E. LAMOYI. 1981. Clin. Immunol. Immunopathol. **21:** 397–406.
42. ROUX, K. H., D. W. METZGER & S. DRAY. 1971. J. Immunol. **122:** 566–574.

DISCUSSION OF THE PAPER

S. EPSTEIN (*National Institutes of Health, Bethesda, Md.*): Instead of postulating that there is such a common idiotype expressed in all responses to anti-allotype, is it possible that this situation is an example of an internal image and that the anti-idiotype actually resembles the allotype. This idea would seem particularly likely because the antigen itself is in an immunoglobulin sequence. The response would not be so simple, and would not require fewer genes.

S. DRAY: An alternate explanation certainly could be an internal image, if that is the way you like to look at it.

UNIDENTIFIED SPEAKER: How do you explain the appearance of the idiotype (Ab1) after immunization with anti-idiotype antibody?

DRAY: We have some earlier data that were obtained in our laboratory by Dr. Roux and Dr. Metzger that I believe is relevant. They worked with a primary immune response system *in vitro* in which the erythrocyte provided the epitope and the anti-allotype antibody provided the paratope. In the presence of a large amount of paratope, synthesis of antibody molecules with the corresponding allotype were suppressed, whereas in the presence of a relatively small amount of paratope, the synthesis of antibody with the corresponding allotype was enhanced. For paratopes that are specific for an idiotype, the situation is probably similar. Thus, whether or not one obtains suppression or enhancement of the idiotype in the presence of anti-idiotype antibody *in vivo* may be concentration dependent, that is, a low concentration of anti-idiotype antibody appears to stimulate the expansion of clones bearing the corresponding idiotype. Because most, if not all, clones that synthesize anti-a2 antibody appear to have a common idiotypic specificity, a low concentration of anti-idiotype antibody (Ab2) would enhance the expansion of these clones, so that relatively large amounts of anti-a2 antibody (Ab1) are produced, as in fact we have observed.

EPSTEIN: My question was quite similar. Could you reiterate what you said about Ab3, because I think it is a key observation in the allotype system? How was Ab3 generated?

DRAY: Ab3, that is, anti-idiotype antibody to antibody (Ab2) specific for the common idiotypic specificity of anti-a2 antibody, was generated by immunization with Ab2.

EPSEIN: You generated with Ab2 a response that consisted of Ab3. Do you have quantitative data on what the response consisted of in terms of the expression of anti-a2?

DRAY: Yes, the antibodies, Ab1 and Ab3, were specifically isolated by immunoadsorption.

EPSTEIN: Did you characterize the antibody that you then got as Ab2?

DRAY: No. We got Ab1 and Ab3.

EPSTEIN: Do you mean that the Ab1 was anti-a2?

DRAY: That is correct.

EPSTEIN: In this case, what percent of anti-a2 reacts with the immunogen? Have you done experiments to distinguish these possibilities? One can not use these terms indiscriminately when the initial immunogen is itself immunoglobulin with V_H determinant.

DRAY: I am not sure how you would distinguish those two possibilities, that is, whether Ab2 has an internal image of a2 or has an antibody combining site for a common idiotypic specificity of anti-a2.

W. J. HORNG: Could I respond to this question? We have induced Ab3 by using Ab2 as immunogen, and the responding molecules—80% of them—are anti-a2, which is Ab1. Therefore this situation looks like a reverse stimulation. Does that answer your question?

EPSTEIN: The way to distinguish these two possibilities has to be by structural features, and if it is an internal image, there is no need to suggest that all the sequences are in fact homologous. They all just recognize a2. So they do not need to share idiotype or V region similarities.

HORNG: An internal image in our Ab2 preparation may have induced Ab1. If we wanted to look into the internal image we should look at the population of anti-idiotype antibody molecules. I hope to have some opportunity to discuss this later and show that some of the molecules are really latent a2 molecules within that anti-idiotype population.

R. MAGE (*National Institutes of Health, Bethesda, Md.*): I have a much more general question. Would you care to speculate on the biological meaning of establishing a fine-tuned pecking order of allotype expression using the idiotype network? What do you think the advantage would be of establishing this order?

DRAY: Thus far, I do not know that there is any clear evidence that a particular allotype has any particular advantage or has a broader spectrum of variability than the other allotype. There is some indication, however, from Dr. Haurowitz's laboratory that there is some preference in response to one of the haptens in the heterozygous rabbit. In a particular colony of rabbits, (I think it was the a3 allotype), the library for one allotype was larger than for another allotype.

MAGE: Are the clones for a particular antigen random?

DRAY: I do not know if that is the case. We really have not worked with the b9s, but certainly that would be an extreme situation where b9 is expressed in relatively small amounts. If you take homozygous rabbits, they do just as well, as far as I know, if they are b9, b5, b6, or b4.

Idiotype-Anti-Idiotype Network. III. Genetic Control of Activation of A48Id Silent Clones Subsequent to Manipulation of the Immune Network[a]

LEONARD J. RUBINSTEIN AND CONSTANTIN A. BONA

Department of Microbiology
Mount Sinai School of Medicine
New York, New York 10029

INTRODUCTION

Immunization of various strains of mice with bacterial levan (BL), a $\beta2{\rightarrow}6$ polyfructosan with $\beta2{\rightarrow}1$ branch points, leads to a vigorous T-independent antibody response.[1] In IghC[a] mice this response is composed of two families of antibodies. One family binds both $\beta2{\rightarrow}6$ and $\beta2{\rightarrow}1$ polyfructosan epitopes and shares the cross-reactive idiotypes (IdX) of several inulin-binding myeloma proteins.[1] The second family binds only $\beta2{\rightarrow}6$ polyfructosan epitopes. This family of antibodies does not express the IdX of inulin-binding myeloma proteins nor of two $\beta2{\rightarrow}6$ polyfructosan-binding myeloma proteins (i.e. ABPC48 and UPC10). The A48Id is a marker of a silent fraction of anti-levan clones.[1]

In previous studies, we have shown that A48Id silent clones can be activated in three experimental conditions: by injection at birth of antibodies bearing the A48 idiotype;[2] by injection at birth of minute amounts of anti-A48Id antibodies;[3] and by hyperimmunization of adult mice with anti-A48-keyhole limpet hemocyanin (KLH) conjugates.[4] In the present communication we show new results that indicate that the activation of A48Id silent clones in these three experimental systems is independent of major histocompatibility complex (MHC) and IghC gene complexes and that this activation is not restricted to IghV[a] genes.

MATERIALS AND METHODS

Animals

BALB/c mice were purchased from the Charles River Breeding Laboratory, Wilmington, Massachusetts. CCB.R4 mice were a gift from Dr. R. Riblet at the Institute for Cancer Research, Philadelphia, Pennsylvania. BALB.B, BALB.K, BAB.14, and CAL.20 mice were a gift from Dr. M. Potter, Laboratory of Cell Biology, National Cancer Institute, National Institutes of Health, Bethesda, Maryland. One day old mice were obtained from breeding in our colony at the Mount Sinai School of Medicine, New York. Characteristics of the mice used are illustrated in TABLE 1.

[a]This work was supported by grant PCN1105788 from the National Science Foundation and by Grant IM-275A from the American Cancer Society, Inc.

Antigens

Bacterial levan from *Aerobacter laevenicum* was prepared according to a previously described technique.[1]

Preparation of Anti-Idiotype Antibody

Syngeneic BALB/c anti-A48Id and anti-U10Id antibodies were prepared by immunization with monoclonal protein-KLH conjugates. Antibodies were purified on Sepharose 4B idiotype columns. Coupling of antibodies to KLH and immunization schedules are as previously described.[5]

Labeling of Sheep Erythrocytes (SRBC) with Bacterial Levan

An *o*-stearoyl derivative of BL was prepared according to the method of Hämmerling and Westphal[6] and was used to coat SRBC as previously described.[1]

TABLE 1. Genetic Characteristics of Mice Used in this Study

Mouse Strain	Major Histocompatibility Complex of the Mouse	IghV	IghC
BALB/c	d	a	a
BALB.B	b	a	a
BALB.K	k	a	a
BAB.14	d	a	b
CCB.R4	d	b	a
CAL.20	d	d	d

Labeling of Antibodies

A48 monoclonal protein was labeled with ^{125}I by the chloramine T method.[7]

Determination of Antibody Titers

Hemagglutination (HA) titers of antibody specific for $\beta2\rightarrow6$ were determined in microtiter plates using SRBC coated with *o*-stearoyl bacterial levan. The titer recorded is $\log_2$ of the highest dilution of antisera giving agglutination.

Radioimmunoassay (RIA) and Determination of Idiotype Titers

The RIA serum level of A48Id was determined by using microtiter plates coated with affinity-purified anti-A48Id antibodies ($50\mu g/ml$) and ^{125}I-A48 as ligand. The concentration of antibody expressing A48Id was determined from a standard inhibition curve obtained with A48 monoclonal protein. This method was described in detail elsewhere.[4,5]

Detection of Plaque-Forming Cells (PFC)

The number of cells secreting antibody specific for BL was determined by a modification of the Jerne plaquing technique as previously described.[5] Anti-BL PFC carrying the A48Id were enumerated by incorporating BALB/c anti-A48 antiserum into the agarose at a final concentration of 1:10,000 and scoring the difference in the number of PFC obtained in the presence and absence of the inhibitor (anti-A48Id).

RESULTS

Genetic Control of Activation of A48Id Silent Clones by Anti-A48Id Antibodies

In previous studies we have shown that either administration of minute amounts of anti-A48Id antibodies at birth[3] or immunization of adult mice with anti-A48-KLH conjugates,[4] leads to the activation of A48Id silent clones. A significant increase of A48Id$^+$ anti-levan antibodies was not found in the sera of mice treated at birth with anti-M460Id antibodies. Therefore, the activation of A48Id silent clones was considered to be an idiotype specific response. Furthermore, in mice treated with anti-A48Id antibodies and not immunized with BL, there was no activation of A48Id clones detected. Thus, this activation was not only idiotype specific, but required antigenic stimulation as well. Until now the expression of A48Id clones has only been studied in BALB/c mice, from which the ABPC48 myeloma originated. For this reason we have been interested in studying whether the expression of the A48Id$^+$ clones is linked only to IghV^a genes. In addition we investigated whether this response is under the control of MHC and/or IghC gene complexes.

In order to study the genetic control of the expression of A48Id, we studied this response in various strains of mice that differ in their MHC, IghC, and IghV haplotypes. These strains were treated at birth with anti-A48Id antibodies, followed one month later by immunization with bacteral levan. Only those mice treated with anti-A48Id, however, developed an A48Id$^+$ response. Activation of A48Id$^+$ silent clones was observed among all the strains. The results depicted in TABLE 2 indicate that all the mouse strains responded to immunization with BL, developing significant HA titers and a vigorous anti-levan PFC response.

A similar A48Id$^+$ anti-levan response was observed in adult mice after hyperimmunization with 75μg of anti-A48-KLH conjugate in Freund's complete adjuvant (FCA), followed by a second injection five days later in Freund's incomplete adjuvant (FIA), and then by six weekly injections of anti-A48-KLH in saline. Every strain of mice hyperimmunized with antiA48-KLH conjugates produced significant HA titers of anti(anti-A48Id) antibodies varying from 2 to 5 log$_2$ units. As expected, these mice developed significant HA anti-levan titers and a significant number of anti-levan PFC in response to immunization with bacterial levan. Furthermore, in these mice the A48Id$^+$ clones were consistently activated subsequent to immunization with BL (TABLE 3). The adult mice that produce anti(anti-A48Id) antibodies, after hyperimmunization with anti-A48-KLH conjugates, were able to develop an A48Id$^+$ anti-levan response following immunization with bacterial levan.

The activation of A48Id silent clones in both experimental models was independent of the MHC gene complex. Indeed BALB/c, BALB.B, and BALB.K mice developed an A48Id$^+$ anti-levan response. In addition, activation was independent of the IghC gene complex. The ability of CAL.20 and BAB.14 mice to develop an A48Id$^+$ response clearly shows that activation is not associated with the IghC gene complex. Interesting-

TABLE 2. Activation of A48Id Silent Clones by the Administration of 10ng Anti-A48Id Monoclonal Protein at Birth

Mouse Strain	Treatment	Antibody Response:Anti-BL HA[a]	Anti-BL PFC/Spleen[c]	A48Id[+] (Percent)	Idiotype Response:A48Id RIA[d]
BALB/c	nil	5.5 ± 0.3	7,833 ± 2,748	8 ± 4	<0.3
	Anti-A48Id	ND[b]	2,700 ± 460	52 ± 7	ND
BALB.B	nil	4.8 ± 1.1	24,067 ± 2,875	13 ± 7	0.7 ± 0.2
	Anti-A48Id	6.0 ± 0.4	4,683 ± 1,816	46 ± 15	20.7 ± 4.6
BALB.K	nil	7.0 ± 3.0	16,100 ± 3,300	ND	ND
	Anti-A48Id	6.3 ± 0.3	44,980 ± 8,985	51 ± 18	15.4 ± 3.5
BAB.14	nil	6.1 ± 0.4	18,975 ± 7,157	5 ± 5	1.4 ± 0.5
	Anti-A48Id	6.4 ± 0.5	34,650 ± 6,895	28 ± 9	36.9 ± 26.0
CCB.R4	nil	>8.0	4,125 ± 3,925	0 ± 0	ND
	Anti-A48Id	2.5 ± 0.9	3,488 ± 1,442	59 ± 17	21.6 ± 10.6
CAL.20	nil	3.4 ± 0.2	7,028 ± 3,225	ND	7.4 ± 3.5
	Anti-A48Id	3.5 ± 0.3	3,668 ± 944	ND	16.7 ± 5.8

[a] Mean log$_2$ units ± SEM
[b] Not determined
[c] Mean ± SEM
[d] RIA expressed as mean μg/ml ± SEM.

TABLE 3. Activation of A48Id Silent Clones by Hyperimmunization of Adult Mice with Anti-A48-Keyhole Limpet Hemocyanin

Mouse Strain	Treatment	Antibody Response:Anti-BL HA[a]	Anti-BL PFC/Spleen[b]	A48Id+ (Percent)	Idiotype Response:A48Id RIA[d]
BALB/c	nil	5.5 ± 0.3	7,833 ± 2,748	8 ± 4	<0.3
	Anti-A48-KLH	7.8 ± 3.2	765 ± 433	32 ± 20	4.8 ± 1.6
BALB.B	nil	4.8 ± 1.1	24,067 ± 2,875	13 ± 7	0.7 ± 0.2
	Anti-A48-KLH	>8.0	183,400 ± 45,061	24 ± 3	36.0 ± 10.0
BALB.K	nil	7.0 ± 3.0	16,100 ± 3,300	ND[c]	ND
	Anti-A48-KLH	6.5 ± 0.5	85,700 ± 5,300	ND	20.1 ± 11.4
BAB.14	nil	6.1 ± 0.4	18,975 ± 7,157	5 ± 5	1.4 ± 0.5
	Anti-A48-KLH	8.0 ± 0.6	69,550 ± 14,663	11 ± 6	27.4 ± 12.2
CCB.R4	nil	>8.0	4,125 ± 3,925	0 ± 0	ND
	Anti-A48-KLH	6.0 ± 0.6	36,933 ± 18,859	12 ± 7	46.6 ± 23.2
CAL.20	nil	3.4 ± 0.2	7,028 ± 3,225	ND	7.4 ± 3.5
	Anti-A48-KLH	5.7 ± 0.3	91,667 ± 24,891	29 ± 14	23.0 ± 15.1

[a] Mean $\log_2$ units ± SEM
[b] Mean ± SEM
[c] Not determined
[d] RIA expressed as mean µg/ml ± SEM

ly, both CAL.20 and CCB.R4 mice developed an A48Id$^+$ response, although they did not express IghV^a genes.

Our results taken collectively indicate that A48Id silent clones can be activated by administration at birth of anti-A48Id monoclonal antibodies or during adult life by hyperimmunization with anti-A48-KLH conjugates. This activation occurs independently of the MHC, IghC, and IghV gene complexes.

Genetic Control of Activation of A48Id Silent Clones by Administration at Birth of A48Id Monoclonal Antibodies

In a recent study, we have shown that BALB/c mice injected at birth with A48Id monoclonal antibodies, led to the activation and dominance of the A48Id$^+$ component of an anti-levan response.[2] In BALB/c mice treated at birth with 10μg of A48Id monoclonal antibody, the majority of anti-levan antibodies expressed the A48Id. The A48Id$^+$ response was both idiotype and antigen specific. Thus, only those mice treated at birth with A48Id monoclonal antibody and challenged one month later with 20μg BL, developed an A48Id$^+$ anti-levan response.

Our data strongly indicated that this idiotype-induced-idiotype response is related to the expansion of A48Id specific T-helper cells. Thus, in transfer experiments we have shown that, the T cell originating from mice treated at birth with A48Id monoclonal antibody were able to help syngeneic B cells to mount an anti-trinitrophenylated (TNP) response subsequent to immunization with TNP-A48 conjugates.

In this communication, we present new results that suggest that the activation of A48Id$^+$ clones is independent of MHC, IghC, and IghV^a gene complexes. The data show that BALB/c, BALB.B, BALB.K, BAB.14, CAL.20, and CCB.R4 were all able to develop an A48Id$^+$ anti-levan response following treatment at birth with A48Id monoclonal antibody and immunization one month later with BL (TABLE 4).

Our results suggest that idiotypes parenterally administered at birth can have a profound influence on the clonal activation during the neonatal period, when the number of B-cell precursors is generally lower and clonotypes are restricted, as compared to the adult.

To extend this observation, we have tested the effects of *in utero* exposure to idiotype on the expansion of silent clones. In order to test this hypothesis, we chose the UPC10 myeloma protein because it exhibits $\beta 2 \rightarrow 6$ polyfructosan binding activity, it shares some of the A48 idiotopes, and it can traverse the placenta. This last fact is true because it is an IgG$_{2a}$ (ABPC48 protein is an IgA immunoglobulin) immunoglobulin, and like A48Id, the U10Id is not expressed during a conventional immune response elicited by bacterial levan. Female mice were intravenously injected during mating and throughout pregnancy with 100μg U10Id monoclonal antibody in saline. The progeny were immunized one month after birth with 20μg BL, and the anti-levan response was measured five days later. The results show that BALB/c, BALB.B, and BAB.14 mice developed a U10Id$^+$ response, whereas CCB.R4 did not (TABLE 5). These preliminary results clearly indicate that the activation of U10Id silent clones subsequent to *in utero* exposure to homologous protein led to an idiotype-induced-idiotype response, similar to that induced by parenteral administration of idiotypes after birth. This idiotype-induced-idiotype response is independent of MHC and IghC gene complexes, but is IghV^a restricted. The IghV^a restriction of this response can be related either to the nature of U10Id or to the specificity of U10Id T-helper cells, which can be IghV restricted. Studies in progress are programmed to elucidate this interesting point.

TABLE 4. Activation of A48Id Silent Clones by the Administration of 10g of A48Id Monoclonal Protein at Birth

Mouse Strain	Treatment	Antibody Response:Anti-BL HA[a]	Anti-BL PFC/Spleen[b]	A48Id+ (Percent)	Idiotype Response:A48Id RIA[d]
BALB/c	nil	5.5 ± 0.3	7,833 ± 2,748	8 ± 4	<0.3
	A48Id	5.7 ± 0.6	21,133 ± 2,245	95 ± 1	82.4 ± 47.6
BALB.B	nil	4.8 ± 1.1	24,067 ± 2,875	13 ± 7	0.7 ± 0.2
	A48Id	4.1 ± 0.7	869 ± 298	55 ± 14	32.0 ± 14.6
BALB.K	nil	7.0 ± 3.0	16,100 ± 3,300	ND[c]	ND
	A48Id	3.0 ± 1.1	ND	ND	18.3 ± 9.0
BAB.14	nil	6.1 ± 0.4	18,975 ± 7,157	5 ± 5	1.4 ± 0.5
	A48Id	3.7 ± 1.2	4,511 ± 1,223	47 ± 12	15.2 ± 4.2
CCB.R4	nil	>8.0	4,125 ± 3,925	0 ± 0	ND
	A48Id	4.6 ± 0.5	1,811 ± 629	26 ± 8	27.1 ± 10.4
CAL.20	nil	3.4 ± 0.2	7,028 ± 3,225	ND	7.4 ± 3.5
	A48Id	4.5 ± 0.5	1,375 ± 125	ND	63.0 ± 22.5

[a] Mean $\log_2$ units ± SEM
[b] Mean ± SEM
[c] Not determined
[d] RIA expressed as mean $\mu g/ml$ ± SEM

DISCUSSION

Soon after the discovery of idiotypes as individual antigenic determinants of human myeloma proteins by Kunkel *et al.*[8] or individual antigenic determinants of rabbit anti-polysaccharide antibodies by Oudin and Michel,[9] it was shown that idiotypes display a great degree of polymorphism. Based on the data accumulated during the last two decades, idiotypes can be described as follows: 1) interspecies cross-reactive idiotypes—those encoded for by germ line genes preserved during evolution such as anti-GAT,[10] anti-Val,[11] anti-acetylcholine receptor antibodies,[12] or anti-phosphoryl-choline antibodies;[13] b) interstrain cross-reactive idiotypes, probably encoded for by germ line genes such as the X24Id of anti-galactan antibodies,[14] anti-allotype antibodies,[15] anti-idiotypic antibodies,[16] or mouse anti-human IgM monoclonal proteins displaying rheumatoid activity;[17] c) cross-reactive idiotypes (CRI or IdX) associated with particular IghC^a genes, such as J558IdX[18] and S117IdX;[19] CRI of anti-arsonate antibodies;[20] CRI of anti-trimethylammonium antibodies;[21] A5AIdX

TABLE 5. Activation of U10Id Silent Clones by *In Utero* Exposure to U10Id Monoclonal Protein

Mouse Strain	Treatment	Anti-BL PFC/Spleen[a]	U10Id$^+$ (Percent)
BALB/c	nil	$40,000 \pm 15,558$	9 ± 9
	U10 females	$13,170 \pm 4,628$	30 ± 15
	offspring	$5,500 \pm 1,622$	93 ± 3
BALB.B	nil	$60,600 \pm 13,500$	10 ± 9
	U10 females	$116,000$	14
	offspring	$16,950 \pm 14,203$	43 ± 28
BAB.14	nil	$15,867 \pm 9,558$	0
	U10 females	$34,575 \pm 15,225$	14 ± 14
	offspring	$5,450 \pm 1,931$	42 ± 11
CCB.R4	nil	$4,125 \pm 3,925$	2 ± 2
	U10 females	$30,833 \pm 7,946$	3 ± 3
	offspring	$7,392 \pm 2,333$	5 ± 2

[a]PFC expressed as mean ± SEM

associated with IghC^e genes[22] or NPV$_h^b$ idiotype associated with IghC^b genes;[23] d) silent idiotypes, which are not expressed during an immune response subsequent to immunization with a conventional antigen. A48 and U10 idiotypes belong to the silent fraction of the anti-β2→6 polyfructosan response. In addition we have shown that the A48Id family belongs to a privileged category of idiotypes that we called regulatory idiotypes. These idiotypes are not normally expressed in the nonimmune animal and can be induced through the manipulation of the steady state immune network. They might represent a feature of those idiotypes that are capable of becoming dominant, because they elicit idiotype specific T-cell regulatory responses.[4,24]

The study of the genetic control of the expression of A48Id has clearly shown that the expression of A48Id is not dependent upon MHC or IghC gene complexes. Indeed, A48Id$^+$ clones were activated in BALB/c as well as in BALB.B and BALB.K mice. These two strains of mice are BALB/c congeneic strains that differ only in the MHC gene complex. The results obtained in BAB.14 and CAL.20 indicated that the activation of A48Id$^+$ clones is not associated with the IghC^a haplotype. Furthermore, the presence of A48Id$^+$ anti-β2→6 polyfructosan antibodies in CAL.20 and CCB.R4 mice clearly indicates that the A48 idiotype is not solely a marker of $IghV^a$ genes. The presence of A48Id in CAL.20 mice is in agreement with the data that showed that the IdX B, A, and G of $\beta 2 \rightarrow 1$ polyfructosan binding myeloma proteins, originating in BALB/c, were expressed on antibodies induced by immunization with BL in CAL.20 mice.[25]

One may ask about the physiological significance of the activation of A48Id silent clones through the manipulation of a steady state network by the administration at birth of idiotype or anti-idiotypic antibodies. One might deduce from our previous studies that the administration of A48Id during the neonatal period is critical for the subsequent dominance of the anti-levan response by A48Id$^+$ clones. Based on these results, we propose the hypothesis that the passive influx of maternal idiotypes to the embryo or newborn across the placenta or through the colostrum, can influence the idiotype distribution in the newborn by favoring the expression of these clones that were dominant in the maternal immune system. The results obtained in the UPC10 system lend strong support to this hypothesis. The parenteral administration of UPC10 monoclonal protein into mice before and during pregnancy led to the activation of U10Id$^+$ clones that otherwise were not expressed during the conventional anti-levan immune response.

The expression of the U10Id$^+$ clones is also independent of MHC and IghC gene complexes. By contrast, however, to the activation of A48Id clones subsequent to parenteral administration of A48Id or anti-A48Id antibodies at birth, the activation of U10Id clones by *in utero* exposure to UPC10 monoclonal protein, is dependent on $IghV^a$ genes. Indeed, the CCB.R4 progeny obtained from females injected with UPC10 did not express the UPC10 idiotype. The lack of UPC10Id$^+$ anti-B2$\rightarrow$6 polyfructosan antibodies in CCB.R4 mice can be related to the induction of suppressor cells specific for 173-UPC10 V_H antigenic determinants borne by several $IghV^a$ proteins belonging to various V_H subgroups that can prevent the activation of UPC10.[26] These determinants can be recognized as foreign antigenic determinants in CCB.R4 mice bearing $IghV^b$ genes. Alternatively, the expression of U10Id can require a light chain of a haplotype that is not provided by the CCB.R4 mice.

The expression of silent clones subsequent to parenteral administration or *in utero* exposure of idiotype have interesting theoretical implications. Actually this data can lead to a redefinition of the concept of acquired immunity, not only as a passive acquisition of maternal antibodies that protect the progeny during the post-natal period, but also a priming of the neonatal immune system for antigens that the mother has previously encountered.

REFERENCES

1. LIEBERMAN, R., M. POTTER, W. HUMPHREY, E. B. MUSHINSKI & M. VRANA. 1975. Multiple individual and cross-specific idiotypes on 13 levan-binding myeloma proteins of BALB/c mice. J. Exp. Med. **142:** 106–119.
2. RUBINSTEIN, L. J., M. YEN & C. A. BONA. 1982. Idiotype-anti-idiotype Network II. Activation of silent clones by treatment at birth with idiotypes is associated with the expansion of idiotype specific helper T cells. J. Exp. Med. **156:** 506–521.
3. HIERNAUX, J., C. BONA & P. J. BAKER. 1981. Neonatal treatment with low doses of anti-idiotypic antibody leads to the expression of a silent clone. J. Exp. Med. **153:** 1004–1008.
4. BONA, C., E. HEBER-KATZ & W. E. PAUL. 1981. Idiotype-anti-idiotype Regulation I. Immunization with a levan-binding myeloma protein leads to the appearance of auto-anti-(anti-idiotype) antibodies and to the activation of silent clones. J. Exp. Med. **153:** 951–967.

5. BONA, C., R. HOOGHE, P. A. GAZENAVE, C. LEGUERN & W. E. PAUL. 1979. Cellular basis of regulation of expression of idiotype. II. Immunity to anti-MOPC-460 idiotype antibodies increases the level of anti-trinitrophenyl antibodies bearing 460 idiotypes. J. Exp. Med. **149**: 815–823.
6. HÄMMERLING, U. & O. WESTPHAL. 1977. Synthesis and use of o-steroyl polysaccharides in passive hemagglutination and hemolysis. Eur. J. Biochem. **1**: 46–50.
7. GREENWOOD, F. C., W. M. HUNTER & J. S. GLOVER. 1963. The preparation of ^{131}I-labelled human growth hormone of high specific radioactivity. Biochem. J. **89**: 114–123.
8. KUNKEL, H. G., M. MANNIK & R. C. WILLIAMS. 1963. Individual antigenic specificities of isolated antibodies. Science **140**: 1218–1219.
9. OUDIN, J. & M. MICHEL. 1963. Une nouvelle forme d' allotypie des globulines γ du serum de lapin, apparemment liée à la function et à la spácificité des anticorps. C. R. Acad. Sci. **257**: 805–808.
10. JU, S. T., B. BENACERRAF & M. E. DORF. 1978. Idiotypic analysis of antibodies to poly(Glu^{60}Ala^{30}Tyr^{10}): Interstrain and interspecies idiotypic crossreactions. Proc. Natl. Acad. Sci. USA **75**: 6192–6196.
11. KAROL, R. A., M. REICHLIN & R. W. NOBLE. 1977. Evolution of an idiotypic determinant: Anti-Val. J. Exp. Med. **146**: 435–444.
12. SCHWARTZ, M., D. NOVICH, D. GIVOL & S. FUCHS. 1978. Induction of anti-idiotypic antibodies by immunization with syngeneic spleen cells educated with acetylcholine receptors. Nature (London) **273**: 543–545.
13. CLAFLIN, J. L. & J. M. DAVIE. 1974. Clonal nature of the immune response to phosphorycholine III. Species-specific binding characteristics of rodent anti-phosphorycholine antibodies. J. Immunol. **113**: 1678–1684.
14. POTTER, M., E. B. MUSHINSKI, S. RUDIKOFF, C. P. J. GLAUDEMANS, E. A. PADLAN & D. R. DAVIES. 1979. Structural and genetic basis of idiotypy in the galactan-binding myeloma proteins. Ann. Immunol. Inst. Pasteur (Paris) **130C**: 263–271.
15. BONA, C., P. K. A. MONGINI, K. E. STEIN & W. E. PAUL. 1980. Anti-immunoglobulin antibodies I. Expression of cross-reactive idiotypes and Ir gene control of the response to IgG$_{2a}$ of the b allotype. J. Exp. Med. **151**: 1334–1348.
16. BONA, C. & J. KEARNEY. 1981. Anti-immunoglobulin antibodies II. Expression of individual and cross-reactive idiotypes on syngeneic and homologous anti-idiotype antibodies. J. Immunol. **127**: 491–495.
17. BONA, C. A., S. FINLEY, S. WATERS & H. G. KUNKEL. 1982. Anti-immunoglobulin antibodies III. Properties of sequential anti-idiotypic antibodies to heterologous anti-γ globulins. Detection of reactivity of anti-idiotype antibodies with epitopes of Fc fragments (homobodies) and with epitopes and idiotopes (epibodies). J. Exp. Med. **156**: 986–999.
18. RIBLET, R., B. BLOMBERG, M. WEIGERT, R. LIEBERMAN, B. A. TAYLOR & M. POTTER. 1975. Genetics of mouse antibodies I. Linkage of the dextran response locus, V_H-DEX, to allotype. Eur. J. Immunol. **5**: 775–777.
19. BEREK, C., B. A. TAYLOR & K. EICHMAN. 1976. Genetics of the idiotype of BALB/c myeloma S117:Multiple chromosomal loci for V_H genes encoding specificity for group A streptococcal carbohydrate. J. Exp. Med. **144**: 1164–1174.
20. NISONOFF, A., S. T. JU & F. L. OWEN. 1977. Studies of structure and immunosuppression of a cross-reactive idiotype in strain A mice. Transplant. Rev. **34**: 89–118.
21. ALEVY, Y. G., C. D. WITHERSPOON, C. A. PRANGE & C. J. BELLONE. 1980. Anti-TMA immunity in mice. I. The appearance of cross-reactive idiotype(s) to the trimethylammonium (TMA) hapten in A/J mice. J. Immunol. **124**: 215–221.
22. EICHMAN, K. 1972. Idiotypic identity of antibodies to streptococcal carbohydrate in inbred mice. Eur. J. Immunol. **2**: 301–307.
23. MAKELA, O. & K. KARJALAINEN. 1977. Inherited immunoglobulin idiotypes of the mouse. Transplant. Rev. **34**: 119–138.
24. PAUL, W. E. & C. BONA. 1982. Regulatory idiotopes and immune networks: a hypothesis. Immunology Today **3**: 230–234.
25. LIEBERMAN, R., C. BONA, C. C. CHIEN, K. E. STEIN & W. E. PAUL. 1979. Genetic and cellular regulation of the expression of specific antibody idiotypes in the anti-polyfructosan immune response. Ann. Immunol. Inst. Pasteur (Paris) **130C**: 247–262.

26. BOSMA, M. J., C. DE WITT, S. J. HAUSMAN, R. MARKS & M. POTTER. 1977. Serological distinction of heavy chain variable regions (V_H subgroups) of mouse immunoglobulins I. Common V_H determinants on the heavy chains of mouse myeloma proteins having different binding sites. J. Exp. Med. **146:** 1041–1053.

DISCUSSION OF THE PAPER

W. E. PAUL (*National Institutes of Health, Bethesda, Md.*): Dr. Bona, in the experiments in which you pretreated mice with the very small amounts of A48 at birth, you showed very clearly that it was necessary to use T cells from such animals to collaborate with B cells in the generation of a response in which A48 dominated. In the experiment, you also drew the B cells from a donor that had been treated with A48 at birth. If you were to have used these cells from a normal donor, would the result have been the same or different?

C. A. BONA: We do not know.

PAUL: I think it would be rather important to know that, and more particularly to know whether the precursor frequency for A48 positive anti-bacterial levan were the same in the two groups. If they were not, then there would be strong evidence that the repertoire of B cells would be shaped by the pretreatment. In this instance one could argue that one had induced a population of regulatory T cells and that they only act after antigen has been introduced into the system.

BONA: We did not do this experiment, and I think you raise a very good point. Thank you.

L. S. RODKEY (*Kansas State University, Manhattan, Kans.*): Dr. Bona, would you predict that if you did the next experiment, that is, with the mother having anti-idiotype rather than transferring idiotype, that you would get an opposite effect?

BONA: Yes. This is what Dr. Nisonoff presented, what Dr. Victor will present, and what Dr. Weiler demonstrated already in SJL. I think that *in utero* exposure to anti-idiotype suppresses the response and induces chronic long-lasting suppression, despite that the exposure induced a very important expansion of both B and Lyt-2 suppressor cells that shared the idiotype. I do not want to anticipate Dr. Victor's presentation.

RODKEY: Is this a new definition of original antigenic sin?

BONA: The definition of original antigenic sin is a sin on antigens or a cross-reactive structure seen by two antibodies.

K. RAJEWSKY (*University of Cologne, Cologne, F.R.G.*): All of these experiments where researchers inject idiotypes or anti-idiotypes into animals and then look for the effects, can be put into a very simple pattern. It is clear that investigators perform these experiments, because when they inject anti-idiotype, they look for the idiotype in the animals. When they inject idiotype, as you do, then they look for the anti-idiotype. In fact, when one puts anti-idiotype into the animal, the analogous experiment is to look for the expression of the anti-idiotype in that same animal. Of course that would be like hunting for the complementary structure. So, in fact all these experiments are exactly the same and show that later on when the animal sees a certain configuration of a variable region, the animal is able to reproduce the configuration in the form of idiotypic memory by just inhibiting the complementary sites.

There is a problem of nomenclature that has confused the issue a lot because of the terms idiotype and anti-idiotype. If one looks at these just as operational terms and looks at the experimental results, one will find that they are all absolutely consistent.

BONA: Dr. Rajewsky, I really thank you for your discussion. I think that there are several problems. The first is a true semantic problem of our terminology. The second is a problem related to the phenomenology, and the third is a theoretical problem related to the functional immune network. I believe that balance between clones, the communication between various regulatory T subsets, based on fragile idiotypic links, can be upset by antigen, idiotype, and anti-idiotypes. In our system, the alteration of the equilibrium between clones that constitute the A48 mini-network has general outcome, namely, the activation of A48 $\beta 2 \rightarrow 6$ fructosan clones. Immunization of nu/nu BALB/c with levan, administration at birth of minute amounts of A48, anti-A48, or injection of the mother with UPC10 during the pregnancy, led to the activation of an A48Id response. Of course, different mechanisms are involved. Dr. Rubinstein has shown that whereas the A48Id response, subsequent to administration at birth of A48Id-bearing monoclonal antibodies, or injection during pregnancy of UPC10 is related to the expansion of Id-specific T-helper cells, the administration of minute amounts of anti-A48Id antibodies is related to the direct interaction of these antibodies with Ig receptor of A48Id precursors.

Of course, that I cannot generalize these data and other parameters as the amount of antibodies injected, the isotype of antibodies, the timing could play an important role. The fact, however, that we can obtain the same effect with antigen idiotype, that is, Ab_1, anti-Id (Ab_2), and certainly with Ab_3 sharing Ab_1 idiotypes, is related to the intriguing dualism of Ig molecules. Their paratope recognize an epitope (nominal antigen or idiotope of other Ig), and by virtue of their idiotopes, function as antigens.

T. MARION (*Yale University School of Medicine, New Haven, Conn.*): I would just like to ask a question about the idiotype specific T-helper cell in your system. Do you know any of the other characteristics about that cell other than its Lyt phenotype?

BONA: They are Thy-1.2 positive.

MARION: Do you know anything about how the T-helper cell interacts with B cells in order to induce its idiotype? Does it act as the classical MHC restricted T-helper cell?

BONA: We do not have data. To answer the question, we did not succeed until the present in obtaining T-cell clones.

H. KOHLER (*Roswell Park Memorial Institute, Buffalo, N.Y.*): Dr. Bona, you obviously reject the idea that you can neutralize T-suppressor cells. Could you affect this induction by free light chains or heavy chains from the A48 proteins?

BONA: We did not perform that experiment.

The Role of Rabbit Immunoglobulin Allotypes in an Immune Network

JOHN A. SOGN, KEVIN L. DREHER, LAURENT J.
EMORINE, EDWARD E. MAX, SUSAN JACKSON, AND
THOMAS J. KINDT

Laboratory of Immunogenetics
National Institute of Allergy and Infectious Diseases
National Institutes of Health
Bethesda, Maryland 20205

INTRODUCTION

The genetics of immunoglobulins (Ig) has been an area of interest for many years. The descriptions of Ig allotypes in the rabbit[1] and the human[2] in 1956, combined with early definitions of idiotypes[3,4] provided the tools needed for a remarkably thorough understanding of the general principles of Ig gene organization and expression. Inevitably, these studies, limited to serology and protein structure, left major gaps in our knowledge of mechanisms operating at the nucleic acid level. The current revolution in molecular biology promises to end the tyranny of serologic inference and permit a molecular appreciation of phenomena that have, to date, remained only partially understood. One problem in immunogenetics that is amenable to analysis by molecular biology is the intriguing and little understood problem of latent allotypes. Latent allotypes are allotypes not detected by qualitative typing procedures and not expected from the genetic background of the animal. They are typically present in very low concentration in serum (often 0.1% of the expected or nominal allotype level) and can be detected only by sensitive assay techniques.

THE CASE FOR LATENT ALLOTYPES

The first reports of unexpected Ig allotypes were by Lobb *et al.*,[5,6] who observed that human cells in culture produced Ig with unanticipated Gm types. Subsequent reports have come from a variety of species, but the majority of studies have been carried out in rabbits. An extensive review of latent allotypes has recently been published.[7] This will not be repeated here, but some points in summary will be made.

First, molecules bearing a latent allotype are serologically indistinguishable from molecules bearing the same specificity as a nominal allotype. Thus, latent allotypes cannot be readily explained by cross-reactivity of a subset of Ig of the nominal allotype or by flaws in anti-allotype reagents. Latent allotypes have been detected in several laboratories using a variety of reagents with a battery of controls sufficient to exclude these trivial explanations. Much of the typing has been done by inhibition assays that impose a fairly strict requirement for serologic identity if a sample is to demonstrate complete inhibition of a complex allotype. In several cases, sufficient amounts of Ig bearing a latent allotype have been present to demonstrate such complete inhibition.[8–11]

Second, in several instances structural evidence has been used to substantiate serologic evidence for latent allotypes. TABLE 1 is a compilation of these studies.

TABLE 1. Structural Studies of Latent Allotypes

Method Used	Latent Allotype	Reference
Acid cleavage	b4	10
Acid cleavage, followed by GGMS sequencing	b9	13
CNBr cleavage	d11	14
CNBr cleavage	d11, d12	15
Peptide mapping	a2	16[a]

[a]Data not shown.

Definitive total amino acid sequence studies have not been possible because of the low amounts of material available, but advantage has been taken of those structural methods that are allotype specific: mild acid cleavage, which bisects light chains of allotypes b4 and b9; CNBr digestion, which yields a smaller fragment from d11 γ chains than from d12; and peptide mapping. Early studies had shown[9,12] that latent allotypes coisolated with Ig (and in some cases with affinity-purified antibody). Upon fragmentation of Ig, the latent allotype reactivity segregated as expected from the known location of the allotypic determinants.

Third, the expression of latent allotypes varies remarkably with time and with genetic background. Latent allotypes are not found in all bleedings from an individual animal that has expressed one or more latent allotypes in the past.[12] When latent allotypes are detected, they may disappear at a rate too great to be explained by the normal lifespan of circulating immunoglobulin.[17]

Fourth, mechanisms such as maternal-fetal or fetal-fetal chimerism are not sufficient to explain latent allotypes, although lymphoid cell chimerism has been experimentally induced in rabbits.[18,19] A strong circumstantial argument against chimerism, as shown in TABLE 2, is that latent allotypes have been found with nearly equal frequency in rabbits whose parents contained or lacked the latent allotypes as nominal allotypes.

CONTROL OF LATENT ALLOTYPE EXPRESSION

Latent allotypes are interesting because of the interdependent questions they raise: how are they (presumably) encoded in the rabbit DNA, and why are they expressed in such low levels. The small amount of data relevant to the control of latent allotype expression suggests that an autologous anti-allotype response plays a key role.

TABLE 2. Frequency of Rabbits Expressing Latent Allotypes That are Present or Absent as Nominal Allotypes in Either Parent

Allotype Group	Latent Allotype in Nominal Genotype of Either Parent[a]	Number Tested	Number Positive	Positive (Percent)	Concentration Range (mg/ml)
a	yes	132	36	28	0.1–29.7
	no	46	15	33	0.5–38.0
b	yes	83	29	35	0.1–26.0
	no	70	16	23	0.8–26.0

[a]Genotypes ascertained by standard genetic techniques. Parental sera were not in every instance subjected to rigorous analysis for allotypes.

The first experiments performed to address this issue were suggested by the unusual rapid clearance kinetics of Ig-bearing latent allotypes. If it is actively cleared by way of an immunologically mediated mechanism, then animals with a history of expression of a particular latent allotype would be expected to be primed for a rapid clearance of passively administered IgG bearing that latent allotype. Animals that had never expressed the latent allotype should be incapable of distinguishing among

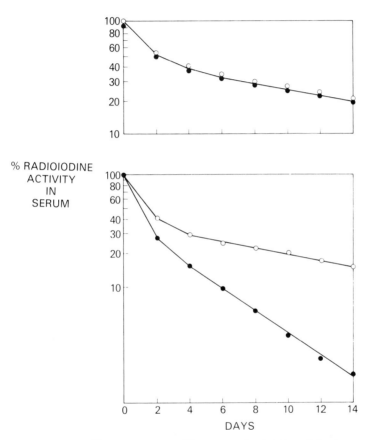

FIGURE 1. Clearance of ^{131}I-a1 IgG (●) and ^{125}I-a3 IgG (○) administered simultaneously by intravenous injection. The upper panel shows results typical of those obtained with all heterozygous a1a3 recipients and with many homozygous a1 or a3 recipients. The lower panel shows results obtained with a homozygous a3 recipient demonstrating selective rapid clearance of a1 IgG.

passively administered IgG samples bearing different allotypes. To test this hypothesis, IgG preparations of different allotypes were radiolabeled with ^{125}I or ^{131}I and ultracentrifuged. Each experimental rabbit received an intravenous injection of 500 μg of labeled IgG matched to the nominal allotypes of the recipient, and an equal amount of labeled IgG unmatched for either a group a or group b allotype. The paired samples were labeled with different isotypes so that their metabolic fates could be individually assessed. In the majority of rabbits, the paired samples were cleared at identical rates, but in several cases the unmatched IgG was cleared more rapidly (FIGURE 1). It was apparent from an analysis of latent allotype expression in the experimental rabbits that an increased rate of clearance for IgG unmatched for a given allotype correlated with a history of expression of that latent allotype. (TABLE 3).

A latent allotype is an autologous antigenic stimulus just as is an idiotype and should be subject to similar control.[16] Neither would be expected to be present while self-tolerance was established during development. With this as a model for latent allotype-anti-allotype interaction, it seemed possible that interfering with the ability to mount an anti-allotype response would increase latent allotype production by removing the system that suppressed it. To test this, five rabbits were immunized with anti-allotype antibodies (three with anti-a2 and two with anti-b6) until an anti-idiotypic response to the anti-allotype antibody was established. To the extent that the antibodies injected shared idiotypes with anti-allotype-producing cells of the recipient,

TABLE 3. Correlation of Rapid Clearance and Latent Allotype Expression[a]

Rabbit	Genotype	Unmatched Allotype	Rapid Clearance	Latent Allotype Expression After Experiment	Latent Allotype Expression Before Experiment
5432	$a^3a^3b^4b^4$	a2	yes	+	+
		b5	yes	+	+
5436	$a^3a^3b^4b^4$	a1	yes	+	+
5441	$a^3a^3b^4b^4$	a2	yes	+	+
		b5	yes	+	+
5453	$a^2a^2b^5b^5$	a3	yes	+	+
		b4	yes	+	+
5	$a^3a^3b^4b^4$	a1	yes	+	+
23	$a^1a^1b^4b^4$	a3	yes	+	+
5455	$a^2a^2b^4b^5$	a3	no	−	±
5456	$a^2a^2b^4b^5$	a3	no	−	−
6	$a^1a^1b^4b^4$	a3	no	−	−

[a]Latent allotypes were determined by radioimmunoassay (RIA). (+) indicates latent allotypes detected in more than half the bleedings examined, (±) indicates latent allotypes detected in fewer than half, and (−) indicates no latent allotypes found.

this response should wholly or partially release the latent allotype from anti-allotype-mediated suppression. This expectation was fulfilled with a steep rise in latent allotype production in all five rabbits (TABLE 4).

A second study implicating cellular control mechanisms in the regulation of latent allotype expression was prompted by results on release from allotype suppression.[20] McCartney-Francis and Mandy[21] treated splenocytes in culture with lipopolysaccharide and an anti-allotype serum directed against the nominal allotype of the splenocytes. This treatment (e.g. b5 anti-b4 serum into a culture of b4 splenocytes) was found to suppress allotype-specific reverse plaque formation of the nominal allotype (b4) and to induce plaques of a latent allotype. In all cases the latent allotype induced was that of the anti-allotype serum used. (In the example given, this would be b5.)

The two studies summarized above are difficult to integrate into a coherent model for control of latent allotype expression, but they do have several features in common. First, they implicate allotype-specific suppression as a major control element. Second,

TABLE 4. Induction of Latent Allotypes by Anti-Allotype Injection

Rabbit	Latent Allotype	Maximum Concentration of Latent Allotype Before Immunization[a]	Maximum Concentration of Latent Allotype After Anti-Allotype Injection	Maximum Concentration of Latent Allotype After Streptococcal Immunization[b]
4805	a2	3.0	12.1	59.0
4806	a2	2.8	10.2	31.7
4809	a2	2.2	9.9	18.6[c]
5455	b6	3.1	9.4	28.0
5456	b6	1.6	7.1	17.8

[a]All concentrations determined by RIA and are given in μg IgG/ml.
[b]Immunization with streptococcal vaccine following anti-allotype immunization was in all cases a secondary immunization. Primary streptococcal immunization was done six months before the beginning of the experiment.
[c]Rabbit died after first injection with streptococcal vaccine.

although they affected only a limited number of rabbits from colonies known to contain animals predisposed to latent allotype expression, no failures of latent allotype induction were reported. If the limited numbers are disregarded, they both suggest that the potential exists for most, if not all, rabbits to produce all of the possible allotypes under appropriate conditions. Third, both studies include rather complex treatments of intact animals or cell cultures and are therefore subject to a variety of potential explanations other than those favored by the authors. A thorough investigation of these systems would require a great deal of work, and the experimental designs could only be optimized if a good model existed for the static Ig gene content of the specific experimental subjects. It is our feeling that such extended studies of latent allotype control are indicated only after direct investigation of the rabbit DNA. Such studies are now relatively easy to do and have already yielded detailed information about rabbit Ig genes. The problem of latent allotypes has not yet been solved, but the definitive experiments can now be done.

THE IMMUNOGLOBULIN GENE COMPLEMENT
AND LATENT ALLOTYPES

Whereas studies of rabbit Ig genes are just beginning to yield detailed results, studies of mouse, rat, and human Ig genes are quite advanced. Latent allotypes have been reported in all of these species,[7] but the observed gene complements provide no evidence for the existence of normally silent genes other than a few pseudogenes. It may be important that latent allotypes in these species have often been observed in limited and unusual circumstances (e.g. in a single congenic mouse strain,[22] in rat radiation chimeras,[23] in human tumor cells during *in vivo* passage,[24] or in a human family carrying a variety of immunological defects[25]). These situations may represent exceptions to the normal rules of gene complement and gene expression. The fact remains that these species show no general tendency to harbor unexpressed genetically unexpected Ig genes in their genomes. A study of the genes encoding the complex rat C_κ allotypes showed no evidence for latent C_κ genes.[35] Whereas results in other species have no necessary bearing on the much better documented rabbit latent allotype data, they provide added incentive for interested workers to demonstrate a structural basis for latent allotypy in the genome of an animal that has a documented history of latent allotypes. The two principal difficulties encountered in studying rabbit Ig genes and especially genes for L chains are the lack of cell lines expressing rabbit Ig and failure of C_κ probes from other species to cross-hybridize with rabbit C_κ genes. To circumvent these problems, our laboratory is using rabbit-mouse hybridomas secreting rabbit Ig chains as starting material for the construction of suitable probes.

RABBIT-MOUSE HYBRIDOMAS

B-cell lines do not exist for the rabbit, eliminating one of the prime resources that exists in other species. Cell lines are an extremely useful resource because they express monoclonal products that can be studied on a continuing basis. Primary tissue, including spleen and peripheral blood, has been used to great effect in many studies, but it is an unrenewable resource, lacks a monoclonal source of an expressed V gene, and may be contaminated with nonlymphoid cells.

In the absence of B-cell lines, hybridomas offer the best substitute.[26-29] Hybridomas expressing rabbit Ig chains must of necessity be interspecies hybrids because there are no rabbit myelomas. This produces several disadvantages as well as a few compensating advantages. Interspecies hybrids are normally subject to selective chromosome loss, and rabbit-mouse hybrids represent an extreme example of this tendency. Hybridoma cells maintained in long-term culture must be recloned frequently to retain secretion of the rabbit immunologulin. In most cases, it appears that these hybridomas reach maximum stability by translocation of the rabbit Ig gene(s) onto a mouse chromosome. This presumption is supported by the presence of few[30] or no[27,28] intact rabbit chromosomes in secreting cells and by the discontinuous manner in which stabilization appears on serial cloning (FIGURE 2).

The instability of the hybridomas makes for more difficulty in obtaining very large numbers of cells. In addition, stable hybrids normally secrete only a single rabbit Ig chain, rather than a functional antibody. Whereas new approaches have made it now

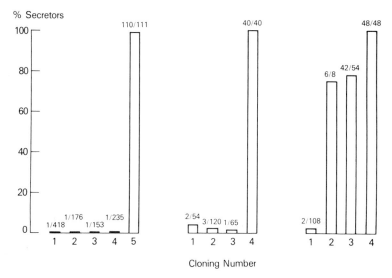

FIGURE 2. Percent secretion of growing clones as a function of sequential cloning number for three RMH cell lines: left–H50; center–H105-131, and right–H105-14. Numbers above the bars indicate the number of clones found positive over the total number tested.

possible to obtain a few lines secreting intact rabbit Ig, some with antibody activity (M-C. Kuo, J.A. Sogn, and T.J. Kindt, manuscript in preparation), rabbit-mouse hybrids remain somewhat difficult to prepare. This disadvantage, however, is partially compensated for by two useful features of these cells. First, the minimal content of rabbit genes in the hybrid makes it possible in some instances to screen efficiently for rabbit Ig genes in clones by differential hybridization to probes prepared from the hybridoma and the parental myeloma. Most of the rabbit genes present are related to the Ig chain(s) secreted by the hybridoma. Second, the rabbit and mouse genes can be distinguished quite easily, so the contributions of the two parental cells to the properties of the hybridoma can be assessed. As mentioned earlier, mouse and rabbit C_κ probes do not cross-hybridize. Also, in a hybridoma secreting an intact rabbit IgM, restriction mapping unambiguously showed the J chain to be of mouse origin (E. Max and J. Sogn, unpublished results). In addition, the presumptive presence of the rabbit genes on mouse chromosomes offers the opportunity to examine, by *in situ* hybridiza-tion,[31] the site of integration of the rabbit genes into the mouse genome. Whereas this translocation may be random, it may also be directed in a manner analogous to the translocation observed in many lymphoid malignancies.[32-34]

GENERATION OF PROBES FOR RABBIT κ CHAIN SEQUENCES

The rabbit group b allotypes of the C_κ region offer the most definitive system in which to look for DNA sequences encoding latent allotypes. Many detailed reports of latent group b allotypes exist, and the amino acid sequences of the various C_κ regions are substantially known and very different. Our initial studies have, therefore, concentrated on a hybridoma (12F2) secreting a rabbit κ chain of the b4 allotype.[36]

Poly(A) RNA was extracted from rabbit-mouse hybridoma 12F2 cells that had been rigorously cloned to ensure maximum rabbit L chain expression. *In vitro* translation analysis of poly(A) RNA, fractionated according to size by sucrose density gradient centrifugation, had confirmed a previous finding,[37] that the rabbit κ mRNA had a size of 12S. The 12S poly(A) RNA was used as a template to prepare duplex cDNA, which was subsequently cloned by dC-dG homopolymer tailing into the PstI site of pBR322. Clones were screened by differential hybridization using [32]P cDNA probes prepared from 12F2 and the parent myeloma P3X63Ag8-U1 and by restriction enzyme analysis. One clone (pB4D5) was isolated from the cDNA library and shown by nucleic acid sequence analysis to code for the entire V, J, and C regions and portions of the leader and 3' untranslated regions of the b4 mRNA produced by the 12F2 cell line (K. L. Dreher, manuscript in preparation).

The translated C_κ sequence from pB4D5 agrees with the b4 amino acid sequence[38] except for a single Asp-Asn interchange. The V_κ sequence agrees with the 25 amino acid residues determined from the amino terminus of the secreted 12F2 light chain. The complete V_κ sequence is very homologous to rabbit V_κ sequences for 3T72 (90% homologous) and 120 (85% homologous).[39] The majority of differences in amino acid sequence among these three V_κ regions were due to single base changes and were confined to the complementarity determining regions. The amino acid sequence encoded by the J_κ region of 12F2 is identical to that observed for all other b4 chains from the Phe at position 98 through the Lys at position 107 (27 sequences have been reported[39]). The three amino acids just before Phe_{98} are of uncertain derivation (L. Emorine, manuscript in preparation).

In order to examine the organization of the κ gene in rabbit germ line DNA, specific probes encoding the V and C regions were prepared from the pB4D5 clone and used in Southern blot analysis of sperm DNA obtained from a homozygous b4 rabbit (FIGURE 3). Many fragments hybridizing to the C_κ region were observed, implying that a number of related sequences exist for this probe in the germ line DNA. The 12F2 DNA yielded two types of fragments that hybridized to the C_κ probe. One set was found also in germ line DNA and was presumed to be unrearranged. A second set was unique to 12F2 and probably includes functionally rearranged sequences. Whether the extra bands represent other C_κ genes is not yet known, but cloning and sequencing will determine their relationship to the principal C_κ b4 gene. A previous study with a b4 C_κ probe[40] produced similar findings. The b4 C_κ probe cross-reacts extensively with multiple fragments in DNA from rabbits of other group b allotypes. Again, further analysis will be required to determine whether the sequences detected are of physiolog-ical significance and whether they can account for latent allotype expression.

Similar studies using a V region probe prepared from pB4D5 revealed a large

Eco R1

b4 12F2 P3U1

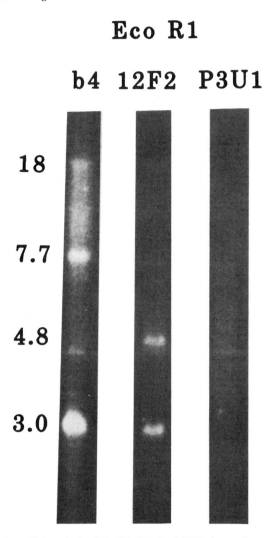

FIGURE 3. Southern Blot analysis of EcoR1 digests of DNA from a homozygous b4 rabbit, rabbit-mouse hybrid cell line 12F2, and mouse myeloma cell line P3X63Ag8-U1. The digests are probed with a labeled fragment of pB4D5 spanning most of the C_κ coding region. Minor bands have not been developed from this blot. The apparent band at 4.4Kb in each lane is an artifact from cutting the filter prior to hybridization.

family of related sequences in germ line b4 DNA. Under conditions used, substantial cross-reaction of the probe with mouse sequences is also seen. Blots done with sperm DNA isolated from rabbits of different group b allotypes give similar but not identical V_κ bands. The hybridization pattern with a J_κ probe is also complex. A principal set of J_κ regions has been identified and studied in detail (L. Emorine, manuscript in preparation). The possible existence of more J_κ regions is under investigation.

SUMMARY

The expression of latent allotypes is a well documented phenomenon in rabbits. Speculation about their molecular genetic basis and the mechanisms that control expression of these unexpected markers lead inevitably to questions about the Ig gene complement of the rabbit. This central question is under current study using probes derived originally from the mRNA of rabbit-mouse hybridomas secreting rabbit Ig chains. Some of the basic features of rabbit Ig genes are already clear from these studies, and DNA fragments that might encode latent allotypes have been identified with the first set of probes. Further gene closing sequencing should shortly provide a definitive answer to the question of latent allotypy and will also provide a detailed understanding of nominal Ig expression in rabbits.

REFERENCES

1. OUDIN, J. 1956. L' "allotypie" de certaines antigenes proteidiques du serum. C. R. Acad. Sci. **242:** 2606–2608.
2. GRUBB, R. 1956. Agglutination of erythrocytes coated with "incomplete" anti-Rh by certain rheumatoid arthritic sera and some other sera. Acta Pathol. Microbiol. Scand. **39:** 195–197.
3. SLATER, R. J., S. M. WARD & H. G. KUNKEL. 1955. Immunological relationships among the myeloma proteins. J. Exp. Med. **101:** 85–108.
4. OUDIN, J. & M. MICHEL. 1963. A new allotype form of rabbit serum γ-globulins, apparently associated with antibody function and specificity. C. R. Acad. Sci. **257:** 805–808.
5. LOBB, N., C. C. CURTAIN & C. KIDSON. 1967. Regulatory genes controlling the synthesis of H chains of human immunoglobulin-G. Nature (London) **214:** 783–785.
6. LOBB, N. 1968. The synthesis of immunoglobulin G by cultured human lymphocytes. Aust. J. Exp. Biol. Med. Sci. **46:** 397–405.
7. KINDT, T. J. & M. YARMUSH. 1981. Expression of latent immunoglobulin allotypes and alien histocompatibility antigens: relevance to models of eukaryotic gene regulation. CRC Crit. Rev. Immunol. **2(4):** 297–348.
8. STROSBERG, A. D., C. HAMERS-CASTERMAN, W. VAN DER LOO & R. HAMERS. 1974. A rabbit with the allotypic phenotype: a1a2a3 b4b5b6. J. Immunol. **113:** 1313–1318.
9. MUDGETT-HUNTER, M., M. L. YARMUSH, B. A. FRASER & T. J. KINDT. 1978. Rabbit latent group a allotypes: characterization and relationship to nominal group a allotypic specificities. J. Immunol. **121:** 1132–1138.
10. MCCARTNEY-FRANCIS, N. & W. J. MANDY. 1979. Serological and chemical studies of latent allotypes in the rabbit. Ann. Immunol. Inst. Pasteur (Paris) **130C:** 115–131.
11. YARMUSH, M. L. & T. J. KINDT. 1978. Isolation and characterization of IgG molecules expressing latent group b allotypes from pedigreed b4b4 rabbits. J. Exp. Med. **148:** 522–533.
12. MUDGETT, M., B. A. FRASER & T. J. KINDT. 1975. Nonallelic behavior of rabbit variable-region allotypes. J. Exp. Med. **141:** 1448–1452.
13. YARMUSH, M. L., H. C. KRUTZSCH & T. J. KINDT. 1980. Amino acid sequence analysis of immunoglobulin light chains by gas chromatographic-mass spectrometric techniques: structural identity of nominal and latent b9 molecules. Mol. Immunol. **17:** 319–326.
14. MANDY, W. J. & A. D. STROSBERG. 1978. Latent expression of a Cγ gene. J. Immunol. **120:** 1160–1163.
15. YARMUSH, M. L., W. J. MANDY & T. J. KINDT. 1980. Evidence for linked expression of latent allotypes of the heavy chain constant and variable regions. J. Immunol. **124:** 2864–2869.
16. STROSBERG, A. D. 1977. Multiple expression of rabbit allotypes: the tip of the iceberg? Immunogenetics **4:** 499–513.

17. YARMUSH, M. L., J. A. SOGN, P. D. KERN & T. J. KINDT. 1981. The role of immune recognition in latent allotype induction and clearance: evidence for an allotype network. J. Exp. Med. **153:** 196–206.
18. ADLER, L. T., F. L. ADLER & A. YAMADA. 1978. Stable chimerism induced in nonbred rabbits by neonatal injection of spleen cells from allotype-suppressed adult donors. II. Distribution of donor and recipient allotypes on blood lymphocytes, in serum immunoglobulins and in specific antibodies. Transplantation **26:** 401–406.
19. ADLER, L. T., F. A. ADLER, C. COHEN & R. G. TISSOT. 1981. Induction of lymphoid cell chimerism in noninbred histocompatible rabbits. A new model for studying allotype suppression in the rabbit. J. Exp. Med. **154:** 1085–1099.
20. ADLER, L. T. & F. L. ADLER. 1978. *In vitro* studies on allotype suppression. IV. Abrogation of waning suppression by normal immunoglobulin of the suppressed allotype. Immunol. Commun. **7:** 269–280.
21. MCCARTNEY-FRANCIS, N. & W. J. MANDY. 1981. Control of latent allotype expression by rabbit splenocytes. J. Immunol. **127:** 352–357.
22. BOSMA, M. J. and G. C. BOSMA. 1974. Congenic mouse strains: the expression of a hidden immunoglobulin allotype in a congenic partner strain of BALB/c mice. J. Exp. Med. **139:** 512–527.
23. HUNT, L. & S. DUVALL. 1976. Rat immunoglobulin allotypes: expression by thymus-independent cells. Biochem. Soc. Trans. **4:** 39–41.
24. POTHIER, L., H. BOREL & R. A. ADAMS. 1974. Expression of IgG allotypes in human lymphoid tumor lines serially transplantable in the neonatal Syrian hamster. J. Immunol. **113:** 1984–1991.
25. SALIER, J. P., L. RIVAT, M. DAVEAU, G. LEFRANC, P. BRETON, C. H. DE MENIBUS & H. H. FUDENBERG. 1980. Quantitative studies of Gm allotypes V. Simultaneous presence of latent Gm allotypes and deficient Gm genes in a family with hypogammaglobulinaemic probands. Immunogenetics **7:** 123–135.
26. YARMUSH, M. L., F. T. GATES III, D. R. WEISFOGEL & T. J. KINDT. 1980. Identification and characterization of rabbit-mouse hybridomas secreting rabbit immunoglobulin chains. Proc. Natl. Acad. Sci. USA **77:** 2899–2903.
27. YARMUSH, M. L., F. T. GATES III, K. L. DREHER & T. J. KINDT. 1981. Serological and structural characterization of immunoglobulin chains secreted by rabbit-mouse hybridomas. J. Immunol. **126:** 2240–2244.
28. BUTTIN, G., C. LEGUERN, L. PHALENTE, E. C. C. LIN. L. MEDRANS & P. A. CAZENAVE. 1978. Production of hybrid lines secreting monoclonal antiidiotypic antibodies by cell fusion on membrane filters. Curr. Top. Microbiol. Immunol. **81:** 27–36.
29. NOTENBOOM, R. H., C-T. CHEN, P. W. GOOD, S. I. DUBISKI, B. CINADER & G. KOHLER. 1980. Isolation and characterization of a rabbit-mouse hybridoma. Immunogenetics **7:** 359–368.
30. MEDRANO, L., L. PHALENTE & G. BUTTIN. 1979. Differential staining and segregation of parental chromosomes in mouse-rabbit hybridomas. Cell. Biol. Intl. Rep. **3:** 503–514.
31. HARPER, M. E. & G. F. SAUNDERS. 1981. Localization of single copy DNA sequences on G-banded human chromosomes by *in situ* hybridization. Chromasoma **83:** 431–439.
32. WIENER, F., S. OHNO, J. SPIRA, N. HARAN-GHERA & G. KLEIN. 1978. Chromosome changes (trisomies number 15 and 17) associated with tumor progression in leukemias induced by radiation leukemia virus. J. Natl. Can. Inst. **62:** 227–237.
33. OHNO, S., M. BABONITS, F. WIENER, J. SPIRA, G. KLEIN & M. POTTER. 1979. Nonrandom chromosome changes involving the Ig gene-carrying chromosome 12 and 6 in pristane-induced plasmacytomas. Cell **18:** 1001–1007.
34. WIENER, F., M. BABONITS, J. SPIRA, G. KLEIN & M. POTTER. 1980. Cytogenetic studies on IgA lambda producing murine plasmacytomas: Regular occurrence of a T (12:15) translocation. Somatic Cell Genet. **6:** 731–738.
35. SHEPPARD, H. W. & G. A. GUTMAN. 1981. Complex allotypes of rat κ chains are encoded by structural alleles. Nature (London) **293:** 669–671.
36. DREHER, K. L., J. A. SOGN, F. T. GATES III, M-C. KUO & T. J. KINDT. 1983. Allotype defined mRNA for rabbit immunoglobulin H and L chains isolated from rabbit-mouse hybridomas. J. Immunol. **130:** 442–448.

37. HEIDMANN, O., C. AUFFRAY, P. A. CAZENAVE & F. ROUGEON. 1981. Nucleotide sequence of constant and 3' untranslated regions of a κ immunoglobulin light chain mRNA of a homozygous b4 rabbit. Proc. Natl. Acad. Sci. USA **78:** 5802–5806.
38. CHEN, K. C. S., T. J. KINDT & R. M. KRAUSE. 1975. Primary structure of the L chain from a rabbit homogenous antibody to streptococcal carbohydrate. II. Sequence determination of peptides from tryptic and peptic digests. J. Biol. Chem. **250:** 3289–3296.
39. KABAT, E. A., T. T. WU & H. BILOFSKY. 1979. Sequences of immunoglobulin chains. NIH Publication No. 80-2008, pp. 51–57.
40. HEIDMANN, O. & F. ROUGEON. 1982. Multiple sequences related to a constant-region kappa light chain gene in the rabbit genome. Cell **28:** 507–513.

DISCUSSION OF THE PAPER

A. D. STROSBERG (*University of Paris, Paris, France*): This Southern Blot that you showed is not very similar to one that was published earlier. Could you comment on the differences?

J. A. SOGN: There was a blot published earlier by Dr. Rougeon using a probe obtained in basically the same way. There are more similarities than there are differences between the various blots. In both cases it is clear that there are a number of sequences—cross-hybridizing with C_κ probes in the rabbit. Some of the exact bands do not exactly correspond, and we are not entirely sure what this is due to. The probes were isolated differently and contain different sequences. That may account for the differences.

R. MAGE (*National Institutes of Health, Bethesda, Md.*): Would you care to tell us exactly what your C_κ probes did consist of? I am particularly interested, because we have found a very high degree of conservation of the three prime UT sequences between b4 and b5. It is only when one gets to the coding sequence that one gets large differences in the nucleic acid sequence.

SOGN: I cannot remember the exact restriction enzymes that were used to produce the probe, but the probe consists entirely of C_κ sequences and goes from very near the J/C junction to very near the 3' junction—very near the end of the coding sequence.

MAGE: I know that the Rougeon blot was with about 71 base pairs of 3' UT, and there are only two base differences between b4 and b5 in that probe.

SOGN: There is no 3' untranslated.

MAGE: That would be the difference between your work and the Rougeon work.

Idiotypic Determinants Used in the Analysis of Antibody Diversification and as Regulatory Targets[a]

K. BEYREUTHER, J. BOVENS, M. BRÜGGEMANN,
R. DILDROP, G. KELSOE, U. KRAWINKEL,
C. MÜLLER, S. NISHIKAWA, A. RADBRUCH,
M. RETH, M. SIEKEVITZ, T. TAKEMORI, H. TESCH,
G. WILDNER, S. ZAISS, AND K. RAJEWSKY[b]

Institute for Genetics
University of Cologne
Cologne, Federal Republic of Germany

INTRODUCTION

In 1973, Imanishi and Mäkelä found that the primary immune response of C57BL/6 mice against the hapten 4-hydroxy-3-nitrophenylacetyl (NP) is dominated by antibodies that bind the cross-reacting hapten 5-iodo-NP (NIP) with higher affinity than the immunizing hapten (heteroclicity).[1] The highly restricted nature of the response was also later demonstrated in isoelectric focusing analysis and was shown to be controlled by the IgH locus.[2,3] The vast majority of primary anti-NP antibodies of IgH^b mice carry λ chains,[4] in contrast to the 95% κ-bearing antibodies in normal mouse immunoglobulin, and express a recurrent idiotype (called NP^b) that is controlled by both the Igh^b and the $Ig\lambda$ locus.[5–7]

The monoclonal antibody technique permitted us to analyze the NP^b idiotype at the level of individual antibody molecules. The idiotype turned out to be expressed by a large family of closely related, but distinct, antibody species, the NP^b antibody family.[8,9] The variable (V) regions of three monoclonal antibodies of our collection were sequenced by A. Bothwell in D. Baltimore's group at the DNA level and the corresponding V genes in the germ line were identified (references 10 and 11, and A. Bothwell, M. Paskind, and D. Baltimore, personal communication). Two of the antibodies, isolated from the primary response and designated B1-8 (IgM, λ1) and B1-48 (IgG$_1$, λ1), carried a V_H sequence identical to that of a germ line V_H gene, V186-2. The third antibody, S43 (IgG$_{2a}$, λ1) had been isolated from a hyperimmune response. Its V_H region was also clearly derived from V186-2, but it carried ten point mutations resulting in seven amino acid substitutions. All three antibodies had drastically different D segments, expressed either JH1 or JH2, and carried λ1 chains. The V_λ region of antibody B1-8 was germ line encoded, whereas that of antibody S43 carried two amino acid substitutions.[10,11] We have recently learned from Dr. H. Sakano and Dr. K. Karjalainen (personal communication) that two further anti-NP antibodies of C57BL/6 origin also carry a V186-2 encoded V_H region. Their D segments are

[a]This work was supported by the Deutsche Forschungsgemeinschaft through SFB 74, the Wissenschaftsministerium des Landes Nordrhein-Westfalen, and the Fazit-Foundation.
[b]Correspondence to: K. Rajewsky, Institut für Genetik, Universität zu Köln, Weyertal 121, D-5000 Köln 41, F.R.G.

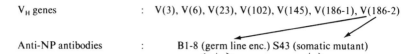

FIGURE 1. Outline of the experimental system. Indicated in the top line is a group of related V_H genes isolated and sequenced by Bothwell *et al.*[10] The monoclonal antibody B1-8 (IgM, λ1) expresses germ line encoded V_L ($V_{\lambda1}$), V_H (V(186-2)), D and J segments. The V_H and V_L regions of antibody S43 (IgG$_{2a}$, λ1) are encoded by the same genes that, however, carry somatic point mutations. The D segments in B1-8 and S43 are also different. Given in the bottom line are some monoclonal anti-idiotope antibodies against B1-8 and S43. Some anti-idiotopes compete with hapten for binding (unbroken arrows), some do not (broken arrows). All anti-idiotopes bear κ light chains and belong to the IgG$_1$ class. In the case of anti-idiotopes Ac146 and A39-40 (underlined), class switch variants of the IgG$_{2a}$ and IgG$_{2b}$ class have been isolated. For details and references see text.

unique, and they express JH2 and JH4 (reviewed in reference 12). Thus, there is clear evidence that a single V_H and a single V_L gene, in combination with a variety of D and J elements, encodes the majority of the NP^b antibody family. Diversity in the family is generated by different combinations of V, D, and J elements and by somatic mutation. Similar results have been obtained in the case of other recurrent idiotypes.[13-17]

We have selected antibody B1-8 with its germ line encoded V region and the somatic mutant S43 and raised monoclonal anti-idiotope antibodies against these proteins.[18] When tested with these antibodies, B1-8 and S43 are non-cross-reactive and thus idiotypically distinct. In FIGURE 1 we depict the components of the experimental system that we discuss in the present paper. Each anti-idiotope recognizes an idiotope on either antibody B1-8 or S43. (We give anti-idiotope and corresponding idiotope the same name, e.g. anti-idiotope Ac38 binds idiotope Ac38.) The idiotopes can be distinguished from each other in several ways. Some can be found expressed on antibodies in the absence of others. Some must be close to or in the NP binding site because hapten competes with the corresponding anti-idiotope. Some are further apart from the hapten binding site.[9,18] FIGURE 1 also lists the group of related V_H genes as identified by Bothwell *et al.*,[10] among them V186-2, the gene encoding most primary

TABLE 1. λ1-Bearing Antibodies (μg/ml)^a

NP-bdg	AC38^{+b}	Ac146^{+b}	8/4^{+c}	20/44^{+c}
493 (1.94)^d	27.5 (2.15)^d	23.7 (2.18)^d	1.1 (1/11)^e	0.40 (1/11)^e

^{a}Eleven mice were immunized with 100 μg alum-precipitated NP chicken gamma globulin and bled 12 days after immunization.

^{b}Idiotopes recognized by anti-idiotope antibodies against the germ line encoded antibody B1-8 (see FIGURE 1).

^{c}Idiotopes recognized by anti-idiotope antibodies against a somatic variant of B1-8, S43 (see FIGURE 1).

^{d}Titers determined in a radioactive binding assay.[19,20] Geometric means of groups of eleven sera, with standard deviations. As described in reference 26, the titers of Ac38$^+$ and Ac146$^+$ antibodies would be substantially higher if determined by absorption on insolubilized anti-idiotopes.

^{e}Idiotope-bearing antibodies were only detectable in one out of eleven sera, at the concentration indicated. In the other sera, idiotope levels were below 0.2 μg/ml.

anti-NP antibodies. As we will show later, some of the B1-8 idiotopes are also expressed on products of other V_H genes in the cluster, when the latter are expressed together with λ chains and certain D and J regions.

We can thus use the anti-idiotopes in FIGURE 1 for an analysis of the antibody repertoire generated directly by the V_H genes in the cluster, and we can analyze the expression of germ line encoded idiotopes and idiotopes of a somatic mutant in anti-NP responses. Furthermore, the system allows us to study the regulatory influence of anti-idiotope antibodies on idiotope expression under quasi-physiological conditions. In the section below, we briefly summarize and interpret our experimental results.

GERM LINE ENCODED IDIOTOPES ARE REGULARLY EXPRESSED IN ANTI-NP RESPONSES. THE EXPRESSION OF IDIOTOPES OF A SOMATIC VARIANT IS IRREGULAR

All idiotopes identified by monoclonal anti-idiotopes on the germ line encoded antibody B1-8 are regularly expressed in primary NP responses of Igh[b] mice.[9,19-22] The level of expression ranges between 5 and 50% of the total NP[b] antibody family, with some variability between individual mice, depending on the assay used (direct inhibition[19,20] or absorption on insolubilized anti-idiotope[26]). Certain idiotopes occur always in association with certain others, whereas other idiotopes are expressed independently of each other (references 18, 19, 21, 22, 26, and unpublished data).

By contrast, idiotopes of somatic mutant S43 were found to be irregularly expressed in primary anti-NP sera. In some sera, they could be detected at low levels. In most sera, they were not detectable at all (G. Wildner, T. Takemori, and K. Rajewsky, to be published). TABLE 1 gives a summary of these results. Thus, the idiotope pattern expressed in the anti-NP responses seems to consist of two components: a set of recurrently expressed idiotopes that are germ line encoded and a set of idiotopes expressed in certain individuals, but not in others. The latter may be specific for somatic mutants, but could also arise from rare V-D-J combinations. So far, there is no evidence in this system for the selection of a recurrently expressed idiotope repertoire generated by somatic mutation.

POINT MUTATION AND RECOMBINATION BETWEEN VARIABLE GENES IN ANTIBODY DIVERSIFICATION

The structural analysis of antibody S43 provided clear evidence for the occurrence of point mutation in somatic antibody diversification,[10,11] in accord with a large body of evidence in other experimental systems (reviewed in reference 12). Subsequent experiments raised the possibility that recombination or gene conversion between V genes may also play a role in the generation of the antibody repertoire. In these experiments, spontaneous idiotope loss variants were isolated by fluorescence activated cell sorting from the hybridoma line secreting antibody B1-8. Two such variants have been isolated so far. Both occurred at low frequency ($\approx 10^{-6}$), and one of them (B1-8.V3) carried a single point mutation in position 103 of the heavy chain (a glycine-arginine exchange) (S. Zaiss, A. Radbruch, K. Beyreuther, and K. Rajewsky, to be published). The second variant (B1-8.V1) had ten amino acid exchanges in the V_H region. Sequence analysis of the latter variant at the protein and the DNA level showed that it was generated by a double recombination or by gene conversion between the V_H gene expressed in antibody B1-8 (V186-2) and a neighboring V_H gene (V102) that exhibits strong homology with V186-2, particularly at the recombination break points.[23-25] It is presently unknown whether recombinations of this type play a role in somatic antibody diversification under physiological conditions. The bulk of the available experimental evidence appears to argue against this possibility (see the article of P. Gearhart et al. in this volume). Variable gene recombinants, however, might well be found when the expression of families of closely related V genes (like the NP^b family) is studied, and when the analysis is not limited to antibodies of a given hapten-binding specificity. Significantly, the B1-8.V1 variant has almost completely lost NP binding specificity.[23]

THE IDIOTOPE REPERTOIRE IS GENETICALLY CONTROLLED AND RESTRICTED BY ANTIBODY STRUCTURAL GENES. V$_H$ REGIONS ENCODED BY RELATED GERM LINE GENES AND DIFFERING IN ANTIGEN BINDING SPECIFICITY CAN SHARE IDIOTOPES.

The somatic variant B1-8.V1 (see above) has largely lost NP binding specificity, and most of its V$_H$ region is encoded by a V$_H$ gene differing from that expressed in the B1-8 wild type. The variant still expresses certain B1-8 idiotopes, however, in particular, idiotope Ac38.[23] Immunization of mice with the anti-idiotope Ac38, cross-linked to keyhole limpet hemocyanin (KLH), has shown that the Ac38 idiotope can be expressed by many members of the NP^{b}V$_H$ gene cluster.[22,26] In the immune sera and in hybridomas derived from the immunized mice, antibodies expressing the Ac38 idiotope were identified by their property of bearing λ1 light chains (this taken as a distinction from anti-anti-idiotopes that are expected to bear κ chains as some 95% of mouse immunoglobulin (Ig)). Indeed, Northern blot analysis of seven out of seven hybridomas characterized in this way revealed strong hybridization of a B1-8 V$_H$ probe with the mRNA expressed by the cells. Partial amino acid sequence analysis of four out of four hybrid cell antibodies showed that their V$_H$ regions are encoded by V$_H$ genes either already identified by Bothwell et al.[10] or closely related to them (R. Dildrop, M. Siekevitz, J. Bovens, K. Beyreuther, and K. Rajewsky, to be published). Only 10% of the induced antibodies expressed NP binding specificity.[22,26] In BALB/c and CBA mice, Ac38 positive antibodies were also induced, but they lacked NP binding specificity altogether. Genetic analysis revealed that the ability to produce Ac38 positive, NP binding antibodies is controlled by the Igh^b haplotype and independent of the H-2 locus. This result is in perfect accord with recent evidence showing that whereas BALB/c mice possess a V$_H$ gene very similar to V186-2, this gene does not encode certain residues that are believed to be responsible for NP binding specificity.[27] The anti-NP response of BALB/c mice appears to make use of another V$_H$ gene.[28] In analogous experiments, it was found that C57BL/6, but not BALB/c or CBA mice, responded to immunization with another anti-idiotope, Ac146, with the production of λ1 chain bearing antibodies expressing the target idiotope. In this case, more than 90% of the Ac146 positive antibodies bound the NP hapten.[26] In accord with the latter result, the Ac146 idiotope had previously been shown by hapten competition studies to be located close to, or possibly within the NP binding site of antibody B1-8.[9] Thus, antibody Ac146 formally functions in this system as the "internal image"[29] of the NP hapten, but the limitations of the view that antibody V regions structurally mimic determinants of conventional antigens is underlined in this case by the fact that many NP antibodies in C57BL/6 mice and all of them in strains BALB/c and CBA lack the Ac146 idiotope.

Taken together, the data summarized in this section demonstrate that the idiotope repertoire is incomplete in a first approximation and controlled by the Igh linkage group. They give a clear example of idiotope sharing between antibodies differing in antigen binding specificity, a phenomenon amply documented in the literature (reviewed in reference 12), and show that the latter phenomenon is in this case due to the participation of a series of V_H, D, and J regions in encoding idiotypically related antibodies.

The participation of a large set of antibody structural genes in encoding the Ac38 idiotope is reflected in a very high frequency of lipopolysaccharide (LPS) reactive B cells expressing this idiotope: such cells occur at a frequency of roughly 1×10^{-3} in bone marrow and spleen. By contrast, B cells expressing the Ac146 idiotope, which appear to depend upon the expression of a single V_H gene in combination with only a few D elements (see reference 12), occur at a 10–100-fold lower frequency.[30] In accord with these data, Ac38 positive antibodies dominate the response to cross-linked Ac38 anti-idiotope in that more than 90% of the induced antibodies express λ light chains. By contrast, animals immunized with Ac146 produce mainly κ-bearing (presumably anti-anti-idiotypic) antibodies (H. Tesch, T. Takemori, and K. Rajewsky, submitted for publication).

REGULATION OF B1-8 IDIOTOPE EXPRESSION BY MONOCLONAL ANTI-IDIOTOPE ANTIBODIES

We have shown that monoclonal anti-idiotope antibodies are potent regulators of the expression of B1-8 idiotopes under quasi-physiological conditions. When doses of 10–100 ng of anti-idiotope were injected into adult mice, and the mice were immunized with the NP hapten 4–8 weeks later, expression of the target idiotope in the population of anti-NP antibodies was enhanced five to ten fold. Microgram doses of anti-idiotope suppressed idiotope expression.[19–21] In the latter situation, T-suppressor cells interfering with idiotope expression were demonstrable in the animals.[31] It was also shown that μg doses of anti-idiotope Ac38 prevent the appearance of Ac38 positive LPS reactive B cells in cultures of bone marrow derived pre-B cells.[30] At the level of serum antibodies, both enhancement and suppression were at the level of the IgG response and only marginally detectable in IgM.[21] Indications that the effector function of the anti-idiotypes may be determined by the constant region of their heavy chain[21,32] could not be verified in recent experiments in which spontaneous class switch variants of two anti-idiotopes (Ac146 and A39-40) were employed. Families of anti-idiotope antibodies were constructed by selection of class switch variants whose members belonged to the IgG_1, IgG_{2a} or IgG_{2b} class and expressed either the V region of antibody Ac146 or A39-40 (see FIGURE 1). In all cases, ng doses of anti-idiotope enhanced, and μg doses suppressed the expression of the target idiotope. We also found variability of the enhancement phenomenon in C57BL/6 (but not (C57BL/6 × BALB/c)F1) animals allowing a reinterpretation of previous results pointing to class-dependent regulation.[21] Finally, the results of this series of experiments reveal an interesting difference in the regulatory function of antibodies recognizing different idiotopes: whereas μg doses of antibody Ac146 suppressed expression of idiotope Ac146 by one or two orders of magnitude, antibody A39-40 affected its target idiotope only slightly. In the same animals, however, the expression of idiotope Ac146 was once again suppressed by one or two orders of magnitude (reference 33, and C. Müller and K. Rajewsky, manuscript in preparation).

A similar phenomenon was also strikingly revealed in experiments of neonatal suppression (T. Takemori and K. Rajewsky, submitted for publication; see also references 12, 22). Mice of strain C57BL/6 were injected with either anti-idiotope Ac146 or Ac38 (1–100 μg per animal) at birth. When such animals were immunized with the NP hapten 8–14 weeks later, idiotope Ac146 was suppressed in both groups, whereas idiotope Ac38 was only suppressed in the latter group. Recovery from suppression started at week 12 in a dose-dependent fashion. So far, these results are not surprising, because idiotope Ac146 is expressed on a subset of Ac38-positive antibodies.[18,22,26] Unexpectedly, however, the recovery of Ac38⁺Ac146⁺ antibodies was slower than that of Ac38⁺Ac146⁻ antibodies. When B cells from the Ac38 suppressed mice were combined with normal T cells in irradiated recipients and the animals immunized with NP coupled to chicken gamma globulin, no Ac38 positive antibody was produced in the IgG$_1$ fraction, although the anti-NP response was the same as in the controls. Thus, despite a normal frequency of Ac38 positive LPS reactive B cells in the suppressed donors, the B-cell population was unable to express the Ac38 idiotype in a T-dependent response. When T cells from the suppressed mice were combined with normal B cells in the irradiated hosts, a normally sized anti-NP response was once again induced. In this response, Ac38⁺Ac146⁻ antibodies were represented at normal

TABLE 2. Cell Source[a] Antibody Response (IgG$_1$)

B cells	T cells	NP-bdg (μg/ml)	Ac38⁺/Ac146⁻ (μg/ml)	Ac38⁺/Ac146⁺ (μg/ml)
Normal	Normal	63 (1.3)[b]	1.5 (2.5)	1.5 (2.6)
Suppressed	Suppressed	47 (2.2)	<0.03	<0.03
Suppressed	Normal	49 (1.8)	<0.03	<0.03
Normal	Suppressed	54 (1.6)	1.0 (4.6)	0.03 (1.7)

[a]Cells were from normal 13 week old C57BL/6 mice ("normal") or age-matched animals injected at birth with 100 μg antibody Ac38 ("suppressed"). The cells were either treated with anti-Thy-1.2, anti-Lyt-2.2 and anti-Lyt-1.2 antibody and complement ("B cells"), or nylon wool purified and panned on petri dishes coated with goat antibodies against mouse IgM ("T cells"). 1×10^7 cells of each type were injected into irradiated (540 r) syngeneic recipients, in the combinations indicated. The recipients were immunized with 100 μg alum-precipitated NP-chicken gamma globulin, and the sera was titrated 12 days later.
[b]Titers determined in a radioactive binding assay.[19,20] Geometric means of groups of 5–8 sera, with standard deviations.

levels: however, Ac38⁺Ac146⁺ antibodies were totally absent. Cell mixing and depletion experiments have so far failed to establish whether the T-cell effect is due to the presence of suppressor cells, the absence of helper cells, or both. A summary of some cell transfer data is given in TABLE 2.

Taking the regulatory experiments in this and in other systems together,[12] there is clear evidence that anti-idiotope antibodies are powerful regulators of idiotope expression under quasi-physiological conditions. This supports the notion that the idiotypic network plays a functional role in the immune system, quite in the sense of the network hypothesis. The regulatory effects are expressed in both the B- and the T-cell compartment by way of mechanisms that remain to be explored. Particularly interesting is the finding that the anti-idiotope antibodies induce T-regulatory cells whose functional specificity seems to differ from that of the inducing antibodies. Whatever anti-idiotope is used for induction, the resulting T-regulatory cells appear to exhibit the same restricted specificity, which we so far fail to understand in detail and can only label by certain marker idiotopes (Ac38⁺, Ac146⁺). Thus, whereas the results clearly support the concept of a functional idiotypic network in T-B interactions, they also raise again the old question of the extent to which T- and B-cell idiotopes resemble each other. In a general way, the results fit into the concept that idiotype sharing between the two cell types is brought about by network-controlled selection in ontogeny of T-cell idiotypes (and anti-idiotypes) by idiotypes expressed in B cells.[12]

CONCLUSION

As discussed elsewhere,[12,34] the regulatory experiments with anti-idiotope antibodies can be interpreted in a coherent fashion if idiotypes and anti-idiotypes are considered operational terms for antibody molecules with complementary binding sites (for the limitations of this view see reference 34). At low antibody concentration (ng range), regulatory mechanisms are set in motion that lead to the recruitment ("enhancement") of complementary binding sites. It is tempting to see this phenomenon as a driving force in the immune system, leading to diversification of the repertoire of binding sites by way of selection of somatic variants through idiotypic interactions. At antibody concentrations in the μg range (typical for those induced in antigen-driven immune responses), the system stabilizes the expressed repertoire by suppressing complementary binding sites. At least two mechanisms seem to produce this effect: the induction of specific T-suppressor cells and the direct interference with the production of B cells expressing complementary ("anti-idiotypic") receptors in the bone marrow.[30,31] Mechanisms of this type have classically been seen as means by which the immune system establishes self tolerance. Once an immune response has been induced, the system tends to stabilize the expression of the corresponding binding-site repertoire. This feature of the immune system, which has been widely observed and discussed,[35] is exemplified in idiotypic research by two types of experiments that are, in fact, strictly analogous. One is the suppression of idiotype by anti-idiotype (see above, and for a review of the literature see reference 12). The second is the enhancement of idiotype expression by the idiotype itself, which has been observed in several instances.[20,36-39] This phenomenon, in which both the elimination of anti-idiotypic suppression and the induction of anti-idiotypic help might often play a role,[20,38] can be seen as idiotypic memory: the immune system sees the idiotypic pattern of an antibody and reproduces this pattern later on, whenever it is suitable in an immune response.

ACKNOWLEDGMENTS

We thank S. Irlenbusch, G. von Hesberg, K. Neifer, G. Zimmer, and G. Zoebelein for expert technical assistance, and Dr. A. Bothwell, Dr. M. Paskind, Dr. D. Baltimore, Dr. H. Sakano, and Dr. K. Karjalainen for giving us unpublished sequence information.

REFERENCES

1. IMANISHI, T. and O. MÄKELÄ. 1973. Eur. J. Immunol. **3**: 323–330.
2. MCMICHAEL, A. J., J. M. PHILLIPS, A. R. WILLIAMSON, T. IMANISHI & O. MÄKELÄ. 1975. Immunogenetics **2**: 161–173.
3. IMANISHI, T. & O. MÄKELÄ. 1974. J. Exp. Med. **140**: 1498–1510.
4. RETH, M., T. IMANISHI-KARI, R. S. JACK, M. CRAMER, U. KRAWINKEL, G. J. HÄMMERLING & K. RAJEWSKY. 1977. *In* Regulatory Genetics of the Immune System, ICN-UCLA Symposia on Molecular and Cellular Biology **6**: 139–149.

5. MÄKELÄ, O. & K. KARJALAINEN. 1977. Immunol. Rev. **34:** 119–138.
6. JACK, R. S., T. IMANISHI-KARI & K. RAJEWSKY. 1977. Eur. J. Immunol. **7:** 559–565.
7. IMANISHI-KARI, T., E. RAJNAVÖLGYI, T. TAKEMORI, R. S. JACK & K. RAJEWSKY. 1979. Eur. J. Immunol. **9:** 324–331.
8. RETH, M., G. J. HÄMMERLING & K. RAJEWSKY. 1978. Eur. J. Immunol. **8:** 393–400.
9. RETH, M., T. IMANISHI-KARI & K. RAJEWSKY. 1979. Eur. J. Immunol. **9:** 1004–1013.
10. BOTHWELL, A. L. M., M. PASKIND, M. RETH, T. IMANISHI-KARI, K. RAJEWSKY & D. BALTIMORE. 1981. Cell **24:** 625–637.
11. BOTHWELL, A. L. M., M. PASKIND, M. RETH, T. IMANISHI-KARI, K. RAJEWSKY & D. BALTIMORE. 1982. Nature (London) **298:** 380–382.
12. RAJEWSKY, K. & T. TAKEMORI. 1983. Ann. Rev. Immunol. **1:** 569–607.
13. CREWS, S., J. GRIFFIN, H. HUANG, K. CALAME & L. HOOD. 1981. Cell **25:** 59–66.
14. GEARHART, P. J., N. D. JOHNSON, R. DOUGLAS & L. HOOD. 1981. Nature (London) **291:** 29–34.
15. SCHILLING, J., B. CLEVINGER, J. M. DAVIE & L. HOOD. 1980. Nature (London) **281:** 35–40.
16. SIEKEVITZ, M., S. Y. HUANG & M. GEFTER. 1983. Eur. J. Immunol. **2:** 123–130.
17. GREENE, M. I., M. J. NELLES, M.-S. SY & A. NISONOFF. 1982. Adv. Immunol. **32:** 253–300.
18. RAJEWSKY, K., T. TAKEMORI & M. RETH. 1981. In Monoclonal Antibody and T Cell Hybridoma: Perspective and Technical Advances. G. J. Hämmerling and J. F. Kearney, Eds.: 399–409. Elsevier/North Holland. Amsterdam.
19. KELSOE, G., M. RETH & K. RAJEWSKY. 1980. Immunol. Rev. **52:** 75–88.
20. KELSOE, G., M. RETH & K. RAJEWSKY. 1981. Eur. J. Immunol. **11:** 418–423.
21. RETH, M., G. KELSOE & K. RAJEWSKY. 1981. Nature (London) **290:** 257–259.
22. RAJEWSKY, K., M. RETH, T. TAKEMORI & G. KELSOE. 1981. In The Immune System. C. M. Steinberg and I. Lefkovitz, Eds.: **2:** 1–11. Karger. Basel.
23. BRÜGGEMANN, M., A. RADBRUCH & K. RAJEWSKY. 1982. Eur. Mol. Biol. Org. J. **1:** 629–634.
24. DILDROP, R., M. BRÜGGEMANN, A. RADBRUCH, K. RAJEWSKY & K. BEYREUTHER. 1982. EMBO J. **1:** 635–640.
25. KRAWINKEL, U., G. ZOEBELEIN, M. BRÜGGEMANN, A. RADBRUCH & K. RAJEWSKY. 1983. Proc. Nat. Acad. Sci. USA. **80:** 4997–5001.
26. TAKEMORI, T., H. TESCH, M. RETH & K. RAJEWSKY. 1982. Eur. J. Immunol. **12:** 1040–1046.
27. RETH, M., A. L. M. BOTHWELL & K. RAJEWSKY. 1981. In Immunoglobulin idiotypes. ICN-UCLA Symposia on Molecular and Cellular Biology. J. Janeway, E. E. Sercarz, and H. Wigzell, Eds.: **XX:** 169–178. Academic Press. New York.
28. LOH, D. Y., A. L. M. BOTHWELL, M. E. WHITE-SCHARF, T. IMANISHI-KARI & D. BALTIMORE. 1983. Cell **33:** 85–93.
29. JERNE, N. K. 1974. Ann. Immunol. Inst. Pasteur (Paris) **125C:** 373–389.
30. NISHIKAWA, S., T. TAKEMORI & K. RAJEWSKY. 1983. Eur. J. Immunol. **13:** 318–325.
31. KELSOE, G., T. TAKEMORI, M. RETH & K. RAJEWSKY. 1981. In B Lymphocytes in the Immune Response: Functional, Developmental and Interactive Properties. Klinman, Mosier, Scher, and Vitetta, Eds.: 423–430. Elsevier/North Holland. Amsterdam.
32. EICHMANN, K. 1974. Eur. J. Immunol. **4:** 296–302.
33. MÜLLER, C. E. 1983. Ph.D. Thesis, University of Cologne.
34. RAJEWSKY, K. 1983. Ann. Immunol. Inst. Pasteur (Paris) **134D:** 133–141.
35. HERZENBERG, L. A., T. TOKUHISA, D. R. PARKS & L. A. HERZENBERG. 1982. J. Exp. Med. **155:** 1741–1753.
36. WIKLER, M., C. DEMEUR, G. DEWASME & J. URBAIN. 1980. J. Exp. Med. **152:** 1024–1035.
37. IVARS, F., D. HOLMBERG, L. FORNI, P.-A. CAZENAVE & A. COUTINHO. 1982. Eur. J. Immunol. **12:** 146–151.
38. RUBINSTEIN, L. J., M. YEH & C. A. BONA. 1982. J. Exp. Med. **156:** 506–521.
39. ORTIZ-ORTIZ, L., W. O. WEIGLE & D. L. PARKS. 1982. J. Exp. Med. **156:** 898–911.

DISCUSSION OF THE PAPER

C. A. BONA (*Mt. Sinai School of Medicine, New York*): You showed that the 8/4 idiotope is a result of the somatic mutation, according to the structure data, and in a very small sample of mice, which means 12, you found this idiotope on 3 out of twelve. Did you think that this somatic mutation was just a very rare event or are there other environmental forces that direct this kind of mutation? In a small sample of 12 you find 3 individuals expressing this idiotope.

K. RAJEWSKY: Dr. Bona, I am grateful for that question, because I want to make a point. When I look at these data, I conclude that there is practically no response in these animals. There may be one weakly positive serum. The rest is just background noise of serology. You can make almost any antibody react with any antigen if you choose the right conditions, and I think that a lot of the problems that come up with respect to genetic control of repertoires come simply from the serological techniques.

BONA: Do you have some information about the role of T cells?

RAJEWSKY: That is not well understood, but work on this question has been done by Takemori who has performed cell mixing experiments. One can take, for example, T cells from injected animals, mix them with normal T cells and see what the response is. One can take T cells from noninjected animals, mix them with normal B cells and see what the response is. The answer to your question is that despite the fact that there is always suppression in these mixing experiments, the situation is not very clear. I think that it is very difficult anyway to separate suppressors and helpers. If there are helpers, then they may be there because the suppressors have been eliminated. There is an interplay between these two cells. I do not think that one will find a situation where one can just induce one of them and then not have the response of the second one. I think the reason why these animals do not respond is that they do not have helpers—suppressors having taken over.

N. R. KLINMAN (*Scripps Clinic and Research Foundation, La Jolla, Calif.*): You say that you think that the T cells learn from the B cells. Why do you not believe that the B cells learn from the T cells?

RAJEWSKY: When the T cells have developed a certain repertoire, they will of course select B cells. In fact, the present experiments, and the experiments of Hetzelberger and Eichmann, showed that T cells from idiotypically manipulated mice will actually now preferentially see B cells that express idiotype. This shows that the two cell types in the animal have been adapted to each other. It is still true that idiotype is controlled by the IgH locus. If you say that the (idiotypically related) T-cell receptor is not encoded by the genes in the IgH locus, then the B-cell idiotypes tell the T-cell idiotypes what they have to see and how they have to look idiotypically. The plasticity must be in the T-cell receptor.

KLINMAN: Could the B cells, however, provide a limit function and just provide limits of variability?

RAJEWSKY: Sure.

The Specificity Repertoire of Prereceptor and Mature B Cells[a]

NORMAN R. KLINMAN, RICHARD L. RILEY,
MARY R. STONE, DWANE WYLIE,
AND DORITH ZHARHARY

Department of Immunology
Scripps Clinic and Research Foundation
La Jolla, California 92037

INTRODUCTION

The expression of the B-cell repertoire of mature individuals represents the product of both complex molecular and differentiating events as well as environmental selection. It is generally assumed that the major environmental selective forces on repertoire expression include both clonal inactivation by way of tolerance induction and immunoregulatory processes such as idiotype specific regulation. In order to assess the relative contribution of differentiating events and environmental selection, we have initiated a detailed comparative analysis of repertoire expression in mature primary splenic B cells, bone marrow B cells, and most importantly, immunoglobulin negative (Ig⁻) B-cell precursors within the bone marrow of adult mice. We anticipate that the analysis of the latter population should provide an assessment of the B-cell repertoire reflective of purely differentiating events, in the absence of specific environmental effects, as well as a starting point for understanding the consequences of positive and negative selection on the ultimate expression of the mature B-cell repertoire.

B-CELL DEVELOPMENT

A considerable amount of current research is attempting to correlate information concerning defined molecular events in immunoglobulin (Ig) expression to stages of B-cell development. As it is now currently perceived (FIGURE 1), a self-replenishing population of stem cells gives rise to cells that upon productive rearrangement of heavy chain variable region genes express cytoplasmic μ heavy chains and are identifiable as "pre-B cells".[1-3] Subsequent to cytoplasmic μ expression, it appears that light chain genes rearrange, and ultimately immunoglobulins are expressed on the cell surface. Although, in *in vitro* cultures, cells at essentially every stage in this developmental process, including pre-B cells and Ig-bearing cells, can proliferate extensively,[4-6] it appears that, *in situ,* little if any cellular division occurs after cytoplasmic μ expression.[7,8]

For purposes of our approach to B-cell repertoire expression, we have arbitrarily defined three functionally identifiable developmental stages of the B-cell lineage (FIGURE 1). The first is the so-called prereceptor B cell that includes all cells that at the

[a]This work was supported by National Institutes of Health Grants AG 01514 and CA 25803. Dr. Zharhary is a recipient of a Chaim Weizmann Postdoctoral Fellowship from the Weizmann Institute of Science.

130

time of isolation are Ig⁻, but that can acquire their Ig receptors and respond to antigen in the culture media within the time frame (4 days) of our fragment culture system. The second are the least mature population of receptor bearing B cells. They represent cells in the stage of development delineated on one end by the first expression of Ig receptors and, on the other end, by loss of tolerance susceptibility.[9] These immature B cells that are susceptible to tolerance induction, possibly represent a stage spanning only a few hours. The third population of cells relevant to these studies include all mature B cells that are beyond the point of being made tolerant both in the bone marrow and in the spleen. The rationale of our approach is that precursor cells, prior to their acquisition of Ig receptors, have not yet interfaced with the environment, insofar as their specific interaction with antigen or anti-idiotypic regulatory mechanisms. These cells should therefore represent the genetically derived repertoire in the absence of environmental selective processes. These cells can be isolated in limiting dilution fragment cultures and can be stimulated uniquely in such cultures by virtue of the

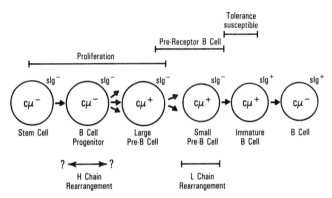

FIGURE 1. Hypothetical lineage relationships of B-cell precursors including presumptive developmental stages associated with rearrangements of immunoglobulin genes, *in situ* proliferation, and tolerance susceptibility. (abstracted from references 3 and 7).

presence of sufficient T-cell help that apparently circumvents the normal tolerance susceptibility of B cells just beginning to express their Ig receptors.[9-12]

PRERECEPTOR B CELLS

Prereceptor B cells are isolated from the bone marrow of mature mice by first rosetting Ig-bearing cells with anti-Ig-coated sheep erythrocytes and subsequently separating Ig⁺ from Ig⁻ cells using a Ficoll gradient.[14,15] The recovery of Ig⁻ cells from this treatment is 35 to 55% of the total bone marrow cell preparation, and the procedure uniformly eliminates over 90% of Ig⁺ cells from the bone marrow preparation. Less than 2% of the remaining cells show any evidence of surface Ig by fluorescence-activated cells-sorter analysis.[15] Prereceptor B cells isolated in this fashion yield characteristic responses in the splenic fragment culture system. Such cells apparently include 20 to 30% of all bone marrow cells responsive to antigenic stimulation in the fragment culture system. The majority of these cells can be made tolerant if treated with tolerogen during the first day of culture,[10] whereas the remaining bone marrow B cells (presumably Ig^+ B cells) are tolerance resistant in the fragment culture system. The clonal progeny of prereceptor B cells invariably give rise to clones of antibody-producing cells yielding only IgM and/or IgA antibodies, and not IgG antibodies, a phenotype typical of immature B cells in general.[15-17]

THE RESPONSES TO 2,4-DINITROPHENOL (DNP)

The first antigen used to analyze the prereceptor B-cell repertoire was the hapten DNP coupled to the carrier limulus polyphemus hemocyanin that had been used to prime the irradiated recipients. The overall frequency of B cells responsive to the DNP determinant per 10^6 injected spleen, bone marrow, and Ig^- bone marrow cells is 2–3, 0.8–1.5, and 0.2–0.5 respectively. In the absence of appropriate markers, it has not yet been possible to firmly establish the proportion of cells in the Ig^- bone marrow population that are at a stage of the B-cell lineage appropriate for their stimulation in the fragment culture system. Thus, it has not been possible to establish how efficiently cells from this population are stimulated in the fragment culture system on a per "prereceptor B cell" basis. Therefore, the frequency of responses to the DNP determinant has been used to normalize responses to other antigenic determinants. Because the ratio of responsive cells from the spleen versus those of the prereceptor B-cell pool is approximately 7:1, we have used this ratio for normalizing other responses. It is understood that this number is arbitrary, because there is no assurance that responses to DNP are typical; however, this assumption has been quite useful for comparative purposes when responses to various antigens have been examined.

The frequency of B cells responsive to DNP in the prereceptor B-cell pool has been found to be relatively consistent in BALB/c mice from the age of two months to over two years.[15] Importantly, the frequency of prereceptor B cells responsive to DNP is unaltered in mice that have been made profoundly tolerant by long-term treatment with DNP coupled to the copolymer of D-glutamic acid and D-lysine (DNP-DGL).[18] Thus, animals depleted of over 80% of their DNP responsive mature splenic and Ig^+ bone marrow B cells reveal no depletion of their prereceptor B cells. This finding serves as strong evidence that prereceptor B cells, as anticipated, represent cells isolated during a stage of B-cell development prior to interaction with environmental antigens.

THE RESPONSES TO INFLUENZA HEMAGGLUTININ (HA)

By far the most useful antigen for delineating repertoire diversity has been the HA molecule of the influenza virus. The existence of a large array of variants of this molecule has permitted extensive fine specificity analyses of monoclonal antibodies on the basis of their characteristic reactivity pattern (RP) of binding to determinants differentially expressed among these HA variants.[19-21] This approach has enabled an extrapolation of over 10^3 recognition phenotypes within the repertoire of mature BALB/c mice for the HA of the PR8 influenza virus.[21-23] Because 1 in 10^5 cells can respond to PR8 HA,[21] the total BALB/c specificity repertoire can be extrapolated to over 10^8 specificities. Importantly, neonatal BALB/c mice of one and two weeks of age, as well as neonates of allotypically distinct murine strains, display reproducibly characteristic and distinctly restricted repertoires of anti-HA antibodies.[24,25] This latter finding has confirmed the concept that repertoire is gradually and reproducibly acquired within a murine strain[16] and has permitted comparative genetic analyses of repertoire acquisition.[25]

Preliminary analyses of the anti-PR8-HA repertoire of BALB/c prereceptor bone marrow B cells has led to several interesting conclusions. First, the frequency of HA-responsive B cells in the prereceptor B-cell pool is approximately one seventh that of the spleen, and is thus consistent with frequencies previously obtained for dinitrophenol.[26] Second, PR8 responsive B cells in the prereceptor pool display considerable diversity, far more diversity than the one- or two-week neonatal repertoire,[24] and a degree of diversity that may ultimately prove to be comparable to that of the repertoire of mature B cells. This finding indicates that a considerable amount of repertoire diversification antedates receptor acquisition and environmental selection. Additionally, it indicates that the repertoire expressed by developing B cells in the bone marrow of mature individuals does not recapitulate expression during early stages of ontogeny and neonatal development. Indeed, the overlap of specificities observed in both the neonatal repertoire and the prereceptor B-cell repertoire represent no more than that anticipated from random repertoire overlap. Finally, as seen in TABLE 1, an investigation of prereceptor B cells derived from individual adult mice reveals an extraordinary degree of repeats of clonotypes expressed within a given individual. This "jackpotting" of clonotypes within an individual, which rarely repeats among individuals, is best explained by the postulate that prereceptor B cells exist within the bone marrow of an

TABLE 1. PR8-HA Specific Responses of Bone Marrow Ig⁻ Cells from Individual Donors[a]

Donor	No. of Clones	Number of RPs	Number of clones of each RP
A	3	3	1,1,1
B	5	2	2,3
C	4	2	3,1
D	5	2	4,1

[a]Donors represent only 4 out of 12 analyzed and include only those yielding more than one anti-PR8-HA specific monoclonal antibody that could discriminate among the tested variant hemagglutinins.

individual as expanded clones. Because approximately 1% of an individual's prereceptor B cells would have been recovered in the isolated Ig⁻ cell population, would have succeeded in homing to the spleen, and would have yielded a clone producing sufficient antibody for extensive examination, it is likely that many clones present within an individual at the prereceptor B-cell level are present as 100 to 800 sister cells. This finding leads to several important conclusions. First, in spite of an enormous potential diversity of the anti-HA repertoire, prereceptor B cells appear already committed to a given specificity. Second, as mentioned above, because the majority of division potential in the B cell lineage antedates light chain rearrangement, it is possible that clonal expansion and specificity commitment may also antedate light chain rearrangement (see FIGURE 1 and DISCUSSION).

THE RESPONSE TO PHOSPHORYLCHOLINE (PC)

The best defined of all immune responses at the clonotype and molecular level is that of BALB/c mice to phosphorylcholine. This response is dominated by a single clonotype identical to the TEPC-15 (T-15) myeloma protein, and somatically derived variants of its germ line encoded light and heavy chain genes.[27-31] The dominant expression of T-15 in this response makes it an excellent candidate for studying the contribution of postreceptor regulatory processes, such as network regulation, on the ultimate expression of the B-cell repertoire. An extensive analysis of the prereceptor bone marrow cells responsive to PC in mature BALB/c mice indicates that the overall frequency of PC responsive cells is in approximately the same proportion as prereceptor B-cells responsive to DNP and PR8-HA. Most striking, is the finding that the proportion and absolute frequency of B cells of the T-15 clonotype is the same in the prereceptor B-cell population as it is in the mature spleen. Thus, B cells whose clonal antibody product is indistinguishable from T-15 by analysis with both rabbit anti-T-15 idiotype[29] and the anti-T-15 hybridoma AB 1-2,[32] represent 60 to 80% of all PC-responsive cells, even at the prereceptor B-cell level. Thus, the high frequency of expression of T-15 (1/50,000 B cells) appears to reflect a high frequency of the expression of this clonotype at the level of generation of precursor cells and does not appear to be the result of postreceptor modulation by positive regulatory mechanisms. Additionally, the frequency of PC reactive B cells that are not of the T-15 idiotype is similar in the prereceptor and mature B-cell pools.

The ability to analyze PC-responsive B cells in the Ig^- bone marrow pool of BALB/c mice has also provided considerable insight into the immunologic deficit of (CBA/N × BALB/c) F1 male mice. These mice have been found to exhibit several X chromosome-linked defects in their immune response mechanisms.[33–37] Among these defects is an absence of the Lyb-5+ B-cell subset, and poor or absent responsiveness to certain antigenic determinants. Thus, (CBA/N × BALB/c) F1 male mice do not respond to PC *per se* and only respond to PC conjugates with immunogenic carriers after prolonged immunization, ultimately making antibodies that recognize *p*-diazophenylphosphorylcholine rather than phosphorylcholine.[37] In order to explain this lack of recognition of PC, investigators have suggested that such mice exhibit a defect in antibody diversification.[37] Alternatively, it has been suggested that such mice lack an entire subset of B cells characterized by the presence of the Lyb-5 surface antigen, and compensate with Lyb-5− cells that are known to remain tolerance susceptible even after being made peripheral.[36] An analysis of $1.5 × 10^8$ spleen cells from (CBA/N × BALB/c) F1 male adults yielded only one responsive precursor cell. The antibody product of this cell did not bear the T-15 idiotype, and its binding was not readily inhibited with phosphorylcholine. An analysis of $3 × 10^8$ Ig^- bone marrow cells, however, displayed a frequency of PC responsive B cells similar to that of normal BALB/c mice. Importantly, the binding of the monoclonal antibody product of most of these cells was PC inhibitable, and some of these antibodies bore the T-15 idiotype. Thus, the prereceptor B-cell pool of (CBA/N × BALB/c) F1 male immunologically defective mice was completely normal with respect to PC responsiveness. This finding is most consistent with tolerance induction within the highly susceptible Lyb-5− cell population due to interaction with environmental PC subsequent to receptor acquisition *in vivo* and argues convincingly against an inherent deficit in repertoire generation in these immunologically defective mice. If the elimination of PC-responsive cells in male defective mice is indeed the result of tolerance due to naturally present antigen, this finding would serve as crucial evidence that tolerance plays an important role in repertoire establishment.

THE RESPONSES TO 4-HYDROXY-3-NITROPHENYLACETYL (NP)

Given the above findings for DNP, PR8-HA, and PC that under normal circumstances clonotype representation in the periphery closely reflects that of the generative pool, it seemed important to extend these studies to another antigen system in which clonal dominance and possibly idiotype regulation may play an important role in repertoire expression. As discussed in detail elsewhere in this volume, mice of the Igh^b allotype display a characteristic repsonse to the NP haptenic determinant wherein a majority of antibodies bear the λ light chain, and demonstrate a characteristically higher affinity for analogues of nitrophenylacetyl.[38-40] At the B-cell repertoire level, it has been shown that, whereas such λ heteroclite specificities represent the majority of mature B cells responsive to NP, B cells are also present that bear the κ light chain. Some of these B cells are heteroclite. Additionally, a small proportion of B cells express the κ light chain on homoclite antibodies, and an even smaller population express λ-bearing antibodies of homoclite specificity.[39] Responses of Ig$^-$ bone marrow cells of CB 20 mice to NP are approximately one seventh the frequency of responses of splenic cells and, therefore, consistent with the relative frequency of responses to all of the above studied antigenic determinants. The prereceptor repertoire for NP in CB 20 mice, however, differs in several important features from the repertoire as expressed in mature B cells. First, κ homoclite clones represent almost half of all responses, and the frequency of such clones is markedly reduced in both the mature bone marrow pool and the splenic B-cell pool. This preliminary finding may imply that a likely explanation for the dominance of heteroclite specificities in mice of the Igh^b haplotype is the elimination of a large proportion of homoclite NP specific B cells during their maturation in the bone marrow. Such a finding would be consistent with mechanisms such as tolerance or idiotype suppression playing an important role in the ultimate expression of the NP specific repertoire by prohibiting the expression in the mature B-cell repertoire of the majority of clonotypes that could have given a homoclite anti-NP response. Second, B cells capable of expressing λ-bearing heteroclite antibodies are relatively lower in frequency in the prereceptor B-cell pool than in the more mature B-cell populations. An analysis of the fine specificity of the λ-heteroclite clonotypes derived from prereceptor B cells reveals that whereas certain reactivity patterns for NP and its analogues are found in similar frequencies in B cells in the prereceptor pool as in the mature B-cell pools, the reactivity pattern most frequently observed in splenic B cells is poorly represented in the prereceptor pool. Among the many potential explanations for this finding is the possibility that clones expressing certain clonotypes are selectively expanded during postreceptor development.

DISCUSSION

The findings in this report represent an overview of our initial assessment of the prereceptor B-cell population present in the bone marrow of mature mice. The anticipation for these studies was that a comprehensive understanding of this cell subpopulation would be pivotal to our understanding of the relative contributions of genetic and differentiative events versus environmental selective events in repertoire establishment. The findings to date have upheld this anticipation and have already provided substantial insights into several previously poorly understood phenomena.

The findings that Ig$^-$ bone marrow cells were incapable of giving rise to IgG production and generally represented the subpopulation of bone marrow precursor cells that are susceptible to tolerance induction are indicative of the immature status of the population of cells used in these studies. Several of the characteristics of the repertoire of Ig$^-$ bone marrow cells serve as confirmation of the concept that cells isolated at the prereceptor stage of development are both representative of the generative B-cell pool and a population that has not yet interacted with environmental antigens. This population of precursor cells remains intact, not only to DNP in overtly DNP-DGL tolerized mice, but also to PC, an environmental antigen, in (CBA/N × BALB/c) F1 male defective mice whose only B cells are of the Lyb-5⁻ subset that may be relatively susceptible to tolerance induction. Additionally, the enormous disparity in κ homoclite and λ heteroclite NP-responsive precursor cells in the prereceptor B-cell pool versus the mature B-cell pools in CB 20 mice is further evidence of the uniqueness of the prereceptor B-cell pool.

The response to PR8-HA indicates that the prereceptor B-cell pool is already highly diversified. These studies also indicate that precursor cell clones within the prereceptor B-cell population are already expanded from 100 to 800 cells within the bone marrow of an individual. Such "jackpotting" of B cells of the same specificity is much less frequently found in analyses of the primary B-cell repertoire of adults, because that population represents an accumulation of clones and is generally far more diverse within a given individual at a given time. The finding that individual precursor-cell clones are expanded within the prereceptor B-cell pool has important implications for considerations of repertoire diversification. First, this finding confirms the commitment of cells to a unique specificity prior to surface Ig expression. Furthermore, light chain gene rearrangement is generally assumed to occur in cells with little division potential *in situ*. Because many members of a clone express the same specificity, and thus presumably the same light chain, it is possible that commitment to a given light chain, or light chain subset, precedes light chain gene rearrangement.

Previous findings from this laboratory have indicated that certain reactivities to murine cytochrome determinants may exist in higher frequency in the prereceptor bone marrow pool than in the mature B-cell pool.[41] Such findings suggest that tolerance induction may play an important role in repertoire establishment. Two of the above findings would be consistent with this interpretation. First, the considerable diminution of the κ homoclite NP specific clones in the CB 20 repertoire as cells progress from prereceptor to mature B cells could be the result of tolerance induction in this highly diversified, but similarly behaving B-cell population. If so, this finding could account for the relatively high level of heteroclite responses found in Igh^b murine strains upon NP immunization. Second, the finding of PC-reactive B cells in the prereceptor B-cell pool of (CBA/N × BALB/c) F1 male mice, but not in their mature B-cell pool, is also potentially the result of tolerance induced by environmental phosphorylcholine.

Because this volume concerns itself with the role of network in immune responses, it is appropriate to conclude with the findings now available concerning the prereceptor B-cell pool and the role that idiotypic recognition may play in repertoire establishment. It should be noted that our experimental approach does not address the role of network regulation, or postantigenic or idiotypic immunization, but rather addresses the question of whether network regulation plays an important role in primary B-cell repertoire expression *per se*. Some of the above findings could be interpreted as implying a relatively minimal role for idiotypic recognition in the expression of the mature B-cell repertoire. Given the diversity of the prereceptor B-cell pool, it is unnecessary to propose a fundamental role for idiotypic recognition in the generation of B-cell repertoire diversity. Additionally, certain unusually high frequency clonotypes, whose dominant expression might have been accounted for by idiotype specific expansion, such as the T-15 idiotype in BALB/c mice and certain λ heteroclite specificities in the NP repertoire of CB 20 mice, are already present in relatively high frequency in the prereceptor B-cell pool. Thus, idiotype specific clonal expansion would not be necessary to account for the high frequency of these clonotypes in the mature peripheral B-cell population. Certain findings, however, could be indicative of a role for idiotype recognition in either the elimination or expansion of specific clones as they emerge into the mature B-cell pool. First, we have found that the frequency of DNP-responsive B cells in aged mice is considerably lower in the splenic B-cell pool than in the bone marrow B-cell subpopulations.[15] This finding could be accounted for by inactivation of B cells by the gradually accumulated antibody specific immunoregulation that has been identified in aged individuals.[42] Second, it is possible that the diminution in both the κ homoclite NP-responsive B cells of CB 20 mice and PC-responsive B cells in (CBA/N × BALB/c) F1 male defective mice could be, in part, due to anti-idiotypic down regulation as opposed to tolerance induction. Finally, the increase in the frequency of representation of some λ heteroclite specificities, particularly the most dominant of these specificities in the NP-responsive splenic B cells of CB 20 mice, might best be explained by idiotype-specific clonal expansion. It is clear that future investigations of the prereceptor B-cell pool should help to clarify the role of both tolerance and network regulation in the expression of the mature B-cell repertoire.

REFERENCES

1. EARLY, P., H. HUANG, M. DAVIS, K. CALAME & L. HOOD. 1980. Cell **19:** 981–992.
2. ALT, F., N. ROSENBERG, S. LEWIS, E. THOMAS & D. BALTIMORE. 1981. Cell **27:** 381–390.
3. KEARNEY, J. F. 1981. *In* B Lymphocytes in the Immune Response: Functional, Developmental, and Interactive Properties. N. R. Klinman, D. E. Mosier, I. Scher and E. S. Vitetta, Eds.: 27–32. Elsevier/North Holland. New York.
4. WHITLOCK, C. A. & O. N. WITTE. 1981. J. Virol. **40:** 577–584.
5. SCOTT, D. W., P. S. PILLAI & S. J. ANDERSON. 1981. *In* B Lymphocytes in the Immune Response: Functional, Developmental, and Interactive Properties. N. R. Klinman, D. E. Mosier, I. Scher and E. S. Vitetta, Eds.: 127–132. Elsevier/North Holland. New York.
6. HOWARD, M., D. W. SCOTT, B. JOHNSON & W. E. PAUL. 1981. *In* B Lymphocytes in the Immune Response: Functional, Developmental, and Interactive Properties. N. R. Klinman, D. E. Mosier, I. Scher and E. S. Vitetta, Eds.: 141–148. Elsevier/North Holland. New York.
7. LANDRETH, K. S., C. ROSSE & J. CLAGETT. 1981. J. Exp. Med. **127:** 2027–2034.
8. OSMOND, D. G., N. SAVERIANO, M. DRINNAN, V. SANTER & M. D. RAHAL. 1981. *In* B Lymphocytes in the Immune Response: Functional, Developmental, and Interactive Properties. N. R. Klinman, D. E. Mosier, I. Scher and E. S. Vitetta, Eds.: 103–110. Elsevier/North Holland. New York.
9. METCALF, E. S. & N. R. KLINMAN. 1976. J. Exp. Med. **143:** 1327–1340.
10. METCALF, E. S. & N. R. KLINMAN. 1977. J. Immunol. **118:** 2111–2116.
11. TEALE, J. M., J. E. LAYTON & G. J. V. NOSSAL. 1979. J. Exp. Med. **150:** 205–217.
12. NOSSAL, G. J. V. & B. L. PIKE. 1975. J. Exp. Med. **141:** 904–917.
13. TEALE, J. M. & N. R. KLINMAN. 1980. Nature (London) **288:** 385–387.
14. WALKER, S. M., G. C. MEINKE & W. O. WEIGLE. 1979. Cell Immunol. **46:** 158–169.
15. ZHARHARY, D. & N. R. KLINMAN. 1983. J. Exp Med. **157:** 1300–1308.
16. KLINMAN, N. R. & J. L. PRESS. 1975. J. Exp. Med. **141:** 1133–1146.
17. TEALE, J. M., D. LAFRENZ, N. KLINMAN & S. STROBER. 1981. J. Immunol. **126:** 1952–1957.
18. KLINMAN, N. R., A. F. SCHRATER & D. H. KATZ. 1981. J. Immunol. **126:** 1970–1973.
19. GERHARD, W., T. J. BRACIALE & N. R. KLINMAN. 1975. Eur. J. Immunol. **5:** 720–725.
20. GERHARD, W. 1977. Top. Infect. Dis. **3:** 15.
21. CANCRO, M. P., W. GERHARD & N. R. KLINMAN. 1978. J. Exp. Med. **147:** 776–787.
22. GERHARD, W., J. YEWDELL, M. D. FRANKEL, A. D. LOPES & L. STAUDT. 1980. *In* Monoclonal Antibodies. R. Kennett, T. McKearn and K. Bechtol, Eds.: 317–333. Plenum Publishing. New York.
23. FAZEKAS DE ST. GROTH, S. 1981. *In* The Immune System. A Festschrift in Honor of Niels Kaj Jerne on the Occasion of his 70th Birthday. C. M. Steinberg and I. Lefkovits, Eds.: **1:** 155–168. Karger. Basel.

24. CANCRO, M. P., D. E. WYLIE, W. GERHARD & N. R. KLINMAN 1979. Proc. Nat. Acad. Sci. USA **76**: 6577–6581.
25. CANCRO, M. P. & N. R. KLINMAN, 1981. J. Immunol. **126**: 1160–1164.
26. WYLIE, D. E. & N. R. KLINMAN. 1981. *In* B Lymphocytes in the Immune Response: Functional, Developmental, and Interactive Properties. N. R. Klinman, D. E. Mosier, I. Scher and E. S. Vitetta, Eds.: 63–68. Elsevier/North Holland. New York.
27. POTTER, M. & R. LEIBERMAN. 1970. J. Exp. Med. **132**: 737–751.
28. KLUSKENS, L. & H. KOHLER. 1974. Proc. Natl. Acad. Sci. USA **71**: 5083–5087.
29. GEARHART, P. J., N. H. SIGAL & N. R. KLINMAN. 1977. J. Exp. Med. **145**: 876–891.
30. GEARHART, P. J., N. D. JOHNSON, R. DOUGLAS & L. HOOD. 1981. Nature (London) **291**: 29–34.
31. CREWS, S., J. GRIFFIN, H. HUANG, K. CALAME & L. HOOD. 1981. Cell **25**: 59–60.
32. KEARNEY, J. F., R. BARIETTA, S. A. QUARE & J. QUINTANS. 1981. Eur. J. Immunol. **11**: 877–883.
33. SCHER, I. 1982. Adv. Immunol. **33**: 2–71.
34. MOND, J. J., R. LIEBERMAN, J. K. INMAN, D. E. MOSIER & W. E. PAUL. 1977. J. Exp. Med. **146**: 1138–1142.
35. QUINTANS, J. J., P. MCKEARN & D. KAPLAN. 1979. J. Immunol. **122**: 1750–1756.
36. METCALF, E. S., I. SCHER & N. R. KLINMAN. 1980. J. Exp. Med. **151**: 486–491.
37. KENNY, J. J. & G. GUELDE. 1981. *In* B Lymphocytes in the Immune Response: Functional, Developmental and Interactive Properties. N. R. Klinman, D. E. Mosier, I. Scher and E. S. Vitetta, Eds.: 77–83. Elsevier/North Holland. New York.
38. IMANISHI-KARI, T., M. RETH, G. J. HAMMERLING & K. RAJEWSKY. 1978. Curr. Top. Microbiol. Immunol. **81**: 20–28.
39. STASHENKO, P. & N. R. KLINMAN. 1980. J. Immunol. **125**: 531–537.
40. KARJALAINEN, K., B. BANG & O. MAKELA. 1980. J. Immunol. **125**: 313–317.
41. JEMMERSON, R. W., P. MORROW & N. R. KLINMAN. 1982. Fed. Proc. Fed. Am. Soc. Exp. Biol. **41**: 420 No. 882.
42. KLINMAN, N. R. 1981. J. Exp. Med. **154**: 547–551.

DISCUSSION OF THE PAPER

W. E. PAUL (*National Institutes of Health, Bethesda, Md.*): I was very fascinated by your point concerning the very large number of dull cells, if you like, that shared the same idiotype in the prereceptor population. This finding would imply, therefore, that the population of prereceptor cells that are derived from an individual progenitor that have not yet expressed light chains was very large. You suggested perhaps as much as 800, which is a very nice point. As I understand it, on the other hand, the finding of people who look at pre-B cells is that most of them do not have the light chains, that is, that they are regarded as μ C, light chain negative. So to put the two together, one would have to postulate that the waste of bad rearrangements must be stupendous. This view, of course, is consistent with how many researchers view of the establishment of allelic exclusion.

N. R. KLINMAN: There are several ways of looking at this problem. One is that there is enormous waste. Another is that there is a limited number of clones. The clones might be much larger at the heavy chain rearranged level than even a thousand. Therefore any of ten light chain rearrangements might be adequate to give you specificity. The most interesting prediction would be that there is no waste at all, but rather that the cell knows precisely what light chain it will express after rearrangement, prior to rearrangement. The prediction would be that the determination of the specificity is set at heavy chain rearrangement or even before heavy chain rearrangement and that the rearrangement event is a *fait accompli* once the clone has expressed itself and is committed. We would also predict that the look of randomness of chain rearrangements is a reflection simply of our ignorance of the events that have taken place.

C. A. BONA (*Mt. Sinai School of Medicine, New York*): You showed in the anti-flu repertoire a number of clonotypes in neonates that were not represented in the pre-B cells. How do you account for this situation? Is this tolerance or only a limited search?

KLINMAN: Actually it is a strange phenomenon. Even in the extensive analysis of the adult B-cell pool, there are still a couple of neonatal clonotypes that have not been seen. I think the best explanation is an incomplete search. I think a second explanation for the mature pool would be that once you express a clone, you are more likely to idiotypically inhibit the expression of that clone later. That does not, of course, explain why we have not seen them yet in the prereceptor pool. We really have looked at a very small sampling, but it could be a very interesting finding.

Detailed Analysis of the Public Idiotype of Anti-Hen Egg-White Lysozyme Antibodies[a]

ALEXANDER MILLER, LEAN-KUAN CH'NG,[b]
CHRISTOPHER BENJAMIN, AND ELI SERCARZ

Department of Microbiology
University of California
Los Angeles, California 90024

PETER BRODEUR[c] AND ROY RIBLET

Institute for Cancer Research
Philadelphia, Pennsylvania 19111

INTRODUCTION

For several years we have studied the idiotypy of the immune response to hen egg-white lysozyme (HEL). We have shown that almost all anti-HEL antibodies, late in the primary response and after secondary immunization, are characterized by the presence of a predominant idiotype, IdXL. This idiotype dominates the anti-HEL response in all animals so far tested: many strains of inbred mice, outbred mice, rats, deermice, and rabbits.[1] IdXL, however, is largely absent on early primary anti-HEL and on monoclonal anti-HEL generated by the hybridoma technique from B cells of mice given a primary immunization nine days previously.[2] IdXL is also absent on antibody raised against human lysozyme (HUL) except for those rare molecules showing cross-reactivity with hen egg-white lysozyme.[1]

On the other hand, monoclonal anti-HEL antibodies produced by hybridomas generated from B cells of mice given a secondary immunization 3 to 5 days previously, universally show the presence of IdXL.[2] These "late" monoclonal antibodies have allowed us to begin an examination of the relation of epitypic specificity and the presence of IdXL. We were able to show that two monoclonal anti-HEL of clearly different specificity (for different regions of HEL) were each reactive with anti-IdXL rabbit sera. Strikingly, each of these antibodies when immobilized on a column was able to completely absorb all anti-IdXL from rabbit sera.[3]

In this report, we more extensively examine the range of epitope specificity of a collection of IdXL positive secondary monoclonal anti-hen egg-white lysozyme. Also examined are the heavy chain variable region gene rearrangements present in hybridomas producing these antibodies.

[a]This work was supported in part by Grant IM-263 from the American Cancer Society and Grants CA-24442, AI-11183, CA-06927, and AI-13797 from the U.S. Public Health Services.
[b]Supported by Tumor Immunology Training Grant CA-09120.
[c]Fellow of the Cancer Research Institute, Inc.

RESULTS
Heterogeneity of Monoclonal Anti-Hen Egg-White Lysozyme Antibodies Bearing IdXL

In a published study of secondary IdXL-positive anti-HEL, it was found that the presence of IdXL was totally independent of the isoelectric point of antibodies as determined by isoelectric focusing (IEF).[1]

In a more recent study,[4] we have examined the IEF patterns of our library of 27 secondary and 17 primary monoclonal anti-hen egg-white lysozymes. Each antibody appears to give a unique IEF pattern. In addition, these antibodies were tested for cross-reactivity with a panel of eight gallinaceous egg-white lysozymes, duck egg-white lysozyme, and human lysozyme. On a qualitative basis, that is, failure to react with a given lysozyme, the antibodies could be placed in 18 distinct groups. Furthermore, on the basis of either restricted or heteroclite reactivity with different lysozymes, many individual members of a group could be distinguished. In a limited number of cases, where differential reactivity was found with closely related lysozymes or with peptide fragments of HEL, some definition of epitypic specificity could be made. In general, these studies supported our previous conclusion based on the properties of secondary anti-HEL, that IdXL-positive anti-HEL antibodies have broad diversity. The recent studies of Gearhart, *et al.*, however, summarized in this volume,[5] raised the possibility that at least part of the diversity we observed might have resulted from a rapid somatic mutation process that would lead to fine specificity differences (and, probably, differences in IEF pattern). We, therefore, turned to an alternative method of analysis that could more clearly establish differences in epitypic specificity.

Noncompetitiveness of Different IdXL-Positive Monoclonal Anti-Hen Egg-White Lysozyme

As has been shown for several groups of monoclonal antibodies of different general specificities,[6,7,8] it is possible to test for nonoverlap of epitypic sites recognized by demonstrating simultaneous binding of two monoclonal antibodies. In the assay we employ, wells of a microtiter plate are coated with affinity-purified antibody. Then, ^{125}I-HEL alone or ^{125}I-HEL preincubated with a 100-fold excess of a second antibody is added and the amount of ^{125}I-HEL bound determined.

Some typical results are shown in TABLE 1. Preincubation of HEL with antibody homologous to the antibody bound on the plates completely blocks binding of HEL to that immobilized antibody. Antibodies 6D7 and 2D10, however, do not block the binding of HEL to immobilized 5E4 or 2F4. Reciprocally, binding of HEL to immobilized 6D7 or 2D10 is little affected by the presence of soluble 5E4 or 2F4. 5E4 and 2F4, however, are mutually inhibitory, as are 6D7 and 2D10, thus forming two nonoverlapping sets. The latter set (6D7, 2D10) is subdivided by 2D1, which prevents binding of HEL to 6D7, but not to 2D10. These results are illustrated in a Venn diagram (FIGURE 1).

A complication of the methodology is indicated by the fact that soluble 6D7 fails to inhibit binding of HEL to 2D1. We attribute this nonreciprocal binding to a relatively low affinity of the soluble antibody for HEL and/or a relatively high affinity of the immobilized antibody, that is, sufficient dissociation of HEL-antibody complexes occurs, even at high antibody excess for binding by an avid immobilized antibody of transiently free hen egg-white lysozyme. Such nonreciprocal binding has, indeed, been

TABLE 1. Noncompetitiveness of Different IdX-L$^+$ Monoclonal Anti-Hen Egg-White Lysozyme

Competing Antibody	Antibody on Plate				
	5E4	2F4	6D7	2D10	2D1
—	65^a	96	51	100	91
5E4	6	7	39	39	48
2F4	6	10	46	52	58
6D7	54	66	3	2	58
2D10	54	65	4	2	61
2D1	56	60	17	47	3

^{a}Percent of added HEL bound (19,500 cpm added)

observed with many of the monoclonal antibodies that are of low affinity. Nevertheless, using the criterion of clear-cut inhibition in at least one direction, we have been able to construct a pattern of cross-reactivity for a larger group of monoclonal antibodies (data will be published separately). These results are summarized in the Venn diagram shown in FIGURE 2. Most monoclonal antibodies can be distinguished in their overlap pattern. Two monoclonal antibodies 1G11 and Hy5, however, (indicated by bold circles) are particularly interesting. Hy5 is a monoclonal anti-HEL isolated and studied in detail by Smith-Gill et al.[9] They have shown that arg-68 is part of the epitope on HEL recognized by this antibody. This antibody overlaps all the other monoclonals tested except for 2F4 and 5E4. We have shown that these two antibodies, of those shown in FIGURE 2, have a reactivity particularly sensitive to removal of the three N-terminal amino acids of hen egg-white lysozyme. The guanidino-carbon of arg-68 and the ε-carbon of Lys-1 are approximately 25Å distant in crystalline hen egg-white lysozyme.[10] Note that one monoclonal antibody, 1G11, overlaps all the other monoclonal antibodies tested, thereby confining the epitopes seen by the monoclonal

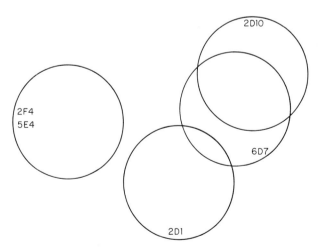

FIGURE 1. A Venn diagram showing competitive binding of HEL by monoclonal anti-HEL antibodies. Based on the data in TABLE 1, competitive binding is represented by overlapping circles. Nonoverlap indicates noncompetitive binding of hen egg-white lysozyme.

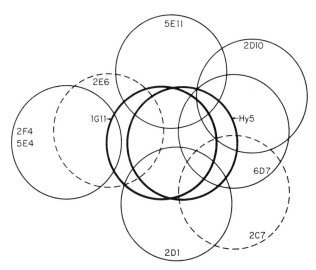

FIGURE 2. A Venn diagram showing competitive binding of HEL by a large group of monoclonal antibodies. The convention used is as in FIGURE 1. The bold circles represent antibodies showing extensive competition with other antibodies. The dashed circles indicate IdXL-negative monoclonal antibodies.

antibodies to a single face of hen egg-white lysozyme. The two antibodies illustrated by dashed lines are "early," primary, and IdXL negative.

Comparison of Serum and Monoclonal Anti-Hen Egg-White Lysozyme

There is some indication that the collection of hybridoma monoclonal antibodies may approximate the secondary serum anti-HEL in overall specificity. First, serum

TABLE 2. Heterogeneous Serum Antibody Versus Monoclonal Anti-Hen Egg-White Lysozyme

| | Antibody on Plate | |
Competing Antibody	A/J	B10.A
—	82[a]	85
A/J	3	1
B10.A	5	2
1G11	19	12
5E4	47	44
2F4	73	64
2D10	64	53
6D7	68	56
2D1	68	56
5E11	68	66
2E6	68	62
2C7	83	71

[a]Percent of added HEL bound (12,100 cpm added)

antibody blocks binding of HEL to any of the immobilized monoclonal antibodies. Second. when serum antibody is immobilized on plastic, binding of HEL to it is blocked very effectively by 1G11—the monoclonal antibody that totally overlaps all the other test monoclonal antibodies (TABLE 2). Other monoclonal antibodies block to a limited extent, which is certainly in part due to their particular specificities. Also, the observed inhibitions may be falsely low because the affinities of some of the monoclonal antibodies are too low to maintain sufficient HEL in the complexed state.

Genetics of Hybridomas Producing Monoclonal Anti-Hen Egg-White Lysozyme

The apparent heterogeneity of IdXL-positive anti-HEL has prompted us to undertake an examination of the heavy chain variable regions (V_H) coding for the different monoclonal antibodies. Our approach has been to use the Southern blot technique. As probes we have used the cloned DNA fragments, pJ_0 and pJ_{11}.[11] The pJ_0

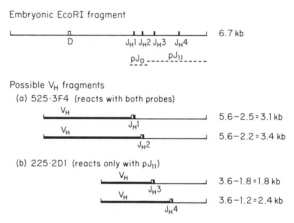

FIGURE 3. Schematic representation of methodology used in analyzing Southern blots of EcoRI fragments hybridized with either a J_H 1-2 probe (pJ_0) or a J_H 3-4 probe (pJ_{11}). See FIGURE 4 for actual blot.

probe overlaps J_H1 and J_H2, whereas the pJ_{11} probe overlaps J_H3 and J_H4 (see FIGURE 3). Embryonic mouse DNA split with the restriction enzyme EcoRI gives a 6.7 Kb fragment that contains the four J_H regions and extends approximately 1 Kb beyond J_H4 at the 3' end (FIGURE 3). After V-D-J_H joining to give a functional gene, the 5' EcoRI site of embryonic DNA is replaced by an EcoRI site related to the rearranged V_H gene. Thus, it is expected that EcoRI cleavage will yield a fragment of length differing from 6.7 Kb. The Southern blot technique[12] was applied to EcoRI-treated DNA from a collection of anti-lysozyme hybridomas with the results illustrated in FIGURE 4. The probe used was pJ_{11}, which overlaps J_H4 and therefore detects all rearranged V-D-J regions. The apparent repeats are almost always from the myeloma used as the hybridizing partner (see legend to FIGURE 4). There is generally more than one band attributable to the hybridized anti-HEL cell. This fact is consistent with the observations of others[13] who have shown that aberrant rearrangements of heavy chain V genes, in addition to the functional rearrangement, are found in the majority of myelomas and

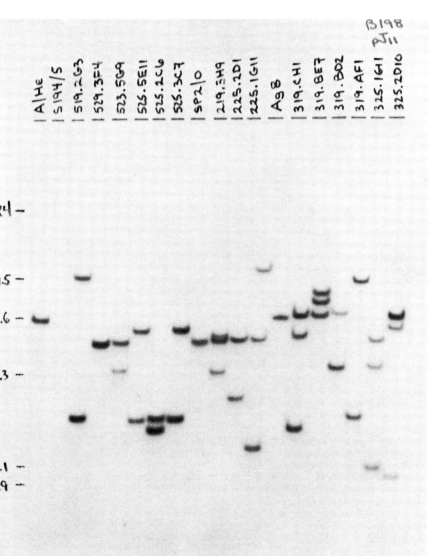

FIGURE 4. A typical Southern blot of EcoRI fragments of the DNA from hybridomas producing anti-HEL hybridized with the pJ₁₁ probe. The numbers on the left indicate the position of molecular weight standards. The first lane (A/He) shows the position of the embryonic DNA fragment. The second lane (S194/5) shows the absence of any J_H-containing fragment in the myeloma cell line S194/5.XXO.BU.1. Hybridomas prepared by fusion with this myeloma contain "5" as the first digit. The lane designated Sp 2/0 shows the EcoRI fragment obtained with the myeloma cell line Sp 2/0-Ag 14. Hybridomas formed by fusion with this myeloma contain "2" as the first digit. The lane designated Ag 8 shows the EcoRI fragment obtained with the myeloma cell line P3X63Ag8. Hybridomas formed by fusion with this myeloma contain "3" as the first digit. Primary IdXL-negative hybridomas are designated by a "1" as the second digit and secondary IdXL-positive hybridomas by a "2" as the second digit.

TABLE 3. Analysis of Southern Blots for Possible V_H Fragments

Secondary, IdXL$^+$ Hybridomas				Primary, IdXL$^-$ Hybridomas			
Hybridoma	Size of Band (Kb)[a]	Reactivity with J_H 1-2 Probe pJ_0	Possible V_H Fragments (Kb)	Hybridoma	Size of Band (Kb)	Reactivity with J_H 1-2 Probe	Possible V_H Fragments (Kb)
525.5E4	1.8		0,0.6	519.2G3	3.1		1.3,1.9
	3.0		1.2,1.8		9.4	+	6.9,7.2
	5.7	+	3.1,3.4	219.3H9	5.9	+	3.4,3.7
	6.1	+	3.6,3.9	319.CH1	2.7	+	0.2,0.5
519.2F4	5.8		4.0,4.6		5.8		4.0,4.6
	6.5	+	4.0,4.3	319.BE7	7.7	+	5.2,5.5
525.6D7	5.1	+	2.6,2.9		8.2		6.4,7.0
	6.3	+	3.8,4.1	319.BD2	4.5		2.7,3.3
529.3F4	5.6	+	3.1,3.4	319.AF1	3.1		1.3,1.9
523.5G9	4.6		2.8,3.4		8.9	+	6.4,6.7
	5.6	+	3.1,3.4				
525.5E11	3.1	+	0.6,0.9				
	6.2	+	3.7,4.0				
525.2C6	2.9		1.1,1.7				
	3.1	+	0.6,0.9				
525.3C7	3.1	+	0.6,0.9				
	6.2	+	3.7,4.0				
225.2D1[b]	3.6		1.8,2.4				
225.1G11	2.6	+	0.1,0.4				
	9.9	+	7.4,7.7				
325.1G11[c]	2.1		0.3,0.9				
	4.7		2.9,3.5				
	5.6	+	3.1,3.4				
325.2D10	2.0		0.2,0.8				
	6.2	+	3.7,4.0				
	6.8	+	4.3,4.6				

[a]Values for 525.5E4, 519.2F4, and 525.6D7 are from another blot.

[b]For hybridomas with the first digit "2," the band at 5.6 Kb is assumed to come from the fusion partner Sp 2/0 and is ignored.

[c]For hybridomas with the first digit "3," the band at 6.8 Kb is assumed to come from the fusion partner Ag8 and is ignored except for the band from 325.2D10 that hybridizes with J_H 1-2 probe unlike the band from Ag8.

TABLE 4. Possible Sets of V_H Coding for IdXL$^+$ Monoclonal Anti-Hen Egg-White Lysozyme

(A) Maximizing Single Set		
0.9 Kb	3.1 Kb	Indeterminant
5E11	3F4	2F4
3C7	6D7	225.1G11
2C6	5G9	2D1
325.1G11		
2D10		
5E4		

(B) Balanced Distribution			
0.3 Kb	1.8 Kb	3.1 Kb	4.0 Kb
325.1G11	2D1	3F4	2F4
2D10	5E4	6D7	5E11
225.1G11	2C6	5G9	3C7

splenic B cells. Because it is not known which band is derived from a functional V_H gene, a complication is introduced in our comparison of different hybridomas.

A simplification, however, is possible. A probe, pJ_0, which hybridizes with J_H2 was used in a second blot (not shown). About half of the bands seen in FIGURE 4 were obtained. Those that did hybridize must have had a V-J joining event at J_H1 or J_H2, whereas those disappearing would have deleted J_H1 and J_H2 during rearrangement. Thus, each band could arise from only two possible V_H as indicated in FIGURE 3. A complete analysis for possible V_H fragments is shown in TABLE 3.

We have attempted to find possible common V_H regions for hybridomas producing IdXL-positive or IdXL-negative anti-hen egg-white lysozyme. There is little indication of a predominant V_H among either set of hybridomas. As shown in TABLE 4(A), the maximum number of hybridomas generating IdXL-positive antibody that can be placed in a single set is five. Of these, 5E11 and 3C7 are probably mutated daughters of the same clone because they uniquely show two common rearrangements. If it is attempted to minimize the total number of sets, then the 12 IdXL-positive hybridomas must be placed in a minimum of four groups using different V_H genes (TABLE 4 (B)).

The hybridomas giving rise to IdXL-negative anti-HEL seem even more heteroge-

TABLE 5. Absence of IdXL on Anti-Lysozyme Antibody Not Cross-Reactive with Hen Egg-White Lysozyme

Immunogen (GEL)[a]	No. of Animals	Percent Inhibition by Anti-IdX[b]		
		^{125}I-Labeled GEL Added	^{125}I-Labeled HEL Added	^{125}I-Labeled GEL (After Removal of Anti-HEL Activity)
JEL	5	67	72	5
REL	5	65	78	5
OEL	3	20	66	9

[a]GEL, JEL, REL, and OEL are gallinaceous, Japanese quail, ringed-neck pheasant, and *Ortalis* egg-white lysozymes, respectively.

[b]Results are expressed as percent inhibition of binding by anti-IdXL under conditions where about 50% of radiolabeled HEL or GEL is bound.

nous. As shown in TABLE 3, DNA from these hybridomas seems unrelated to that from hybridomas producing either IdXL-positive or IdXL-negative antibody.

Specificity Restriction of IdXL-Positive Anti-Hen Egg-White Lysozyme

The data presented above are consistent with the idea that IdXL-positive anti-HEL consists of a highly heterogeneous collection of antibodies. There is indeed, however, one important element of restriction. All our IdXL-positive antibodies react specifically with hen egg-white lysozyme. The first anti-IdXL sera generated in our laboratory were generated against rare HEL-HUL cross-reactive antibodies from an anti-HUL response. This approach would have failed if any appreciable part of the non-HEL-cross-reactive anti-HUL was IdXL-positive, because this non-cross-reactive antibody was used to absorb the generated anti-IdXL.

In TABLE 5, it can be seen that even for more closely related lysozymes such as those from Japanese quail or ringed-neck pheasant egg-white, which are highly cross-reactive with HEL, the non-cross-reactive molecules are all idiotype negative.

Only the HEL-cross-reactive antibody appears idiotype positive. These results are discussed below.

DISCUSSION

The results presented above confirm and extend our previous experiments,[2,3] indicating that the presence of IdXL on anti-HEL is independent of the epitope specificity of the antibody. Furthermore, the results summarized in FIGURES 1 and 2 show that epitope specificities for individual monoclonal antibodies are quite diverse and make unlikely the possibility that these antibodies have in common a recognition element for some subsite of different epitopes. Presumably, each monoclonal antibody is specific for an epitope that may be thought of as a constellation of five or six amino acid residues on the surface of hen egg-white lysozyme. If there were a common restriction in recognition, that is, recognition of a single amino acid in a unique manner, or recognition of two amino acids in a specific position, then there would be an expectation of relatively few sets as defined by FIGURES 1 and 2 rather than the result found in which almost every antibody defines a unique overlap specificity.

Nevertheless, there is clear evidence for spatial relatedness of the epitopes seen by the different monoclonal antibodies. As illustrated in FIGURE 2, the monoclonal antibody 325.1G11 interferes with the binding of HEL of each of the other monoclonal antibodies. Furthermore, this monoclonal antibody strongly competes with secondary serum anti-HEL for binding to HEL (TABLE 2). It appears that epitopes on HEL recognized by the B-cell precursors of the hybridomas and the B cells producing serum anti-HEL are largely restricted to one face of the HEL molecule. This restriction in epitope recognition can not be attributed to differential "foreignness" of one region of the surface of HEL relative to mouse lysozyme. Hen egg-white lysozyme and the other bird lysozymes differ from sequenced mammalian lysozymes (rat, baboon, man) at approximately 50 amino acid residues that are distributed over the entire surface of the molecules, exclusive of the conserved catalytic site. Thus, it seems likely that the restriction is a reflection of limitation in B-T collaboration. It should be noted that two IdXL-negative monoclonal antibodies, 2E6 and 2C7, compete with 1G11 for binding to HEL (FIGURE 3). We are currently testing other IdXL-negative monoclonal antibodies as well as early primary anti-HEL sera for competitive binding with 1G11. Such studies may allow a decision as to whether the observed restriction can be dissociated from idiotypy.

Consistent with the determination of heterogeneity with regard to epitope specificity are the results obtained regarding possible V_H genes coding for the monoclonal antibodies. The results shown in FIGURE 4 and TABLE 3 indicate that a minimum of four V_H genes code for the V_H regions of the 12 hybridomas tested (TABLE 4). Furthermore, there is no indication of correlation of V_H genes with apparent epitope specificity.

These results suggest a model in which the common idiotypy reflects a selection process dictated by an element present prior to immunization. We postulate that there exists in the preimmune animal a set of T cells that recognize an epitope that is ubiquitous in mammals and highly conserved. This intrinsic epitope (E_i) is fortuitously present on the immunoglobulin receptors of a subpopulation of B cells. These B cells are assumed to be of diverse genetic origin, that is, they are coded for by at least several, and perhaps many, different V_H genes. Within this subpopulation there are B cells whose immunoglobulin receptors recognize certain epitopes on hen egg-white lysozyme.

When a mouse (or other animals) is immunized with HEL, there is an activation of antigen-specific T cells (AgTh) that, in turn, collaborate with a set of B cells specific for epitopes on hen egg-white lysozyme. (We had previously shown that the epitypic specificity of AgTh was highly restricted and had postulated that this led to a restriction in activation of B cells with regard to their epitypic specificity.[14]) The B cells activated and the immunoglobulins produced early in the primary response are epitypically restricted, but do not in general bear any recognized idiotypic coherence. Among these B cells, however, there is some number that bears immunoglobulins that have on their variable region a conformation approximating the specific intrinsic epitope. These activated B cells stimulate the E_i-recognizing T cells, thus beginning a positive Servo mechanism. Antigen-specific T cells and activated E_i-recognizing T cells collaborate to strongly select a population of HEL-recognizing E_i-bearing B cells, with the selection being especially strong for the generation of a B-memory population. It is E_i that is recognized as a commonality (or public idiotype, IdXL) on secondary anti-HEL and monoclonal antibodies derived from secondary HEL-specific B cells.

The above model leaves unanswered the question of why a single idiotype predominates in the secondary anti-HEL response. Unlike the usual polysaccharides or haptens used for most idiotype studies, protein antigens provide a plethora of different potential epitopes that would greatly facilitate the dual selection mechanism described above. Thus, a process in which a relatively rare B-cell receptor is selected seems plausible. On the other hand, it is not possible to rule out hierarchical mechanisms where a single idiotype becomes dominant and masks other potential idiotype expressions. Indeed, such dominance has been found in several systems manipulated with anti-idiotypic antibodies.[15]

Finally, we think that further experimentation is required before an interpretation is attempted of the results given in TABLE 5. At face value, it would appear that in an animal that has never seen HEL, there is a dual selection among antibodies generated by a cross-reactive lysozyme for anti-HEL activity and IdXL. This finding is true, despite the fact that positive idiotypy is not restricted to antibodies specific for a given epitope or particular pattern of cross-reactivity with regard to lysozymes other than hen egg-white lysozyme. The breadth of epitope recognition, however, associated with IdXL-positive anti-HEL is based on studies with monoclonal antibodies. It may be, at least quantitatively, that serum antibody is far more restricted. Were this so, the apparent paradox of restriction to HEL cross-reactivity accompanied by lack of epitope restriction would disappear; that is, if serum anti-HEL is mainly directed at a single epitope (or even on a highly restricted determinant region), the association of idiotypy and HEL cross-reactvity may be inevitable.

ACKNOWLEDGMENTS

It is a pleasure to acknowledge the contribution of Dr. Dennis Metzger who generated the anti-HEL-producing hybridomas used in the present study and who first studied many of the properties of these monoclonal antibodies. We also wish to thank Margaret Kowakzyk for preparation of the figures and Vicky Godoy for preparation of the manuscript.

REFERENCES

1. BENJAMIN, C., A. MILLER, E. E. SERCARZ & M. HARVEY. 1980. J. Immunol. **125:** 1017.
2. METZGER, D. W., A. FURMAN, A. MILLER & E. E. SERCARZ. 1981. J. Exp. Med. **154:** 701.

3. METZGER, D. W., A. MILLER & E. E. SERCARZ. 1980. Nature (London) **287:** 541.
4. METZGER, D. W., L.-K. CH'NG, A. MILLER & E. SERCARZ. 1983. Eur. J. Immunol. In press.
5. GEARHART, P. J. 1983. N. Y. Acad. Sci. This volume.
6. SCHROER, J. A. & T. P. BENDER. 1982. Fed. Proc. Fed. Am. Soc. Exp. Biol. **41:** 594.
7. KOHNO, Y., I. BERKOWER, J. MINNA & J. A. BERZOFSKY. 1982. J. Immunol. **128:** 1742.
8. MALISSEN, B., N. REBAI, A. LIABEUF & C. MAWAS. 1982. Eur. J. Immunol. **12:** 739.
9. SMITH-GILL, S. J., A. C. WILSON, M. POTTER, E. M. PRAGER, R. J. FELDMAN & C. R. MAINHART. J. Immunol. 1982. **128:** 314.
10. NORTH, A. C. T. & D. C. PHILLIPS. 1969. Prog. Biophys. Mol. Biol. **19:** 5.
11. MARCU, K. B., J. BANESJI, N. A. PENNCAVAGE, R. LANG & N. ARNHEIM. 1980. Cell **22:** 187.
12. SOUTHERN, E. M. 1975. J. Mol. Biol. **98:** 503.
13. COLECLOUGH, C., R. P. PERRY, K. KARJALAINEN, M. WEIGERT. 1981. Nature (London) **290:** 372.
14. SERCARZ, E. E. & D. W. METZGER. 1980. Springer Semin. Immunopathology **3:** 145.
15. HART, D. A., A. L. WANG, L. A. PAWLAK & A. NISANOFF. 1972. J. Exp. Med. **135:** 1293.

DISCUSSION OF THE PAPER

G. W. SISKIND (*Cornell University Medical College, New York*): While you had this very broad idiotype representation, could your anti-idiotype be an internal image looking like hen egg-white lysozyme?

A. MILLER: This is the sort of idea that has recently been published in the *EMBO Journal* by Jerne *et al.* and by Bona and Kunkel in the *Journal of Experimental Medicine*. That is why I emphasized the fact that there was no overlap of the epitopes on monoclonal antibodies that were able to completely remove the idiotypic activity. These results would require a rather strange kind of recognition. The internal image idea works quite well, I think, if you have a unique epitope or a cluster of epitopes, or if you only remove part of the anti-idiotype with each of the specific monoclonals. That, however, is not what we find.

A. AUGUSTIN (*University of Colorado, Denver*): If the anti-id is the internal image, then anything would bind; the HEL would also bind the internal image, the anti-id. The anti-id looks like the HEL, structurally.

MILLER: So?

A. AUGUSTIN: Then anything that binds HEL would also bind the anti-id.

MILLER: It is not HEL that is recognized, it is a single epitope on HEL. I mean, it is not fair to talk about HEL; one part of HEL is as different from another part as any two unrelated proteins are different.

B. PERNIS (*Columbia University, New York*): It seems to me that your phenomenon is very reminiscent of the Oudin phenomenon.

MILLER: Yes, absolutely. Oudin described the same thing almost twenty years ago with ovalbumin and duck and turkey albumin. There are many cases. I think that people just have not dealt with them, and there has been much more emphasis on some of the anti-hapten idiotypes that have a different character.

Analysis of Idiotypic Heterogeneity in the Anti-α1-3 Dextran and Anti-Phosphorylcholine Responses Using Monoclonal Anti-Idiotype Antibodies[a]

JOHN F. KEARNEY, BRIAN A. POLLOK, AND
ROBERT STOHRER

Department of Microbiology
The Cellular Immunobiology Unit of the Tumor Institute
and
The Comprehensive Cancer Center
University of Alabama in Birmingham
Birmingham, Alabama 35294

INTRODUCTION

The antibody responses of BALB/c mice to the antigens α1-3 dextran (DEX) and phosphorylcholine (PC) have been used as models for studying mechanisms used in generation and regulation of antibody diversity.[1-3] Although these responses are relatively restricted, from the small number of B-cell clones that participate, recent molecular studies have shown that anti-DEX and anti-PC antibodies consist of families of closely related antibodies, with a remarkable degree of diversity within each family.[4-6] These systems have provided a great deal of information on the molecular basis for V region diversity including the multiplicity of germ line genes coding for V, D, and J regions, the combinatorial association of these gene segments for formation of a complete V_H domain, and the role of somatic mutation in further increasing V region diversity within these families.[7,8]

Little is known, concerning the mechanisms used in the regulation of expression of these clones, for example, why one particular member of an antibody family dominates the humoral response to a given antigen. This situation that is reflected in both the DEX and PC systems, provides model systems for determining why certain V regions are more frequently expressed and, in particular, why during development of a particular antibody response somatic mutation occurs within these families of antibodies.

We have constructed panels of murine monoclonal anti-idiotype (Id) antibodies (MAIDs) to the prototype BALB/c DEX-binding proteins J558 ($\alpha\lambda$), MOPC-104E ($\mu\lambda$), and the PC-binding antibody HOPC-8 ($\alpha\kappa$). These MAIDs have been used to study the individual idiotopes (IdI) and cross-reactive idiotopes (IdX) expressed by serum antibodies after immunization with the appropriate antigen. Various monoclonal anti-Id and anti-(anti-idiotype) antibodies have been used to modulate the expression of these idiotopes *in vivo,* and some of the regulatory mechanisms involved

[a]The results reported in this manuscript were supported by Grants CA 16673 and CA 13148, awarded by the National Cancer Institue, and AI 14782, awarded by the National Institute of Allergy and Infectious Diseases. Dr. John F. Kearney is the recipient of Research Career Development Award AI 00338.

151

in the control of these antibody responses have been examined. We have also used the collection of distinct monoclonal anti-Id antibodies specific for idiotopes on myeloma and hybridoma anti-DEX proteins to study the heterogeneity in Id expression by different immunoglobulin isotypes secreted by clonal precursors in the splenic focus assay.

MONOCLONAL ANTI-IDIOTYPE ANTIBODIES

A/J, SJL/J, or idiotype suppressed BALB/c mice were immunized with purified myeloma proteins according to protocols previously described.[9,10] Briefly, mice were

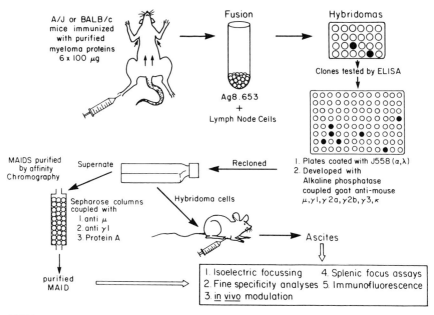

FIGURE 1. Schematic outline of methods used in immunization, production, and characterization of monoclonal anti-Id antibodies.

given multiple subcutaneous injections of 100–500 μg of native purified protein at three-day intervals into the rear footpad, the inguinal, and the axillary regions. The first injection was given in complete Freund's adjuvant and the remainder in saline. One day after the last injection, lymphocytes from the popliteal, inguinal, axillary, and brachial lymph nodes were fused with the nonsecreting myeloma NS1 (for MAIDs GB4-10, AB1-2, and EB3-7-2) or P3x63Ag8.653 for all other hybridoma antibodies described.[10–12] Hybridomas secreting MAIDs were screened, cloned, and tested according to the scheme described in FIGURE 1.

SPECIFICITY OF MONOCLONAL ANTI-IDIOTYPIC ANTIBODIES

Monoclonal anti-idiotypic antibodies were tested in an enzyme-linked immunosorbent assay (ELISA) by direct binding to the immunizing protein as an initial screen for

TABLE 1. List of MAIDs Used to Analyze Heterogeneity of Anti-Dextran Responses

| MAID | MAIDS specific for DEX-binding proteins | | |
	Specificity	Isotype	Strain of Derivation
EB3-7	J558 IdI	$IgG_{1\kappa}$	A/J
B6-10	J558 IdI	IgG_1	BALB/c
EB3-16	J558 IdI	IgG_1	A/J
TD6-4	J558 IdI	IgG_1	A/J
LA4-8	J558 IdI	$IgG_{2a\kappa}$	A/J
RD3-2	J558 IdI	$IgG_{2a\kappa}$	A/J
JB2-2	J558 IdI	$IgG_{2a\kappa}$	A/J
SJL18-1	M104 IdI	IgM,κ	SJL
CD3-2	DEX IdX	$IgG_1\lambda$	A/J

antibodies with anti-Id activitity and then tested by ELISA or radioimmunoassay (RIA) inhibition assays for fine specificity.[10,13] TABLE 1 lists the selected monoclonal antibodies prepared against the DEX binding proteins J558 and MOPC-104E that were used in these studies. TABLE 2 lists those antibodies reactive with PC-binding proteins. It should be noted that purified myeloma proteins were used in all cases, except in the case of antibody DB1-1 for which isolated HOPC-8 heavy chain was used as the immunogen. Neither denaturation nor chemical modifications by attachment of foreign carrier protein or haptens was necessary for production of MAIDs using the methods outlined above.

The large proportion of MAIDs with anti-Id activity against DEX binding antibodies were of the IgG_1 class in agreement with the isotype predominance reported previously for allo-(anti-Id) antibodies.[1] The next most frequent isotype obtained was IgG_{2a} followed by IgM. Monoclonal anti-idiotypic antibodies with IdI specificities (63%) were obtained more frequently than IdX specific antibodies (31%). These results differ from those reported previously where IdX specific antibodies were found to predominate in alloantisera preparations. These differences may indicate that the potential repertoire of anti-Id antibodies may not be expressed in sera.[15] The reactivity of all MAIDs with IdX and IdI specificities for the DEX-binding proteins, was inhibited by the trisaccharide nigerotriose, indicating that idiotopes detected by these MAIDs were associated with the binding site (data not shown).

By constrast, the binding of T15$^+$ proteins by MAIDs AB1-2 and GB4-10, was inhibited by PC bovine serum albumin (BSA) conjugates but not by free PC hapten. DB1-1 antibody was strongly reactive with HOPC-8 heavy chain, and recognized a V_H-associated Id on most anti-PC antibodies, but did not bind readily to intact immunoglobulin; thus antigen or hapten inhibition effects on the binding specificity of DB1-1 were not detectable.

TABLE 2. List of MAIDs Used to Analyze Heterogeneity of Anti-Dextran and Anti-Phosphorylcholine Responses

| MAID | MAIDs specific for PC/T15 system | | |
	Specificity	Isotype	Strain of Derivation
AB1-2	T15	$IgG_{1\kappa}$	A/J
GB4-10	T15	$IgG_{1\kappa}$	A/J
DB1-1	T15 (V_H)	$IgG_{2a\kappa}$	A/J
MM-60	GB4-10	$IgM\lambda$	BALB/c

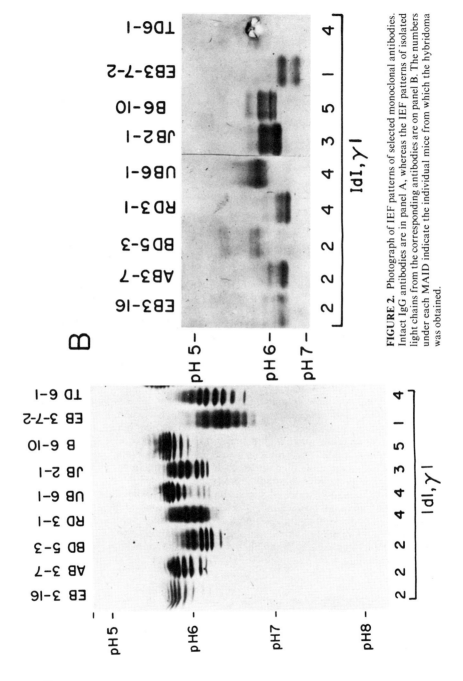

FIGURE 2. Photograph of IEF patterns of selected monoclonal antibodies. Intact IgG antibodies are in panel A, whereas the IEF patterns of isolated light chains from the corresponding antibodies are on panel B. The numbers under each MAID indicate the individual mice from which the hybridoma was obtained.

The MAIDs specific for DEX-binding antibodies were considerably diverse as determined by their isoelectric focusing (IEF) spectra. FIGURE 2 shows the IEF patterns of a representative selection of IgG_1 IdI-specific antibodies derived from six independent fusions of lymph node cells from individual mice. Although the intact antibodies focused at a similar pI, no duplicate patterns were observed (FIGURE 2A). Isolated light chains from these hybridomas also showed heterogeneous IEF patterns (FIGURE 2B). These results suggest that although the epitopes to which these IdI-specific MAIDs bind are closely associated on anti-DEX antibodies, a highly heterogeneous anti-Id response results from immunization with myeloma proteins as previously observed in the production of syngeneic anti-Id sera.[14,15] Although λ chains of the DEX group of proteins have been shown to exhibit identical IEF patterns,[4] they may have undetected V region amino acid substitutions that would affect DEX idiotypes. Therefore, some of the idiotope heterogeneity described below could possibly

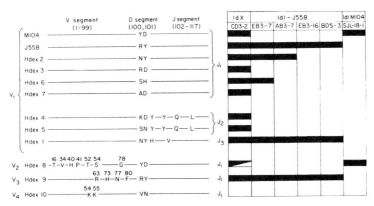

FIGURE 3. A comparison of the reactivities of selected monoclonal anti-Id antibodies with anti-DEX proteins and their V_H amino acid sequences as described in reference 5.

be due to variability in V_λ structure within the DEX-binding group of myeloma and hybridoma proteins.

FINE SPECIFICITY OF MONOCLONAL ANTI-IDIOTYPIC ANTIBODIES

Because the goal behind the construction of these MAIDs was to use them as clonal markers to study Id expression by cells or serum antibodies, their epitope specificity and structural associations were determined. In collaboration with Dr. Brian Clevinger, some of these MAIDs were selected and tested for binding to DEX-specific proteins with known V_H sequences. In FIGURE 3, a comparison is made between the V_H amino acid sequences of a series of anti-DEX proteins and the reactivity of the MAIDs as determined by binding inhibition analysis.

It can be seen that CD3-2 (γ_1, λ) appears to have the same specificity as previously described for a heterologous goat anti-IdX antiserum.[5] This idiotope appears to be associated with amino acid residues 54, 55, and possibly the carbohydrate moiety associated with the asparagine residue at position 55. This conclusion can be drawn by its failure to react with HDEX10, which has substitutions at these positions. The syngeneic BALB/c monoclonal antibody [N-20 ($\mu\kappa$)] shows similar specificity. SJL18-1 appears to distinguish precisely between MOPC-104E (M104E) and J558, which have identical light chain amino acid sequences and which differ only at D region amino acid residues 100 and 101.[5] This antibody, however, also shows some reactivity with HDEX7, which like M104E has an asparagine residue at position 101. EB3-7-2 antibody, which precisely defines the D region differences between M104E and J558 and appears to be specific for the latter, also reacts with HDEX9, which has a different V_H, and also HDEX1, which has a different D segment. This MAID therefore appears to define a broader group of anti-DEX proteins than SJL18-1. Intermediate in specificity are the proteins AB3-7, BD5-3, and EB3-16 that define different sets of anti-DEX molecules, depending on substitutions at position 100, but appear to react with molecules that have tyrosine at position 101. EB3-16 and BD5-3 also react with proteins with similar D regions as J558 and HDEX-25. The other MAIDs specific for anti-DEX antibodies have not been tested in this assay, but as shown later, all exhibit fine differences in their binding specificities.

In FIGURE 4, the reactivities of the MAIDs specific for T15$^+$ molecules are correlated with known amino acid sequences. It can be seen that AB1-2 reacts with all proteins defined as T15$^+$ by an heterologous A/J anti-T15 idiotype serum. It does not react with anti-PC antibodies that have either an inappropriate light chain (non-T15 V_L) or an abnormally long D region in the heavy chain. GB4-10 antibody reacts with most T15$^+$ antibodies, but does not react with proteins where there are amino acid substitutions at the beginning or middle of the D region. Whereas it is difficult to assign a structural correlate to the AB1-2-defined idiotope, specificity depends on an idiotope associated with a native D region structure. In testing the fine specificity of the anti-T15 V_H antibody DB1-1, it was found to react with a much broader spectrum of PC-binding proteins; it did not, however, bind to MOPC-167, which has a large number of V_H substitutions compared to the germ line T15 V_H sequence. This antibody also did not bind to the anti-PC proteins 6G6 and HPCG15 that appear to use a different V_H gene from T15 (L. Claflin, personal communication). The usefulness of DB1-1 antibody in the following studies was limited, however, because the DB1-1 idiotope appears to be hidden in the native intact molecule, and DB1-1 reacts only with the isolated heavy chain or the whole immunoglobulin molecule if partially denatured, for example, by binding the antibody to plastic. In summary, AB1-2 defines a larger population of monoclonal anti-PC antibodies within the T15$^+$ set than does GB4-10, and anti-T15 MAIDs recognize an overlapping group of immunoglobulins all using the same V_H and V_L genes.

IDIOTYPE EXPRESSION IN SERUM

Mice were immunized with 100 μg doses of α1-3 dextran (B13555) or 2×10^8 heat-killed *Streptococcus pneumoniae* (R36A) organisms, and bled 7 days and 12 days respectively after immunization. Sera were assayed for the content of IdX and IdI antibodies. The levels of λ bearing anti-DEX antibody and the percentage of IdI$^+$ antibodies varied considerably among litters and individual mice as shown by the saline controls representative of antibody levels in normal mice (FIGURE 5). B6-10, a syngeneic BALB/c anti-IdI J558 that is clearly IdI-specific for J558, did not bind to BALB/c serum anti-DEX antibody. When a series of strains and F$_1$ hybrids of these strains were tested for expression of the B6-10 idiotope, it was detected in the serum of

V_L group		V region (1–95)	D region (96–100)	J region (100–113)	Reactivity vs: AB1-2	GB4-10	DB1-1
TEPC 15	T15		YYGSS	—	+	+	+
HOPC 8	"		N	—	+	+	+
HPCG 8	"	F (53)	R	—	+	+	+
HPCG II	"	I (28), S (53)		—	+	+	+
C3	"	S-R (14 16), R-G (40 44)		T	+	+	+
7C6	"	S-R (14 16), A-G (40 44)	-DG- H		+	−	+
HPCM6	"		-DYP H		+	−	+
HPCG 14	"	A (31), F (71)	-V-YD ()		−	−	+
HPCM 3	M603				−	−	+

FIGURE 4. A comparison of the reactivities of MAIDs AB1-2, GB4-10, and DB1-1 with anti-PC proteins and their V_H sequences.

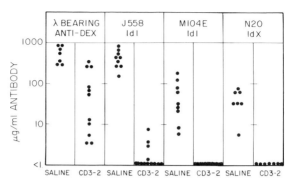

FIGURE 5. Levels of λ- and Id-positive anti-DEX antibodies in mice neonatally suppressed with IdX-specific MAID CD3-2. Mice were challenged at 6 weeks after birth.

only a small proportion of DEX immunized F_1 hybrids at concentrations ranging from 10–80 µg/ml (TABLE 3). The failure to detect this idiotope in normal BALB/c mice is puzzling, and its emergence in some but not all F_1 hybrids may represent an example of a hidden or very rare idiotope, because it was also occasionally detected in supernatants from BALB/c splenic focus assays (R. Stohrer and J. Kearney, unpublished).

The λ-bearing anti-DEX response has been shown to be linked genetically to the Igh-a allotype.[16] Because it is probable that different V, D, or J segments are involved in the generation of the major idiotype that shows this genetic linkage, we studied the expression of λ^+ anti-DEX IdI and IdX-bearing antibodies in several murine inbred strains, F_1 hybrids, and a set of sera from DEX-primed recombinant strains kindly provided by Dr. Roy Riblet. As can be seen in FIGURE 6, λ-bearing anti-DEX IdX-positive antibody was detectable in rare individual mice of the Igh-b allotype, for example, C57BL/6. Analysis of IdI and IdX expression in the λ^+ anti-DEX antibody produced by this panel of strains, however, showed that both IdI and IdX monoclonally-defined idiotopes are linked to allotype, as was the case for sera from recombinant strains (data not shown). These results suggest that at least with the monoclonal anti-Id tested, which are directed towards V_H-IdX or D region-associated IdI, that expression of a particular V_H-D-J_H complex of anti-DEX specificity is linked to expression of the appropriate immunoglobulin heavy chain allotype.

In the PC system, the proportions of anti-PC antibodies expressing the AB1-2 and GB4-10-defined Id were represented at very constant levels in the serum of R36A-

TABLE 3. Distribution of the B6-10 Idiotope in Various Mouse Strains

Strain	B6-10⁺	Amount in µg/ml
BALB/c	0/87[a]	—
C57BL/6	0/13	—
SJL/J	0/11	—
A/HEN	0/10	—
BAB/14	0/14	—
CB6F₁	1/7	32[b]
CSF₁	2/8	10,20
CAF₁	1/10	89

[a]Number of mice tested for the expression of the B6-10 idiotope.
[b]Detectable antibody levels (>0.2 µg/ml) in individual B6-10⁺ mice.

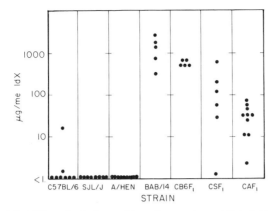

FIGURE 6. Lambda IdX$^+$ antibody detected in various strains and F_1 hybrids after intraperitoneal immunization with 100 μg of α1-3 DEX.

immunized mice. TABLE 4 shows the mean values for expression of the various idiotypic phenotypes among BALB/c anti-PC antibody populations. Although the physiological basis for the dominance of the AB1$^+$GB4$^+$ phenotype is unknown, perhaps exposure to normal environmental antigens preferentially selects B cells with that phenotype for expansion, resulting in its predominant expression among anti-PC serum antibodies.[17] Nevertheless, it is possible by administration of suppressive amounts of GB4-10 antibody in adult mice, followed by continued antigen boosting, to force the AB1$^+$GB4$^-$ phenotype to dominate the anti-PC antibody response, just as it is possible to suppress completely the T15$^+$ portion of the anti-PC response by administering AB1-2 antibody.[10]

BIOLOGICAL ACTIVITIES OF MONOCLONAL ANTI-IDIOTYPIC ANTIBODIES

Many diverse effects on specific immune responses have been described following *in vivo* administration of anti-Id antibodies.[18] In the case of the DEX system, we have produced MAIDs with differing epitope specificities and of different isotypes, thus making it possible to study modulatory effects of these MAIDs on the level of total anti-DEX antibody as well as on the level of expression of various IdI and IdX components of this response. Administration of MAIDs specific for anti-DEX antibodies suppressed the appropriate response when given to both adult and neonatal BALB/c mice. Injection of IdI-specific antibodies EB3-7 and SJL18-1 into adult mice

TABLE 4. Expression of T15-Associated Idiotopes among BALB/c Anti-Phosphorylcholine Hybridomas, Splenic Foci, and Serum Antibody

MAID	Isotype	Percent Id Positive Anti-PC IgM		
		Hybridoma	Spleen foci	Serum Ab
AB1-2	IgG$_1$	85	77	86–100
GB4-10	IgG$_1$	80	66	83–100

completely ablated the corresponding idiotope-bearing portion of the antibody response after DEX challenge, without significantly diminishing the overall λ^+ anti-DEX response. Adult mice remained totally suppressed until 6 weeks after MAID treatment, when some began to escape from suppression. By contrast, neonatal suppression of this kind was complete and permanent, with deletion of functional IdI$^+$ B-cell activity. Neonatal administration of IdX-specific MAIDs drastically depleted the overall anti-DEX antibody responses including both IdI and IdX levels as shown for neonatally suppressed mice (FIGURE 5).

In summary, we have shown that by using appropriate antibodies of IdI specificity, it was possible to precisely inactivate clones expressing a specific idiotope without affecting expression of other IdI determinants. By contrast, administration of anti-IdX MAIDs produced a severe decrease in total λ^+ anti-DEX serum antibody and ablated the IdX portion of the response. This pattern of suppression differs from the arsonate system where administration of a heterologous IdI-specific antibody effected a suppression of IdX.[19] Suppression could be accomplished using a wide range of doses of MAIDs prepared from ascites as well as those purified from tissue culture supernatants. The latter were isolated in such a way that they did not contain other T- and B-cell-derived humoral components or exogenous Ab1, Ab2, Ab3 antibodies that may have been present in antisera and ascites fluids, nor did they contain idiotope-bearing material that may have copurified with antigen affinity column-prepared material.

Monoclonal anti-idiotype antibodies of IgM and IgG isotypes were equally effective in eliciting suppression of the appropriate idiotopes when used in suppressive doses. In many experiments using variable doses of MAIDs of IgM and IgG isotype (concentrations of 100 ng–1 mg), we could not produce enhancement of a particular IdI or an increase in the total λ^+ anti-DEX response (results not shown). This situation is in contrast to that observed in other systems (notably the NP^b system) where idiotope levels can be increased substantially by appropriate treatment of mice with certain monoclonal anti-idiotype antibodies.[20] The obvious differences between the two types of systems may depend on the thymus-independent nature of anti-PC and anti-DEX responses, or may be due to the dominance of certain IdI and IdX levels in these responses, or possibly reflect stimulation of these B-cell clones by environmental antigens that result in relatively high levels of preformed serum antibodies. In the latter instance, the antibody responses studied would be secondary in nature and might already be under tight regulation by appropriate control mechanisms. Alternatively, differences in the specificities of MAIDs used may account for these results.

IDIOTYPE-ISOTYPE ANALYSIS OF SPLENIC FOCI WITH ANTI-DEXTRAN ACTIVITY

It is apparent from the structural correlation of Id in this system (FIGURE 3) and the above *in vivo* studies, that these MAIDs probably do not act as clonal markers for DEX-specific B cells. The specificity of these antibodies, however, may be used to advantage to detect fine V region differences between two similar, but distinct, immunoglobulin molecules. A panel of eight hybridomas with anti-DEX activity was tested against the panel of seven hybridomas with anti-Id activity (FIGURE 7). These MAIDs were shown to be unique, at least by their IEF patterns and by their specificity as shown in FIGURE 3. It can be seen that each monoclonal anti-DEX hybridoma or myeloma protein exhibited a distinct pattern of reactivity when tested against the panel of monoclonal anti-idiotypic antibodies. From these studies, a panel of MAIDs was selected that detected the greatest degree of heterogeneity within the family of anti-DEX hybridomas.

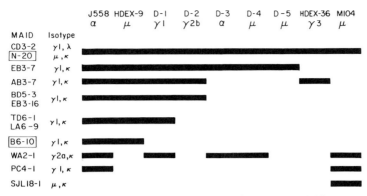

FIGURE 7. Reactivities of various MAIDs with a panel of anti-DEX hybridoma proteins of differing heavy chain isotypes.

The objective of these experiments was to study the idiotope heterogeneity of immunoglobulins secreted in the splenic focus assay. Because one of our primary goals was to determine whether the idiotype profile was identical in clones secreting multiple isotypes, we tested a panel of MAIDs against anti-DEX hybridomas of different isotypes. The immunoglobulin isotypes expressed by a panel of 38 different hybridomas derived from the fusion of DEX-immunized BALB/c spleen cells with the nonsecreting myeloma P3x63Ag8.653 are listed in TABLE 5. The large majority of the hybridomas were of the μ isotype, whereas others occurred in the descending order of frequency of $\alpha > \gamma_3 > \gamma_{2b}$. No hybridomas were obtained of the ϵ or γ_{2a} isotypes. TABLE 6 illustrates the Id profile of these hybridomas and shows that the cross-reactive idiotopes CD3-2 and N-20 were expressed by an overlapping population of hybridomas (constituting 73% and 81% of those obtained, respectively). SJL18-1[+] and EB3-7-2[+] populations were the next most frequently obtained and comprised (except for one example) nonoverlapping populations. J558 IdI determinants were expressed on a heterogeneous group of proteins, most of which were EB3-7-positive. From this analysis, it can be seen that the anti-Id chosen for this study reacted with a heterogeneous group of purified hybridoma proteins of differing Id that were at least as heterogeneous in their idiotope profile as the antibodies in normal anti-DEX immune serum. Within the panel selected, there did not appear to be a preferential association

TABLE 5. Isotype Distribution of Anti-Dextran Hybridomas From BALB/c Mice[a]

Isotype	Number	Percent
μ	25	66
IgG$_1$	1	3
IgG$_{2a}$	0	—
IgG$_{2b}$	1	3
IgG$_3$	5	13
α	6	16
ϵ	0	—

[a]Mice were immunized intravenously with 100 μg of α1-3 DEX (B1355S), and spleen cells were fused with P3X63Ag8.653 5 days later.

TABLE 6. Idiotypic Analysis of Anti-Dextran Hybridomas[a]

Anti-Idiotype	Number	Percent
IdX		
CD3-2	30	81
N-20	27	73
M104-IdI		
SJL18-1	13	35
J558-IdI		
EB-7-2	21	57
EB3-16	2	5
B6-10	0	—
IdI Negative	1	3

[a]See footnote for TABLE 5.

of any particular MAID-determined idiotope with a particular immunoglobulin heavy chain isotype, but there is, in these studies, a complete association of these idiotopes with the λ light chain.

Having defined a panel of anti-Id antibodies that can detect a variety of fine structural differences in anti-DEX antibodies, we than began to analyze anti-DEX-positive splenic foci. T-independent responses using unprimed donor B cells and recipients were studied using dextran B1355S as antigen. T-dependent responses were studied using limulus hemocyanin primed recipients and DEX-hemocyanin (DEX-Hy) as antigen. The splenic foci were screened by ELISA for anti-DEX activity on DEX-BSA-coated plates for λ-positive antibody. These clones were then tested for isotype expression by a similar ELISA with isotype-specific antibodies. To determine the idiotopes associated with each immunoglobulin class of anti-DEX antibody, an ELISA assay was used as described in FIGURE 8. In this assay, MAIDs (purified from hybridoma tissue culture supernatants on anti-mouse immunoglobulin affinity columns) were coated to plastic plates. Foci supernatants were added and enzyme-labeled goat or rat monoclonal anti-mouse isotype antibodies were used to develop the assay.

The positive foci analyzed from the T-independent assays in TABLE 7 and the

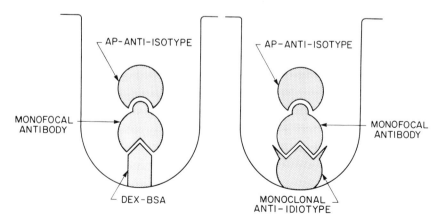

FIGURE 8. Diagram of ELISA assays for isotype and idiotype determinations of DEX-positive antibodies from splenic foci.

TABLE 7. Isotype Analysis of Splenic Foci Obtained with the T-Independent Assay

Isotype	Positives	Frequency	Expected Double Frequency[a]
μ	200	90%	—
$\gamma2b$	4	1.8%	—
$\gamma3$	6	2.7%	—
α	30	13%	—
ϵ	5	2.2%	—
$\mu,\gamma2b$	1	0.5%	0.3%
$\mu,\gamma3$	1	0.5%	0.5%
μ,α	20	9%	1%

[a]Calculated frequencies of double isotype-producing clones results from random association of two independent precursors.

isotypes detected within each anti-DEX positive focus were either single or IgM with one other non-IgM isotype. In general, the isotype representation obtained in the T-independent foci was similar to that obtained in hybridomas, except that some IgE-secreting clones were obtained. In the T-independent assays, only 2 clones out of 200 tested were obtained that expressed more than one non-μ isotype. When the T-dependent assays were analyzed, there was no significant increase in the overall frequency of DEX positive clones obtained (data not shown). These results suggest that there was no further recruitment of DEX positive precursors secreting λ antibody in the T-dependent assays. The isotype profile observed, however, was quite different with a very large increase in the number of IgA-containing foci and a corresponding decrease in the number of IgM-containing foci (FIGURE 9). Large increases in the frequency of foci secreting multiple isotypes were also seen in T-dependent responses compared to T-independent foci (FIGURE 10).

The idiotypic analysis of splenic foci T-independent responses are described in

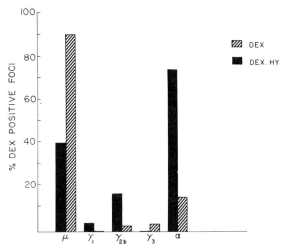

FIGURE 9. Comparison of isotypes expressed by DEX-positive antibodies in splenic foci from T-dependent and T-independent responses.

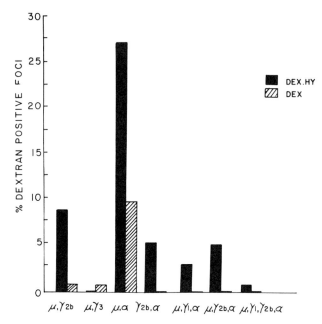

FIGURE 10. A comparison isotype expression in foci from T-independent and T-dependent assays, showing an increase in foci producing multiple isotypes in the latter assay where DEX-Hy was used as immunogen.

TABLE 8. In general, the idiotope profiles and frequencies of idiotope expression by both T-dependent and T-independent foci and hybridomas were very similar. Again, no preferential association of idiotype with a particular isotype was noted.

IgM antibodies in anti-DEX containing foci showed considerable heterogeneity with respect to the idiotopes expressed, and within limits (due to the relatively small number of non-IgM producing clones), no large differences were detected between IgM and non-IgM clones in the degree of heterogeneity of idiotopes expressed by each isotype.

Because it was possible to analyze independently idiotopes expressed by IgM and

TABLE 8. Idiotypic Analysis of Splenic Foci

Anti-idiotype	Number[a]	Percent
IDX		
CD3-2	185	83
N-20	157	70
M104 IdI		
SJL18-1	58	26
J558 IdI		
EB37-2	165	74
EB3-16	13	6
B6-10	4	2

[a]Supernatants from 2928 individual splenic fragments were tested for anti-DEX activity. The 223 DEX-positive supernatants were analyzed for idiotype expression as described in the text.

non-IgM isotypes within the same clone, we could then determine whether the antibody-secreting progeny within a clone could give rise to antibodies with slightly different V regions. In 50% of clones containing two isotypes, the Id profiles did not differ from each other. In those instances where the number of double isotype-producing clones was greater than expected by chance alone, there were different idiotopes expressed by IgM and IgG or IgA. Some examples of these combinations are shown in TABLE 9. These results suggest that during the development of isotype-restricted antibody-secreting cells from IgM-, IgM/IgG, or IgM/IgA-expressing precursor B cells, some variation occurs in the V regions of IgM and non-IgM antibodies that is reflected by fine differences in Id expression by the two classes of molecules. These could, of course, result from L chain differences, although previous data from analysis of hybridomas suggests that the DEX λ chains are structurally identical.[15] The genetic mechanisms responsible for the production of these idiotypically distinct molecules is, of course, open to speculation. Evidence, however, has been produced recently that shows that a high degree of somatic mutation occurs during B-cell differentiation that results in an extraordinary amount of diversity even in restricted responses such as anti-PC and anti-dextran.[7,8] The results that we have

TABLE 9. Idiotype-Isotype Associations in Representative Foci Producing Anti-α1-3 Dextran Antibodies of Differing Isotypes in Response to Dextran-Hemocyanin

Foci	Isotype Detected in Focus	Monoclonal anti-Id antibodies							
		EB3	B610	3-16	TD6	LA4	RD3	JB2	CD3
D7	μ	+	−	+	+	+	−	−	+
	γ2b	+	−	−	−	−	−	−	+
	α	+	−	−	−	−	−	−	+
F6	γ2b	+	−	+	−	+	−	−	+
	α	+	−	−	−	−	−	−	−
E5	μ	+	−	−	+	+	−	−	+
	α	+	−	+	+	+	−	−	+
B7	μ	+	−	−	−	+	−	−	+
	α	+	−	−	−	−	−	−	+

described here support this data obtained from molecular studies and, furthermore, places in perspective the point that at least some of this mutation can occur quite rapidly within the time frame of the antigen-driven expansion of clonal precursors in this essay.

CHARACTERIZATION OF AN AUTO-ANTI-(ANTI-IDIOTYPE) ANTIBODY

In models of immunoregulation affecting proposed idiotype/anti-idiotype interactions, it is frequently necessary to use nonphysiological means to induce the production of antibody populations (Ab$_1$, Ab$_2$, and Ab$_3$, etcetera) proposed to be involved in immunoregulatory networks.[21] The existence of such antibodies and their physiological role in regulating and maintaining normal immune equilibrium has been questioned for these reasons. We have been attempting to isolate by cell-fusion techniques the clones of B cells involved in these putative regulatory processes (during normal *in vivo* anti-DEX and anti-PC in BALB/c mice). In this final section, we describe the biological properties of a monoclonal hybridoma that secretes the anti-(anti-T15 Id) antibody MM60 ($\mu\lambda$). This hybridoma was isolated from the spleen of a normal BALB/c mouse undergoing an anti-PC response due to immunization with the rough strain *Streptococcus pneumococcus* R36A. Details of the isolation of MM60 and some of its properties have been previously described.[22]

This antibody was first detected by its reactivity with the monoclonal anti-Id antibody GB4-10.[10] General characteristics of this antibody are described in TABLE 10. It is highly specific in that it reacts only with GB4-10, but not with other anti-T15 monoclonal anti-idiotypic antibodies. Because MM60 uses a distinct V_H (as determined by amino acid sequence) and expresses a λ light chain, it is probably not a molecule that uses a distinct V region that also expresses the GB4-10-defined idiotope.[22] This idiotope is determined by a D region-related structure in combination with a T15 light chain as is shown in FIGURE 4. It reacts with a surface immunoglobulin of B cells ($1-4/10^4$) from adult spleens. This binding can be inhibited by 50-fold excess of the anti-PC antibody HOPC8 (AB1-2^+ GB4-10^+). In an exquisite test for specificity, the MM60-defined B cells behave very similarly to the specificity of the anti-Id GB4-10 antibody in that staining by MM60 was not inhibited by PC12-3 anti-PC protein (which is AB1-2^+GB4-10^-). In summary, the immunochemical and

TABLE 10. Characteristics of the Monoclonal Auto-Anti-(Anti-Idiotype) Antibody MM-60

Immunochemistry
- Specific for GB4-10 MAID, no other anti-T15 antibodies
- Does not bind PC, R36A
- V_H and V_L distinct from T15$^+$ Ig, not a GB4-10$^+$ antibody
- Binds to $2/10^4$ BALB/c spleen cells, no T cells stained

Biological activity
- Suppresses anti-PC response in idiotype-specific manner
- Activates MM-60 Id$^+$ B cells of anti-T15 specificity
- Suppressive in *nu/nu* mice, no evidence for T-cell involvement

Ontogeny
- MM-60 Id$^+$ B cells arise in parallel with GB4-10$^+$Id$^+$ B cells; Id and anti-Id B cells appear to develop independently.

---

cell-binding data suggest that MM60 defines a population of antibodies and B cells that have anti-idiotypic activities similar to that possessed by the MAID GB4-10.

BIOLOGICAL ACTIVITIES OF MM60

Because this antibody is a syngeneic antibody isolated from fusion of cells from BALB/c mice undergoing a normal immune response to R36A, we examined its effect on the PC response by *in vivo* administration of MM60. It was found that injection of 10ng–10μg of MM60 suppressed that proportion of the anti-PC serum antibody response in BALB/c and CAF$_1$ mice that is normally T15$^+$, permitting increased production of anti-PC antibody that is non-T15$^+$. The suppression was shown to be idiotype specific in that MM60 had no effect on the anti-PC responses of AB1-2 neonatally suppressed mice (T15$^-$). Furthermore, MM60 treatment had no effect on the anti-PC responses of GB4-10-negative strains of mice (CBA/J) or experimentally induced GB4-10$^-$ mice (neonatally suppressed with GB4-10 MAID) that have an anti-PC response that is mainly AB1-2$^+$ GB4-10$^-$. These results suggest that the suppression induced by MM60 is highly idiotope specific and that the MM60 target cells that mediate the suppression act specifically on the GB4-10 idiotope-bearing portion of the anti-PC response. Administration of MM60 appears to expand a population of MM60$^+$ B cells when given *in vivo*, because there is a 10-fold increase in MM60 Id-bearing cells in suppressed mice ($2.8/10^3$ versus 2.2×10^4). In neither normal or MM60-suppressed mice were T cells stained, and because the suppression occurred equally as efficiently in *nu/nu* mice as normal mice, T cells did not appear to be involved in MM60-induced suppression of T15$^+$ antibody production.

We have studied the ontogeny of MM60$^+$ B cells in spleen and found that the frequency of these B cells increases in parallel with GB4$^+$ B cells, suggesting that development of anti-Id B cells as defined by MM60 is not dependent on the previous development of T15 Id$^+$ B cells. Similarly CBA/N mice that cannot make a T15$^+$ anti-PC response have normal frequencies of both GB4-10$^+$ and MM60$^+$ B cells (Id and anti-Id, respectively). These results suggest that the development of Id and anti-Id cells may be independent of each other during B-cell development, although it cannot be excluded that maternally derived immunoglobulins are involved in the induction and maintenance of these clones of cells.

Isolation of hybridoma clone MM60 that has potent specific suppressive activities on the T15 portion of the anti-PC response suggests that further clones may be isolated by similar experimentation from mice making normal antibody responses. The probable mechanism of its suppressive activity appears to be independent of T cells and may result from an expansion of "GB4-10-like" idiotope-specific anti-T15 B cells. Because it is only GB4-10$^+$ anti-PC cells that are suppressed, it is logical to assume that the expanded anti-T15 B cells are responsible for inactivation of GB4-10$^+$ positive B cells that are normally responsible for the majority of the anti-PC response in BALB/c mice. These results indicate that the regulation of the fine idiotope heterogeneity of anti-PC antibodies may be mediated physiologically by anti-T15 and anti-(anti-T15) clones of B cells.

SUMMARY

Panels of monoclonal anti-idiotype antibodies (MAIDs) specific for individual (IdI) and cross-reactive (IdX) idiotopes were prepared and used to study the expression of these idiotopes on anti-DEX and anti-PC antibodies produced in response to antigenic stimulation *in vivo*, clonal expression of idiotopes in an *in vitro* splenic focus assay, and the alterations in the idiotypic profile of these responses after *in vivo* administration of monoclonal anti-Id antibodies. Using these panels of MAIDs, it was possible to inactivate IdI-bearing B cells both in neonates and adult mice without affecting the responsiveness of IdI$^-$ B cells. By contrast, suppression with IdX-specific antibodies resulted in greatly reduced antibody responses. By studying the idiotypic profile of anti-DEX clones in the splenic focus assay, it was shown that IgM, IgG, and IgA antibody Id were diverse and paralleled those expressed in serum. Within some clones there was evidence that idiotope-isotype associations differed, suggesting that V region variants may have been generated within the progeny of a clone following stimulation by dextran. An anti-anti-Id antibody isolated from a BALB/c mouse undergoing a normal immune response to R36A was shown to have a T-cell independent highly idiotope-specific regulatory effect on the T15$^+$ anti-PC response, apparently affecting induction of anti-idiotypic B cells.

ACKNOWLEDGMENTS

We wish to acknowledge the advice, criticism, and help of Dr. H. Kubagawa, Dr. M. D. Cooper, Dr. D. Briles, and Dr. Ming Chou Lee. We thank Mrs. Ann Brookshire for the preparation of this manuscript.

REFERENCES

1. WEIGERT, M., W. C. RASCHKE, D. CARSON & M. COHN. 1974. Immunochemical analysis of the idiotypes of mouse myeloma proteins with specificity for levan or dextran. J. Exp. Med. **139**: 137–147.
2. KOHLER, H. 1975. The response to phosphorylcholine: dissecting an immune response. Transplant. Rev. **27**: 24–56.
3. COSENZA, H., M. JULIUS & A. AUGUSTIN. 1977. Idiotypes as variable region markers: analogies between receptors on phosphorylcholine-specific T and B lymphocytes. Immunol. Rev. **34**: 3–33.
4. SCHILLING, J., B. CLEVINGER, J. M. DAVIE & L. HOOD. 1980. Amino acid sequence of homogeneous antibodies to dextran and DNA arrangements in heavy chain V-region gene segments. Nature (London) **283**: 35–40.
5. CLEVINGER, B., J. SCHILLING, L. HOOD & J. DAVIE. 1980. Structural correlates of cross-reactive and individual idiotypic determinants on murine antibodies to α1-3 dextran. J. Exp. Med. **151**: 1059–1070.
6. GEARHART, P., N. JOHNSON, R. DOUGLAS & L. HOOD. 1981. IgG antibodies to phosphorylcholine exhibit more diversity than their IgM counterparts. Nature (London) **291**: 20–34.
7. EARLY, P., H. HUANG, M. DAVIS, K. CALAME & L. HOOD. 1980. An immunoglobulin heavy chain variable region is generated from three segments of DNA: V_H, D and J. Cell **19**: 981–992.
8. CREWS, S., J. GRIFFIN, H. HUANG, K. CALAME & L. HOOD. 1981. A single V_H gene segment encodes the immune response to phosphorylcholine: somatic mutation is correlated with the class of the antibody. Cell **25**: 59–66.
9. LIEBERMAN, R., S. RUDIKOFF, W. HUMPHREY & M. POTTER. 1981. Allelic forms of anti-phosphorylcholine antibodies. J. Immunol. **126**: 172–176.
10. KEARNEY, J. F., R. BARLETTA, Z. S. QUAN & J. QUINTANS. 1981. Monoclonal versus heterogeneous anti-H-8 antibodies in the analysis of the anti-phosphorylcholine response in BALB/c mice. Eur. J. Immunol. **11**: 877–883.
11. KOHLER, G. & C. MILSTEIN. 1976. Derivation of specific antibody producing tissue culture and tumor lines by cell fusion. Eur. J. Immunol. **6**: 511–519.
12. KEARNEY, J. F., A. RADBRUCH, B. LIESEGANG & K. RAJEWSKY. 1979. A new mouse myeloma cell line that has lost immunoglobulin expression but permits the construction of antibody-secreting hybrid cell lines. J. Immunol. **123**: 1548–1550.
13. CLEVINGER, B., J. THOMAS, J. DAVIE, J. SCHILLING, M. BOND, L. HOOD & J. KEARNEY. 1981. Anti-dextran antibodies; sequences and idiotypes. *In* Immunoglobulin Idiotypes. C. Janeway, E. Sercarz & H. Wigzell, Eds.: 159–168. Academic Press. New York.
14. SCHULER, W., E. WEILER & H. KOLB. 1977. Characterization of syngeneic anti-idiotype antibody against the idiotype of BALB/c myeloma protein J558. Eur. J. Immunol. **7**: 649–654.
15. SCHULER, W., E. WEILER & J. J. WEILER. 1981. Biological and serological comparison of syngeneic and allogeneic anti-idiotypic antibodies. Mol. Immunol. **18**: 1095–1105.
16. RIBLET, R., B. BLOMBERG, M. WEIGERT, R. LIEBERMANN, B. A. TAYLOR & M. POTTER. 1975. Genetics of mouse antibodies. I. Linkage of the dextran response locus V_H DEX to allotype. Eur. J. Immunol. **5**: 775–777.
17. BRILES, D. E., C. FORMAN, S. HUDAK & J. L. CLAFLIN. 1982. Anti-phosphorylcholine antibodies of the T15 idiotype are optimally protective against *Streptococcus pneumoniae*. J. Exp. Med. **156**: 1177–1185.

18. C. BONA. 1981. Idiotypes and Lymphocytes. Academic Press. New York.
19. HIRAI, Y., E. LAMOYI, Y. DOHI & A. NISONOFF. 1981. Regulation of expression of a fan. of cross-reactive idiotypes. J. Immunol. **126:** 71–74.
20. KELSOE, G., M. RETH & K. RAJEWSKY. 1980. Control of idiotope expression by monoclonal anti-idiotope antibody. Immunol. Rev. **52:** 75–88.
21. JERNE, N. K. 1974. Towards a network theory of the immune system. Ann. Immunol. Inst. Pasteur (Paris) **125**(C):373–389.
22. POLLOK, B., A. BHOWN & J. KEARNEY. 1982. Structural and biological properties of a monoclonal auto-anti-(anti-idiotype) antibody. Nature (London) **299:** 447–449.

DISCUSSION OF THE PAPER

D. E. MOSIER (*Institute for Cancer Research, Philadelphia, Pa.*): The clones that make both μ and α are divided into classes that are idiotypically identical and those that are idiotypically distinct. The question arises as to whether the idiotypically distinct populations exist because of somatic diversification, or the chance capture of two B cells in the same fragment. Your data should allow one to make that distinction, because if the idiotypic profile is as diverse in the double expressors as it is in the individual single expressors, it would argue heavily for the chance capture of two independent B cells. If there is very limited heterogeneity, however, one might argue for somatic mutation.

J. K. KEARNEY: We have done one calculation like that in the μ-α double—in the ones that are idiotypically different by statistical evidence. I know that is all we can do. I think 20% of them can be accounted for by chance; 80% of them presumably were not double precursors. That is all that I can say to that question.

G. W. SISKIND (*Cornell University Medical College, New York*): Eighty percent of them could not be accounted for by capture of two cells. Is that what your conclusion is?

KEARNEY: By statistical analysis, yes, that is correct.

SISKIND: There could be, however, a selective pressure to get two into the same site, especially in the T-dependent assay where there is a T cell in there with which they might interact.

KEARNEY: Exactly. We found no difference in the idiotype profile of T independent versus T dependent.

SISKIND: Did you find more doubles in the T-dependent assay that would or could favor a capture hypothesis?

KEARNEY: We found more doubles that could favor a capture.

SISKIND: It could be consistent with a capture.

KEARNEY: I am sure many in the audience would not agree with that conclusion.

A. MILLER (*University of California, Los Angeles*): Would you tell us your methods for detecting mixture mu.

KEARNEY: Our method is to coat a panel of ten or so monoclonals, coat with one idiotype, put on the serum, and μ presumably would have enough free binding sites. One puts on a panel of other anti-idiotope antibodies, and you should be able to detect a clone that has two populations of μ, unless of course they are on the same molecule. I presume, however, that they are not.

MILLER: Haven't you done the experiment?

KEARNEY: We are doing it at the moment.

UNIDENTIFIED SPEAKER: Dr. Kearney, this GB10 anti-idiotope detects only the heavy and light.

KEARNEY: Yes.

D. A. ROWLEY (*University of Chicago, Chicago, Ill.*): You have generated in an immunized mouse the cells that are producing an anti-idiotype that is demonstrably regulatory. Would it be impossible to go back and see that clone arise again spontaneously?

KEARNEY: That is what we would hope.

ROWLEY: The problem, it seems to me, is not whether they appear; it is whether they ever expand or can be expanded. How do you go about finding that out? That is my question.

KEARNEY: How these antibodies expand is an explanation for why these kinds of antibodies are not found more frequently. The possibility exists that they may not have to be activated or proliferate. They may secrete antibody in a microenvironment.

ROWLEY: This occurs in the presence of great excesses of idiotype.

R. KALISH (*Downstate Medical Center, Brooklyn, N.Y.*): If I understand you correctly your MM60 that is an anti-(anti-idiotype) antibody—which would be an Ab3, if you put it into your system—induces higher levels of Ab2 activity that suppress the immune response.

KEARNEY: That is an interpretation.

KALISH: Earlier this morning you said that anti-idiotype antibody can either suppress or enhance the immune response within a given idiotope, depending on the concentration. If you put it in nanogram amounts it will cause stimulation; if you put in higher amounts it will cause suppression. So given this, is it not possible that the suppression of the immune response you see now is dose dependent, whereas if you gave it at a high level of your MM60, it would cause suppression of Ab2 and enhance the immune response? If you gave a low level of your MM60, would it cause enhancement of Ab2 and a suppressed immune response?

KEARNEY: We have done the experiment from very wide-ranging doses of MM60, and all we have obtained, if anything, is suppression. We have not seen enhancement.

KALISH: Thank you.

D. SACHS (*National Institutes of Health, Bethesda, Md.*): Was your answer to Dr. Mosier's question on a statistical basis, that the 80% of your 50% of your clones would have come from a single precursor as opposed to two separate cells? Was that statement made on the basis of a statistical argument sequence or from idiotypic profile?

KEARNEY: It was from comparing the idiotypic profile of different clones.

SACHS: Was the comparison with the monoclonal anti-idiotypes?

KEARNEY: Yes.

SACHS: Dr. Rajewsky had an example where a single point mutation led to loss of all of these monoclonal anti-idiotypic reactivities. He cited another case where he had a gene conversion and a massive difference of sequence and yet retained all of the idiotypic specificities. So I think without sequence data, it would be very hard to make that statistical argument.

SISKIND: I think the message that it is hard to use monoclonal anti-Id as clonal markers has come across clear enough from many different sources. Monoclonal anti-Id just do not turn out to be the poor man's sequencer.

The Effect of Somatic Mutation on Antibody Affinity[a]

PATRICIA J. GEARHART

Department of Biochemistry
School of Hygiene and Public Health
The Johns Hopkins University
Baltimore, Maryland 21205

Antibody variable region diversity is produced by a variety of mechanisms acting on genes during the developmental stages of B cells. In early B cells, multiple variable (V), diversity (D), and joining (J) gene segments join to produce complete variable regions. This phenomenon represents the germ line repertoire of V regions for heavy and light chains, which is expressed in IgM molecules. At a later stage in B-cell development, a mutational mechanism mutates V genes. This somatically generated repertoire is frequently expressed in IgG and IgA molecules.[1] Thus, the repertoire of secondary B cells contains both germ line-encoded and variant antibodies. To determine the effect of somatic mutation on the affinity of antibodies, we compared the affinities of several germ line and variant anti-phosphorylcholine antibodies taken from immunized mice. The hybridoma protein sequences were defined by nucleotide and amino acid sequencing, and association constants for diazophenylphosphorylcholine were obtained by fluorescence quenching. The affinities of the variant immunoglobulins were fivefold higher than their germ line-encoded counterparts.

GERM LINE AND VARIANT ANTIBODIES DERIVED FROM ONE V_K GENE AND ONE V_H GENE

To directly compare the affinities of both germ line and variant antibodies, a series of hybridoma proteins derived from one V_K gene, V_{K167}, and one V_H gene, V_{HT15}, were studied. In the V_{K167} light chain group, Selsing and Storb[2] and Gershenfeld et al.[3] have shown that only one germ line gene encodes these V regions. We found that the V_{K167} gene consistently rearranges next to the J_{K5} gene in anti-phosphorylcholine antibodies. The protein sequences of V_{K167} light chains derived from antibody-secreting cells were compared to the published germ line nucleotide sequences of the V_{K167} and J_{K5} gene segments to identify variant antibodies. As shown in FIGURE 1, three V_K regions are germ line: HPCM27, HPCG9, and HPCG10; and one is variant: HPCG13. Although HPCG10 does not have amino acid substitutions, it does have extensive nucleotide substitutions in the noncoding flanking regions surrounding the gene.[5] The amino acid substitution in HPCG13 is due to a single nucleotide substitution.

In the V_{HT15} group of heavy chains, Crews et al.[6] showed that only one gene, V_{HT15}, codes for anti-phosphorylcholine heavy chains. The V_{HT15} gene rearranges next to the J_{H1} gene in anti-phosphorylcholine antibodies. Therefore the sequences of hybridoma V_H regions were compared to the germ line nucleotide sequences of the V_{HT15} gene, J_{H1} gene, and a prototype D segment.[1,6,7] As shown in FIGURE 2, two V_H regions are germ line: HPCM27 and HPCG9, and two have substitutions: HPCG10 and HPCG13.

[a]This work was supported in part by National Institutes of Health Grant CA25507.

171

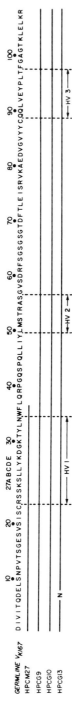

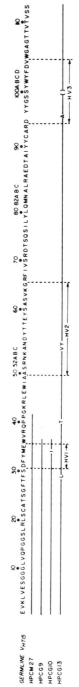

FIGURE 1. Protein sequences of V$_{K167}$-J$_{K5}$ light chain variable regions. The one-letter code for amino acids is used. The horizontal lines signify identity with the germ line sequence shown at the top. HV designates the hypervariable regions. The sequence of HPCM27 was determined by amino acid sequencing. The sequences of HPCG9, HPCG10, and HPCG13 were determined from nucleotide sequencing.[5]

FIGURE 2. Protein sequences of heavy chains with the V$_{HT15}$, D, and J$_{H1}$ gene segments. [ ] indicates a deletion. Sequences were determined by amino acid sequencing.[1]

Substitutions in both variants are found in the hypervariable regions that bind antigen. The isoleucine substitution in HPCG10 and the four amino acid substitutions in HPCG13 are due to somatic mutation of the V_{HT15} gene segment. The insertion and deletion in the third hypervariable region of HPCG13 is due to imprecise joining of V_H, D, and J_H gene segments.

VARIANT ANTIBODIES HAVE HIGHER AFFINITY FOR ANTIGEN THAN THEIR GERM LINE-ENCODED COUNTERPARTS

Antigen binding by the intact antibody molecule affects both the heavy and light chains. FIGURES 1 and 2 show that HPCM27 and HPCG9 have germ line-encoded heavy and light chains, and HPCG10 and HPCG13 have variant heavy and light chains. Both variants have amino acid substitutions in hypervariable regions of the heavy chain, which may affect antigen binding. If B cells express variant antibodies with higher affinity for antigen than the germ line-encoded antibody, they may be preferentially stimulated by antigen and clonally expanded.

The affinities of the variant antibodies were initially measured with the phosphorylcholine hapten, and no difference in affinity was found.[1] The mice from which the hybridoma cells were derived, however, were immunized with a derivative of phospho-

TABLE 1. Increased Affinity of Variant Antibodies for Diazophenylphosphorylcholine[a]

	Class	Sequence	$K \times 10^5$ (M^{-1})
HPCM27	IgM	germ line	4.7
HPCG9	IgG_3	germ line	3.4
HPCG10	IgG_3	variant	20.6
HPCG13	IgG_1	variant	25.6

[a]Data from Rodwell et al.[8]

rylcholine diazophenylphosphorylcholine, linked to a protein carrier. The association constants of the germ line and variant antibodies for diazophenylphosphorylcholine were measured by fluorescence quenching with John Rodwell and Fred Karush.[8] The results in TABLE 1 show that the variant antibodies HPCG10 and HPCG13 have a fivefold increase in affinity compared to the germ line-encoded antibodies, HPCM27 and HPCG9. Therefore, mutation, presumably followed by antigen selection *in vivo,* can produce antibodies with higher affinity than their germ line-encoded counterparts.

SELECTION CANNOT ACCOUNT FOR SILENT MUTATIONS

Although selection may contribute to the mutation frequency, it is unlikely that selection accounts for all of the genetically silent mutations found around antibody genes. Nucleotide sequencing of genomic, rearranged V_{k167} genes from HPCG10 and HPCG13 has revealed that mutations occur as frequently in the 5' and 3' flanking sequences of the gene (0.8%) as in the coding region (0.6%).[5] Extensive mutation in the flanking regions of several rearranged V_{HT15} genes is also found.[9] No mutations were found in or around the constant C_K or C_H genes. Thus, there is no strong selection for mutations to accumulate in the coding region of the V gene. When a nucleotide substitution in the coding region causes an amino acid substitution that changes the affinity of the molecule, selection of the variant cell by antigen may occur in an immunized animal.

The rate of mutation around the rearranged V gene must be very high to produce a frequency of 0.8% unselected mutations. The elucidation of this very unusual mutational mechanism that produces extensive base substitutions around the rearranged V-J gene will require additional studies of a more dynamic character.

ACKNOWLEDGMENTS

I am grateful to the many collaborators who contributed to this study: Dan Bogenhagen, Richard Douglas, Lee Hood, Nelson Johnson, Fred Karush, and John Rodwell. I thank Nadine Nivera and Allison Patterson for technical help.

REFERENCES

1. GEARHART, P. J., N. D. JOHNSON, R. DOUGLAS & L. HOOD. 1981. IgG antibodies to phosphorylcholine exhibit more diversity than their IgM counterparts. Nature (London) **291:** 29–34.
2. SELSING, E. & U. STORB. 1981. Somatic mutation of immunoglobulin light-chain variable-region genes. Cell **25:** 47–58.
3. GERSHENFELD, H. K., A. TSUKAMOTO, I. L. WEISSMAN & R. JOHO. 1981. Somatic diversification is required to generate the V_K genes of MOPC 511 and MOPC 167 myeloma proteins. Proc. Natl. Acad. Sci. USA 78:7674–7678.
4. MAX, E. E., J. G. SEIDMAN & P. LEDER. 1979. Sequences of five potential recombination sites encoded close to an immunoglobulin K constant region gene. Proc. Nat. Acad. Sci. USA **76:** 3450–3454.
5. GEARHART, P. J. & D. F. BOGENHAGEN. 1983. Clusters of point mutations are found exclusively around rearranged antibody variable genes. Proc. Natl. Acad. Sci. USA **80:** 3439–3443.
6. CREWS, S., J. GRIFFIN, H. HUANG, K. CALAME & L. HOOD. 1981. A single V_H gene segment encodes the immune response to phosphorylcholine: Somatic mutation is correlated with the class of the antibody. Cell **25:** 59–66.
7. EARLY, P., H. HUANG, M. DAVIS, K. CALAME & L. HOOD. 1980. An immunoglobulin heavy chain variable region gene is generated from three segments of DNA: V_H, D and J_H. Cell **19:** 981–992.
8. RODWELL, J. D., P. J. GEARHART & F. KARUSH. 1983. Restriction in IgM expression. IV. Affinity analysis of monoclonal anti-phosphorylcholine antibodies. J. Immunol. **130:** 313–316.
9. KIM, S., M. DAVIS, E. SINN, P. PATTEN & L. HOOD. 1981. Antibody diversity: Somatic hypermutation of rearranged V_H genes. Cell **27:** 573–581.

DISCUSSION OF THE PAPER

A. MARKS (*University of Toronto, Toronto, Ontario, Canada*): Referring to Dr. Scharff's data where he finds an extraordinarily high rate of antigen-binding mutation, that is, one of seven cells, how can you deal with the paradox that what you may be seeing is a phenomenon that occurs during the isolation of your hybridoma (or essentially of myeloma in culture) and does not reflect what occurs in lymphocytes *in vivo*?

P. J. GEARHART: We do not see any mutations in the IgM hybridomas that are maintained the same way as the IgGs and the IgAs, and, second, I think it would be very interesting if mutation were to occur in culture, because that is how we could study the mechanism of mutation.

K. RAJEWSKY (*University of Cologne, Cologne, F.R.G.*): Dr. Gearhart, surely one would not argue with you that the mutations that you see are due to point mutations, but I think the extrapolation that you make, that in the system it is only point mutations that occur and that generate variants, is not based on any evidence. In fact, the mutations that you described could be interpreted as a mechanism that is only important at the end of a given immune response to make antibodies a little bit more specific than they originally are. That observation may be important or not, depending on the antigen one uses. Take for example, the situation Dr. Klinman was describing this morning, where the pre-B cells are expanding and the single clone is going from 1 cell to 800 cells in the repertoire that would then be expressed later in the immune system. I think one should be careful in extrapolating too much from a particular mechanism.

GEARHART: One cannot argue against the possibility of recombination or gene conversion going on among unrearranged genes during evolution to generate the germ line repertoire. In most cases, however, where the sequence of the germline gene is known and the sequences of the variant antibodies are known, mutation is due to single point mutations.

RAJEWSKY: I was talking about rearranged genes in the early B-cell populations that Dr. Klinman has just studied, for example. I really do not want to argue with the data you present. Surely they cannot be due to recombination, because you have the mutations downstream from the J segment. Let us not extrapolate too much. That is all I want to say.

G. W. SISKIND (*Cornell University Medical College, New York*): I think your point is essentially that the demonstration of one model is not evidence for ruling out another.

GEARHART: I think, Dr. Rajewsky, that you should look at your 3' sequences, because then you would have to say that some mutations might be due to point mutations.

RAJEWSKY: I think the argument is actually an important one, because the question deals with what the somatic mutations contribute to the antibody repertoire. It may very well be that the kinds of mutation that Dr. Gearhart is describing do not really contribute anything. In fact, you could look at the situation as a really new emergence of a germ line theory, because when you immunize a mouse with phosphorylcholine, it is not actually using lots of somatic mutants to generate a response. In fact the mouse is always using the same gene and is making a lot of mutation at the end of it. When you think about other possibilities of somatic processes in generating the antibody repertoire, then early processes in the repertoire might be much more important. In fact, whether there are processes of gene conversion or recombination occurring at these stages, is a very interesting question, which is completely untouched by these kinds of experiments.

J. CERNY (*University of Texas Medical Branch, Galveston, Tex.*): I would like to hear your comment about the apparent homogeneity of the sequences of IgM variable region phosphorylcholine hybridomas. I realize that the molecular probing and cytological probing are two different things, but surely the argument does not have the same power in both directions. I really do not see, as the people working with serology have seen, exactly how the same sequences of all IgM antibodies would result in such a remarkable heterogeneity.

GEARHART: Well, Dr. Cerny, it is hard to say without the structural data. Heterogeneity could be due to different germline D and J gene segments, and to diversity caused during VJ joining. It is hard to analyze your data without a structural basis.

D. SACHS (*National Institutes of Health, Bethesda, Md.*): How does your mechanism explain the failure to see mutations in IgM antibodies?

GEARHART: We think the mutational mechanism has not been activated yet. B cells producing IgM antibodies have a very short half-life, and unless they are recognized by antigen and either proliferate or become secondary cells, they die within a few days. A rearranged gene may act as a substrate for mutational enzymes within a cell. The enzymes may be developmentally activated at a later time.

SACHS: Do you believe that mutations occur before or after antigen exposure?

GEARHART: I do not know.

D. E. MOSIER (*Institute for Cancer Research, Philadelphia, Pa.*): I wanted to make a brief comment about some work that Dr. Luedtke is doing with anti-influenza hybridomas. These hybridomas were originally made by Dr. Walter Gerhard, and Dr. Luedtke has been analyzing both the DNA and the protein sequence of these hybridomas. What he finds is variability between IgM and IgG hybridomas. There is clear clonal evolution going on before the fusion process, that is, one can organize the hybridomas into families: those clearly derived from one early variant, those that gave rise to subsequent variants, and those that were captured by the fusion process. As one might predict, if you fuse early after immunization, the antibody structures are closer to germ line sequences than if you fuse later. One can calculate a mutation rate from this data, and it is close to the rate that you quote. In trying to calculate the data, however, one has to add the denominator of the time over which the events occur. We presume that these events begin with antigen exposure and are captured at the time of fusion. I wonder how you can derive a mutation rate that does not have a time factor.

GEARHART: I was careful not to mention the word rate. You are absolutely right. We can not measure rates, because we have not really kept track of how many divisions the cells have undergone. We refer to the data in terms of frequency.

MOSIER: How much does your data change if you exclude M511 and M167 myeloma proteins, which may have arisen long after antigen stimulation?

GEARHART: Both hybridomas taken a month after immunization had just as high a rate of mutation as M167 and M511.

SISKIND: I presume that when you showed us two hybridomas or two proteins that had somatic mutations that led to a higher affinity, that you were assuming that these had to occur randomly and that there would also be ones that were of lower affinity, and that you did not happen to sample them or that they were not expanded by antigen. Is that correct?

GEARHART: That is correct.

Antibody-Specific Regulation of Primary and Secondary B-Cell Responses

SUSAN K. PIERCE AND NANCY A. SPECK

Department of Biochemistry, Molecular Biology, and Cell Biology
Northwestern University
Evanston, Illinois 60201

Since its initial proposal by Neils Jerne,[1] certain elements of the network theory of immunoregulation have gained considerable experimental support. It has been shown that lymphocytes within an individual have the capability of recognizing their own antibody idiotypes. Idiotype-recognizing T cells and B cells have been demonstrated following various procedures that might be viewed as having the net effect of perturbing the homeostasis of the immune system. These include immunization of adult animals with antibody bearing the idiotype,[2-5] anti-idiotypic antibodies,[6] the antigen for which the idiotype is specific,[7-10] or by induction of neonatal tolerance to the idiotype.[11] Whereas the evidence for the existence of idiotype-specific T and B cells is strong, a functional role for such cells in regulating immune responses is not well established. Consequently, workers in this field are often left with the unsettling notion that the observation of idiotype-specific lymphocytes may be more an artifact of laboratory experiments than a manifestation of an important regulatory mechanism.

Several years ago, we carried out experiments to test the postulate that subsequent to primary immunization, an individual develops the ability to regulate the synthesis of antibody, specific for the stimulating antigen, through the recognition of the B-cell receptor.[12] If such a regulatory function does indeed develop, several predictions could be made concerning its specificity and target. First, such a regulatory function should be highly specific for the antibody idiotypes that are synthesized in the initial immune response, leaving antibody responses to unrelated antigens unaffected. Second, as secondary or memory humoral immune responses, by definition, occur in previously immunized animals, such a regulatory function must not effect memory B-cell responses.

To test this postulate, we evaluated the ability of hapten-specific B cells to respond to antigenic challenge following transfer to immune (hapten-carrier immunized) or nonimmune (carrier immunized) irradiated recipients.[12] If an immunoregulatory function did develop following immunization, we predicted that the response of nonimmune (primary) B cells in immune spleens should be quantitatively or qualitatively different than their response in nonimmune recipients. These studies were carried out using the splenic fragment culture system, as it enabled the quantitation of the primary B cells that were able to respond to an antigen in an immune versus a nonimmune splenic environment. The results of this study are summarized in TABLE 1. As shown, only approximately 30% of 2,4-dinitrophenyl (DNP) specific B cells from nonimmune mice are able to respond to DNP-hemocyanin (DNP-Hy) in DNP-Hy immunized irradiated recipients as compared to Hy immunized recipients. The inhibition of responses appeared to be specific for B cells that recognized the immunizing antigen, as the B-cell response to an unrelated antigen, fluorescein, was unaffected in DNP-Hy immunized recipients. The induction of the regulatory function following immunization appeared to be a general phenomenon, as subsequent studies demonstrated similar inhibition of antigen-specific primary B-cell responses following

177

TABLE 1. The Response of Primary and Secondary Hapten-Specific B Cells in Carrier versus Hapten-Carrier Immunized Recipients

| Donor B-Cell[a] Source | Recipient | Donor/Recipient Syngeny at Igh[b] | Recipient Immunization | In vitro Antigen[c] | | | |
| | | | | DNP-Hy | | F1-Hy | |
				Number Anti-DNP Specific Foci per 10^6 Cells Analyzed	Percent Control[d]	Number Anti-F1 Specific Foci per 10^6 Cells Analyzed	Percent Control
BALB/c	BALB/c	+	Hy	1.83	100	1.40	100
BALB/c	BALB/c	+	DNP-Hy	0.54	29	1.50	107
CB20	BALB/c	−	Hy	1.87	100		
CB20	BALB/c	−	DNP-Hy	2.00	107		
DNP-Hy BALB/c	BALB/c	+	Hy	3.48	100		
DNP-Hy BALB/c	BALB/c	+	DNP-Hy	3.39	97		

[a]B cells were obtained from spleens of nonimmune mice or mice that had been immunized 4 to 8 weeks earlier with 0.1 mg DNP-Hy is complete Freund's adjuvant (CFA).

[b]Donor and recipient animals are congeneic inbred strains that are either identical or dissimilar at the Igh gene locus.

[c]Fragment cultures prepared from recipient spleens were stimulated with either DNP-Hy or F1-Hy in vitro at $10^{-6}M$ hapten concentration. Culture fluids were assayed for the presence of anti-DNP and anti-F1 antibody respectively.

[d]The percent control is percent of B-cell responses in Hy-immunized mice.

transfer to recipients immunized to a wide variety of antigens including influenza virus, phosphorylcholine (PC) and (4-hydroxy-3 nitrophenyl) acetyl (NP).

The specificity of the antigen-induced regulation suggested that the target molecule of the regulatory function may be the immunogobulin receptor of the B cell. To test this, donor and recipient strains were selected that were congeneic at the immunoglobulin heavy chain locus (Igh). As shown in TABLE 1, the majority of DNP-specific primary B cells of the BALB/c strain (Igh^a) were suppressed in DNP-Hy immunized BALB/c recipients, whereas primary B cells of the CB20 strain (Igh^b) were not. Thus, the target of the antigen-induced regulatory function appeared to be the immunoglobulin of the B cell.

Not all B-cell subpopulations, however, appeared to be susceptible to regulation. As shown in TABLE 1, in contrast to the observation using primary B cells, the response of B cells from DNP-Hy primed mice (secondary B cells) were similar in Hy and DNP-Hy primed recipients. Thus, the B lymphocytes obtained from immunized animals that had developed an antibody-specific regulatory function were not susceptible to its regulation. The time course of the induction of antibody-specific suppression and the induction of B cells that were refractory to its effects are presented in TABLE 2. As shown, both appear as early as can be measured, approximately 1 to 2 weeks following immunization.[12,13]

In order to determine which cells in the immunized recipients were required to mediate the suppressive function, adoptive transfer experiments were carried out.[14] To do so, T- and B-cell populations were purified from immunized mice and transferred to irradiated (700R) Hy-primed recipients. Reconstituted animals were given a second dose of radiation (600R) and used as recipients of donor B cells in the splenic fragment culture system. It was determined that suppression of primary B-cell responses required the transfer of Ly-2.2$^+$ T cells from hapten-carrier primed mice and that equivalent numbers of B cells from immune mice did not transfer suppression (TABLE 3).

To further characterize this T-cell population, we determined if its function

TABLE 2. The Induction of Antibody-Specific Regulation is Coincident with the Induction of Refractory B Cells

Weeks Following Hapten-Carrier, Immunization^a	Antibody-Specific Regulation Induced^b	Percent Hapten-Specific B Cells Refractory to Regulation^c
0	−	14
1	NT^d	17
2	+	54
3	+	72
4–6	+	94
>12	+	97

^{a}Animals were immunized with a hapten-carrier conjugate in CFA and analyzed at various times following immunization to determine if the antibody-specific regulatory function has developed, and if the B-cell population has become refractory to suppression.

^{b}The ability of an animal to suppress a primary B-cell response is scored as + when less than 30% of primary B cells transferred to it are able to respond, as compared to the response of the same B-cell population in carrier-immunized animals.

^{c}The percent B cells refractory to regulation is determined by the ability of the B-cell population to respond in a hapten-carrier versus carrier-primed environment.

^{d}This point not tested.

TABLE 3. Suppression of Hapten-Specific Primary B-Cell Responses Can Be Adoptively Transferred by T Lymphocytes but Not by B Lymphocytes

Adoptive Host Immunization	Adoptive Host Reconstitution[a]	Total Number Donor Cells Analyzed $\times 10^{-6}$	Number NP-Specific Foci per 10^6 Cells Analyzed	Percent Control
Hy	—	20	1.2	100
NP-Hy	—	20	0.3	25
Hy	3×10^7 NP-Hy T	10	0.4	33
Hy	3×10^7 NP-Hy T Anti-Ly 2.2 + C	10	1.0	83
Hy	3×10^7 NP-Hy B	10	1.0	83

[a]Irradiated recipients (700R) received 3×10^7 purified T cells, purified B cells, or anti-Lyt-2.2 and complement (C)-treated T cells from NP-Hy immunized BALB/c donors. T cells were purified by panning on anti-Fab'$_2$ coated plates, and B cells were purified by treating donor cells with anti-Thy-1.2 and C.[14] Recipient animals subsequently received an additional 600R radiation and were used as the recipients of primary B cells in the fragment culture system.

required the joint recognition of both Igh and major histocompatibility complex (MHC) gene products in a manner similar to T cells that recognized conventional antigens.[14] These experiments were feasible as we had previously demonstrated that collaborative interactions can occur between MHC dissimilar T cells and B cells in the fragment culture system.[15,16] At the same time, collaborative interactions in this system do manifest an MHC restriction that is demonstrable by the isotype of the resulting antibody.[15,16] The question concerning the MHC restriction of antibody-specific T cells has recently become a rather important issue as several laboratories have presented evidence that suggests that T cells that function through the recognition of antibody idiotypes do not require the joint recognition of the MHC gene products.[17-19] By contrast to these reports, the results of our studies demonstrated that only donor B cells that shared both MHC and Igh genetic identity with hapten-carrier primed recipients were suppressed, whereas responses of either MHC dissimilar or Igh dissimilar B cells were unaffected. Thus, at least in this system, the T-cell mediated antibody-specific function was dependent on the presence of both the appropriate Igh and MHC encoded molecules on the target B cells. As these studies were carried out using whole splenic T-cell populations, it is not possible to determine which cell interactions were MHC restricted. It is possible, for example, that there were several T-cell interactions that were essential for suppression of the B-cell responses. Certain of these may be restricted only by Igh, others by major histocompatibility complex. Studies to dissect these are in progress (TABLE 4).

Thus far, these studies have demonstrated two parallel events that occur following immunization. The first was the generation of an antibody-recognizing T-cell function that served to suppress primary B-cell responses. The second was the induction of a B-cell population that was refractory to its effects. As the immune potential of an individual in which an antibody-specific function is induced is presumably maintained through the generation of a refractory B-cell population, it is important to understand the condition under which refractory secondary B cells are generated. Of particular interest is the role of T cells in the generation of a refractory B-cell population. As shown in TABLE 5, we have determined that refractory B-cell populations can be generated in the absence of T cells in athymic BALB/c nude mice by immunization with either the T-dependent antigen DNP-Hy or the T-independent antigen DNP-Ficoll.[13] In both instances, the frequency of DNP-specific B cells increased and the majority of B cells became refractory to antibody-specific regulation. Whereas, by this

TABLE 4. Syngeny at Both Major Histocompatibility Complex and Igh Is Necessary for Effective Suppression of Hapten-Specific Primary B-Cell Responses

Donor[a]	Donor Priming	Recipient	Donor-Recipient Syngeny		Recipient Immunization[b]	Total Number Cells Analyzed $\times 10^{-6}$	Foci per 10^6 Donor Cells Analyzed[c]	Percent Control
			MHC	Igh				
B10.D2	—	B10.D2	+	+	Hy	12	3.0	100
					NP-Hy	12	1.1	36
BALB/c	—	B10.D2	+	−	Hy	8	2.7	100
					NP-Hy	12	2.3	84
B6	—	B10.D2	−	+	Hy	20	2.0	100
					NP-Hy	10	2.1	105
B6	—	B6	+	+	Hy	20	2.3	100
					NP-Hy	15	0.7	30
B10.D2	—	B6	−	+	Hy	12	5.0	100
					NP-Hy	15	1.6	123
B6	NP-Hy	B6	+	+	Hy	12	5.0	100
					NP-Hy	12	5.0	100
B10.D2	NP-Hy	B10.D2	+	+	Hy	4	8.8	100
					NP-Hy	4	8.1	92

[a]Donor cells were obtained from either nonimmune animals or animals immunized with 0.1 mg NP-Hy 6 weeks prior to use. Between 1 and 3×10^6 donor cells were transferred to each recipient.

[b]Animals to be used as recipients recieved one injection of 0.1 mg Hy in CFA 8 weeks prior to use followed by 0.1 mg of either Hy or NP-Hy in saline 4 weeks prior to use.

[c]Fragment cultures were stimulated *in vitro* with NP-Hy (10^{-6} M NP), and culture fluids were assayed for the presence of NP-specific antibodies.

TABLE 5. The Role of T Cells in the Induction of a Refractory B-Cell Population

Donor Cells[a]	Donor Immunization[b]	Recipient Immunization	Number Donor Cells Analyzed $\times 10^{-6}$	Number Foci per 10^6 Cells Transferred[c]	Percent Response in Hy-primed Recipients	Percent Response IgG[d]
BALB/c	—	Hy	45	1.35	100	60
	DNP-Hy	DNP-Hy	32	0.18	14	—
BALB/c	DNP-Hy	Hy	30	3.50	100	95
	DNP-Hy	DNP-Hy	22	3.30	94	—
BALB/c	DNP-Ficoll	Hy	69	2.00	100	50
	DNP-Ficoll	DNP-Hy	47	1.10	54	—
BALB/c nude	—	Hy	85	1.10	100	35
	—	DNP-Hy	117	0.43	39	—
BALB/c nude	DNP-Hy	Hy	67	0.91	100	75
	DNP-Hy	DNP-Hy	37	0.85	93	—
BALB/c nude	DNP-Ficoll	Hy	30	4.76	100	84
	DNP-Ficoll	DNP-Hy	13	4.92	103	—

[a]Between 2×10^6 and 5×10^6 donor spleen cells were transferred to each irradiated (1300 r) recipient.
[b]Donor mice received one intraperitoneal injection of 0.1 mg DNP-Hy or DNP-Ficoll 4–6 weeks before use.
[c]The number of DNP-specific foci was determined.
[d]The percent of antibody-producing clones synthesizing antibody of the IgG_1 heavy chain isotype is shown. These clones may also synthesize IgM antibody. Clones not synthesizing IgG_1 antibody were demonstrated to synthesize IgM or IgA antibody.

criteria, the generation of refractory B-cell populations did not require T cells, the event can apparently be regulated by T cells if they are present during immunization, but not actively involved in promoting B-cell responses. This phenomenon is observed in the B-cell population of DNP-Ficoll immunized euthymic mice (TABLE 5). As compared to the DNP-specific B cells of DNP-Ficoll immunized athymic nude mice, the B cells of DNP-Ficoll immunized euthymic mice did not increase in frequency, and the majority of B cells were sensitive to regulation. Thus, although the B-cell population has the potential to both expand and acquire a refractory character in the absence of T cells, neither occurs in the presence of T cells following T-independent immunization. As is also summarized in TABLE 5, the immunization of athymic nude mice with either DNP-Hy or DNP-Ficoll induced a shift in the predominant secreted isotype to IgG from IgM or IgA.[20] Whereas a similar shift in the secreted isotype expression also occurred in DNP-Hy immunized euthymic mice, it did not occur in DNP-Ficoll immunized euthymic mice as shown in TABLE 5. Thus, there appears to be a cell, presumably a T cell, present in euthymic mice that has the potential to regulate the expansion, isotype expression, and acquisition of a refractory character by the B-cell population. Studies are in progress to determine the nature of this cell population.

Having defined a B-cell population that is refractory to T-cell antibody-specific regulation, it was important to attempt to determine the molecular basis of this refractory state. From a very simplistic point of view, the refractoriness could be accounted for in one of two ways. First, the secondary B-cell idiotype repertoire specific for a particular hapten may not have been identical to the primary B-cell repertoire specific for the same hapten. If this were the case, a T-cell regulatory function generated in response to the primary B-cell repertoire would not recognize the secondary B-cell repertoire. The refractory character would then be a consequence of the B cell's escaping surveillance by idiotype-specific T cells. Alternatively, the secondary B cells may have borne receptors that were a subset of those expressed by the primary B-cell repertoire. The secondary B cell, however, may have differentiated such that it was no longer susceptible to a T-cell signal delivered through its receptor. This finding could be thought of as analogous to the relative susceptibility to tolerance induction of neonatal as compared to adult B cells bearing the same immunoglobulin idiotype.[21] We have initiated studies to begin to test these alternatives. It is important to stress that these analyses are in the initial stages, and whereas certain interesting results have been obtained, these are not conclusive.

In the first case, it is difficult to determine if the primary and secondary idiotype repertoires are identical, as probes to identify all expressed V regions do not exist. Consequently, we approached the question in a somewhat different fashion and asked how extensive the T-cell recognition of antibody was following immunization. Were all possible antibody V regions recognized by the T-cell population within an immune individual even when the V regions were generated by somatic mutational mechanisms? We were able to approach this question as a series of PC-binding hybridoma and myeloma proteins became available for which the amino acid sequence of the proteins[22] and the genes encoding these sequences[23] had been determined. The analysis of these antibody heavy chain V regions provided very strong evidence that they represented a germ line encoded V region and somatic mutants of these V regions. In addition, an analysis of the heavy chain isotypes of these antibodies demonstrated a striking correlation between the expression of the germ line encoded sequence and the IgM heavy chain isotype.[22] By contrast, somatic variants of the germ line encoded sequence were expressed with heavy chain constant regions other than IgM, notably the IgG isotypes. This correlation had very interesting implications concerning the expression of these antibodies during conventional immune responses.

We carried out experiments to determine if the T-cell population within PC-Hy immunized animals was able to recognize both the germ line encoded and somatic variant antibodies.[10] To measure recognition, we asked that the T-cell population provide a helper function to 2,4,6-trinitrophenyl (TNP)-specific B cells in response to the antigen TNP coupled antibodies. These studies were carried out in the fragment culture system and are summarized in TABLE 6. As shown, the T-cell population's recognition of PC-binding antibodies in PC-Hy immunized mice was quite extensive and included both germ line encoded and somatic variant antibodies. By contrast, there was no recognition of the DNP-binding antibody M460 in PC-Hy primed mice and no recognition of PC-binding antibodies in Hy primed mice. At least a portion of T cells recognized a determinant shared in common between germ line encoded, and somatic variant antibodies as immunization with one antibody, T15, induced recognition of all other antibodies tested. Whereas this analysis does not allow us to draw conclusions

TABLE 6. T Cells in Phosphorylcholine-Hemocyanin Immunized Animals Recognize both Germ Line Encoded Antibodies and the Somatically Generated Variants of These Antibodies[a]

In Vitro Antigens	Antigen-Binding Specificity	Heavy Chain Isotype	Germ Line Encoded IgVh	T15 Idiotype Positive	Helper Function Provided in Recipients Primed to:		
					PC-Hy	Hy	T15
TNP-T15	PC	IgA	+	+	+	−	+
TNP-M460	DNP	IgA	NT	−	−	−	NT
TNP-M167	PC	IgA	−	−	+	−	NT
TNP-HPCM2	PC	IgM	+	+	+	−	+
TNP-HPCG8	PC	IgG_3	−	+	+	−	+
TNP-HPCG11	PC	IgG_3	−	+	+	−	+
TNP-HPCG15	PC	IgG_1	−	−	+	−	+
TNP-HPCG9	PC	IgG_3	−	−	+	−	+
TNP-HPCG13	PC	IgG_1	−	−	+	−	+

[a]Primary B cells were transferred to irradiated recipient animals that had been immunized with either PC-Hy, Hy, or the affinity-purified T15 antibody 6 to 8 weeks prior to use. Spleen fragment cultures were subsequently prepared from recipient spleens and stimulated in vitro with the TNP-coupled antibodies listed. Culture fluids were analyzed for the presence of TNP-specific antibody. A positive response was scored when the frequency of B-cell responses was >0.5 per 10^6 cells analyzed. Negative responses were <0.1 foci per 10^6 cells analyzed, which in all cases indicated undetectable B-cell responses.

concerning the function of these antibody-recognizing T cells in regulating the response of B cells bearing these receptors, it does demonstrate that there are no obvious holes in the T-cell repertoire specific for PC-binding antibodies that might allow secondary B cells to escape surveillance.

To approach the second possibility, that the refractory secondary B cells had differentiated such that they were no longer sensitive to a regulatory signal delivered through their immunoglobulin receptor, we attempted to correlate the induction of an independent character of secondary B cells, with the induction of the refractory character. Whereas there are few defined characteristics of secondary B cells, one possible correlation was that of the cell's isotype expression, both cell surface and secreted. As stated earlier, we did observe that the generation of the refractory character correlated with the preference for IgG_1 antibody secretion in vitro (TABLE 5). To determine if the refractory character was correlated with the expression of cell

TABLE 7. An Analysis of Isotype Expression under Conditions That Induce Refractory B Cells

Donor[a]	Donor Immunization[b]	B-Cell Population Refractory to Regulation	Panning Reagent[c]	Total Number Cells Analyzed $\times 10^{-6}$	Number Foci per 10^6 Cells Transferred	Percent Response IgG[d]
BALB/c	—	—	—	96	1.60	47.5
			anti-μ	93	.29	41.5
BALB/c	DNP-Hy	+	—	30	3.50	58.5
			anti-μ	126	.54	92.6
BALB/c	DNP-Ficoll	—	—	44	1.60	33.3
			anti-μ	42	1.08	13.2
BALB/c nude	—	—	—	76	.82	34.6
			anti-μ	130	.40	2.5
BALB/c nude	DNP-Hy	+	—	18	1.74	42.5
			anti-μ	100	.57	64.9
BALB/c nude	DNP-Ficoll	+	—	30	4.76	84.3
			anti-μ	43	1.67	84.5

[a]Between 2 and 6×10^6 donor cells were transferred to each carrier-primed irradiated (1300R) recipient.

[b]Donor mice were immunized 6 to 8 weeks prior to cell transfer with 0.1 mg DNP-Hy in CFA intraperitoneally.

[c]Donor cell populations were panned for μ-bearing cells. This was accomplished according to the method of Wysocki and Sato (24). Petri dishes were coated with affinity-purified goat-anti-rabbit Ig. Spleen cell populations were incubated at 4° C with rabbit anti-mouse IgM antibody for 30 minutes, washed twice, and incubated at 4° C on the antibody coated plates. Nonabsorbed cells were removed from the plate and analyzed in the fragment culture system.

[d]Antibody producing foci not synthesizing antibody of the IgG$_1$ heavy chain isotype synthesized either IgM or IgA antibody.

surface IgG, we attempted to remove IgG synthesizing cells by "panning," using anti-IgM antibody. We analyzed the B cells derived from DNP-Ficoll or DNP-Hy immunized euthymic and athymic mice. A summary of these experiments is shown in TABLE 7. It appears that panning B lymphocytes using anti-IgM antibody has the potential to remove the majority of IgG_1 secreting B cells from susceptible but not refractory populations. This suggests that the IgG_1 antibody response in refractory populations is due to B cells that bear receptor isotypes other than IgM, presumably IgG_1. Whereas this analysis must be confirmed using techniques to directly recover IgM- and IgG-bearing B cells, it suggests that the shift to IgG expression occurs in parallel to the acquisition of refractory B cells. Experiments are in progress to directly test if IgG expression is necessary for the refractory state.

The finding of a B-cell population that is insensitive to an antibody-specific regulatory function is important to the consideration of the role of such regulatory functions in conventional immune responses. In this instance, an antibody-specific regulatory function was induced following immunization that persisted in the animal for months after immunization, and was capable of suppressing the response of primary B cells. At the same time the induction of antibody-specific regulation did not adversely affect the ability to mount a secondary antibody response, as there was a concomitant generation of a B-cell population that was insensitive to suppression. The results of these experiments[12,13] and others[20] have indicated that the vast majority of B cells in an immune individual have the characteristics of secondary B cells, and few, if any, primary B cells persist in the immune individual. It may be that once a memory B-cell population has been established, the observed antibody-specific regulatory function serves to regulate the expression of primary B cells that continue to rise from bone marrow precursor cells during an individual's lifetime. Consistent with this notion is the observation that a primary like B-cell population persists in immunized athymic nude mice, which do not develop antibody-specific regulation, but do acquire a secondary like B-cell population.[20] Thus, in the absence of T cells, B cells with primary and secondary characteristics coexist. In the presence of T cells, the vast majority of B cells are secondary, and few if any primary B cells are maintained.

Whereas these experiments demonstrate that secondary B cells are not sensitive to the suppressive effects of the antibody-specific immunoregulation, we do not want to rule out the possibility that antibody-specific regulatory cells may play an active role in the promotion or maintenance of the memory B-cell population. The results of Woodland and Cantor[25] and Bottomly and coworkers[26] have suggested that idiotype-recognizing T cells are required for the promotion of B-cell responses. Our own analysis of T-helper cell functions have demonstrated that a single antigen specific T cell is capable of promoting primary B-cell responses and that the helper function is not restricted to a single isotype or idiotype.[27,28] It is possible, however, that such restrictions occur in T-helper cell–memory B-cell collaborative interaction. Studies to test this possibility are in progress.

In summary, we have described two parallel and interrelated events that occur following immunization. The first is the generation of antibody-specific T cells that serve to suppress primary B-cell responses. The second is the induction of a secondary B-cell population that is refractory to its effects. Studies in progress should further elucidate the specificity and nature of the regulatory T cells and the refractory B-cell population.

REFERENCES

1. JERNE, N. K. 1974. Ann. Immunol. Inst. Pastuer (Paris) 12SC: 373.
2. GLEASON, K., S. PIERCE & H. KOHLER. 1981. J. Exp. Med. 153: 924.

3. Bona, C. & W. E. Paul. 1979. J. Exp. Med. **149:** 592.
4. McKearn, J. P. & J. Quintans. 1980. Fed. Proc. Fed. Am. Soc. Exp. Biol. **39** (Suppl. 3): 1607.
5. Sy, M. S., B. A. Bach, A. Brown, A. Nisonoff, B. Benacerraf & M. I. Greene. 1979. J. Exp. Med. **150:** 1229.
6. Hetzelberger, D. & K. Eichmann. 1978. Eur. J. Immunol. **8:** 846.
7. Kluskens, L. & H. Kohler. 1974. Proc. Nat. Acad. Sci. USA **71:** 5083.
8. Goidl, E. A., A. F. Schrater, G. W. Siskind & G. J. Thorbecke. 1979. J. Exp. Med. **150:** 138.
9. Kelsoe, G. & J. Cerny. 1979. Nature (London) **279:** 333.
10. Pierce, S. K., N. A. Speck, K. Gleason, P. Gearhart & H. Kohler. 1981. J. Exp. Med. **154:** 1178.
11. Strayer, D. S., W. M. F. Lee, D. A. Rowley & H. Kohler. 1975. J. Immunol. **114:** 728.
12. Pierce, S. K. & N. R. Klinman. 1977. J. Exp. Med. **146:** 509.
13. Speck, N. A. & S. K. Pierce. 1982. Eur. J. Immunol. **12:** 449.
14. Speck, N. A. & S. K. Pierce. 1982. Eur. J. Immunol. **12:** 972.
15. Pierce, S. K. & N. R. Klinman. 1976. J. Exp. Med. **144:** 1254.
16. Pierce, S. K., N. R. Klinman, P. H. Maurer & C. F. Merryman. 1980. J. Exp. Med. **152:** 336.
17. Bottomly, K. & P. H. Maurer. 1980. J. Exp. Med. **152:** 1571.
18. Yamauchi, K., D. Murphy, H. Cantor & R. K. Gershon. 1981. Eur. J. Immunol. **11:** 905.
19. Juy, D., D. Primo, P. Sanchez & P. Cazenave. 1982. Eur. J. Immunol. **12:** 24.
20. Speck, N. A. & S. K. Pierce. 1981 J. Exp. Med. **155:** 574.
21. Metcalf, E. S. & N. R. Klinman. 1976. J. Exp. Med. **143:** 1327.
22. Gearhart, P., N. D. Johnson, R. Douglas & L. Hood, 1981. Nature (London) **291:** 29.
23. Crews, S., J. Griffin, H. Huang, K. Calome & Hood. 1981. Cell **25:** 59.
24. Wysocki, L. G. & V. L. Sato. 1978. Proc. Nat. Acad. Sci. USA **75:** 2844.
25. Woodland, R. & H. Cantor. 1978. Eur. J. Immunol. **8:** 606.
26. Bottomly, K. & D. E. Mosier. 1979. J. Exp. Med. **150:** 1344.
27. Pierce, S. K., M. P. Cancro & N. R. Klinman. 1978. J. Exp. Med. **148:** 759.
28. Pierce, S. K., & N. R. Klinman. 1980. Eur. J. Immunol. **11:** 71.

DISCUSSION OF THE PAPER

J. Cerny (*University of Texas Medical Branch, Galveston, Tex.*): I would like to ask you about the apparent restriction of your T-suppressor cells that presumably are directed against idiotypic determinants. Both the Ig locus and H2 locus regulate expression of idiotypes, as several laboratories have shown. Is it possible that instead of restriction, that you are looking at absence of the target molecule?

S. K. Pierce: That is exactly right. We worried that, in fact, in an MHC dissimilar animal, the primary B-cell repertoire would be different. We analyzed the ability of F1 animals to suppress parent and reciprocal combinations, and we eliminated that as an obvious explanation for the escape of the majority of cells.

A. Augustin (*University of Colorado, Denver*): I understand that the first population of B cells seems to be restricted. Did you try to map the restriction?

Pierce: That was not measured.

Augustin: I ask this question because it appears that the function of the assay in the PC binding myeloma and the function for the first set of idiotype specific T cells are different.

PIERCE: Absolutely.

AUGUSTIN: If you do not have restriction data and you assay also for a different function, then you cannot make an equation between these two types of cells. The second one is obviously a T-helper cell population.

PIERCE: The analysis has been done with the recognition of the soluble antibody, and that is similarly MHC restricted. In that case, we used an I region congeneic, but we do not have the precise restriction data. You saw the recombinant that we used. This, however, does not get to your more important point, that until we actually do the experiment, we cannot relate these antibody-recognizing cells in this experiment to the functional cell. I think it was the only way to ask one question, which was, is there any glaring hole in the T-cell repertoire for recognition of germ line versus somatic variants. And I think we have somewhat of an answer to that, but we clearly do not yet want to make an extrapolation to the function of those antibody-recognizing cells.

AUGUSTIN: I would propose an answer to that question, and I will elaborate tomorrow about this point. We have data in our laboratory that suggest very strongly that T-helper cells that recognize T15-like idiotypes exhibit structures that mimic phosphorylcholine. Could that be compatible with your data? I am going to bring evidence tomorrow about that topic.

PIERCE: If it is actually PC-like epilope T cells, then that is right.

AUGUSTIN: What you assay on are myelomas that bind for phosphorylcholine. Is that what all of them definitely have in common?

PIERCE: That they bear a phosphorylcholine determinant is what they also have in common.

Restricting Elements in the Immunological Circuitry: the Role of I Region-Controlled Determinants

TOMIO TADA, KO OKUMURA, SEIJI MIYATANI,
ATSUO OCHI, HIROMITSU NAKAUCHI, AND
HAJIME KARASUYAMA

Department of Immunology
Faculty of Medicine
University of Tokyo
Tokyo, Japan

INTRODUCTION

Unlike the network concept that applies to the regulation mediated by the variable region of antigen-recognition molecules regardless of the cell types carrying such variable region structures, the circuit idea is primarily concerned with the sequential activation of different types of immunocompetent cells, regardless of the structure responsible for such selective interactions. Two major restricting elements have been proposed in the circuit type regulation based on the fact that the matching of either immunoglobulin V_H or major histocompatibility complex (MHC) between two different cell types was necessary for an effective and meaningful cell interaction. We have reported in the carrier-specific regulation of the antibody response by T cells that MHC products play important roles in the sequential activation of the suppressor or augmenting pathway.[1] In the suppressor circuit, the antigen-specific T-suppressor cell factor ($T_S F$) derived from the Lyt-2^+ T-suppressor cell (T_S) carries I region determinants controlled by an I-J subregion gene and acts on the responding cells derived from strains sharing the same I-J subregion haplotype.[2] In the case of augmentation, the augmenting factor ($T_A F$) derived from the Lyt-1^+ T cell (T_A) has determinants controlled by an I-A subregion gene and augments the response of I-A subregion compatible strains.[3] The treatment of responding cells with conventional anti-I-J and anti-I-A results in the inability of acceptance of $T_S F$ and $T_A F$ effects. In addition, some but not all T-helper cells ($T_H 2$) carry an I-J determinant, which is serologically distinguishable from that expressed on T-suppressor cells.[4] These results suggested that the I region controls a series of determinants selectively expressed on T cells and that they are the major elements that restrict the cell interaction to lead to the suppression or augmentation of the immune response.

In order to delineate the mechanism of such restrictions, we have attempted to study the immunochemical properties of I region-controlled (Iat) determinants on T cells. Thus, we made a number of functional hybridomas and T-cell clones with T_S and Ta nature expressing different I region determinants distinguishable serologically with I region-specific alloantibodies.[5-7] We also developed several monoclonal antibodies that define such I region determinants with their exquisite specificites.[8] This paper deals with the serological and immunochemical analysis of Iat structures on hybridomas and cell lines, and considers the roles of such polymorphic determinants in the restricted interactions among the members in the immunological circuit.

HYBRIDOMAS AND T-CELL LINES

A T-cell hybridoma (FL10) of A/J (H-2^a) mouse origin producing a keyhole limpet hemocyanin (KLH)-specific $T_A F$ was described elsewhere.[6] This hybridoma has been known to possess the following characteristics: chromosome number 68 ± 6; positive for Thy-1.1 and Thy-1.2; IgV_H (framework structure of the heavy chain variable portion as detectable by rabbit anti-V_H[9]); and Lyt-1.2. Although an anti-Ia antiserum (B10.S(9R) × ATFR-5) Fl anti-A.TL (anti-I-A^k subregion) reacted with this hybridoma, neither of the monoclonal anti-Ia.17 or anti-Ia.2 was able to stain or kill this cell line. In addition, A.TH anti-A.TL, which was preabsorbed with H-2^k B cells, could stain FL10. It has recently been found that this T-cell hybridoma expresses an allotypic determinant associated with the constant structure of IgT (Tind^d) as stained by a monoclonal antibody (clone 9IIIA2), provided by Dr. F. L. Owen.[10] The extract from FL10 was able to augment the antibody response to dinitrophenylated (DNP)-KLH of H-2 compatible spleen cells from DNP-KLH-primed mice.

Another T-cell hybridoma (7C3-13) with a suppressor function was derived from B10.BR (H-2^k, Igh^b) spleen cells primed with a hapten, 4-hydroxy-3-nitrophenylacetyl (NP). This hybridoma expresses NP^b idiotype, heteroclite fine specificity for a cross-reactive hapten NIP (4-hydroxy-5-iodo-3-nitrophenylacetyl), Qa-1 and I-J^k determinants. The factor extracted from 7C3–13 could suppress the total and idiotype positive anti-NP antibody response of mice of Igh-1^b, but not Igh-1^a strains. Otherwise, physicochemical properties of the 7C3-13-derived T-cell factor are quite the same as those of KLH-specific T-suppressor cell factor (R. Abe *et al.*, manuscript in preparation). The cell line also expresses an Igh allotype-linked constant structure of the T-cell receptor molecule (Karasuyama *et al.*, manuscript in preparation). In some experiments, another NP-specific T-cell hybridoma (7F4) of the same series was used. This cell line also expressed I-J and NP-binding ability, whereas the expression of NP^b idiotype was ambiguous.

A continuous cell line of C3H origin, 3D10, was established two years ago from KLH-binding splenic T cells. The cell line is dependent on the T-cell growth factor and has been recloned several times. 3D10 produces a KLH-specific suppressor factor in the culture supernatant only in the presence of the T-cell growth factor. The factor suppresses directly the Lyt-1$^+$ T-helper cell and is regarded as a suppressor effector factor. The epitopes detected on these three different clones and their factors are listed in TABLE 1.

MONOCLONAL ANTIBODIES

Monoclonal antibodies reactive with I region products on T cells and T-cell factors were produced by the method described previously.[8] In brief, A.TH spleen cells immunized by A.TL lymphoid cells were fused with P3-X63-Ag8-653 by the method of Köhler and Milstein.[11] Monoclonals were screened with C3H nu/nu spleen cells, and those that reacted with H-2^k B cells and macrophages were excluded. They were further selected by their reactivity with I-A$^+$ FL10 and KLH-binding T cells of A/J that were generally enriched with Ia$^+$ T cells. Several clones were established on the criteria that they did not react with B cells while being able to stain selected T cells and T-cell clones. By a similar procedure, anti-I-J^k monoclonals were established from 3R spleen cells immune to 5R lymphoid cells. It has been found that there are at least three different types of monoclonal anti-I-J^k that react with inducer type T_S (prototype cell line: 7C3-13), effector Type T_S (3D10), and some of the T_H2 (Kurata *et al.*,

TABLE 1. Three Prototypic Cell Lines Producing Different T-Cell Factors

Prototype cell line (origin)	Category	Target	Iat (m Ab)	C_T (m Ab)	Factor	Polypeptide
FL10 (A/J)	$T_A(i)$	Lyt-1,2,3	I-A (1L9)	Tind^d (9IIIA2)	$T_AF(KLH)$ (V_H^+,Iat^+,C_T^+)	2
7C3-13 (B10.BR)	$T_S(i)$	Lyt-1,2,3	I-J (1G8)	Tsu^b (KL79)	$T_SF(NP)$ (Id^+,Iat^+,C_T^+)	2
3D10 (C3H/He)	$T_S(e)$	Lyt-1	I-J (KN34)	Tsu$_a$ (HA7)	$T_SF(KLH)$ (V_H^+,Iat^+,C_T^+)	?

manuscript in preparation). Because these Iat determinants have been detected only on T cells and not on B cells and macrophages, they are designated as Iat antigens.

Monoclonal antibodies against Igh-linked allotypic determinants on putative antigen receptors of T cells were made by fusion of a myeloma cell line with SJL (Igh-1^b) or SJA (Igh-1^a) spleen cells that were immunized reciprocally with their spleen cells containing naturally developed blast cells. The monoclonals were selected by their ability to kill T_S or T_A (or T_H). The detailed description of these monoclonals will be published elsewhere (Okumura *et al.*, manuscript in preparation). Monoclonal anti-Tsu^d and anti-Tind^d were kindly provided by Dr. F. Owen.

EXPRESSION OF I REGION-CONTROLLED AND IgH-LINKED (C_T) DETERMINANTS ON T-CELL LINES

As depicted in TABLE 1, all the cell lines were characterized by the expression of different Iat and C_T determinants. Noteworthy is the fact that 7C3-13 and 3D10, both derived from H-2^k mice, carry different I-J controlled determinants. A monoclonal anti-I-J, 1G8, was able to stain 7C3-13, while being unable to react with 3D10. The other anti-I-J, KN34, stained 3D10, but not 7C3-13. These results reflect the fact that 7C3-13 is an inducer (or transducer) type T_S that activates Lyt-1$^+$2$^+$3$^+$ intermediary T cells to induce the effector type T_S, the latter of which corresponds to 3D10. In fact, when the primed whole spleen cells were treated with these monoclonals and complement (C), 1G8 suppressed the antibody response, whereas KN34 always enhanced the response, indicating that different cell types were affected by these monoclonal anti-I-J.

These two suppressor-cell lines showed expression of different C_T determinants being linked to Igh allotype. 3D10 carry determinants HA7 and HA16, both of which are linked to Igh^a. 7C3-13 was stained with a monoclonal KL79 that was raised against Igh^b T cells. The augmenting T-cell hybridoma, FL10, expressed Tind^d determinant as determined by a monoclonal antibody, 9IIIA2, which was provided by Dr. F. Owen.

The biochemical properties of the antigen-specific molecule produced by FL10 were extensively studied (Miyatani *et al.*, submitted for publication). In summary, T_AF is a heterodimer composed of two polypeptide chains, one being the product of an I-A subregion and the other carrying the Tind^d determinant and antigen-binding site. Both polypeptides have a molecular weight of 33,000.

Although all the monoclonal anti-I-A antibodies derived from A.TH immune to A.TL reacted with I-A$^+$ T-cell hybridoma FL10, there was a considerable heterogeneity observed when they were used to treat functional T cells. Some of the monoclonals were capable of killing all the T_H, whereas others affected only T_H2 that helps B cells through the production of antigen-nonspecific helper factors.[4] It was also found that the ability to kill $T_A F$-producing cells was not evenly distributed among monoclonals.[8] All these results indicate that Iat antigens heretofore described are heterogeneous molecules expressed on functionally distinct subsets of T cells. We suggest that each monoclonal reacts with a particular epitope expressed only on certain functional subsets probably being associated with molecules involved in the antigen-recognition and restricted-cell interactions.

COMMON AND DISTINCT I REGION CONTROLLED EPITOPES ASSOCIATED WITH AUGMENTING FACTOR AND T-SUPPRESSOR CELL FACTOR

In the course of this study, we found that one of the anti-I-A monoclonals (2L2) unexpectedly stained 7C3-13 that had been characterized by the expression of I-J subregion product and T_S function. This finding suggested to us that Iat molecules that are controlled by different I subregions had previously unknown cross-reactive determinants.

To ascertain this fact, $T_A F$ from FL10 and $T_S F$ from 7F4 (comparable to 7C3-13) hybridomas were absorbed with immunoadsorbents of different monoclonal anti-Iat antibodies (TABLE 2). It was demonstrated that some monoclonal anti-I-A (e.g. 1L9), derived from A.TH anti-A.TL, were capable of absorbing the $T_A F$ activity from the extract of FL10, but not the I-J$^+$ $T_S F$ obtained from 7F4. On the other hand, another monoclonal anti-I-A (e.g. 2L2), which originated similarly from A.TH anti-A.TL spleen cells and originally assigned its specificity to the I-A subregion, was capable of absorbing both $T_A F$ and $T_S F$ from augmenting (FL10) and suppressive (7F4)

TABLE 2. Presence of Common and Individual Epitopes on Iat Polypeptides Associated with T_A and $T_S F$

T-Cell Factors Added	Anti-DNP IgG PFC/Culture	Percent Response
$T_A F$ from FL10		
Not added	1395 ± 211	100
Unabsorbed $T_A F$	2839 ± 250	205
Absorbed with 1L9[a]	1210 ± 122	87
Eluted from 1L9	2371 ± 155	170
Absorbed with 2L2[a]	1429 ± 148	102
Eluted from 2L2	2637 ± 189	189
Absorbed with 1G8[b]	2571 ± 233	184
Eluted from 1G8	1320 ± 49	95
$T_S F$ from 7F4		
Not added	2579 ± 139	100
Unabsorbed $T_S F$	814 ± 190	31
Absorbed with 1L9[a]	827 ± 117	32
Eluted from 1L9	2349 ± 108	91
Absorbed with 2L2[a]	2427 ± 527	94
Eluted from 2L2	628 ± 289	24
Absorbed with 1G8[b]	2195 ± 319	85
Eluted from 1G8	1078 ± 48	42

[a]Derived from A.TH anti-A.TL, originally screened with I-A$^+$ hybridoma.
[b]Derived from 3R anti-5R, originally screened with I-J$^+$ hybridoma.

hybridomas. Both activities were eluted in the acid eluate from the column. By contrast, the immunoadsorbent column of an anti-I-J monoclonal (1G8) was unable to absorb FL10-derived T_AF while removing the suppressor activity from I-J$^+$ 7F4 extract. These antigenic epitopes are of polypeptide nature, because the massive treatment with Tunicamycin, a potent inhibitor of glycosylation, did not alter the expression of the determinant. The results indicate that the epitope 1L9 is present only on T_AF, but not on T_SF, and is mapped in the I-A subregion; that the epitope 1G8 is present on T_SF, but not T_AF, and is mapped in I-J; and that the epitope 2L2 is present on both T_AF and T_SF and therefore cannot be mapped in a single subregion.

By repeating the above experiments, we found that a number of epitopes detected by our monoclonals are shared by both these T-cell factors, T_AF and T_SF, whereas some epitopes are unique to either one factor with a different I subregion assignment. By the inhibition of binding of a radioactive monoclonal by others, we can tentatively assign at least two separate clusters of epitopes on Iat polypeptides associated with T_AF and T_SF as depicted in FIGURE 1. The schemas in FIGURE 1 represent epitope organizations on Iat polypeptides of the augmenting factor and the T-suppressor cell

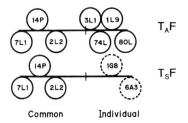

O defined by m. anti-I-A
◌ defined by m. anti-I-J

FIGURE 1. Separate clusters of common and individual epitopes on Iat polypeptide chains associated with T_AF and T_SF. Epitopes detected by monoclonal anti-I-A and anti-I-J antibodies are assigned on two polypeptides from T_AF and T_SF. Topography was estimated by the competitive inhibition of binding of radioactive monoclonals to a hybridoma FL10.

factor. We have also attempted to find similar common and individual epitopes on I-J$^+$ and I-A$^+$ T_H2 and have found that some common epitopes do exist among Iat antigens on various functional T-cell subsets. Thus, it was concluded that Iat polypeptides have a prototypic structure composed of common and individual epitopes. In view of the second antigen-binding polypeptide associated with T_SF and T_AF linked to Igh loci, the presence of such a polymorphic structure on Iat polypeptide may be of importance for the restriction specificities of T cells in the regulatory circuit.

QUESTIONS AND INTERPRETATIONS

We have previously described two general pathways of suppressive-cell interactions in which either MHC or IgV$_H$ were the restricting elements.[12] The IgV$_H$ restricted pathways were simply interpreted as the idiotype-anti-idiotype interaction, in which T_S expressed an allotype-linked major cross-reactive idiotype (NP^b) that activated anti-idiotypic sets of T cells. Such anti-idiotypic or paratopic sets that may exist inherently in the relevant Igh allotype strains can manifest the IgV_H restricted suppression of the idiotype positive antibody response by B cells (Abe *et al.*, submitted for publication). Such a simple concept may have to be reconsidered in the light of well-known difficulties in identifying the V_H gene rearrangements in such idiotype-positive T cells with B-cell derived genetic probes.

More controversy was brought about by the present findings. The second polypeptide chain of the antigen-specific T-cell factors, that is, Iat polypeptide, has a considerable heterogeneity and unexpected cross-reactivity within the member products. Such a heterogeneity may be important for the complementary interaction between different products that determine the consequence of cell interaction. The presence of common and individual structures may indicate that such heterogeneous products are derived from a new multigene family distinct from known class II genes. These implications are apparently correct, as we can indeed detect such multiple products on functionally different subsets.

This concept is, however, being seriously criticized again by the recent molecular genetic studies in which molecule geneticists had difficulty in locating such Iat genes within the I region of the major histocompatibility complex.[13] Under the situation where molecular geneticists cannot find the I-J subregion, how can we allocate multiple genes for multiple Iat determinants for T cells?

One possibility at the present time is that the major portion (common structure) of T-cell factors is encoded by a gene in the I-A subregion regardless of the T_S and T_A functions. The I-J subregion that is close to the E_β gene may contain a few small DNA segments that cannot be detected by the usual hybridization analysis, as was the case of the D region in the Ig gene segment. Both I-A and I-J (and even other subregions) may contain such mini genes that can modify the structure and function of the products that are encoded by undetermined loci.

The second possibility that we are now exploring is that these apparent Iat determinants are not encoded in the major histocompatibility complex. Let us assume that self MHC determinants stimulate T cells with anti-self nature under the physiologic condition. This is well substantiated by the fact that T cells recognize antigen only in association with self MHC products. Thus, we can postulate a frequent occurrence of T-cell receptors for class I and class II antigens. For class I antigens, responding T cells may be dominated by Lyt-2 T cells. By contrast, Lyt-1 T cells may have receptors for class II antigens. If such receptors carry idiotype-like structures that are shared by certain functional cell types (such as Lyt-1$^+$ cells that recognize A or E molecules), these receptors can induce antibodies reactive to them (anti-T-cell receptor for Ia). Because self-recognizing receptors occur only when self MHC products are present, their existence is apparently linked to the MHC haplotype (pseudo linkage). If this postulate is true, Iat antigens are not the direct products of I region genes, but are induced in response to self Ia. The anti-Iat antibodies are then anti-anti-Ia antibodies. We are now exploring this possibility by analyzing the idiotypes on both anti-Ia and anti-Iat antibodies.

If the latter situation holds true, we are confronted with unexpected possibilities that may explain several other unsolved phenomena. T cells have self-recognizing structures evolved from unknown origin with prototypic idiotype-like structure. We say prototypic, as the structures on Ia molecules recognizable by self T cells should be very limited and commonly used by a particular T-cell subset. Such a structure (we want to designate it as a prototype) continuously stimulates T cells that carry anti-prototype receptors. The prototypes on self-recognizing T-cell receptors may be easily altered in the chimeric situation where the stimulating self is different. This may also explain the fact that both idiotypic and anti-idiotypic T cells are present only in strains where the stimulating idiotype originally existed. Thus, T-cell receptors for self Ia and idiotypes are induced only in the presence of original Ia or the idiotype, creating the situation where idiotype and Iat specificities are apparently linked to Igh or MHC loci.

Although every postulate is based on an assumption, we are indeed confronted with enormous problems that we have never before seriously approached. Are the Iat antigens anti-Ia? Are the idiotypes and anti-idiotypes on T cells results of inductive processes by preexisting idiotype positive B cells? Are the restriction specificities imposed by anti-self? And finally, where can we locate the genes coding for such anti-self-receptors on T cells? These questions are of utmost importance at this moment. We feel that we are like Jonah expelled from the stomach of a giant fish, who is the semiotic symbol of Captain Ahab who crazily chased for Moby Dick.

REFERENCES

1. TADA, T., M. TANIGUCHI & C. S. DAVID. 1977. Cold Spring Harbor Symp. Quant. Biol. **41:** 119–127.
2. TADA, T., M. TANIGUCHI & K. OKUMURA. 1977. Prog. Immunol. **3:** 369–377.
3. TOKUHISA, T., M. TANIGUCHI, K. OKUMURA & T. TADA. 1978. J. Immunol. **120:** 414–421.
4. OCHI, A., M. NONAKA, K. HAYAKAWA, K. OKUMURA & T. TADA. 1982. J. Immunol. **129:** 227–231.
5. TANIGUCHI, M., T. SAITO & T. TADA. 1979. Nature (London) **278:** 555–558.
6. HIRAMATSU, K., S. MIYATANI, M. KIM, S. YAMADA, K. OKUMURA & T. TADA. 1981. J. Immunol. **127:** 1118–1122.
7. TADA, T. & M. NONAKA. 1982. *In* Isolation, Characterization and Utilization of T Lymphocyte Clones. F. Fitch and S. Fathman, Eds. 95–107. Academic Press. New York.
8. HIRAMATSU, K., A. OCHI, S. MIYATANI, A. SEGAWA & T. TADA. 1982. Nature (London) **296:** 666–668.
9. BEN-NERIAH, Y., C. WUILMART, P. LONAI & D. GIVOL. 1978. Euro. J. Immunol. **8:** 797–801.
10. OWEN, F. L. 1982. J. Exp. Med. **156:** 703–718.
11. KÖHLER, G. & C. MILSTEIN. 1976. Eur. J. Immunol. **6:** 511–519.
12. TADA, T., K. OKUMURA, K. HAYAKAWA, G. SUZUKI, R. ABE & Y. KUMAGAI. 1981. *In* Immunoglobulin Idiotypes. C. Janeway, E. E. Sercarz and H. Wigzell, Eds. 563–572. Academc Press. New York.
13. STEINMETZ, M., K. MINARD, S. HORVATH, J. McNICHOLAS, J. FRELINGER, C. WAKE, E. LONG, B. MACH & L. HOOD. 1982. Nature (London). In press.

DISCUSSION OF THE PAPER

W. E. PAUL (*National Institutes of Health, Bethesda, Md.*): Dr. Tada, the concept that the Iat antigens were associated with the cell receptors for Ia would, of course, imply that the expression of these antigenic determinants was not, in fact, a genotypic property of the T cells that expressed them, but, in fact, an altered form through some type of selection within the thymus. I imagine that you are busily trying to examine Fl. Do you have any data that you could share with us now?

T. TADA: We do not have any data. We are now exploring this possibility.

A. AUGUSTIN (*University of Colorado, Denver*): Referring to your first set of data where you had the inhibition with anti-Ia monoclonal generating in ATL anti-ATH, can you explain to us how you did these experiments practically? Did you have the cultures?

TADA: Yes.

AUGUSTIN: Did you then put the antibody in the culture?

TADA: Yes. We have done a few different experiments, but we can, of course, just add monoclonals to block the T/B cell interaction.

AUGUSTIN: The interaction is restricted, however. If you have anti-Ia, you would block the interaction by blocking the interaction with your restriction element with the final epitope. Did you take the precautions to make sure that you had such controls?

TADA: I do not understand your question.

AUGUSTIN: The B cells or macrophages have Ia. If you put anti-Ia, how do you know that the target is the B cell and not the T cells?

TADA: We can take the T-cell population and treat them with anti-Ia and complement and then mix them with B cells.

AUGUSTIN: In that case, when you use a panel of anti-Ia monoclonal antisera, you would expect that situation, if you had, let's say, a different population of T cells. This one will kill this; this one will kill that. Is that how it is happening, or does it just wipe out all of them? Do you have a pattern of activities or not?

TADA: Perhaps it is the quantitative problem, but we have selected these monoclonals that can kill T-helper cells. Is that all right?

AUGUSTIN: Yes and no, and I will tell you why. You proposed two hypotheses at the end of your paper. One of them, because we are on the grounds of network, is extremely attractive. This hypothesis has been attractive to me and to my experiments. The idea is that T cells actually represent clonally distributed internal images of the I region and coded determinants. This is the jargon that we would use for naming those particular determinants that would have T-cell receptor determinants that mimic I region encoded determinants present conventionally on class II molecules. If this is possible—an objective reality—then the implications of such a fact are tremendous for the development of a T-cell repertoire. I personally have the impression that that is the correct way to view this situation. If this finding is true, although you would have this type of internal image, you would not expect that a T-cell receptor would copy the whole series of Ia encoded determinants, which is very large for one duplex, one α-plus-β chain. One T cell will have this, one of them will have that, so then you have a clonal distribution of these more or less perfect copies. Do you have any data on this topic?

TADA: No. If we take F1 T cells and ask whether one of our monoclonals can affect the response (B cell response of one parent but not the other), then, in fact, the monoclonal can eliminate one response, but not the other. So I think these determinants that we are detecting are recognizing one particular epitope fraction of Ia antigen, but not the other.

C. A. BONA (*Mt. Sinai School of Medicine, New York*): Related to this regulatory structure that can be shared, I would like to ask you if the specificity of 2L2 was defined by absorption with effluent from columns of enhancing and suppressor factors, or also with absorption with cells with congeneic strain or inbred recombinant—to define if it is possible to absorb this activity with the cells.

TADA: We mapped the specificity to I-A at first, but by absorption with ATH. Later on we tried to absorb anti-Iat with recombinant mice, and found that we could not map it in a single subregion.

K. RAJEWSKY (*University of Cologne, Cologne, F.R.G.*): I wanted to clarify something that I did not quite understand. You proposed two possibilities for these I-J determinants on T cells. One is minigene rearrangements that one might not see, and the other one is that, in fact, these are cell self-recognizing receptors. First of all, these two things do not seem to be exclusive. These are two completely different models that do not exclude each other.

TADA: That is right.

RAJEWSKY: The point that I do not quite understand is how any of those results solve the problem of the I-J region. Do you want to say that there may be no I-J region and that the 5R-3R combination is showing that they are just gigantic artifacts?

TADA: I am quite sure that the I-J subregion does exist, but not like we expected. So there should not be the complete gene, but there should be something that is different between the 3R and the 5R at this point—at exactly that point—and this may modify the product, even though they are not the structured genes.

RAJEWSKY: What you say is basically the same thing that was said about the presence of idiotypes on T cells this morning.

TADA: Exactly. This assumption is based on the fact that T cells are so plastic that they can adapt themselves very easily.

The Design of Regulatory Circuitry: Predominant Idiotypy and the Idea of Regulatory Parsimony[a]

ELI E. SERCARZ, BARBARA ARANEO,
CHRISTOPHER D. BENJAMIN, MICHAEL HARVEY,
DENNIS METZGER, ALEXANDER MILLER,
LINDA WICKER, AND ROBERT YOWELL

Department of Microbiology
University of California
Los Angeles, California 90024

In this past decade of considerations about the role of idiotypy in defining and shaping immune repertoires, so presciently formulated by Niels Jerne,[1] we have learned how certain members of the B-cell repertoire became especially well represented. All idiotypes are equal, but some idiotopes become more equal than others, to paraphrase George Orwell.[2]

The thesis of this report is that it is in the design of intercellular regulatory circuitry that the importance of idiotypic connectance is paramount. The ease of organizing regulation based on predominant idiotypic motifs must have been a major force in their evolution. Recently, the notion of regulatory idiotopes has been enunciated, clearly delineating a set of predominant idiotopes that are not intimately associated with active site residues, but essential for regulation. Accordingly, a dissociation exists between the substance of the specificity repertoire encompassed by the residues making contact with the antigen, and the control of the expression of this repertoire that is modulated by idiotypic forces.

We assume here that the crucial idiotypic forces of regulatory significance are the T-helper (T_H) and T-suppressor (T_S) cells that at the Ab_2 stage can recognize regulatory idiotopes on antibodies of various specificities. The internal image set of Ab_2 antibodies, which through complementarity with Ab_1 receptor sites can mimic epitopes on the antigen, represent an entirely different consequence of the system. The concept of internal images has intriguing aspects, for example, in relation to repertoire development.[3]

SECONDARY ANTI-HEN EGG-WHITE LYSOZYME AS AB_3

The remarkable situation first described by Oudin and Cazenave,[4] that rabbit antibodies directed towards separate epitopes on the same protein could share idiotypy, was studied within the lysozyme response system of mice as presented earlier in this volume.[5] In that paper several sets of monoclonal antibodies bearing a single idiotype (IdXL) were enumerated that could simultaneously bind to HEL without mutual interference. These different antibodies not only had specificity for unique peptides,

[a]This work was supported in part by Grant IM-263 from the American Cancer Society and Grants CA-24442 and AI-11183 from the United States National Institutes of Health.

but could also be shown to belong to a variety of V_H subgroups. Whereas secondary response antibodies are almost exclusively $IdXL^+$, a large majority of the IgG_1 antibodies appearing during the primary response to HEL do not bear IdXL. With an abundance of initial idiotypic possibilities, what could it be that causes the system to eventually favor IdXL over subordinate idiotopes?

The key selective element seems to be an IdXL-recognizing T_H (IdXL-T_H) that is not optimally activated until the primary response has run its course.[6] Initially, the antigen-specific T-helper cell (AgT$_H$) triggers B cells with broad idiotypic heterogeneity. Subsequently, we assume that IdXL displayed on antigen-stimulated B cells, activates the IdXL-T_H, which in turn will positively select $IdXL^+$ cells. Accordingly, the late primary and secondary responses become overwhelmingly IdXL positive. We thus visualize the secondary response to HEL as representing an "Ab_3" stage of intrinsic idiotypic development, in a sequence in which the IdXL-T_H functions at the

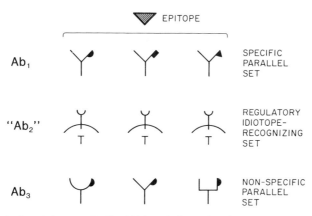

FIGURE 1. Antigen induces antibodies (Ab_1) each directed against a particular epitope. These Ab_1 represent a specific set of molecules with differing idiotopes, shown by the filled geometric shapes. Only the semi-circular structure is a "regulatory idiotope" that is recognized by a particular set of T cells, the $T(Ab_2)$. Finally, a nonspecific parallel set of B cells, bearing the regulatory idiotope, will be activated by $T(Ab_2)$. Of course, in the case of the protein antigen considered here, the Ab_3 that are lysozyme reactive need not be specific for the same epitope.

Ab_2, idiotype-recognizing level, as depicted in FIGURE 1. The resultant response to this multideterminant protein is heterogeneous in specificity for antigen but homogeneous in idiotypy. Although the essential interplay of the IdXL-T_H and B cells is considered to reflectively maintain the dominance of the IdXL idiotope, anti-idiotypic antibody molecules may also play a role.

SINGLE VERSUS MULTIPLE PREDOMINANT IDIOTYPES

It might seem a simple design in a regulatory system for a single idiotypic motif to be either recognized or carried by every lymphocyte in the circuit. On the one hand, focus on a single set of recognition motifs can unite a system by providing an integrated and simplified recognition scheme that allows for unambiguous partnerships between effectors and their targets. On the other hand, such a unitary requirement might lead to possibly unwanted interactions, because of the complementarity of an antigen-specific idiotype-bearing T_H and an idiotype-recognizing T_H, for example. This may be the state of affairs in the phosphocholine idiotypic system,[7] and surely is true for the anti-Streptococcal carbohydrate A5A system,[8] although both of these antigens can be AgT_H independent. Therefore, in monomeric protein antigen systems, since the specificity of AgT_H and B cell are different, it may be a better premise for regulatory system design for a multi-idiotypic, or at least a bi-idiotypic arrangement to prevail.

This arrangement would be rationalized as a principle of minimal ambiguity, an optimal form of regulation that uses independent idiotypic universes for the helpful and suppressive elements of the system. Such dual idiotypy seems to characterize the lysozyme system. The idiotype(s) of the AgT_H T proliferating are not cross-reactive with IdXL. The same rabbit or guinea pig anti-IdXL that eliminated T_S had no effect on T_H activity (reference 9 and unpublished results); likewise these anti-IdXL do not eliminate clones of major histocompatibility complex (MHC) restricted AgT_H of varying epitope specificity. Furthermore, when the AgT_H and AgT_S are positively selected on HEL-pulsed syngeneic monolayers, only the AgT_S selection is inhibited by anti-IdXL; the AgT_H can still be positively selected even in the presence of excess anti-IdXL[10] (see FIGURE 2). Within these experiments, it was shown that the ability of the HEL-pulsed macrophage monolayers to select AgT_S was MHC restricted. Thus, by all the criteria we have employed, the idiotype of the AgT_H belongs to a distinct universe from the AgT_S, the $IdXT_H$, and the B cell, all of which interact around the IdXL motif. This "asymmetry" in the system can be seen, *ex post facto* at least, as permitting independent regulation of AgT_H activity, and engaging a maximal degree of helpful interaction between AgT_H of a variety of specificities and B cells. Not circumscribed by an idiotypic connection, a much larger set of the antigen-activated AgT_H should be usable for triggering specific B cells by way of an antigen-bridging element than if idiotypic complementarity were required.

IS THERE A PREDOMINANT AgT_H IDIOTYPE?

What is not known is whether AgT_H bear a separate predominant idiotype, rather than displaying heterogeneous idiotypy. A certain homogeneity will result from the fact that for each haplotype, a severely limited number of sites on a protein are recognized by the AgT_H. This is another example of an apparent evolutionary principle of the immune system, which we have interpreted to be: "Keep the regulation simplified."

FIGURE 2. HEL-pulsed antigen-presenting cells (APC) can positively select antigen-specific T_H as well as antigen-specific T_S, each subpopulation specific for a distinct HEL epitope. In the experiments cited[10] enhanced recovery of AgT_S, for example, requires that the APC be syngeneic as well as HEL pulsed. Because anti-IdX interfered with lysozyme-specific T_S selection, but had no effect on positive selection of AgT_H, it is assumed that the AgT_H belong to a separate idiotypic family.

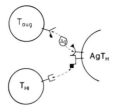

FIGURE 3. Two hypothetically different types of interactions between amplifying T cells whose function it is to augment or induce AgT_H activity. T_{HI} (a T helper-inducer cell) bears a receptor complementary to the square idiotope on the AgT_H receptor. This receptor is pictured here as having two separate subsites on two peptide chains. The T_{aug} (T_H augmenting cell) is $IdXL^+$, and in this instance representatives from the two distinct idiotypic universes interact over an antigen bridge.

In parallel with the intricate maneuvers that the immune system uses to regulate its suppressor arm, it might be predicted that there would be a comparable complexity to the AgT_H system. Helper-inducer cells[11] and contrasuppressor cells[12] have been described that directly seem to interact with the AgT_H set, although by which specificity or idiotypic element remains unexplored. Invoking symmetry, we could expect to find interactions between AgT_H and a helper-inducer T cell based upon idiotypic complementarity, as in FIGURE 3. We can envision an alternative relationship also depicted in FIGURE 3 in which a member of the $IdXL$ universe is portrayed as an augmenting cell, (T_{aug}), relating to the AgT_H by an antigen bridge rather than through idiotypic homology.

It is particularly interesting that the idiotypy of AgT_H seems to be distinct in the lysozyme system, because it might have been possible, considering the diversity of $IdXL$ antigen specificities, that the AgT_H would have been included within the $IdXL$ universe.

RELATIONSHIP BETWEEN $IdXL^+$ T-SUPPRESSOR CELLS AND $IdXL^+$ B CELLS

To return to the IdXL-bearing T-suppressor cell, it should now be asked what maintains the connection between the similar idiotype on the B cell and T-suppressor cell.

B Cells

In earlier work, we demonstrated that at least in the $H-2^a$ mouse, a majority of the secondary antibodies are directed against the N-terminal-C-terminal peptide of the molecule (N-C = 1-17:cys 6-cys 127:120-129) and are IdXL positive. Surprisingly, an extremely large proportion, 30 to 70% of the early and peak primary response antibody, requires the presence of the three amino-terminal acids (lys-val-phe = TIP). This was determined using two distinct types of plaque-forming cell (PFC) analysis: inhibition with aminopeptidase-treated HEL, (AP-HEL, which is missing the TIP), and mixed-monolayer lysis with HEL and AP-HEL coated red cell monolayers, in which TIP-specific PFC can only lyse the HEL-coated erythrocytes and therefore result in turbid plaques. Interestingly, the significant preference for TIP in the primary antibody response is later lost in the secondary response, to be replaced by a preference for epitopes occupying nearby position(s) on HEL, on the N-C peptide, but not requiring TIP.

Because there is a concomitant switch from IdXL$^-$ to IdXL$^+$ in idiotypy and from TIP-requiring to 95% TIP-independent in specificity, it would seem that the display of the predominant idiotype is not TIP associated.

T-Suppressor Cell Specificity

On the other hand, all functional antigen-specific T_S that we have detected in the nonresponder B10 strain can be inactivated by anti-IdXL + C treatment. Apparently for the IdXL$^+$ T_S to be induced, the TIP must be present on hen egg-white lysozyme. An experiment indicating this point is shown in TABLE 1. Either AP-HEL or HEL in complete Freund's adjuvant (CFA) was employed *in vivo* to attempt to induce T_S that would subsequently abrogate or reduce the subsequent response to HEL-coupled to red blood cells. Whereas HEL-CFA induced strong suppression by this criterion, AP-HEL-CFA actually caused an enhancement. This dramatic loss of suppression by simple removal of 3 of the 129 amino acid residues indicated that suppressor-inducing determinants on HEL are very limited, perhaps to a single site at the N-terminus of lysozyme. Likewise, determination of the number of T_S-inducing sites on the β-galactosidase tetramer (monomer MW = 116,250) employed in suppressing subsequent responses to fluorescein-coupled β-galactosidase has indicated that, at least functionally, only two such epitopes exist even on such a large molecule.

The importance of TIP for the T_S might have been predicted from two other lines of evidence: amino acid residue 3 seemed to be critical in determining whether a lysozyme was immunogenic or nonimmunogenic for H-2^b strains; and the N-C peptide, or the N-terminal dodecapeptide alone, was able to induce T-suppressor cells.

Therefore, it seemed logical, when we first learned that T_S were IdXL$^+$, to assume that there was a critical association between the TIP epitope on HEL and "IdXL-ness." In fact, this supposition was first contradicted at the B-cell level by the information that monoclonal antibody of a wide variety of specificities could still be IdXL positive. Besides, a large proportion of TIP-specific antibodies in the primary response do not seem to bear IdXL (L. Wicker, unpublished data).

It is apparent that the large majority of IdXL$^+$ antibody-producing cells constituting the secondary response display specificities for epitopes on N-C that are different from TIP. Nevertheless, the idiotypy is shared with a T_S population that seems to be uniquely specific for the TIP epitope.

TABLE 1. The Role of TIP in Suppression[a]

Priming	Response to HEL-Red Blood Cells
None	+ +
AP-HEL	+ + +
HEL	±

[a]Groups of B10 nonresponder mice were primed with 100 μg of antigen, or saline in CFA. Four weeks later, an injection of HEL-coupled sheep erythrocytes was used as a challenge to test for suppression. Whereas saline-primed mice responded well, AP-HEL primed mice did not suppress, but rather enhanced the anti-HEL-RBC response.

TABLE 2. Markers on Cells Involved in Suppression[a]

	I-A	I-J	IdXL
T_{SI}	−	+	−
AgT_H	−	−	−
AgT_S	+[b]	−	+

[a]Each of the cell types involved in demonstrating suppression in the nonresponder B10 strain has a distinctive array of the three markers shown. The 10-day antigen-primed footpad-draining popliteal lymph node serves as the source of AgT_H and T_{SI}, whereas the 10-day antigen-primed spleen provides T-suppressor cells.
[b]B. Araneo, and R. Yowell, unpublished results.

REGULATORY PARSIMONY IN THE SUPPRESSIVE ARM

The conclusion seems inescapable that the sharing of IdXL between predominant B cells in the secondary response and all of the T_S, but none of the AgT_H, is not an accident, but at the very basis of a coordinated regulatory strategy. According to this view of "regulatory parsimony," it is necessary to design the system with a single focus—IdXL. When the secondary B-cell response has progressed along the stage where IdXL$^+$ PFC are numerous, it is time to turn off the system by triggering either an idiotype-recognizing T-suppressor inducer cell that will then activate the IdXL$^+$-bearing T_S or an idiotype-recognizing T-suppressor cell (IdT_S) that may then shut down IdXL$^+$ PFC synthesis and possibly prevent the activation of more IdXL. (Such an IdT_S has not yet been sought in the HEL system.) The possibility that hundreds of idiotypes on B cells could impinge on the regulatory system by triggering hundreds of cognate helper or suppressor cells seems incredibly chaotic. Rather than a Tower of Babel, what is required is that all the cells speak the same idiom.

There is no doubt that the T_S and the secondary B cells demonstrate different specificity repertoires, and yet share IdXL. According to one view, suppressor determinants are rare because they arise as a direct result of the limited degree of interaction between a T_S cell-restricting element coded for within the MHC and a site on the antigen.[13] With HEL, the sole site of attachment is close to the N-terminus, and therefore TIP is presented to T_S precursor cells. Whether or not there is MHC restriction of T_S cell initiation, a variety of IdXL$^+$, TIP specific T_S arise, and only those that are activated by suppressor-inducer (T_{SI}) cells (presumably IdXL-recognizing) are allowed to mature. The influence of the T_{SI} on T_S may be analogous to the influence of Id-recognizing T_H on the maturing B cell.

The evidence is still fragmentary that the T_{SI} cell recognizes the idiotype, because we have only shown that the T_{SI} does not bear IdXL. Although the complete phenotype of the T_{SI} and the T_S in the lysozyme system is still unknown, our current information is summarized in TABLE 2.

THE BIRTH OF IdXT_H

A continuing puzzle has been the origin of the predominance in IdX systems. What is the primitive IdX, the UrIdX? Although it usually is considered to arise from the B-cell repertoire, one suggestion is that, in fact, it is the T_S that establishes the predominance. The developmental scenario would begin as follows. T-helper cells receive their imprinting from I region encoded (Ia) molecules or some other prominent epitope on the thymic epithelium, or from cells in their environs. One of these ambient cells could be a T_S that bears IdXL. The UrIdXT$_H$ would recognize the T_S and start to proliferate, giving rise to a predominant set of IdXT$_H$. After maturation, the IdXT$_H$ could then select developing B cells displaying this idiotype in its role as a helper cell. The idiotopes on the T_S and B cell could therefore have quite a disparate structural basis. Although the UrIdXT$_H$ would have first experienced the crucial idiotope on a regulatory T_S cell, the expression of its activity on B cells would depend on a broad distribution of IdXL on antibody molecules. Formally, this might represent the initiation of UrIdXT$_H$ maturation by way of recognition of an internal image in the thymus that later becomes expressed by a second recognition of the same idiotope on the B-cell surface as a "regulatory idiotope."

PARALLEL PREDOMINANT IDIOTYPES FOR T- SUPPRESSOR AND T-HELPER CELLS

Thinking globally, there may be two quite disparate objectives in the design of T-cell circuitry. An important guiding principle is the necessity to establish regulatory circuits in order to keep a lid on responsiveness, and to maintain a streamlined focus on a minimal number (*e.g.* one) of cellular recognition motifs. Evolution of single predominant idiotypic control accomplishes this and avoids the anarchy to which a multiplicity of idiotypic systems might lead.

Is it desirable, however, to extrapolate this type of unitary suppressive control to the situation within the antigen-specific helper-cell universe? We have shown that the idiotypy of these AgT$_H$ is distinct, but it is unnecessary to argue that a coordinated, single idiotypic framework paralleling the T_S, IdXL$^+$ universe must exist. It may rather be preferable, given the success of suppressive control, for a completely different principle to be operative in the helper universe: let a thousand flowers bloom. Amplification circuitry working by way of antigen bridging may provide a suitable signal to AgT$_H$ bearing a diversity of idiotypes. The principle might be that to get a response started, no possibility should be overlooked, as long as the response can eventually be turned off. Whether this is the *modus operandi* in the system remains to be established.

REFERENCES

1. JERNE, N. K. 1974. Ann. Immunol. **125C:** 373–389.
2. ORWELL, G. 1946. Animal Farm. Harcourt, Brace, Jovanovich, Inc. New York.
3. SIM, G. K. & A. A. AUGUSTIN. 1983. N.Y. Acad. Sci. This Volume.
4. OUDIN, J. & P.-A. CAZENAVE. 1971. Proc. Natl. Acad. Sci. USA **68:** 2616–2620.
5. MILLER, A., L.-K. CH'NG, C. D. BENJAMIN, E. SERCARZ, P. BRODEUR & R. RIBLET. 1983. N.Y. Acad. Sci. This Volume.
6. SERCARZ, E., L. WICKER, J. STRATTON, A. MILLER, D. METZGER, R. MAIZELS, M. KATZ, M. HARVEY & C. BENJAMIN. 1981. *In* Immunoglobulin Idiotypes. C. Janeway, E. E. Sercarz and H. Wigzell. Eds.: 533–546. Academic Press. New York.
7. JULIUS, M. H., H. COSENZA & A. A. AUGUSTIN. 1980. Eur. J. Immunol. **10:** 112.
8. EICHMANN, K. 1978. Adv. Immunol. **26:** 196.
9. HARVEY, M. A., L. ADORINI, A. MILLER & E. E. SERCARZ. 1979. Nature (London) **281:** 594–596.

10. ARANEO, B. A., D. W. METZGER, R. L. YOWELL & E. E. SERCARZ. Proc. Natl. Acad. Sci. USA **78:** 499–503.

11. TADA, T. 1983. *In* Immunogenetics. B. Benacerraf, Ed. Masson. Paris. In press.

12. GERSHON, R. K., D. D. EARDLEY, S. DURUM, D. R. GREEN, F. W. SHEN, K. YAMAUCHI, H. CANTOR & D. B. MURPHY. 1981. J. Exp. Med. **153:** 1533.

13. GOODMAN, J. W. & E. E. SERCARZ. 1983. Ann. Rev. Immunol. **1:** 465–498.

Similarities between Transplantation Antigens on Methylcholanthrene-Induced Sarcomas and T-Cell Regulatory Molecules

PATRICK M. FLOOD,[a] ALBERT B. DELEO,[b]
LLOYD J. OLD,[b] AND RICHARD K. GERSHON[c]

[a]Department of Pathology
Yale University School of Medicine
New Haven, Connecticut 06510
and
[b]Department of Tumor Biology
Sloan-Kettering Institute
New York, New York 10021
and
[c]Department of Pathology
Howard Hughes Medical Institute
Yale University School of Medicine
New Haven, Connecticut 06510

INTRODUCTION

Cells of the immune system have learned to communicate with one another by expressing a series of very specialized gene products that can recognize and interact to alter the functional programming of these cells. One such set of products are encoded by a cluster of genes called the major histocompatibility complex (MHC) found on the 17th chromosome in mice. Molecular products of the MHC can act as cellular interaction molecules (CIM) for a great number of intercellular communications, including the activation of T and B cells, the restricting element of suppressor circuits, and as a target for the rejection of transplanted tissue grafts. In addition to MHC, there are other CIM that are also used by the immune system as an intercellular message system. These other CIM, including the immunoglobulin heavy chain complex (Igh) gene cluster, may also act as targets for the regulation of certain subsets of cells under control of the immune system. These CIM can also activate tissue rejection in strains of mice that express different genetic polymorphisms at these loci. It may be that transplantation resistance in genetically disparate members of a species is a general characteristic of all cellular interaction molecules.

Many chemically induced tumors, including those induced by the carcinogen 3-methylcholanthrene (MC) express antigens that act as transplantation antigens in that they can act as targets for the immune system, although often these immune rejection mechanisms are not sufficient to cause rejection of a primary inoculum. Secondary responses, however, (those elicited after primary exposure and excision of the tumor mass) appear to be quite potent and exquisitely specific for the immunizing tumor. The nature of the highly polymorphic individually distinct tumor-associated transplantation antigens is not known. They may represent products of genes mutated by the chemical carcinogen, the expression of previously silent and highly polymorphic normal gene products, or the monoclonal expansion of ectopically expressed but rare antigens that are products of highly polymorphic regions that cells use as CIM, such as the case where myeloma protein can act as a tumor-specific transplantation antigen.[1]

In general, attempts to answer these questions have proved unsuccessful because of the difficulty in producing antisera that recognized the individually distinct antigens that acted as transplantation antigens on chemically induced sarcomas. Recently, DeLeo *et al.*[2] have produced antisera that recognize a unique transplantation antigen on the surface of the BALB/c MC-induced sarcoma Meth A. Using this serum and a series of somatic cell hybrids between Meth A and the Chinese Hamster cell line E36, the structural gene for the Meth A unique antigen was mapped to a region on the 12th chromosome, indistinguishable from the Igh gene complex.[3] This region is of particular interest because it codes for at least two minor histocompatibility loci[4,5] as well as both B[6] and T[7] CIM involved in immunoregulatory interactions.

Taken together, all of these bits of information lead to the exciting possibility that the functional similarity of individual antigens on MC-induced tumors and Igh-linked gene products, as well as their proximity in DNA, may not be fortuitous. Therefore, we tested the hypothesis that antisera against MC-induced tumors might identify normal or abnormal variants of Igh-linked gene products that are used to communicate by cells of the immune system. We asked whether these antibodies could inhibit interactions between T-cell subsets that were known to require shared Igh-linked polymorphisms for biological activity. We found that many of these sera could block Igh variable region (Igh-V) restricted T-cell interactions, but only when the cells involved in the interaction shared Igh^a gene products. Further, this activity could be absorbed on tumor cells, identified a 12th chromosome product, and bound to the Igh-V restricting element found in Ly-1 TsiF, a T-cell derived suppressor inducer factor from Ly-1$^+$2$^-$ cells.

MATERIALS AND METHODS

Mice

BALB/c, C57Bl/6, and (BALB/c × C57Bl/6)F$_1$ (CB6F$_1$) mice, 6 to 10 weeks of age were obtained from the Jackson Laboratory, Bar Harbor, Maine, the Breeding Colonies at the Sloan Kettering Institute, and Yale University School of Medicine.

Tumors

The chemically induced sarcomas, (cell lines were derived from the m), and leukemias used in these studies have been described in previous publications.[2,8]

Antisera

The syngeneic and semi-syngeneic antisera to tumors of BALB/c and B6 origin were prepared according to procedures described by DeLeo *et al.*[8] Individual bleedings as well as pooled antisera were tested. Sera of tumor bearing mice (TBS) were obtained 7 to 10 days following intraperitoneal injection of 5×10^6 cells. Normal mouse serum (NMS) was obtained from both male and female mice 6 to 8 weeks of age. All sera were tested as coded samples. Rabbit anti-gp70 was a generous gift of Dr. Hans Schreiber from the University of Chicago. Anti-I-J^b serum was prepareed by hyperimmunizing B10.A(5R) cells with a mixture of B10.A(3R) spleen and lymph node cells. (We thank Dr. D.B. Murphy of Yale University for preparing these sera.) Monoclonal anti-Ly-2.2 was prepared and used[9] as described previously, and was a generous gift of Dr. F.W. Shen, Sloan-Kettering Institute, New York. Briefly, 10^7 cells/ml in an appropriately diluted antisera were incubated for 45 minutes on ice, followed by an incubation with rabbit complement (1:5) for 45 minutes at 37° C. Rabbit complement used in these experiments was serum from animals selected for low natural cytotoxicity to mouse spleen cells and subsequently absorbed with 80 mg of agar/ml of serum.

Absorption Tests

Antisera were absorbed according to procedures described in reference two.

Antigens

Sheep erythrocytes (SRBC) were obtained from Colorado Serum Company Laboratories, Denver, Colorado.

Preparation of the Ly-1 Derived Suppressor Inducer (Ly-1 TsiF) Material

Preparation of Ly-1 TsiF has been previously described.[7] Briefly, a suspension of spleen cells from mice hyperimmunized with SRBC was treated with anti-Ly-2 and rabbit complement, and subsequently cultivated *in vitro* for 48 hours at a concentration of 10^7 cells/ml. After 48 hours, supernatant fluids were cleared and passed through millipore filters.

In Vitro *Primary Anti-Sheep-Erythrocyte Response*

Anti-SRBC responses were generated *in vitro* using a modification of a cell-culture technique described initially by Mishell and Dutton.[10] The number of plaque-forming cells (PFC) were determined by using the Cummingham modification of the Jerne-Nordin plaque assay as previously described.[11] Results are given as the means ± S.E.M. for three individual values of each culture condition. Ly-1 TisF was added at a final concentration of 1:10 on day 0 of culture. Plaque-forming cell responses were measured 5 days after initiation of culture.

Blocking Assays

The blocking activity of the antisera was measured by addition of antisera at a final concentration of 1% to *in vitro* primary SRBC cell cultures. Either T-suppressor cells or suppressor-inducer factors from them were also added to some of the cultures.

Percent blocking was determined using the formula:

$$1 - \frac{\text{percent suppression of T-suppressor factor (T}_S\text{F)}}{\text{percent suppression of T}_S\text{F in cultures of NMS}} \times 100$$

Cultures that contained test antisera alone never showed any significant difference in the PFC response to SRBC when compared with the effect of NMS alone. Further, NMS alone did not cause any significant changes from normal.

Somatic Cell Hybrids

Production of somatic cell hybrids and their use in absorbing test antisera has been detailed elsewhere.[3]

Cell Preparations

Spleens were harvested from mice, and single cell suspensions were made by gently pressing minced spleen fragments between the frosted ends of sterile glass slides.

Absorption of Soluble Factors

Immunosorbent columns were prepared by conjugation of the antisera (anti-I-J or anti-MC tumor) to cyanogen bromide-activated Sepharose 4B. Supernatants containing Ly-1 TsiF were then passed over the appropriate immunosorbent column, and after extensive washing, the column was eluted with $0.2M$ sodium carbonate (Na_2CO_3), pH 11, and immediately neutralized in $0.3M$ borate buffer, pH 8.3. The eluted material was then concentrated to original volume and dialyzed overnight first against phosphate-buffered saline (PBS), the RPMI 1640.

RESULTS

Antisera to BALB/c 3-Methylcholanthrene Induced Sarcomas Block Immunosuppressive Interactions between Regulatory T-Cell Subsets (TABLES 1 and 2)

Antisera raised against BALB/c MC-induced sarcoma Meth A in BALB/c or (BALB/c × C57B1/6) (CB6F[1]) mice were tested for their ability to inhibit the action of Ly-1 TsiF in inducing suppression. Antiserum was added to cultures of Ly-1 TsiF and spleen cells, and the anti-SRBC PFC response was measured on day five. Although the antisera had no significant effect on primary anti-SRBC *in vitro* responses, they were very effective in blocking the induction of suppression by Ly-1 TsiF (TABLE 1). Syngeneic antisera to other MC-induced sarcomas, CMS 1, CMS 3, CMS 4, and CMS 5 as well as CB6F$_1$ anti-CMS 4 had similar effects on the induction of suppression in BALB/c mice. Identical results were obtained when BALB/c anti-SRBC Ly-1$^+$,2$^-$ T-suppressor inducer cells were used in place of Ly-1 TsiF to induce suppression (data not shown).

TABLE 1. Antisera to Methylcholanthrene-Induced Tumors in BALB/c Mice Block the Induction of Suppression by Ly-1 TsiF

Antiserum added to BALB/c culture[a]	Anti-SRBC PFC/culture		
	−Ly-1 TsiF	+Ly-1 TsiF[b]	Percent Suppression
BALB/c NMS	3100	600	80
BALB/c anti-Meth A	3300	2500	25
BALB/c anti-CMS 1	2700	3100	0
BALB/c anti-CMS 4	3400	2500	25
BALB/c anti-CMS 5	3300	4200	0
CB6F$_1$ NMS	3000	200	95
CB6F$_1$ anti-Meth A	3100	2700	15
CB6F$_1$ anti-CMS 4	3000	2600	15

[a]Serum was added at a final concentration of 1% on day 0 of culture.
[b]Ly-1 TsiF was added at a final concentration of 10% to 10^7 unprimed spleen cells on day 0 of a primary in vitro anti-SRBC culture.

TABLE 2. List of Mouse Antisera Tested for Blocking the Induction of Suppression by Ly-1$^+$,2$^-$ Cells or Ly-1 TsiF in Mice that Share Igh-Linked Polymorphisms with BALB/c Mice

Antisera with high blocking activity[a]	Antisera with intermediate blocking activity[a]	Antisera with no blocking activity[a]
BALB/c anti-Meth A[b] (13)	CB6F$_1$ anti-Meth A (4)	BALB/c Meth A TBS (1)
BALB/c anti-CMS 1 (2)	CB6F$_1$ anti-CMS 4 (6)	BALB/c CMS 4 TBS (2)
BALB/c anti CMS 3 (2)	BALB/c Meth A TBS (1)	BALB/c anti-CMS 5 (1)
BALB/c anti-CMS 4 (11)	BALB/c CI4 TBS (2)	BALB/c CI4 TBS (1)
BALB/c anti-CMS 5 (2)		CB6F$_1$ anti-BALB/c-RVd (1)
CB6F$_1$ anti-Meth A (2)		CB6F$_1$ anti-B6 RV1 (2)
CB6F$_1$ anti-CMS 1 (1)		B6: B6 RV-TCl TBS (1)
CB6F$_1$ anti-CMS 4 (2)		B6 anti-B6MS 2 (2)
BALB/c Meth A TBS (3)		HD200-47 (anti-P53) (1)
BALB/c CMS 4 TBS (5)		Rabbit anti-gp70 (1)
BALB/c BALB/c RV1 TBS (1)		BALB/c NMS (6)
BALB/c BALB/c RV2 TBS (1)		B6 NMS (2)
BALB/c (anti MoV-trans. BALB/c 3T3) (1)		CB6F$_1$ NMS (2)

[a]High blocking activity: reduction of suppression by more than 75%; Intermediate activity: reduction of suppression between 25–50%; No blocking activity: reduction of suppression by less than 25%. The formula for percent of blocking is given in MATERIALS AND METHODS. All sera were added at a final concentration of 1 percent.
[b]Meth A, SMC, and CI are all BALB/c methylcholanthrene-induced firbrosarcomas. Different tumor lines are identified by number. RV are radiation leukemia virus-induced tumors. Numbers given in parentheses were the number of individual bleeds or pools of antiserum tested.

A battery of sera were tested for their ability to block the induction of suppression in this system (TABLE 2). From the results, it is evident that blocking activity is not restricted to sera from highly immunized mice. Sera from animals with progressively growing sarcoma transplants also blocked TsiF action. Blocking activity was also found in the sera of mice with transplants of BALB/c leukemia cells, indicating that induction of blocking activity is not an exclusive property of sarcoma cells. The results with sera from tumor-bearing mice were more variable than they were with hyperimmune sera, possibly indicating that the titers of blocking factor were lower. Sera that showed no blocking activity included antisera against C57B1/6 MC-induced tumors, a monoclonal antibody against the P53 tumor antigen, antisera specific for the viral

TABLE 3. List of Tumor Cell Lines Tested for their Ability to Absorb Blocking Activity of Anti-3-Methylcholanthrene-Induced Sarcoma Sera

	Tumor cell lines that absorbed blocking activity[a]	Tumor cell lines that did not absorb blocking activity
Experiment I:	Meth A ascites sarcoma Meth A(a) *in vitro* line CMS 4 *in vitro* line CI4 ascites sarcoma	AKR leukemia cells B6 Rad LV leukemia BALB/c Rad LV leukemia CII10 ascites sarcoma BALB/c spleen cells
Experiment II:	Meth A ascites sarcoma Meth A(a) CMS 3 ascites sarcoma CMS 4 *in vitro* line	B6MS 3 ascites sarcoma BALB/c 3T3 cells BALB/c SV-40 trans. 3T3 cells
Experiment III:	Meth A/C36 hybrid mAE 28	Meth A/E36 hybrid mAE 4 Chinese hamster cell line E36

[a]Experiments I, II, and III were done by absorbing CB6F$_1$ anti-CMS 4 sera with the various cell lines as described.[9] Cell lines that absorbed out more than 80% of the blocking activity were regarded as positive. Cell lines that did not absorb out blocking activity reduced the blocking activity of the serum by less than 20 percent.

specific glycoprotein gp70 (indicating the blocking activity was not due to any antiviral activity that may have been present in the test antisera), as well as all batches of normal mouse sera tested.

The Specificity in the Anti-3-Methylcholanthrene Induced Sarcoma Sera That Blocks the Interactions between T-cell Subsets is Directed to Determinants Expressed on BALB/c 3-Methylcholanthrene-Induced Sarcomas that Are Coded on the Same Portion of Chromosome 12 as the Immunoglobulin-Heavy Chain Complex

In order to determine whether the relevant activity of the anti-MC-antisera in blocking the Ly-1 TsiF was directed against antigens on the BALB/c MC-induced sarcomas, CB6F$_1$ anti-CMS 4 antiserum was absorbed with a variety of cell populations and then tested for its ability to block the action of the Ly-1 TsiF *in vitro* (TABLE

TABLE 4. Anti-3-Methylcholanthrene-Immunosorbent Binds to I-J$^+$ chain of Ly-1 TsiF^a

Assay cells in culture	Ly-1 TsiF factor preparation		Percent suppression of anti-SRBC PFC
	anti-Meth A column	anti-I-J column	
BALB/c	—	—	standard
	whole TsiF	—	75
	Filtrate	—	15
	Eluate	—	15
	Filtrate + Eluate	—	65
	—	Filtrate	0
	—	Eluate	25
	—	Filtrate + Eluate	60
	Filtrate	Filtrate	20
	Filtrate	Eluate	65
	Eluate	Filtrate	60
	Eluate	Eluate	30

^{a}Ly-1 TsiF column fractions were added to 10^7 normal BALB/c spleen cells at a final concentration of 10% on day 0 of a primary *in vitro* anti-SRBC culture.

3). Cells that were able to absorb out the blocking activity included the Meth A ascites sarcoma cells and the *in vitro* line derived from it, Meth A(a). Additionally, absorption of the antiserum with CI4, CMS 3, and CMS 4 tumor cell lines removed the ability of anti-MC antiserum to block the activity of Ly-1 TsiF. Cell lines that did not remove the blocking activity of the antiserum included AKR leukemia cells, CII10 ascites sarcoma, B6MS 3 cells, B6 or BALB/c radiation virus (RadLV)-induced leukemias, BALB/c 3T3, and SV-40 transformed 3T3 cells. We then used somatic cell hybrids to absorb the blocking activity of the antiserum in order to determine if the relevant antigen was a structural product of the 12th chromosome. These hybrid cells had been used in the chromosomal assignment of the gene responsible for the Meth A tumor specific transplantation antigen[3] expression. Positive absorption of the antiserum was accomplished only by the somatic cell hybrid that expresses both the Meth A unique antigen, and the Igh gene locus (mAE 28). Cell lines that showed no absorption capability included the parental Chinese Hamster cell line E36, and the somatic cell hybrid that expresses neither the Meth A antigen nor the Igh gene cluster (mAE 4). Interestingly, absorption of antiserum with normal BALB/c spleen cells did not remove the majority of the activity, even though the relevant activity appeared to be against a subset of T cells normally found in the spleen. This may be because anti-MC antiserum binds only a very small fraction of splenic T cells (less than 5 percent).

Antiserum That Blocks Ly-1 TsiF Activity Binds to the Igh Variable Region Restricting Element of Ly-1 TsiF

Because anti-MC-induced sarcoma antiserum (Pool XIV) blocked the interaction between Ly-1 TsiF and its acceptor cell, we investigated whether the activity of the antiserum was directed against determinants found on the Ly-1 TsiF molecular complex. Ly-1 TsiF was passed over an immunosorbent column made from Pool XIV antiserum. The data in TABLE 4 show that whereas whole Ly-1 TsiF showed significant suppressive activity, filtrate or eluate from the Pool XIV immunosorbent column had no suppressive activity. When filtrate and eluate were mixed together, suppressive activity returned. If Ly-1 TsiF was passed over an anti-I-J immunosorbent, a similar result was seen: no suppressive activity in filtrate or eluate fractions, but a mixture of filtrate and eluate returned suppression. These results recapitulate our earlier findings that the Ly-1 TsiF is two chains, one of which is I-J$^+$, and suggests that Pool XIV antiserum binds to one of the two chains of the Ly-1 TsiF. Therefore, filtrates or eluates from anti-I-J columns were added to filtrates and eluates from Pool XIV columns to determine which chain of the Ly-1 TsiF was binding to the anti-MC antiserum. We found that filtrates from anti-I-J columns mixed with eluates from Pool XIV columns or vice versa (eluates from anti-I-J columns mixed with filtrates from Pool XIV columns) had potent suppressive activity, whereas anti-I-J filtrates mixed with Pool XIV filtrates (or anti-I-J eluates mixed with Pool XIV eluates) had no suppressive ability. These findings suggest that the anti-MC-induced sarcoma antiserum binds to one of the two chains of Ly-1 TsiF, the I-J$^+$ chain that is the chain responsible for the Igh-V restriction exhibited by the Ly-1 TsiF.[12]

The Ability of the Anti-3-Methylcholanthrene-Induced Sarcoma Antiserum to Bind to Ly-1 TsiF is Restricted to Strains Expressing the Igh^a Gene Locus

Because the antisera against MC-induced fibrosarcomas is restricted in its activity to block an Igh-V restricted interaction between T cells (or their products),[13] we investigated whether the ability of Pool XIV antiserum to bind to the I-J$^+$ chain of Ly-1 TsiF was itself restricted to genes linked to the polymorphism of the Igh region of the BALB/c mouse (Igh^a). Ly-1 TsiF from BALB/c, B6, and congeneic mice that express different polymorphisms at Igh were passed over an immunosorbent column made from Pool XIV antiserum. The filtrate, eluate, and mixtures of both were then tested for the ability to suppress CB6F$_1$ spleen cell cultures. The results in TABLE 5 show that the ability to bind the I-J$^+$ portion of the Ly-1 TsiF was related to the Igh haplotype of the cells that produced the factor. Ly-1 TsiF from BALB/c or Igh

TABLE 5. Binding Activity of Anti-3-Methylcholanthrene-Antiserum for Ly-1 TsiF is Restricted to Factors from Igh^a Mice

Assay cells in culture	Source of Ly-1 TsiF^a	Column fraction	Percent suppression of anti-SRBC PFC
	—	—	standard
	BALB/c	Filtrate	15
	BALB/c	Eluate	15
	BALB/c	Filtrate + Eluate	60
	C57Bl/6	Filtrate	95
	C57Bl/6	Eluate	20
CB6F$_1$	C57Bl/6	Filtrate + Eluate	80
	C.B20	Filtrate	80
	C.B20	Eluate	20
	C.B20	Filtrate + Eluate	70
	B.C9	Filtrate	20
	B.C9	Eluate	30
	B.C9	Filtrate + Eluate	70

^{a}Column fractions of Ly-1 TsiF were added at a final concentration of 10% to 5×10^6 unprimed (BALB/c $\times$ C57Bl/6)F$_1$ spleen cells on day 0 of a primary *in vitro* anti-SRBC culture.

congeneic B.C9 mice were retained when passed over the column, whereas B6 and C.B20 (a mouse that shares its entire genome save for the Igh gene complex with BALB/c) Ly-1 TsiF were unaffected by passage through Pool XIV column. Identical binding patterns as BALB/c Ly-1 TsiF were obtained when Ly-1 TsiF from BALB.B and BALB.K were passed over the Pool XIV column, whereas Ly-1 TsiF from C.AL20 mice was similarly unaffected by the Pool XIV column as C.B20 (data not shown). These findings argue strongly for the fact that the antiserum was reacting against a gene product controlled by genes linked to the Igh locus.

DISCUSSION

We have earlier shown an activity in antisera against MC-induced sarcomas of BALB/c origin that blocks the induction of suppression by a T cell-derived suppressor factor *in vitro*.[13] Absorption of these antisera with MC-induced sarcoma cells removes this activity, suggesting that a tumor-associated surface antigen on these cells may have determinants that are cross-reactive with these T-cell regulatory molecules. Because the cell-surface antigen on MC-induced sarcomas and the immunoregulatory structure found on T-cell derived factors have both been mapped to the Igh region of the 12th chromosome,[3,7] and the blocking activity of the antiserum is itself restricted to the Igh^a gene locus, we took this as evidence that the antiserum was blocking a T-cell regulatory activity by interfering with the Igh-V restricted interaction between the Ly-1 cells and their acceptor cells. We tested this hypothesis by investigating whether there was any physical association between the anti-MC antiserum and a determinant found on a small subset of T cells and their biologically active soluble mediators. We found that not only does the antiserum bind to the T-cell regulatory molecule, but has exquisite specificity for the portion of the molecule that imparts the Igh-V-linked genetic restriction exhibited between the factor and its acceptor cell.

The ability of anti-MC antisera to block Igh-V-linked T-cell regulatory activities, and to bind to T-cell regulatory molecules, allows us now to investigate the nature of the Igh restriction exhibited by T-T interactions. It has now been found that the anti-MC antisera has at least three separate activities, each one being capable of blocking a very specific Igh-linked T-T interaction[13] (manuscript in preparation). All of these blocking activities are confined solely to the Igh^a haplotype; animals that do not share this polymorphism at Igh with BALB/c are unaffected by the anti-Meth A sera. Because it is very unlikely that MC-induced sarcomas carry the entire array of "idiotypes" expressed by BALB/c mice, one can postulate that these cross-reactive determinants represent constant regions that are independent of V_H-encoded determinants used by B and (perhaps) T cells to recognize antigen. This finding introduces the possibility that V_H restriction is not dependent on individual recognition of a wide variety of idiotypic determinants. Investigations into this matter were facilitated greatly by the nature of the Ly-1 TisF. The factor consists of two chains: one binds nominal antigen, and the other is I-J$^+$.[12] There are no physical or functional restrictions between the two chains, so this situation allows us to determine which chain is reactive with the anti-MC-antisera. This possibility becomes more believable in light of the fact that the anti-MC-induced sarcoma antisera binds to a non-antigen-binding I-J$^+$ molecule. This I-J$^+$ molecule is the source of the Igh restriction.[12] We have found in a number of systems that T-cell factors require two chains for functional activity[12,14] (manuscripts in preparation), including the response to SRBC, horse red blood cells, burro red blood cells and trinitrophenol. The I-J$^+$ molecule from our SRBC-specific

T-cell factor has functional activity in all of these systems. Therefore, because the I-J$^+$ molecule is the source of the Igh restriction, bears a 12th chromosome region product, but has no antigen specificity, then the V_H restriction we see with our T-cell factors has nothing to do with the unique hypervariable regions of B- and T-cell molecules used to recognize and bind antigen, and hence has nothing to do with idiotype-anti-idiotype interactions in the classical sense.[15]

These results, however, lead us into a quandary. How does one get a product of the 12th chromosome and the 17th chromosome on the same molecule? These speculations are further complicated by observations made in F_1 animals that show that whereas Ly-1 TsiF from CB6F$_1$ mice is composed of both I-J^{b+} and I-J^{d+} molecules, the I-J^{b+} molecules have specificity only for Igh^{b+} cells, and I-J^{d+} molecules have specificity only for Igh^{a+} cells.[16] Furthermore, anti-MC antiserum can only bind to the I-J^{d+} molecule from CB6F$_1$ animals (Flood, unpublished observations). The reason for this is at present unknown, but represents a very perplexing and exciting genetic mechanism at work, one that can selectively unite molecular complexes controlled by two different chromosomes in a preferential manner depending on the genetic background of the mice.

One must strongly consider then, that the antigen being expressed by both the tumor and the T cells are on the same gene product. Further, this gene product is used by at least some sets of T cells to communicate by way of the Igh-linked gene products. We have tested a number of other T-T interactions, and found that other Igh-V-linked interactions are blocked by this serum, whereas other interactions not restricted by gene products of the Igh region are unaffected.[13] The nature of these antigens on sarcoma cells remains a mystery, but may represent either normal (or modified) differentiation products present on normal T cells as well as the tumor-precursor cells, or the ectopic expression of a normal (or modified) gene product used by normal cells (T cells that use Igh gene products to communicate), but represent an "abnormal" expression on tumor cells as a consequence of the malignant transformation. These possibilities are currently under investigation.

Whatever the nature of these antigens, they represent molecules that are identical or very similar to normal T-cell cellular interaction molecules. How can tumor cells induce antibody against such antigens? Two possibilities exist. Either these antigens are relatively rare under normal conditions (and under clonal expansion—as in the case of malignancy—a solid state of self tolerance cannot be maintained) and autoimmunity against self antigens is induced, or tumors have a specialized capacity to break self tolerance. Tolerance may be broken because of the following circumstances. Tumor antigens represent modified products of CIM, and modification of normally nonimmunogenic antigens can lead to the breakdown of immunologic tolerance.

Another possible mechanism worth considering because of the present studies, which is related to the breaking of self tolerance, is that this particular group of tumors, BALB/c MC-induced sarcomas, have the specialized capacity for interfering with normal immune regulatory interactions. The parasitic use of CIM that are encoded by or linked to the Igh complex is not only an optimal way of generating diversity (since the Igh complex is a "hot bed" of gene rearrangement and other mechanisms for generating diversity), but also provides an ideal way of "deregulating" suppressor-cell interactions that use these or similar antigens to communicate. Conversely, use of suppressor cell CIM may be an optimal way of generating massive amounts of systemic suppression by way of a type of "pseudoactivation" of suppressor-cell circuits. In addition, it now appears that cellular interactions between other cell circuits may also be disrupted by anti-MC-antisera. Antisera raised in CB6F$_1$ but not BALB/c mice can block the induction of contrasuppression, (a cellular activity that can overcome the effects of suppression), and this activity correlates with an increased incidence of metastasis in the F_1 animal compared to the parent (manuscript in preparation). By disrupting a number of different cellular interactions that use Igh-linked CIM to communicate, the tumor cells can increase their chance for survival.

This brings us to another important question: Why do so many MC-induced sarcomas in BALB/c mice express a 12th chromosome product, which was normally absent (or at a much reduced level) on the tumor-cell precursor after malignant transformation with 3-methylcholanthrene? Although many explanations could be advanced, two seen most likely. 1) Methylcholanthrene can randomly alter DNA, but only mutations at certain "transformation sights" can lead to a malignantly transformed cell. One (and perhaps the only one) of these transforming sights exists near or in the Igh region complex and causes the expression of abnormally high levels of these particular antigens. 2) Methylcholanthrene can transform anywhere in the genome, but there exists translocation "hotspots" where either oncogenes or promoter genes activated by the carcinogenic process are translocated. One of these "hotspots" may exist in or near the Igh gene locus. Precedence for these sorts of translocations and DNA rearrangements exist for both myeloma and B-cell lymphomas (for review, see reference 17). Investigations of other tumor-cell types may turn up similar translocations and may represent a "normal" consequence of malignant transformation for all cell types.

Thus, the network, in its much broader sense, involves a complex intertwining of phylogenetically related molecules from many different systems that serve to facilitate cellular communication within and between functionally related cell sets. In this sense, the immunologic system is not special, because the CIM used by these cells is no longer restricted to cells within this set, but has now been found on cells whose ontogenic and functional basis is quite different. Why these molecules appear on these cells, and how this relates to recognition and communication mechanisms remains to be seen. These findings may lead us to some very important discoveries not only in the mechanisms of tumor evasion of host immunologic defenses, but also in understanding the very mechanisms by which cells of the immune system regulate themselves.

SUMMARY

Successful interaction among T-cell subsets requires, among other things, homology at certain genetic loci that code for cellular interaction molecules (CIM). One such interaction, the induction of an acceptor-cell population by an Ly-1 T-suppressor-inducer cell, is controlled by genes that map to the variable region of the immunoglobulin heavy chain (Igh) complex. If the suppressor-induced cells (or their cell-free products) do not share Igh-V polymorphisms with their acceptor cells, the induction event fails to take place. Recently, structural genes of a transplantation antigen on the methylcholanthrene-induced sarcoma Meth A were mapped to the same region of chromosome 12 as the Igh gene complex.[3] We tested whether there was any relationship between the Meth A transplantation antigen and T-cell regulatory molecules by using antisera against the Meth A antigen to block this particular Igh-linked T-T interaction. We found that isoantisera against a large number of methylcholanthrene-induced sarcomas tested were capable of blocking the induction of T-suppressor cells so long as the inducer and acceptor cells bore the Igh[a] polymorphism. Further, we found a structural gene on MC-induced tumors that could absorb out this activity, and the structural gene for this antigen is coded for the same region as the Igh gene loci. The antisera binds to the I-J$^+$ portion of a T-cell regulatory molecule Ly-1 TsiF, the portion of the molecule that has no specificity for antigen and imparts the Igh-linked genetic restriction. The implications of these findings for both oncology and immunology were discussed.

REFERENCES

1. LYNCH, R. G., R. J. GRAFF, S. SIRISINHA & H. N. EISEN. 1972. Myeloma Proteins as tumor-specific transplantation antigens. Proc. Natl. Acad. Sci. USA. **69**: 1540–1544.
2. DELEO, A. B., H. SHIKU, T. TAKAHASHI, M. JOHN & L. J. OLD. 1977. Cell surface antigens of chemically induced sarcomas of the mouse. I. Murine Leukemia virus-related antigens and alloantigens on cultures fibroblasts and sarcoma cells: Description of a unique antigen on BALB/c Meth A sarcoma. J. Exp. Med. **146**: 720–734.
3. PRAVTCHEVA, D. D., A. B. DELEO, F. H. RUDDLE & L. J. OLD. 1981. Chromosome assignment of the tumor-specific antigen of a 3-Methylcholanthrene-induced mouse sarcoma. J. Exp. Med. **154**: 964–977.
4. ROLINK, T., K. EICHMANN & M. H. SIMON. 1978. Detection of two allotype (Ig1)-linked minor H-loci by use of H-2 restricted cytotoxic T cells in congenic mice. Immunogenetics **7**: 321–336.
5. RIBLET, R. & C. CONGLETON. 1977. A possible allotype-linked H-gene. Immunogenetics **5**: 511–518.
6. HENGARTNER, H., T. MEO & E. MULLER. 1978. Assignment of genes for immunoglobulin and heavy chains to chromosome 6 and 12 in the mouse. Proc. Natl. Acad. Sci. USA **75**: 4494–4498.
7. YAMAUCHI, K., D. B. MURPHY, H. CANTOR & R. K. GERSHON. 1981. Analysis of antigen-specific, Ig-restricted cell-free material made by I-J$^+$ Lyl cells (Ly-1 TsiF) that induces Ly2$^+$ cells to express suppressive activity. J. Immunol. **11**: 905–912.
8. DELEO, A. B., G. JAY, E. APELLA, G. C. DUBOIS, L. W. LAW & L. J. OLD. 1979. Detection of a transformation-related antigen in chemically induced sarcomas and other transformed cells in the mouse. Proc. Nat. Acad. Sci. USA **76**: 2420–2424.
9. YAMAUCHI, K., D. B. MURPHY, H. CANTOR & R. K. GERSHON. 1981. Analysis of an antigen-restricted H-2 restricted cell-free product(s) made by "I-J" Ly2 cells (Ly-2 TsF) that suppresses Ly2 cell-depleted spleen cell activity. Eur. J. Immunol. **11**: 913–918.
10. GERSHON, R. K., D. D. EARDLEY, S. DURUM, D. R. GREEN, F. W. SHEN, K. YAMAUCHI, H. CANTOR & R. K. GERSHON. 1981. Contrasuppression: A novel immunoregulatory activity. J. Exp. Med. **153**: 1533–1546.
11. CUNNINGHAM, A. J. & A. SZENBERG. 1968. Further improvements in the plaque technique for detecting single antibody-forming cells. Immunology **14**: 599–600.
12. YAMAUCHI, K., N. CHAO, D. B. MURPHY & R. K. GERSHON. 1982. Moleculear composition of an antigen-specific, Lyl T suppressor-induced factor: One molecule binds antigen and is I-J; another is I-J$^+$, does not bind antigen, and imparts an Igh-variable region-linked restriction. J. Exp. Med. **155**: 655–667.
13. FLOOD, P. M., A. B. DELEO, L. J. OLD & R. K. GERSHON. 1983. The relation of cell surface antigens on methylcholanthrene-induced fibrosarcomas to Igh-V-linked T cell interaction molecules. Proc. Natl. Acad. Sci. USA. **80**: 1683–1687.
14. FLOOD, P. M., K. YAMAUCHI & R. K. GERSHON. 1982. Analysis of the interaction between two molecules that is required for the expression of Ly2 suppressor cell activity: Three Different Types of Focusing Events May Be Needed to Deliver the Suppressive Signal. J. Exp. Med. **156**: 361–371.
15. JERNE, N. K. 1974. Towards a Network Theory of the Immune System. Ann. Immunol. Inst. Pasteur (Paris) **125C**: 373–389.
16. KLEIN, G. 1981. The role of gene dosage and genetic transpositions in carcinogenesis. Nature (London) **294**: 313–318.
17. CHAO, N. 1981. Analysis of an antigen-specific Ig restricted cell free material made by I-J$^+$ F$_1$ Lyl cells. Thesis, Yale University School of Medicine, New Haven, Connecticut.

DISCUSSION OF THE PAPER

W. E. PAUL (*National Institutes of Health, Bethesda, Md.*): Dr. Flood, one cannot help but wonder about the relationship of the expression of the methane antigen and the recent attention that has been paid to the idea that oncogenes are rearranged into the V_H region in, for example, both mouse myelomas and Epstein Barr virus-induced (EB) tumors. Although I do not have any obvious way to put that together, I am nonetheless wondering if you have given any thought to the possibility that the Meth-A induced antigen may in fact perhaps be the product of some prototypic oncogene.

P. M. FLOOD: We have given thought to the idea that perhaps there is a specific activation site where methylcholanthrene attacks, that is, near the IgH region, which gives us a transformed phenotype in the cell. It may well be a rearrangement of other transformed products that just jump to the 12th chromosome and then get expressed by a promoter gene, for example. We do not really have any other way of explaining it. I must have confused everybody.

PAUL: No, I do not think so. I think, in fact, that your explanation was a model of clarity.

UNIDENTIFIED SPEAKER: On your slide, the antigen-binding peptide did not have a second anti-IJ site on it.

FLOOD: The antigen-binding peptide is non-IJ positive.

UNIDENTIFIED SPEAKER: No, anti-IJ. In your paper you had two sites on the antigen.

FLOOD: That is the Lyt-2TsiF. In order to function, it works by way of an induction of an IJ positive molecule in its final target cells. There is no evidence to suggest in the Lyl story that there is a J/anti-J interreaction between the two chains. It is a little confusing, so I do not want to get into it too much.

R. KALISH (*Downstate Medical Center, Brooklyn, N.Y.*): You have shown that anti-sera to various methylcholanthrene-induced tumors is able to absorb out this tumor cell and this T-cell suppressive factor. Have you investigated the possibility that this is because the tumor cell antigen is equivalent to such a factor? There is much literature on the topic of tumor cells making suppressive factors.

FLOOD: That is a possibility and we have done a number of studies to see if, for example, extracted tumor antigen or supernatant from tumors can do suppression in the Meth A system. It does not seem to be the case in this particular system. I do not know if that is simply because we do not have enough of it or if it does not shed enough. Perhaps it means that some other molecule is needed. It is just an incomplete molecule. For example, we do not know if the Meth A is J positive, and we know that J is required on this molecule for its suppressive activity. So it may well be that it is a product of the 12th chromosome but lacks something else needed on that molecule to affect suppression.

J. A. BLUESTONE (*National Cancer Institute, Bethesda, Md.*): If I understand correctly, the determinant that you are seeing is not clonally restricted at all and is present on other factors as well.

FLOOD: That is right.

BLUESTONE: Therefore it would represent some more constant region type of marker. Yet it maps to the variable region that is unlike, for instance, the Francis Owen type markers that are mapping to the other side. Have you attempted to put together those two pieces of data with regard for how the molecule fits together?

FLOOD: Well, the way we look at it is that the molecule that we are identifying is a V_H constant region-like marker. That molecule of the anti-Meth A does not change, so it seems to me nonrelated to any IgH restricting element as such. It just seems to be an allotype-like marker on the VH region, as Francis Owen would describe for the C_H region.

Idiotype Determined Circuits in Maternally Suppressed Mice[a]

C. VICTOR, C. BONA, and B. PERNIS[b]

Department of Microbiology
Mount Sinai School of Medicine
New York, New York 10029
and
[b]Department of Microbiology
College of Physicians and Surgeons
Columbia University
New York, New York, 10032

The developing immune system of a newborn is exquisitely susceptible to the suppressive effects of antibodies directed against idiotypic determinants. Exposure to anti-idiotypic (anti-Id) antibodies in utero or immediately after birth renders that animal incapable of using that specificity as part of its immune repertoire.[1] Significant aberrations occur in the clonal distribution that manifest themselves by profound qualitative as well as quantitative changes in the immune response related to this idiotype.[2,3] In order to gain a greater understanding of the cellular basis for idiotypic suppression, the membrane expression of the J558 idiotype on the lymphocytes of mice who were maternally suppressed was studied.

The J558 idiotype is a predominant constituent of the anti-α 1,3 dextran response of BALB/c mice.[4] The response to this polysaccharide is so clonally restricted that its idiotypic profile can be described in terms of two BALB/c α 1,3 dextran binding myeloma proteins; that is J558 (α, λ) and MOPC 104E (μ, λ). Both myelomas express a cross-reactive idiotype (IdX) that is consistently displayed by 80% of anti-α 1,3 dextran antibodies. In addition, each myeloma bears its own private idiotype (IdI), the J558 IdI or 104E IdI respectively, that is expressed by a lower and variable percentage of the anti-α 1,3 dextran antibodies. The expression of IdX depends on amino acids in position 54 and 55 of hypervariable region (HV) II of the heavy chain, and for the IdI amino acids in position 100 and 101 of the D segment of the V_H as well.[5] The ability to produce antibodies bearing these idiotypes is linked to the IgCh locus, because it segregates with, and is observed only in, those mice expressing the IgCh^a allele. Furthermore, the ability to express this idiotype is a dominant trait because it is observed in F$_1$s made between a producer and a nonproducer strain of mouse.[6] This dominant inheritance of idiotype production was exploited as the basis of our system for generating maternally suppressed mice, which in fact was first described by Weiler *et al.*[7] Females of the A/J (IgCh^e) strain, who do not produce this idiotype, but are known for their vigorous production of anti-Id antibodies were hyperimmunized with J558 until anti-idiotypic activity was detectable in their sera. Then, they were mated to BALB/c males, and the progeny of these matings were the putative maternally J558 idiotype suppressed CAF$_1$ mice.

Indeed, the suppression of the J558 idiotype positive component of the anti-α 1,3 dextran response in these mice was verified by challenging them with the dextran at

[a]C. Victor is an Anna Fuller Fund research fellow. This work was supported by Grant PCN1105788 from the National Science Foundation.

220

various intervals after birth. Dextran responsiveness was assayed by direct plaque forming cells (PFC) on day 5 after immunization, and idiotype expression was evaluated by radioimmunoassay (RIA) on the spleens and sera respectively of individual mice. The IdX determinant was identified by affinity-purified heterologous goat anti-MOPC 104E IdX antibodies and the J558 IdI by the monoclonal EB 3-7-2, a gift of John Kearney (University of Alabama, Birmingham, Alabama). The results of this experiment are depicted in TABLE 1. The maternally suppressed CAF₁ mice show a chronic suppression of the $\alpha 1,3$ dextran specific PFC response with a concomitant decrease of the serum idiotype levels. This situation is to be contrasted to the normal CAF₁ mice who in fact show an age dependent increase in the PFC response with the display of the expected idiotypes. Clearly, CAF₁ mice born of mothers with anti-J558 Id immunity are suppressed for both anti-α 1–3 dextran antibody response and its J558 idiotypic component.

TABLE 1. Anti-Dextran Plaque-Forming Cell Response in Normal and Idiotype Suppressed CAF₁ Mice

Animal	Age (weeks)	PFC/$10^{6a,b}$	RIA (μg/ml)	
			IdX	IdI
Normal[c]	1	35 ± 3	nd	nd
CAF₁	2	175 ± 23	nd	nd
	3	525 ± 79	nd	nd
	4	1300 ± 125	nd	nd
	6	1839 ± 240	nd	nd
	8	2440 ± 560	40 ± 5	5 ± 0.3
	12	2465 ± 370	41 ± 3	4 ± 0.8
Suppressed[c]	3	3 ± 2	3 ± 0.2	<1
CAF₁	4	27 ± 10	1.5 ± 0.4	<1
	8	5 ± 0.4	1.8 ± 0.8	<1
	12	9 ± 1	<1	<1
Normal	4	0	<1	<1
CAF₁	8	0	<1	<1
(nonim-	12	0	<1	<1
mune)				

[a]Represents the average of six mice per group
[b]Sheep erythrocyte background is subtracted off.
[c]Immunized with 100 μg dextran B1355 intraperitoneally; spleen cells for PFC test and serum for idiotype RIA collected 5 days after immunization

It remained necessary, however, to demonstrate that this observed suppression was indeed idiotype specific and not related to allotype suppression, a possible consequence of immunizing IgCh[e] mice with a BALB/c myeloma protein bearing "a" allotype determinants. At 4 and 6 weeks after birth, CAF₁ mice from J558 immune A/J females, were challenged with trinitrophenylated Ficoll (TNP-Ficoll) as well as α 1,3 dextran. On day 5 after immunization, antigen responsiveness was assessed by a direct PFC assay to the appropriate antigen. The idiotype expression was studied by inhibition of the PFC with anti-Id antibodies. Goat anti-IdX and EB 3-7-2 were used to study the idiotypic profile of dextran specific PFC, whereas A/J anti-MOPC 460Id, a minor idiotypic component of TNP specific antibodies of BALB/c mice, was used to study the TNP PFC response. These results, which are depicted in TABLE 2, show that in spite of the fact that maternally suppressed CAF₁s mount no detectable anti-α 1,3

TABLE 2. Specificity of the Suppression in Maternally Suppressed CAF_1 Mice

| Animal | Age | Dex PFC^a/ 10^6 Cells | Percentage Inhibition by: | | TNP PFC^a/ 10^6 Cells | Percentage Inhibition by: anti-M460 Id |
			EB3-7-2	GT anti-IdX		
I Normal-CAF_1	4 weeks	315 ± 79	—	—	3300 ± 420	13
	6 weeks	565 ± 165	39	78	5120 ± 980	11
II Maternally suppressed CAF_1	4 weeks	0	—	—	4310 ± 300	9
	6 weeks	0	—	—	3720 ± 500	14

^{a}Mice were immunized with 100 μg Dextran B1355 and 20 μg TNP-Ficoll intraperitoneally. Spleens were removed on day 5 after immunization for direct PFC determinations.

dextran response, their anti-TNP response is quantitatively and qualitatively equivalent to their nonsuppressed CAF_1 counterparts. Hence, the observed suppression of the J558 idiotype in maternally suppressed mice is not a consequence of any allotype suppression.

Therefore, the question of the clonal expression of the J558 idiotype in the maternally suppressed mice could now be addressed. The J558 IdX and IdI were identified by goat anti-IdX and EB 3-7-2 respectively on the membranes of splenic lymphocytes using the technique of immunofluorescence.[8] Stainings were performed on freshly prepared whole spleen cells, with B and T cells being identified by a concomitant anti-IgM(μ), anti-IgD(δ) staining or anti-Thy-1.2 staining, respectively. The results of four individual experiments are depicted in TABLE 3. Regarding the B-cell compartment, the maternally suppressed animals demonstrate a 3- to 4-fold

TABLE 3. Frequency of B and T Lymphocytes with Membrane Expression of Idiotypes of the Anti-Dextran System in Suppressed and Normal CAF_1 Mice at Four Weeks of Age

	Percent IdI^+/Ig^{+b}	Percent IdX^+/Ig^{+c}	Percent $IdI/Thy\text{-}1.2^{+d}$	Percent $IdX^+/Thy\text{-}1.2^+$
Experiment 1:				
Normal CAF_1	$0.7 (0.7)^a$	0.8	$0^{(0)a}$	0
Suppressed CAF_1	$2.2 (1.7)^a$	1.1	$2.6 (3.2)^a$	0
Experiment 2:				
Normal CAF_1	0.9	0.85	0	0
Suppressed CAF_1	2.5	0.9	3.0	0
Experiment 3:				
Normal CAF_1	0.75	0.7	0	0
Suppressed CAF_1	3.1	1.5	2.75	0
Experiment 4:				
Normal CAF_1	$1.0 (0.7)^a$	1.1	$0^{(0)a}$	0
Suppressed CAF_1	$4.0 (3.3)^a$	1.9	$4.0 (3.8)^a$	0

[a]Value obtained after culturing cells for 24 hours at 37° C
[b]Number of cells reacting with the monoclonal anti-J558 IdI antibody, among 100 B spleen lymphocytes assessed by membrane immunoglobulin staining
[c]Number of cells reacting with the polyclonal anti-IdX antibodies among 100 spleen B lymphocytes
[d]Number of cells reacting with the monoclonal anti-J558 IdI among 100 T spleen cells detected by anti-Thy-1.2 staining

increase in the percentage of B cells displaying the J558 IdI, whereas the IdX bearing B cells do not seem to be significantly increased. The idiotypes detected here are entirely immunoglobulin in nature, as assessed by complete cocapping with anti-μ plus anti-δ antibodies. These idiotypes are not passively acquired from the cells, because reculturing the cells for 24 hours *in vitro* gave results comparable to those obtained with the freshly prepared cells. Finally, the staining of the idiotypes is specific because the appropriate myeloma proteins inhibit the staining.

In maternally suppressed mice, we have observed a new subpopulation of T cells exclusively bearing the J558 IdI, in absence of the cross-reactive idiotype. The endogenous origin of the J558 IdI on the T cells from the maternally idiotype suppressed mice is suggested by the fact that the same results were obtained with freshly prepared nylon wool purified T cells as with the same cells cultured for 24 hours *in vitro*. It should be mentioned that this staining was inhibited with J558.

TABLE 4. T Cells from Idiotype Suppressed Mice Transfer the Suppression in Naive Syngeneic Mice[a]

Donor Cells	Direct Dextran PFC/10⁶	Percent Inhibition	RIA (μg/ml)	
			IdX	IdI
None	1000 ± 151	0	30 ± 6	2.5 ± 0.3
15×10^6 Normal F$_1$ T cells	905 ± 87	9.5	21 ± 3	1.2 ± 0.5
15×10^6 suppressed[b] F$_1$ T cells	460 ± 51	54	4.2 ± 0.3	<1.0
Idiotype suppressed T cells absorbed on EB 3-7-2 plate	1099 ± 125	0	35 ± 8	3.2 ± 0.8
Idiotype suppressed T cells recovered from EB 3-7-2 plate	370 ± 22	63	1.5 ± 1	<1.0

[a]Recipient CAF$_1$ mice were immunized with 100 μg Dextran B1355 intraperitoneally 24 hours after transfer of cells; spleen cells of recipient mice and their serum were collected 5 days after immunization.
[b]Donors were suppressed CAF$_1$ mice, 4 weeks of age.

Because these IdI-bearing T cells were identified only in the suppressed mice, the experimentation was now directed towards elucidating the role of these cells in inducing and maintaining the suppressed state. Fifteen million nylon wool purified T cells from the maternally suppressed CAF$_1$ were infused into age-matched syngeneic recipients. The recipients were challenged 24 hours later with α 1,3 dextran. Dextran responsiveness was measured by PFC assay, whereas the level of the J558 Id was measured by RIA on the sera of these animals. As can be seen in TABLE 4, the T cells from the maternally suppressed CAF$_1$ animals can transfer the suppression to naive recipients. Furthermore, the entire suppressive population is contained within the IdI-bearing cells because the suppressive ability of these T cells is contained within the fraction of cells adhering to anti-J558 Id coated dishes, that is with EB 3-7-2 monoclonal antibody.

The Lyt phenotype of these putative suppressor cells was studied next by pretreating with either Lyt-1.2 or -2.2 specific reagents plus complement, prior to

TABLE 5. T Cells Responsible for Idiotype Suppression Bear Lyt-2.2 Alloantigens

Donor of T Cells	Direct Dextran PFC/10⁶[a]	Percent Inhibition
None	940 ± 120	0
5×10^6 Idiotype Suppressed T Cells[b] plus Complement	285 ± 40	70
5×10^6 Idiotype Suppressed T Cells Treated with anti-Lyt-2.2 plus Complement	900 ± 100	4

[a]Recipient CAF$_1$ mice were immunized with 100 μg Dextran B1355 intraperitoneally 24 hours after transfer of cells; spleen cells of recipient mice for PFC determination were collected 5 days after immunization.
[b]Donors were suppressed CAF$_1$ mice, 4 weeks of age.

TABLE 6. Expression of IdI and IdX in Mice Treated at Birth with 10 ng of EB 3-7-2

Treatment at Birth	Challenge one month later	Percent IdI/Ig$^+$	Percent IdX/Ig$^+$	Percent λ/Ig$^+$	Percent IdI/Thy-1.2$^+$	Dextran PFC response/10^6	RIA (μg/ml) IdX	IdI
10 ng EB 3-7-2	None	7.4 ± 1.0 (0.08 ± 0.02)[a] (0.80 ± 0.12)[b]	6.5 ± 0.5	7.2 ± 1.6	0	0.5	5.6 ± 0.8	<1.0
10 ng EB 3-7-2	Dextran	7.2 ± 0.8	4.1 ± 0.5		0	2886 ± 311	200 ± 55	60 ± 10
10 ng EB 3-7-2	Inulin-BA	9.2 ± 1.5	3.4 ± 1.0		0	3	2.3 ± 0.4	<1.0
None	Dextran	3.6 ± 0.9	6.6 ± 0.8		0	1155 ± 211	40 ± 4	6 ± 0.8
None	None	0.9 ± 0.1	1.2 ± 0.3		0	2	1.2 ± 0.1	<1.0

[a]Staining in the presence of 1.0 mg/ml of J558
[b]Staining in the presence of 1.0 mg/ml of α1–3 Dextran, B1355S

infusing them into normal recipients, as described in TABLE 4. The results shown in TABLE 5 demonstrate that these IdI-bearing T cells exhibit the Lyt-2.2 phenotype.

The results obtained in maternally suppressed mice prompted a similar study of the effect of treatment with anti-J558 IdI administered at the time of birth. In these experiments normal CAF$_1$ animals were injected with 10 ng EB 3-7-2 within 24 hours of birth. One month later, the expression of the IdI and IdX on the membranes of B and T cells, in addition to the magnitude of the α 1,3 response, was studied. As can be seen in TABLE 6, mice treated at birth with 10 ng EB 3-7-2 showed an increased number of IdI and IdX-bearing B cells. In spite of their increased number, these B lymphocytes did not secrete antibody unless the animal was immunized with α 1,3 dextran. Furthermore, challenge with antigen did not induce any further expansion of the Id-bearing clones. In these mice no IdI-bearing T cells were observed.

DISCUSSION

Our results have shown that mice that are idiotype suppressed by maternal immunization had a surprisingly high level of T cells expressing J558 IdI, but not J558 cross-reactive idiotype. These T cells have the suppressor Lyt phenotype and indeed can transfer the suppression into naive animals. Two main points require discussion. One is the mechanism whereby these T cells mediate Id suppression, and the other is the nature of membrane molecules carrying the private idiotype.

With regard to the first point, our findings parallel those of Nisonoff, et al.[9] that have shown that idiotype suppression in the arsonate system is related to both idiotypic and anti-Id T-suppressor cell factors. It is conceivable that in our system as well, the IdI-bearing T cells may have been accompanied by other T cells with anti-Id receptors. We are currently examining this possibility that would provide further elements in this complex circuit of idiotype suppression.

The second point is quite interesting because it appears that the IdI idiotope was synthesized by the T-suppressor cells and therefore was presumably part of the T-suppressor cell molecules. In this regard, two elements of our observations are striking: the brightness of the immunofluorescent staining, indicating that the corresponding molecules were in high numbers on the membrane of the T cells, and the high percentage of IdI T cells. (In fact we have seen up to 4% of the T cells scoring with the anti-J558 IdI antibody in the suppressed animals.) This value is comparable with that of 7% of all T cells reported by Owen and Nisonoff in adult idiotype suppressed mice.[10] It appears that under some conditions of idiotype suppression, extensive segments of the T-cell system can be involved.

Another point concerns the presence on T cells of molecules bearing only J558 IdI idiotope in total exclusion of the cross-reactive idiotypes. Immunoglobulin molecules with this dissociation of idiotype expression are rare in the anti-α 1,3 dextran response.[11] This is in itself an indication that Id-bearing molecules observed on T-cell membranes in suppressed animals were not passively bound immunoglobulin.

The structural basis of the IdI expression on T-cell molecules remains to be established. In particular, it could be that similar determinants are generated in T and B cells through the use of the same genetic information (such as one of the D "mini-gene" segments), or alternatively convergent evolution may have provided B and T cells with related specificities and with related structures even in the absence of common genetic information for these molecules.

REFERENCES

1. PAWLAK, L., D. HART & A. NISONOFF. 1973. Requirements for prolonged suppression of an idiotypic specificity in adult mice. J. Exp. Med. **137:** 1442–1458.
2. KOHLER, H. 1975. The response to phosphorylcholine: dissecting an immune response. Transplant. Rev. **27:** 24–57.
3. NISONOFF, A., T. J. SHYR & T. L. OWEN. 1977. Studies of structure and immunosuppression of a cross-reactive idiotype in strain A mice. Immunol. Rev. **34:** 89–116.
4. CARSON, D. & M. WEIGERT. 1973. Immunochemical analysis of the cross-reacting idiotypes of mouse myeloma proteins with anti-dextran activity and normal anti-dextran antibody. Proc. Natl. Acad. Sci. USA **70:** 235–239.
5. SCHILLING, J., B. CLEVINGER, J. M. DAVIE & L. HOOD. 1980. Amino acid sequence of homogeneous antibodies to dextran and DNA rearrangements in heavy chain V region gene segments. Nature (London) **238:** 35–40.
6. RIBLET, R., B. BLOMBERG, M. WEIGERT, R. LIEBERMAN, B. A. TAYLOR & M. POTTER. 1975. Genetics of mouse antibodies. I. Linkage of the dextran response locus, V_H-dex, to allotype. Eur. J. Immunol. **5:** 775–777.
7. WEILER, I. J., E. WEILLER, R. SPRINGER & H. COSENZA. 1977. Idiotype suppression by maternal influence. Eur. J. Immunol. **7:** 591–597.
8. VICTOR, C., C. BONA & B. PERNIS. 1983. Idiotypes on B lymphocytes: association with immunoglobulins. J. Immunol. **130:** 1819–1825.
9. HIRAI, Y. & A. NISONOFF. 1980. Selective suppression of the major idiotypic component of an anti-hapten response by soluble T cell derived factors with idiotypic or anti-idiotypic receptors. J. Exp. Med. **151:** 1213–1221.
10. OWEN, F. L., T. J. SHYR & A. NISONOFF. 1977. Binding to idiotypic determinants of large proportions of thymus derived lymphocytes in idiotypically suppressed mice. Proc. Natl. Acad. Sci. USA **74:** 2084–2088.
11. Hansburg, D., R. M. PERLMUTTER, D. E. BRILES & J. M. DAVIE. 1978. Analysis of the diversity of murine antibodies to dextran B1355. III. Idiotypic and spectrotypic correlations. Eur. J. Immunol. **6:** 532–539.

DISCUSSION OF THE PAPER

J. MESTECKY (*University of Alabama in Birmingham*): Have you excluded the possibility that there are T-suppressor cells present in the milk of these animals? Have you looked in the milk lymphocytes?

C. VICTOR: No.

MESTECKY: Milk is a very rich source of T-suppressor cells.

VICTOR: We are not ruling out that the suppression came as a level of *in utero* exposure or milk; we are keeping both of those in mind.

W. E. PAUL (*National Institutes of Health, Bethesda, Md.*): The B-cell population of the maternally suppressed animals is expanded in the frequency of cells that express the idiotypes, and yet there is no response. You attribute that lack of response obviously to the action of the suppressor cells or the T cells, at the very least, that are coexistent. If you prepare B-cell populations and test them either *in vitro* or *in vivo*, can you demonstrate that the cells will proliferate when exposed to, let us say, anti-Id antibody or to dextran. Will they secrete antibodies?

VICTOR: We have not done those experiments yet.

D. W. SCOTT (*Duke Medical Center, Durham, N.C.*): We have some analogous results in our laboratory, and some experiments done by Brigitte Grouix from my laboratory. (The results are partially similar.) She used a modified cell system in which she coupled MOPC 104-E to syngeneic spleen cells and was able to generate specific suppressor cells that were Lyt-2 positive that would suppress the private Id using similar monoclonal reagents generously provided by John Kearney, whose mark is all over this session. The difference, though, that we observed was that the total anti-dextran response was unaffected in her experiments, and we could not find any increase in other idiotypes in the small sample we had to use. So there is that difference, and at least we are getting private Id specific suppression, which is analogous to your system.

In your maternally suppressed system, you are immunizing the mother with the idiotype, with the J558, and you are generating Id positive T cells eventually in your suppressor population. Can you give an explanation for it? Is there another T cell in this circuit that you are leaving out for simplicity?

VICTOR: That is one of two explanations. Obviously the T cell we are detecting, first of all, cannot act directly on the B cell, unless it is by way of an antigen bridge, or as you suggest, by an intermediary T cell, which to date we in this system have not yet identified, although the precedent does exist in the NP [(4-hydroxy-3-nitrophenyl) acetyl hapten] as well as the Ars (arsonate) system.

D. E. MOSIER (*Institute for Cancer Research, Philadelphia, Pa.*): First of all, would you clarify what the absolute number of B cells and T cells expressing the Id in suppressed mice are? You showed a ratio. Was that a percentage of total cells or was that a ratio of suppressed and nonsuppressed mice?

VICTOR: The way the data was depicted, first of all, was percentage of total B cells or percentage of total T cells.

MOSIER: Those are very high numbers.

VICTOR: Yes, they are.

MOSIER: The second comment has to do with Dr. Mestecky's question. Eberhart Weiler showed that these suppressive effects of neonatal immunization with idiotype or with antigen could be transferred by foster nursing. Presumably the suppressive effects did not depend upon prenatal transfer of idiotype or anti-idiotype. With regard to that observation, have you attempted to directly measure the circulating Id levels or anti-J558 antibodies in newborn mice born to immunized mothers?

VICTOR: What I can tell you about that is that in the suppressed F1 mice, I have measured the levels of anti-idiotype. We do not know whether it is endogenous, or whether it comes from the mother, but it does show a steady decrease with increasing age of the animal and does not correlate at all with the chronic suppression that we see.

MOSIER: If there is anti-idiotype, as one might expect, there is even more of a surprise to find anti-idiotype bearing T cells.

VICTOR: These animals, however, were studied for T cells at 4 weeks of age. That is where we saw the peak number of T cells. What I did not tell you is that we were looking at week 1, week 2, and week three. At week 1 there was a higher level of anti-idiotype than there was at week four. Week 4 is practically nondetectable, and that is where we see the peak number of Id-bearing T cells.

J. CERNY (*University of Texas Medical Branch, Galveston, Tex.*): I have a question with regard to the implications of your findings for a T-cell (idiotype) structure. I might have misunderstood, but is it possible that what is happening in these animals is in fact a selection of what would be a nonspecific parallel set, if I can use the analogy, from B cells, and that in fact you have selected T cells bearing that Id, but not necessarily having paratopic qualities? Therefore, is this really representative of the structure of the really specific B-cell receptor?

VICTOR: We do not know yet; we have not tested whether in fact they can directly bind dextran. I can tell you, however, that the suppression that we see is absolutely dextran specific, comparing it to trinitrophenol. There was absolutely no suppression of the TNP response in these animals, if that can be used as an irrelevant test antigen.

CERNY: I understand, but we do not know what the effective pathway of the separation really is.

VICTOR: I cannot say it is 100% dex-specific. No, we do not know.

H. KOHLER (*Roswell Park Memorial Institute, Buffalo, N.Y.*): Are the Id positive T cells equally negative by conventional anti-Ig antibody?

VICTOR: Yes.

KOHLER: Can you induce, with your reagent, capping of the Id, and can you clear the surface and demonstrate re-expression on the T cells?

VICTOR: We did not do those experiments. We just did the overnight culture, the 24-hour culture, to answer the question of passive uptake.

KOHLER: So does there remain the possibility of absorbed idiotype?

VICTOR: The possibility is highly unlikely, extremely unlikely, because they were cultured in the total absence of B cells, in the total absence of any mouse serum.

PAUL: One always learns caution in immunology.

VICTOR: That is true.

B. PERNIS: The reason I was absolutely convinced of our data is that passive immunoglobulin would have given IdX, together with idiotype.

VICTOR: I agree.

PAUL: If you could induce a parallel set, it might, in principle, be possible to introduce Id positive/IdX negative antibody that was not dextran-specific. Is that your point, Dr. Kohler?

PERNIS: We have looked at dextran precursors, B cells, of course, and we have seen segregation of Id and IdX, so it is possible to have Id without IdX.

PAUL: I think we are all very impressed with the evidence. We agree, on the other hand, that we would not be quite as bold as Dr. Victor and say that there was no possibility.

The Role of B-Cell I Region Encoded Antigens in T-Cell Dependent B-Cell Activation: I Region Encoded Antigen Density Correlates With Idiotype Expression

KIM BOTTOMLY[a] AND EILEEN DUNN

Howard Hughes Medical Institute
and
Department of Pathology
Yale University School of Medicine
New Haven, Connecticut 06510

INTRODUCTION

T-helper cells activate antigen-specific B cells by recognizing both the foreign antigen and, in most instances, major histocompatibility complex (MHC), in this case, I region (Ia) glycoprotein antigen on the B-cell surface.[1-2] Whereas all B cells express cell surface Ia glycoprotein antigens, the range of Ia antigen densities expressed on B cells from an individual animal is heterogeneous.[3] Furthermore, subsets of B cells have been defined by means of B cell surface Ia expression.[3] It has been shown that, in contrast to normal mice, CBA/N mice, that are missing a subset of B cells expressing the B-cell surface antigens Lyb-3 and Lyb-5, are also relatively deficient in B cells bearing low to moderate amounts of Ia glycoproteins. These studies suggest that B cells with low to intermediate density Ia may express the Lyb-3 and Lyb-5 alloantigens. It has been shown previously in studies using strains of mice differing in cell-surface density of a particular Ia glycoprotein that relatively small changes in cell-surface Ia density have profound effects on recognition of antigen in the content of that Ia glycoprotein.[4] Whereas this has been clearly demonstrated for T-cell interactions with antigen-bearing antigen presenting cells, few studies have focused on the effect of B-cell Ia density, and none have examined the expression of idiotype as a function of B-cell surface Ia antigen expression.

The role of T-helper cells in the response to the hapten phosphorylcholine (PC) in mice has been examined. Previous studies have shown that in adoptive secondary antibody responses, two distinct sets of T-helper cells appear to synergize in the production of the TEPC 15 (T15) idiotype. One of the T-helper cell sets recognizes Ia glycoproteins on the B-cell surface and is most effective in collaboration with the B cell if the hapten and carrier are physically linked. This T- cell set appears to be identical to the "classical" T-helper cell. The second cell appears to interact selectively with B cells bearing the T15 idiotype by recognizing the T15 determinant directly on the B cell.[5,6] The T-dependent response to PC requires the presence of the classical Ia-recognizing T-helper cell, and this helper cell alone is sufficient to generate an anti-PC plaque-

---

[a]Associate Investigator, Howard Hughes Medical Institute.

forming cell (PFC) response. The presence of two T-helper cells has also been demonstrated by Woodland and Cantor for the response to the arsonate hapten,[7] by Hetzelberger and Eichmann in response to strep A carbohydrate,[8] by Adorini, Harvey, and Sercarz in response to hen's egg lysozyme,[9] by Jayaraman and Bellone in response to trimethylammonium hapten,[10] and by Rohrer, Kemp, and Gershon in the response of the MOPC 315 myeloma to haptenated erythrocytes (personal communication).

In order to more accurately analyze cell interactions in this experimental system, an *in vitro* T-dependent anti-PC response to PC conjugated to ovalbumin (OVA) has been established, using purified B cells and, as a source of classical T_H cells, cloned, OVA-specific, self-Ia recognizing T-helper cells.[11] This has allowed an analysis of the role of B-cell Ia antigens in the *in vitro* response to phosphorylcholine. This response is strictly dependent on the presence of the cloned T-helper cells at all antigen doses, and the interaction between T and B cells requires that the cloned T-helper cell recognize Ia on the B-cell surface. The response generated by cloned, OVA-specific T-helper cells and unprimed B cells in response to PC-OVA was idiotypically heterogeneous. Between 12 and 50% of the anti-PC PFC bear the T15 idiotype. To test for the importance of Ia density in B-cell activation by an Ia-recognizing T-cell clone, an attempt was made to eliminate high density B cells with limiting amounts of anti-Ia monoclonal antibody and complement. These studies demonstrated that T15-bearing B cells express low to intermediate amounts of Ia and may be difficult to activate *in vitro* using an Ia-recognizing T-cell clone. If a source of idiotype-specific T-helper cells, purified by specific binding to T15-coated plastic dishes, is added to the *in vitro* cultures, the number of B cells secreting T15-bearing antibody increases. It might be suggested that the idiotype-specific T-helper cells function by selectively increasing Ia density of T15-bearing B cells, making them more susceptible to influences by Ia-recognizing T-helper cells.

RESULTS

Cloned, Ovalbumin-Specific T Cells Can Activate Syngeneic B Cells to Respond to Phosphorylcholine-Ovalbumin

Approximately 40 cloned, OVA-specific, Ia recognizing T-cell lines have been analyzed for their ability to induce the secretion of anti-PC antibody in response to phosphorylcholine-ovalbumin. All of the clones but one have induced substantial anti-PC PFC responses using unprimed syngeneic B cells. The *in vitro* response is T-dependent in that no response is observed in the absence of the cloned T-helper cells, and the magnitude of the response is proportional to the number of cloned T-helper cells added to the culture (TABLE 1). As few as 100 cloned T-helper cells will induce a measurable response in 2.5×10^5 B cells. This response requires that the hapten be linked physically to the carrier protein, with an optimal antigen dose between 0.01 and 0.1 $\mu g/ml$.

Cloned, Ovalbumin-Specific T-Helper Cells Recognize I Region Encoded Glycoproteins on the B-Cell Surface

When cloned T-helper cell lines were analyzed for their ability to stimulate B cells of various genotypes, identity at MHC was found to be required for successful activation of B cells (TABLE 2). To determine if the T-cell clones recognized B-cell Ia

TABLE 1. Helper Activity of Cloned Ovalbumin-Specific T Cells

T_{OVA} Cell Number[a]	Antigen[b]	Geometric Mean $(x/\div$ Relative S.E.) PC-PFC[c]
0		
10^2	PC-OVA	372 (1.06)
3×10^3	PC-OVA	513 (1.03)
10^4	PC-OVA	667 (1.09)
3×10^4	PC-OVA	565 (1.05)
10^3	PC-Keyhole limpet hemocyanin + OVA	42 (1.42)

[a]2.5×10^5 B cells from unprimed mice were cultured with varying numbers of OVA-specific T-cell clones (T_{OVA}) in 96 well Costar plates. B cells were prepared by treatment with anti-Thy-1, anti-Lyt-1, anti-Lyt-2 plus rabbit complement.

[b]The final concentration of PC-OVA and PC-keyhole limpet hemocyanin + OVA in each well is 0.1 μg/ml.

[c]The number of anti-PC PFC was determined after 5 days. Each group consisted of 3 to 5 wells, and the data was expressed as the geometric mean (relative standard error) of the wells.

TABLE 2. Cloned Ovalbumin-Specific T-Helper Cells Recognize Ia on the B-Cell Surface

B-Cell Haplotype	T_{OVA} Haplotype	Antigen[a] PC-OVA (μg/ml)	PC-Specific PFC Response	Percent of PFC Response Eliminated by Y3 + C[b]
d × b	b	0.1	+	100
d × b	b	20	+	100
d × b	d	0.1	+	100
d × b	d	20	+	90
b	b	0.1	+	100
b	b	20	+	97
b	d	0.1	−	
b	d	20	−	
d	b	0.1	−	
d	b	20	−	
d	d	0.1	+	0
d	d	20	+	3
d + b	b	0.1	+	100
d + b	b	20	+	100
d + b	d	0.1	+	0
d + b	d	20	+	0

[a]10^5 T_{OVA} clones (B6d.D2/B2 = "d" haplotype or B6B5/B2 = "b" haplotype) were added to 3 million B cells prepared as described in TABLE 1. B cells were taken from CB6F1 (d × b), BALB/c (d) and BALB.B (b) unprimed donors. B cells, T_{OVA} clones and 0.1 μg/ml or 20 μg/ml of PC-OVA were cultured in 24 well Costar plates.

[b]Plaques were assayed on day 5 of the response, and the PFC bearing H-2[b] were determined by killing the PFC either with complement alone or with monoclonal anti-K[b] antibody (Y3) plus complement. The percent of PFC eliminated is indicated.

rather than antigen presenting cell Ia, purified B cells from BALB/c (d) and BALB.B (b) were cultured with either Ia^d-recognizing or Ia^b-recognizing T-cell clones. Antigen presenting cells of both haplotypes were present in all wells. All of the anti-PC PFC in such an experiment were syngeneic to the cloned T-helper cell, suggesting that B-cell Ia is critical for B-cell activation to antibody secretion in these experiments. Furthermore, the requirement for a restricted interaction between cloned T-helper cells and unprimed B cells occurs at both 0.1 μg/ml and at the higher antigen dose of 30 μg/ml.

Expression of the TEPC 15 Idiotype in the Response of Unprimed B Cells and Cloned T-Helper Cells to Phosphorylcholine-Ovalbumin

Previous studies have shown that the antibody response to T-dependent and T-independent forms of the hapten PC in BALB/c mice is characterized by the production of antibody bearing the T15 idiotype.[12-15] Eighty-five to 100% of anti-PC PFC are T15 bearing.

TABLE 3. TEPC 15 Idiotype Expression Using Cloned Ovalbumin-Specific T-Helper Cells

T-Cell Clone[a]	Haplotype	Induces B-Cell Secretion of Anti-PC Antibody	Percent T15 Expression[b]
B6d.D2.B2	d	+	20–47
D4b	b	+	17–54
B6B5/B2	b	+	23–50
D10G4	k	+	12–40

[a]For details of the in vitro culture system, see TABLES 1 and 2.
[b]Represents data from 10–36 experiments

In the present studies, OVA-specific T-helper cells in the presence of PC-OVA, induce an anti-PC PFC response of which 12 to 54% is T15 bearing (TABLE 3). By contrast, unseparated populations of T cells activate predominantly a T15-bearing PFC response (90 to 100%), data not shown. The failure of the OVA-specific T-cell clones to induce a T15 dominated response was not due to a direct effect of the clones on idiotype expression, because the expression of T15 in response to PC-Brucella abortus, a T-independent antigen, was not affected by the presence of the cloned T-helper cells. These data suggest that T15-bearing B cells may have different activation requirements from other PC-specific B cells.

Evidence that B Cells with the Highest Cell Surface I Region Encoded Glycoprotein Antigen Density Preferentially Express Anti-Phosphorylcholine Receptors Lacking the TEPC 15 Idiotype

Because the cloned T-helper cells recognize B-cell surface Ia, and because there are differences between B cells in density of Ia expressed, it might be suggested that the activation of a B cell by the cloned T-helper cells may depend on a threshold level of Ia on the surface of the B cell. Thus, it seems logical to examine the possibility that the cloned T-helper cells act selectively on B cells expressing higher amounts of cell-surface Ia glycoprotein antigens. Furthermore, as noted above, CBA/N mice, which do not express the T15 idiotype, also have B cells with relatively high cell-surface Ia antigen density.[3]

In order to separate B cells by virture of their cell-surface Ia antigen density, advantage was taken of the observation that the monoclonal anti-A_e:E_α antibody Y-17 killed a subpopulation of B cells in (BALB/cxC57BL/6)F1 (CB6F1) mice.[16,17] This was subsequently shown to be the subpopulation of B cells expressing the greatest density of cell-surface A_e^b:E_α complexes. Thus, this monoclonal antibody can be used at plateau titers, and will kill only 20 to 50% of B cells, reflecting cell-surface Ia density. Although it is not clear that antigens encoded in I-A are expressed in exact proportion to A_e^b:E_α complexes, we have preliminary data using the cell sorter that this is true. This antibody has the added advantage over the use of graded doses of anti-I-A antibodies that it can not interfere with collaboration between the clones used here, which recognize I-A^d on CB6F1 B cells, as shown by blocking studies (data not shown).

In the experiment in TABLE 4, CB6F1 B cells were divided into two groups, one of which was treated with Y-17 and complement. Both populations of B cells were cultured at the same density of viable cells along with cloned T-helper cells from BALB/c mice. The data show that elimination of B cells that are sensitive to Y-17 and complement markedly reduces the T15 negative component of the anti-PC PFC response, whereas the T15 positive component is relatively unaffected. Because about 20 to 50% of B cells are killed in such experiments, and because the cell numbers are restored to control levels before culturing, it is likely that some T15 positive B cells are also killed by this treatment. There is clearly a distinction, however, in Ia antigen density between T15 positive and T15 negative B cells capable of responding to PC-OVA in the presence of Ia recognizing, cloned, OVA-specific T-helper cells. Thus, selective activation of B cells lacking the T15 idiotype in this system likely reflects a higher density of Ia glycoproteins on this subset of B cells. Pretreatment of B cells with limiting concentrations of anti-I-A monoclonal antibodies and complement also gives similar results (data not shown).

Augmentation of the TEPC 15 Positive Anti-Phosphorylcholine Antibody Response by Antigen-Primed Ly-1 T Cells Purified by Binding to TEPC 15 Coated Plastic Plates

In vivo studies have demonstrated that selective activation of T15 bearing PFC could be obtained by adding a source of Ly-1 T cells that act selectively on T15-bearing B cells in anti-PC antibody responses.[5,6] Because of this selectivity, and because several other studies have appeared in which cells resembling idiotype-specific T-helper cells could be purified by binding to idiotype coated plastic plates, we attempted to enrich for idiotype-recognizing T cells by adherence to T15-coated plastic petri dishes. The cells were eluted and added to cultures of B cells and cloned T-helper cells, as shown in TABLE 5. The results indicate that the T15 adherent population of Ly-1 T cells selectively increased the T15 positive PFC response, without affecting the T15 negative component of the response, as previously observed in adoptive transfer studies. These studies show that such cells can bind T15, strongly supporting the concept that there is a recognition unit on such cells for T15-bearing anti-PC antibody. Specificity for T15 was shown by inhibition of binding with free T15, but not with free MOPC 460 myeloma proteins (both are IgA,K BALB/c myelomas; data not shown). Whereas these cells have not been examined directly for antigen specificity, other studies have shown that Ly-1 cells from mice primed with antigens, for which they are genetic nonresponders, can also selectively augment the T15 component of this *in vitro* response.

TABLE 4. Importance of Ia in B-Cell Activation: Pretreatment of B Cells With Anti-I Region Encoded Antigens and Complement

Pretreatment of B-Cell Donor[a]	T_{OVA}	Antigen	Percent Reduction of the[b]:		
			Total PFC	T15$^+$PFC	T15$^-$PFC
Complement only	+	PC-OVA	0	0	0
Y17 + C	+	PC-OVA	50	10	80
Complement only	+	PC-BA	0	0	0
Y17 + C	+	PC-BA	35	35	35

[a]B cells from CB6F1 donors are treated as described in TABLE 1 and subsequently treated with monoclonal anti-A_eE_α antibody (Y17) plus complement or complement alone. The residual cells are then cultured as described in TABLE 2. Forty-five percent of B cell are killed by this procedure.

[b]The percent reduction of PFC = number of PFC generated by pretreated B cells/number of PFC generated by untreated B cells × 100. The proportion of anti-PC PFC shown to be T15$^-$ was determined by plaque inhibition with monoclonal anti-T15 antibody. The number of T15$^+$ PFC was determined by subtracting the T15$^-$ PFC response from the total anti-PC PFC response.

DISCUSSION

These studies have explored the interaction of purified B cells with cloned, Ia-recognizing T-helper cells. They demonstrate that T-cell clones alone will help B cells to secrete antibody. This helper effect requires a physical linkage between the hapten PC and the protein carrier to which the clone is specific. The clones recognize the B cells binding the hapten carrier conjugate in the context of the appropriate Ia glycoprotein antigen at the B-cell surface. Hence, two properties of the B cell appear to be of paramount importance for the response to occur: it must bind the antigen by way of its immunoglobulin receptor, and it must express the appropriate Ia glycoprotein. The expression of the T15 idiotype in these responses was lower than had been found in previous experiments using unselected populations of T cells *in vitro*. This appears to be due to the selective activation of a subpopulation of B cells having a high density of cell-surface Ia antigens and expressing predominantly anti-PC receptors having idiotypes other than TEPC 15. Finally, activation of the T15 positive, low Ia-density subpopulation could be augmented by adding a population of antigen-primed, idiotype binding Ly-1 T cells purified on idiotype-bearing petri dishes.

TABLE 5. Helper-Cell Activity of TEPC 15 Plate Adherent Ly-1$^+$ T Cells

Source of Ly-1$^+$ T Cells Added to T_{OVA} Clones and Unprimed B Cells[a]	Geometric Mean PC-PFC (x/ ÷ relative standard error)	
	Total PC-PFC	T15$^+$-PFC
None	54 (1.41)	32 (1.73)
T15 plate adherent[b]	437 (1.18)	420 (1.16)
T15 plate nonadherent	89 (1.16)	43 (1.46)
Bovine serum albumin plate adherent	95 (1.03)	66 (1.15)

[a]The plate adherent population were from BALB/c donors primed with 100 μg for 7 days; inguinal and popliteal lymph nodes were removed and minced. The cells were passed over nylon wool and treated with anti-Lyt-2 plus complement. 30×10^6 Ly-1$^+$ cells were put on T15 coated petri dishes, and after 1 hour the adherent and nonadherent populations were collected. The recovery off the plate for this experiment was .06 percent.

[b]Twelve thousand T15 plate adherent cells were added to each well. The culture were set up as described in TABLE 2 except 0.5×10^5 T_{OVA} cells were used.

One implication of these results is that B cells must express a certain threshold level of Ia in order to be activated by classical T-helper cells and antigen, and that B cells with Ia-antigen densities lower than this threshold may require additional mechanisms to become activated to secrete antibody. Because the presence of T15-recognizing T-helper cells *in vitro* activates significantly more PC-specific B cells bearing the T15 idiotype to secrete antibody, it is important to understand how this T-cell set succeeds in activating B cells. One obvious possibility is that contact with T15-bearing immunoglobulin receptor on the B cell leads to an increase in the density of Ia molecules on the B-cell surface. It has been shown that stimulation with anti-immunoglobulin antibodies leads to an increase in surface Ia antigen density, and it would seem possible that idiotype-recognizing T-helper cells may have a similar effect on B cells. This increased Ia antigen density would then allow these T15 positive B cells to be activated by cloned Ia-recognizing T cells *in vitro*. This mechanism is being tested in a two-step culture procedure with an intervening anti-Ia antibody and complement treatment step.

One may ask why there is high Ia density expressed selectively on idiotype-negative B cells? It seems possible that T-independent forms of PC selectively stimulate T15-positive B cells because they are best fit for the antigen; such B cells would not be constrained in Ia density, because their activation *in vivo* appears not to require T cells. Furthermore, because the presence of T-helper cells that act on activated, idiotype-bearing B cells, in what is probably an Ia-restricted fashion, has been suggested by the studies of Cerny and Caulfield,[18] it may be necessary to have T15 expressed only on low Ia-density B cells to avoid auto-activation of these two cell circuits in the absence of antigen. Such a situation could be maintained by T-suppressor cells. Alternatively, many studies have suggested that the state of B-cell activation may influence what signals are necessary to induce immunoglobulin secretion. It is possible that Ia density may correlate with activation state, and we are exploring this possibility at the present time.

REFERENCES

1. Katz, D. H., M. Graves, M. E. Dorf, H. Dimuzio & B. Benacerraf. 1975. J. Exp. Med. **141:** 263.
2. Sprent, J. 1978. J. Exp. Med. **147:** 1159.
3. Mond, J. J., S. Kessler, F. D. Finkelman, W. E. Paul & I. Scher. 1980. J. Immunol. **124:** 1675.
4. Matis, L. A., P. P. Jones, D. B. Murphy, J. M. Hedrick, E. A. Lerner, C. A. Janeway, Jr., J. M. McNicholas & R. H. Schwartz. 1982. J. Exp. Med. **155:** 508.
5. Bottomly, K., C. A. Janeway, Jr., B. J. Mathieson & D. E. Mosier. 1980. Eur. J. Immunol. **10:** 159.
6. Bottomly, K. & D. E. Mosier. 1981. J. Exp. Med. **154:** 411.
7. Woodland, R. & H. Cantor. 1978. Eur. J. Immunol. **8:** 600.
8. Hetzelberger, D. & K. Eichmann. 1978. Eur. J. Immunol. **8:** 846.
9. Adorini, L., M. Harvey & E. E. Sercarz. 1979. Eur. J. Immunol. **8:** 600.
10. Jayaraman, S., J. E. Swierkosz & C. J. Bellone. 1982. J. Exp. Med. **155:** 641.
11. Bottomly, K. & F. Jones, III. 1981. Idiotypic dominance manifested during a T-dependent anti-phosphorylcholine response requires a distinct helper T cell. *In* B Lymphocytes in the Immune Response: Functional Developmental and Interactive Properties. N. Linman, D. Mosier, I. Scher and E. Vitetta. Eds.: 415. Elsevier North Holland. New York.
12. Lee, W., H. Cosenza & H. Kohler. 1974. Nature (London) **247:** 55.
13. Claflin, J. L., R. Lieberman & J. M. Davie. 1974. J. Immunol. **112:** 1747.
14. Quintans, J. & H. Cosenza. 1976. Eur. J. Immunol. **6:** 399.

15. COSENZA, H., M. H. JULIUS & A. A. AUGUSTIN. 1977. Immunol. Rev. **34:** 3.
16. LERNER, E. A., L. A. MATIS C. A. JANEWAY, JR., P. P. JONES, R. H. SCHWARTZ & D. B. MURPHY. 1980. J. Exp. Med. **152:** 1085.
17. MCNICHOLAS, J. M., D. B. MURPHY, L. A. MATIS, R. H. SCHWARTZ, E. A. LERNER, C. A. JANEWAY, JR. & P. JONES. 1982. J. Exp. Med. **155:** 490.
18. CERNY, J. & M. J. CAULFIELD. 1981. J. Immunol. **126:** 2262.

DISCUSSION OF THE PAPER

W. E. PAUL (*National Institutes of Health, Bethesda, Md.*): There are several points, Dr. Bottomly, that fascinate me. First, it has been the general expectation, based on studies of mice with the xid determined defect, that the bulk of the response to PC, particularly the T15 positive component of it, would be a feature of so-called Lyb-5 positive B cells. By contrast, Hodes and their colleagues have emphasized that T-B restriction at the level of B cells was certainly a feature of Lyb-5 negative cells, and they really were unable to directly test the question of whether Lyb-5 positive cells could also participate in restricted interactions. They, however, could show that they could participate in unrestricted reactions.

Your data suggest that a large number of your T cell (OVA) clones have the property of histocompatibility restricted interactions with PC specific B cells, which by inference were all Lyb-5 positive. Therefore, we can conclude that you demonstrated that Lyb-5 positive B cells can participate in T-B restricted interactions.

K. BOTTOMLY: I would like to make that conclusion, but I think it is fair to say that there is nothing in this data to support the idea that the T dependent response is all Lyb-5 "positive." There may be T15 bearing and non-T15 bearing B cells in the B cell pool. So we cannot really address the question. The response that we augment by the helper cell for idiotype effect may, in fact, be all Lyb-5 positive, but we have not tested the H-2 restriction with the add-back used.

J. KENNY (*Uniformed Services University of the Health Sciences, Bethesda, Md.*): As Dr. Klinman pointed out this morning, as Dr. Paul just pointed out, and as we have shown in several publications, the T15-positive precursors are totally restricted to the Lyb-5 positive B-cell subset.

The second point that I would like to make is that Dr. Mond showed that xid B cells had a different level of Ia. When one looks at a series of mice with xid, this particular pattern does not hold up, and the level of Ia on Lyb-5 positive and Lyb-5 negative varies from strain to strain. That is the finding of Dr. Steven Kessler.

My third point, which is a question, is, Have you sorted your cells in terms of their Ia intensity using the cell sorter and put those cells into your system, showing where the T15 positive precursors fall?

BOTTOMLY: Let me answer the last one first. We have not sorted yet. We have not had the machine that allows us to get sterile cells out again. I think, however, that this procedure is really worthwhile doing, and we hope to be able to do it in the near future. With regard to your comments that T15 is found in the Lyb-5 positive population, am I to understand that you do not find T15 expressed in Lyb-5 negative populations in normal mice?

KENNY: That is right. If we treat normal mice with anti-Lyb-5 plus complement and then assay those cells at least in a primary assay using the splenic fragment assay, we cannot find any precursors remaining in that animal. That finding may be flawed. It may not totally answer your question.

BOTTOMLY: This point is a very important one because it says that the data that we see depends on the activation of Lyb-5 positive B cells and appears to be in direct conflict with the results of Singer and Hodes.

KENNY: We have shown and Dr. Wicker has shown, using chymeric restricted animals, that one can turn on the Lyb-5 positive subset in an MHC restricted fashion and B cells expressing the T15 idiotype. Dr. Metcalf and Dr. Singer, using the splenic fragment assay, have also shown that essentially five positive cells can also be turned on in a MHC-restricted fashion.

BOTTOMLY: That might suggest that the state of activation may play a very big role here. One might be able to activate B cells if they are in a certain state of differentiation in an H-2 restricted fashion, whereas other B cells in a different state of differentiation may not require the same signal.

PAUL: It should be emphasized, at least if I recall the Singer-Hodes set of studies properly, that what they were able to say was that five negative cells required restricted activation, but that five positive cells could be activated unrestrictively. I do not think they were able to demonstrate that they could not be activated restrictively, and this data to which you are both alluding suggests they can. What determines the set of circumstances under which they can use restricted or unrestricted activation still remains to be elucidated.

I would like to address another question to you, Dr. Bottomly. You show that if you added the population of idiotype specific T_H cells *in vitro* that you could get T15 expressed to a substantially greater degree. By the way, it seems to me that your demonstration must be one of the first examples of the direct action of these cells *in vitro*. This point must be emphasized in terms of the power that it will provide for the analysis of the system. What happens if you use one or another of the soluble factors that we all know and love? Will they also have the property of aiding the activation of this subpopulation of B cells?

BOTTOMLY: The strength of my evidence is all negative data, but we have tried. T-cell replacing factor (TRF) and a variety of soluble factors that one can derive from stimulated T cells will show an augmentation in the total response, but not a selective augmentation of the idiotype positive portion of it.

PAUL: I noticed that you could enhance the PC-OVA response quite substantially by the addition of cells from your clone without apparent stimulation, because it seemed to me you were not adding ovalbumin. So I had to assume that cloned T cells had some type of constitutive action.

BOTTOMLY: Ovalbumin is always present with the clone.

PAUL: You did show, however, a group of studies in which you added PC-*Brucella abortus* and showed that an additional number of T cells caused about a four-fold enhancement in the response.

BOTTOMLY: Yes, that is an interesting point. Just to reiterate the point: if one adds ovalbumin specific helper cells and B cells and looks at the response to PC on *Brucella abortus,* there is no added ovalbumin. One can get four- to ten-fold enhancement of that response. We do not know why that is true, but it appears to be true for all T-independent antigens that we have looked at so far.

PAUL: Do you think that situation is due to some spontaneous factor production?

BOTTOMLY: Yes.

J. CERNY (*University of Texas Medical Branch, Galveston, Tex.*): I would just like to utter a comment of caution for those who will be comparing the effects of T-cell replacing factor (TRF) and syngeneic whole T cells in reconstitution of idiotype clones. The T-cell clone supernatant is a mixture of specific factors, and depending on the background activity of anti-idiotype T cells and the source of the factor, you may or may not see certain reconstitution with the factor. That has been our problem, and I think one should look for that kind of variability.

PAUL: Your point is very well taken. I was simply alluding to the question of whether the nonspecific factors might have this function, but that certainly is an added level of complexity.

KENNY: We have done five experiments where we have sorted Ia-positive cells for bright and dull cells and then analyzed those cells in the splenic fragment in collaboration with Dr. Metcalf. The T15 positive precursors in these experiments have fallen into both subsets, into the bright Ia and the low Ia.

BOTTOMLY: I would point out that the splenic fragment assay, while being very powerful, is not the same as looking at a response generated by a cloned T cell. There are many possibilities for T cell influence in the splenic focus assay, and it is not possible to reconcile the data at this point.

KENNY: The splenic focus assay is an equivalent system because the T cells that are activating those cells are functioning in an MHC-restricted fashion in which hapten and the carrier linkage are required to turn those cells on. Those cells are all Lyb-5 positive.

BOTTOMLY: I would agree, but that does not rule out the fact that there may not, in fact, be other T cells that are acting in that particular situation, which may be influencing the expression of the T15 idiotype.

KENNY: I agree that other T cells certainly can augment the response.

The Internal Image of Catecholamines: Expression and Regulation of a Functional Network[a]

B.-Z. LÜ, P.-O. COURAUD, A. SCHMUTZ,
AND A. D. STROSBERG

Molecular Immunology Laboratory
The Jacques Monod Institute
The National Center for Scientific Research
and University of Paris
Paris, France

INTRODUCTION

Antibodies and hormone sensitive cyclase systems present attractive conceptual analogies that may well be reflected in molecular similarities.[2] In both systems, a ligand-binding recognition component, the variable region in antibodies, the hormone receptor in the cyclase complex, interacts with a signal transmitter component, CH_1, and the hinge region in antibodies, the guanosine triphosphate (GTP) binding regulatory component in the cyclase system. Effector functions reside in the crystallizable fragment (Fc) of immunoglobulins and in the adenylate cyclase catalytic subunit.[2] Whereas final proof for this conceptual homology may rely on molecular studies, immunological approaches have proved to be of considerable importance in elucidating interactions in the hormone sensitive complex.

Interactions between the hormone and the receptor can be compared to those between the hormone and the antibody on the one hand, and the receptor and an anti-receptor antibody on the other hand (FIGURE 1). If the receptor itself bears analogies to an antibody, then antibodies against the receptor should somehow be comparable to anti-idiotypic antibodies raised against anti-hormone antibodies. Some of these antibodies will actually function as the "internal image" of the hormone. We have analyzed each of these possibilities in the catecholamine-sensitive adenylate cyclase complex. In addition, we have shown that the expression of the anti-idiotypic antibodies is regulated by autoantibodies that bind the ligand.

HORMONE, RECEPTOR, AND ANTI-RECEPTOR ANTIBODIES

We will first consider the interaction that occurs between the hormone, the receptor, and the anti-receptor antibodies. Extensive studies have been carried out on the binding of catecholamine ligands, agonists, and antagonists to the β-adrenergic receptor.[3] This binding is rapid, reversible, stereospecific, and of high affinity. Displacement studies of the radiolabeled antagonist dihydroalprenolol reveal an order

[a]This work was supported by Grants from the National Center for Scientific Research, the National Institute for Health and Medical Research (No. 80.1017), the Association for the Development of Cancer Research (No. 6110), and the Foundation for Medical Research.

of potencies in which antagonists such as propranolol bind considerably better than agonists such as isoproterenol or adrenaline.

Antibodies were raised against affinity purified β-adrenergic catecholamine receptor and were shown by immunofluorescence or enzyme-linked detection systems to specifically stain receptor-bearing cells and membranes.[4,5] These antibodies, whether polyclonal or monoclonal, could immunoprecipitate a major 60,000 dalton component of the iodinated receptor. In addition they mimicked the catecholamine agonists in their ability to activate adenylate cyclase to produce cyclic adenosine monophosphate (AMP).[1,6] These findings establish the fact that the biological information that modulates this hormonal system resides in the receptor rather than in the ligand. Once the hormone has triggered the complex by binding to the receptor, its role is apparently over.

HORMONE, ANTI-HORMONE, AND ANTI-ANTI-HORMONE ANTIBODIES

The second type of interaction to be discussed concerns hormones, antibodies, and anti-antibodies. Immunization of rabbits or mice with a derivative of dihydroalprenolol

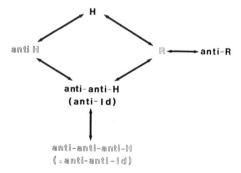

FIGURE 1. A network of immunological interactions involving a hormone and its specific receptor and antibodies. The symmetrical positions of the anti-hormone antibodies (anti-H) and the receptor (R) around the hormone (H) are mirrored by those of the anti-R and the anti-anti-H antibodies around R. The network of interactions is extended by the emergence of anti-anti-anti-H antibodies that are anti-idiotypic (anti-Id) towards the anti-anti-H immunoglobulins.

results in the production of antibodies (Ab_1) that bind various catecholamine ligands with an order of potency very similar to that seen for the receptor: again propranolol binds the best, the agonists considerably less.[1,7] Anti-idiotypic antibodies (Ab_2) were raised in allotypically matched rabbits by immunization with Ab_1 containing IgG fractions. Some of the Ab_2 completely inhibited binding of the ligand to Ab_1.

INTERACTION OF ANTI-IDIOTYPIC ANTIBODIES (Ab_2) WITH THE HORMONE RECEPTOR

The effect of the anti-anti-hormone antibodies toward the receptor was compared with that of the anti-receptor antibodies. If indeed some Ab_2 antibodies were complementary to the combining site of the anti-hormone antibodies, then perhaps they could behave as an internal image of hormone itself in binding to the receptor.

We first used an immunofluorescence test to show that some of the Ab_2 specifically stained β-adrenergic receptor-bearing cells or purified membranes. Cells lacking these receptors were, however, not recognized. This binding of the anti-idiotypes to the receptor could be quantitated using radioiodinated goat anti-rabbit antibodies as a tracer. The amount of labeling using either preimmune IgG or cells without receptors did not exceed a third of the specific labeling at saturation.[1]

More interestingly, the interaction of anti-idiotypic Ab_2 antibodies with the receptor could interfere with the binding of the hormone. Turkey erythrocyte membranes, which possess β-adrenergic receptors, were preincubated with Ab_2 for one hour at 30°C, after which their binding capacity for [^{3}H]dihydroalprenolol (DHA) was measured. FIGURE 2 shows that the Ab_2 antibodies were able to inhibit the ligand binding to the receptor to a considerable extent. The remaining [^{3}H]DHA binding sites conserved their initial binding affinity for the ligand.[1] Thus Ab_2 anti-idiotypic antibodies appeared to recognize the hormone binding site of the receptor, even though their characteristics of interaction seemed to be different from those of the catecholamine ligand (apparent, noncompetitive interactions of Ab_2). These differences might have been due, at least partially, to the very different sizes of immunoglobulins and hormones that could have, in turn, influenced the size of the respective interaction sites on the receptor molecule.

STIMULATION OF BASAL AND CATECHOLAMINE SENSITIVE ADENYLATE CYCLASE BY Ab₂

The comparison between the anti-idiotypic and the anti-receptor antibodies also included interaction with the cyclase. Adenylate cyclase activity of turkey erythrocyte membranes was measured after preincubation with increasing amounts of Ab_2 IgG or preimmune IgG as control. It appeared that Ab_2 was able to stimulate basal activity in a dose-dependent and saturable fashion (FIGURE 3). The observed stimulation (300%) was comparable with the hormone stimulation.

The comparison of Ab_2 and catecholamine actions on the β-adrenergic receptor-coupled adenylate cyclase was further investigated. Ab_2 and levo stereoisomer [(−)-] (−)-isoproterenol, a potent catecholamine agonist, were compared for their ability to stimulate turkey erythrocyte membrane adenylate cyclase activity in the presence of either a maximally stimulating concentration of (−)-adrenaline, or a high concentration of the nonmetabolizable analog of GTP, 5'-guanylyl imidodiphosphate [Gpp(NH)p]. Despite their similar effect on the basal activity of the enzyme, Ab_2 and (−)-isoproterenol had opposite actions in the presence of hormone or Gpp(NH)p: Ab_2 could overstimulate adenylate cyclase in the presence of a saturating dose of hormone,

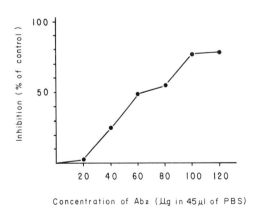

FIGURE 2. Inhibition of [^{3}H]DHA binding to β-adrenergic receptor by anti-idiotypic antibodies. Turkey erythrocyte membranes were preincubated in 75 mM Tris HCl buffer, pH 7.4/25 mM MgCl$_2$, with increasing amounts of purified anti-idiotypic antibodies (Ab_2) for 1 hour at 30°C. After further incubation for 8 minutes at 30°C and filtration on glass fiber filters, they were then tested for their ability to bind [^{3}H]DHA. Control binding capacity was measured with membranes preincubated with equivalent amounts of normal rabbit IgG. Results are expressed as the percentage of [^{3}H]DHA binding inhibition due to Ab_2.[8]

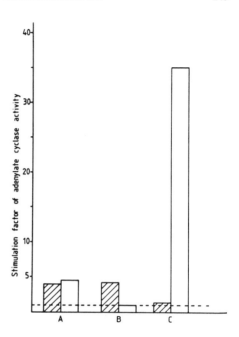

FIGURE 3. Comparison of stimulation of adenylate cylase activity by Ab_1 and by $(-)$-isoproterenol. Adenylate cyclase activity was measured with either Ab_2 (5 mg/ml) (▨) or $(-)$-isoproterenol $(10^{-4} M)$ (☐), under three different experimental conditions: (A) no addition; (B) $+10^{-4} M$ $(-)$-epinephrine; and (C) $+10^{-4}$ Gpp(NH)p. The percentage stimulation of adenylate cyclase activity due to Ab_2 or $(-)$-isoproterenol was plotted under each of these experimental conditions. The control levels of enzymatic activity (with neither Ab_2 nor $(-)$-isoproterenol) were the following: (A) 6.5 pmol/mg; (B) 29.1 pmol/mg; (C) 34.7 pmol/mg.

but had no effect on Gpp(NH)p-stimulated enzyme,[6] whereas $(-)$-isoproterenol was shown to compete with $(-)$-adrenaline and to act in synergy with Gpp(NH)p for the stimulation of adenylate cyclase.

REGULATION OF Ab_2 SYNTHESIS BY INDUCTION OF ANTI-ANTI-IDIOTYPIC ANTIBODIES (Ab_3)

As shown schematically in FIGURE 1, the hormone interacts with both receptor and anti-hormone antibodies; the receptor also combines with anti-receptor antibodies and anti-anti-hormone antibodies. The production, however, of the Ab_2 molecules was observed to be quite irregular. In six rabbits studied thus far, five, at one time or another, made anti-idiotypic antibodies that interacted with the receptor. Only in two animals could this be shown with serum immunoglobulin (Ig). In the other three animals it was necessary to first absorb the Ig fraction on an anti-hormone Ab_1 affinity gel.[8] The acid eluate that contained the anti-idiotypic antibodies did indeed bind to the receptor. The effluent, however, also displayed interesting activity: it could be shown to bind the ligand, suggesting the presence of Ab_3 antibodies. The autologous Ab_3 were anti-idiotypic towards the Ab_2 receptor-binding antibodies. Their expression was transient, and could actually be detected directly in the complete Ig fraction.[8] If we superimpose the time course of both types of activities, the expression of Ab_2 and Ab_3 is seen to alternate with time, as if one stimulates the production of the other (FIGURE 4).

It thus appears that Ab_1 resembles receptor (R), that some Ab_2 resemble the hormone, and that some Ab_3 resemble Ab_1, binding both Ab_2 and the hormone. The differences between Ab_1 and Ab_3 must be emphasized: Ab_3 arose spontaneously and appeared to neutralize Ab_2, while binding the hormone with affinities that were different from those of Ab_1. This finding was initially observed in the sera of the nonresponding animals and could be verified by adding Ab$_3$ antibodies purified over an alprenolol-agarose column affinity to Ab$_2$ purified over an Ab$_1$ agarose gel. Ab$_3$ initially bound the ligand better than Ab$_1$, but in the successive weeks, antibodies were made that had affinities lower than those of Ab$_1$, as if they were drifting away from the initial model.[8]

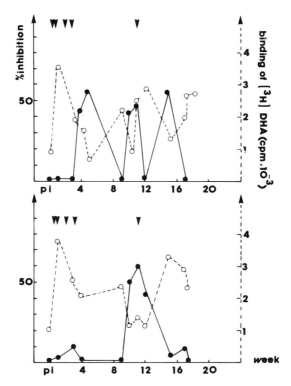

FIGURE 4. Superimposition of time courses of Ab$_2$ and Ab$_3$ activities. Upper frame: Rabbit 58; Lower frame: Rabbit 57. Ab$_2$ activity (●——●) was expressed as inhibition of [³H]DHA binding to turkey erythrocyte membranes. Ab$_2$ was purified from each bleeding by affinity chromatography on an Ab$_1$-Sepharose gel. Ab$_3$ activity (○——○) was expressed as [³H]DHA binding capacity of the corresponding effluents, not retained on the Ab$_1$-Sepharose gel. Ab$_3$ binding capacity was measured in phosphate buffered saline containing 0.25% bovine IgG. After an overnight incubation of effluents with [³H]DHA at 4°C, IgG was precipitated with 50% ammonium sulfate and filtered on glass fiber filters. Nonspecific binding was determined by addition of a 200-fold excess of (d,l)-alprenolol. In control experiments, an apparent specific binding of [³H]DHA to bovine IgG was observed (approximately 10³ cpm in our test conditions). This value has not been subtracted in the results described here.[8]

DISCUSSION

The existence of a network of interactions between idiotypic and anti-idiotypic antibodies has been demonstrated in the studies of numerous investigators (recently reviewed by Urbain *et al.*[9]). Our discussion will be restricted to the networks involving hormones, neurotransmitters, and their receptors and antibodies. In these systems, physiological constraints may considerably influence the dynamic equilibrium between the various components, leading to an increased instability and hence to cyclical responses not generally reported for systems involving synthetic haptens or antigens for which no function has yet been defined.

As recently as 1978, Sege and Peterson[10] had shown that the injection into rabbits of anti-insulin antibodies resulted in the synthesis of anti-idiotype(Id) antibodies that mimicked the action of the hormone by binding to the insulin receptors and by simulating some of the physiological effects of insulin. The production of these anti-Id antibodies was, however, short-lived. These data were confirmed and expanded recently by Shechter *et al.*[11] who suggested that the simple injection of insulin stimulated the production of anti-insulin antibodies (Id) rapidly followed by the synthesis of anti-Id antibodies that competed with insulin both for binding to the receptor and stimulation of glucose uptake by insulin-sensitive cells.

Our own work (Schreiber *et al.*[1], Couraud *et al.*[6], and the present paper) has shown that similar hormone mimicking anti-Id antibodies can be raised even though the original ligand (alprenolol) does not have a peptide-like structure. Wasserman *et al.*[12] raised anti-Id antibodies against anti-trans-3,3′-bisα-(trimethylammonio)methyl azo-benzene bromide(BisQ) antibodies. BisQ is an agonist of the acetylcholine receptor, and is even further removed from a peptide-like structure than alprenolol. The anti-Id BisQ antibodies do, however, display acetylcholine-like properties. These data and those of others[13,14] then suggest that anti-Id antibodies can adopt conformations that are complementary to the Id antibodies as well as to the receptors, even though the structural resemblance with the original ligands may be hard to grasp.

Emergence of these anti-Id antibodies is, however, not necessarily considered innocuous by the individual: the binding to the receptor of large molecules may trigger either receptor aggregation, receptor internalization, or complement activation. These effects may have detrimental physiological consequences manifested by desensitization or permanent stimulation, observed in autoimmune diseases such as myasthenia gravis or Graves' hyperthyroidism, which are characterized respectively by antibodies against the nicotinic acetylcholine receptor and against the thyrotrophin receptor. In fact, Wasserman *et al.*[12] have indeed described Myasthenia Gravis in rabbits that make anti-Id antibodies against the anti-BisQ antibodies. These considerations would therefore explain the transient character of the synthesis of internal image anti-Id antibodies in studies involving hormones and hormone receptors. Our data clearly suggest that these antibodies are quickly neutralized by a third kind of antibody that, in turn, binds the ligand.

In conclusion, the data presented here support the existence of a network of functional interactions between idiotypic and anti-idiotypic antibodies.[15,16] When these interactions involve hormones and receptors, additional constraints are imposed on the regulation of the system, leading to important physiopathological modifications.

ACKNOWLEDGMENTS

The authors acknowledge the invaluable help of Dr. A. B. Schreiber in the initial stages of this work and the contributions of Dr. J. Hoebeke and Dr. B. Vray.

REFERENCES

1. SCHREIBER, A. B., P. O. COURAUD, C. ANDRE, B. VRAY & A. D. STROSBERG. 1980. Proc. Natl. Acad. Sci. USA **77:** 7385–7389.
2. STROSBERG, A. D., P. O. COURAUD & A. B. SCHREIBER. 1981. Immunol. Today **2:** 75–79.

3. STROSBERG, A. D., P. O. COURAUD, O. DURIEU-TRAUTMANN & C. DELAVIER-KLUTCHKO. 1982. Trends Pharmacol. Sci. **3**: 272–285.
4. COURAUD, P. O., C. DELAVIER–KLUTCHKO, O. DURIEU-TRAUTMANN & A. D. STROSBERG. 1981. Biochem. Biophys. Res. Comm. **99**: 1295–1302.
5. COURAUD, P. O., B. Z. LÜ, A. SCHMUTZ, O. DURIEU-TRAUTMANN, C. KLUTCHKO-DELAVIER & A. D. STROSBERG. 1983. J. Cell Biochem. In press.
6. COURAUD, P. O., A. B. SCHREIBER, C. DELAVIER-KLUTCHKO, C. ANDRE, O. DURIEU-TRAUTMANN, B. VRAY, A. SCHMUTZ & A. D. STROSBERG. 1982. Proc. 29th Coll. Prot. Biol. Fluids: H. Peeters, Ed.: 493–496. Pergamon Press. New York.
7. HOEBEKE, J., G. VAUQUELIN & A. D. STROSBERG. 1978. Biochem. Pharmacol. **27**: 1527–1532.
8. COURAUD, P.-O, B.-Z. LÜ & A. D. STROSBERG. 1983. J. Exp. Med. **157**: 1369–1378.
9. URBAIN, J., C. WUILMART & P.-A. CAZENAVE. 1981. Contemp. Top. Mol. Immunol. **8**: 113–148.
10. SEGE, K. & P. PETERSON. 1978. Proc. Natl. Acad. Sci. USA **75**: 2443–2447.
11. SHECHTER, Y., R. MARON, D. ELIAS & I. R. COHEN. 1982. Science. **216**: 542–545.
12. WASSERMAN, N. H., S. PENN, P. I. FREIMUTH, N. TREPTOW, S. WENTZEL, W. L. CLEVELAND & B. F. ERLANGER. 1982. Proc. Natl. Acad. Sci. USA **79**: 4810–4814.
13. MARASCO, W. A., H. J. SHOWELL, R. J. FREER & E. L. BECKER. 1982. Anti-f Met-Leu-Phe: J. Immunol. **128**: 956–962.
14. FARID, N. R., B. PEPPER, R. URBINA-BRIONES & N. R. ISLAM. 1982. J. Cell. Biochem. **19**: 305.
15. JERNE, N. K. 1974. Ann. Immunol. Inst. Pasteur (Paris) **125C**: 373–389.
16. JERNE, N. K., J. POLAND & P. A. CAZENAVE. 1982. Eur. Mol. Biol. Org. J. **1**: 243–247.

DISCUSSION OF THE PAPER

J. CERNY (*University of Texas Medical Branch, Galveston, Tex*): I am fascinated by what you said with regard to Ab₃ and Ab₁. I am not sure I agree with you. I do not know if you compared the first peak for affinity with the second or third. I am fascinated because that peak precedes the anti-Id peak. I think that is what Dr. Jerne has seen. We have seen the peak also, but did not know how to handle it, because it did not make any sense to us—the idea that the complementary response would precede the idiotypic response. Could you comment on that? I think it is a fantastic point.

A. D. STROSBERG: Yes. It is of course difficult to explain. My feeling, however, is that indeed we are uncovering antibodies that were there. This finding suggests to us that the role of these antibodies, which we do not understand, might be completely different. They may not be limited to interacting with Ab₂.

UNIDENTIFIED SPEAKER: Have you considered the possibility that the variable region of the hormone receptor might actually be structurally related to the variable regions of the antibodies by evolution?

STROSBERG: Yes. This, of course, is what we set out to show. Ten years ago, we decided that immunology was getting too difficult, so we turned our attention to hormone receptors. So far, no hormone receptor has been purified sufficiently to allow sequence work to be done. This work is, of course, in progress. We have already seen that hormone receptors for many different hormones have a molecular weight that is often 70,000. This finding is reminiscent of membrane μ chain. So far that is the only evidence, and I would not build anything on it. It is, of course, a very interesting concept.

UNIDENTIFIED SPEAKER: Perhaps you could test the hypothesis by making a monoclonal correlate of an antibody of Ab₁ and then to each of the monoclonal correlates producing polyclonal sera, finding out which one of these polyclonal sera has the property that you are looking for. You could then go back to the original Ab_1 and isolate the DNA, looking at the sequence of V region.

STROSBERG: This research is being done right now.

A. R. PACKNER (*Yale University, New Haven, Conn.*): Did any of these manipulations of the adrenergic receptor have any physiological effects on the animal?

STROSBERG: This question is a recurrent one. So far we have not observed anything clear-cut, except that the rabbits die rather quickly.

PACKNER: Something subtle like that!

C. A. BONA (*Mt. Sinai School of Medicine, New York*): I would like to know your opinion on two aspects of your study—and the other studies, if you like. The first is this Ab_3 with high cross-reactivity. Actually, I think that it belongs to the Ab_1 family, and if you make an anti-anti-anti, this means an Ab_4. Probably you will not have the same idiotype expressed on Ab_1.

STROSBERG: This question is going to be tested with murine monoclonal antibodies, because all this research has been done in rabbits. It is extremely difficult to have a clear-cut phenomenon if you have heterogeneous molecules. So we have started to make monoclonal anti-alprenolol and monoclonal anti-idiotype, and we will work the whole way through.

BONA: I would like to know your opinion on my second question. The majority of anti-idiotypes that display internal images were obtained, generally, in a system in which one of the immunogens or one of the antibodies was obtained across a heterologous or homologous barrier. There are very rare examples in which anti-idiotypes were obtained in the syngeneic system. For example, our homobody that displays rheumatoid activity like human rheumatoid factor, again, was obtained across the heterologous barrier—namely in mice. Do you think that this kind of manipulation plays a very important role in the ability to pick up this kind of Ab_2, carrying the internal images of the antigens?

STROSBERG: I am not convinced. What you are saying is that often one goes from a mouse antibody to a rabbit anti-antibody and so on. Up to the present, we have worked in the rabbit system. Ab_1 is rabbit, Ab_2 is rabbit, and Ab_3 is rabbit, but, of course, as you said, the receptor that we studied is not a rabbit receptor. It is a turkey erythrocyte receptor, a human receptor, or a rat receptor, but of course, it is a different species. There, you might be right. Although, some people now start to say that, for instance, in Graves' disease, where you have spontaneous antibody, that you indeed have antibodies that are made. They say that the antibodies are anti-idiotypic as well. So there you have a homologous situation.

Cross-Reactivity of Anti-Idiotypic Antibodies as a Tool to Study Nonimmunoglobulin Proteins[a]

KARIN SEGE

Department of Cell Research
The Wallenberg Laboratory
University of Uppsala
S-751 22 Uppsala, Sweden

Antibodies can be raised to a vast variety of foreign substances, each antigen usually inducing hundreds of antibody-forming clones. The idiotype of the antibody molecule harbors the antigen combining site and is unique to each clone of antibodies.[1] The great number of different antibody-producing clones, activated by an antigen, suggested to us that the idiotypes of the antibodies possibly accounted for a sizable fraction of all the possible molecular interactions in which nature could engage the antigen. Antibodies can be elicited to the idiotype of another antibody molecule.[2,3] Furthermore, it has been proposed that the immune system comprises a network in which antigen induces production of idiotypes that in turn induce anti-idiotypes that can regulate the initial response.[4] We were interested to know whether the idiotype-recognizing antibodies, in addition, could substitute for the antigen, against which the idiotype carrying antibodies were raised. The very naive reasoning that we wanted to study is schematically described in FIGURE 1.

In an antibody population directed towards, for example a hormone, some antibodies might bind to the hormone in a way similar to that of the receptor for this hormone. Anti-idiotypic antibodies raised against the "receptor-like" antibodies may in turn interact with these antibodies very similarly to the way they bind to the hormone molecule. If so, some of the anti-idiotypic antibodies may be similar enough to the hormone to mimic its effect in certain situations. To test this reasoning, we raised anti-idiotypic antibodies to two different sets of antibodies, namely, anti-retinol-binding protein (RBP) antibodies and anti-insulin antibodies. Many aspects of this work have been discussed elsewhere.[5-8]

ANTI-IDIOTYPIC ANTIBODIES TO ANTI-RETINOL-BINDING PROTEIN ANTIBODIES

The vitamin A transport system in serum consists of two proteins, the actual vitamin A binding protein, RBP, and the thyroxine-binding prealbumin (PA).[9] Under physiological conditions one molecule of RBP is bound to one molecule of prealbumin.

Antibodies to highly purified human RBP were raised in ten Sprague-Dawley rats. Each animal was given 0.3 mg of antigen emulsified in complete Freund's adjuvant. The animals were boosted repeatedly with the same amount of antigen dissolved in

[a]This work was supported by grants from the Swedish Medical Research Council and Nordisk Insulinfond.

incomplete Freund's adjuvant. The rats were finally exsanguinated, and their sera were pooled. Specific antibodies to human RBP were isolated by immunosorbent purification on a Sepharose 4B column to which RBP had been covalently coupled.[10] The antibodies were eluted with 0.2 M glycine-HCl buffer pH 2.9, containing 0.5 M NaCl. The specific antibodies were subjected to a second purification step on a Sephadex G-100 gel filtration column equilibrated with propionic acid pH 2.8. This removed any traces of human RBP or rat PA from the antibody preparation.

The specific antibodies were dialyzed against phosphate buffered saline pH 7.4. To ascertain that the specific antibody preparation was free of any contaminating human RBP or rat PA, the antibody fraction was labeled with ^{125}I and incubated with a specific anti-human RBP antiserum and a specific anti-rat PA antiserum. The immune complexes were collected as described.[11] These tests did not reveal the presence of any human RBP or rat prealbumin.

The specific rat anti-RBP antibodies were used to immunize two rabbits. The primary immunization was given intranodally using 0.3 mg of antigen emulsified in complete Freund's adjuvant. Intradermal booster injections were given repeatedly using the same amount of antigen dissolved in incomplete Freund's adjuvant. The rabbits were bled 12 days following each boost, and the sera were collected. IgG was isolated from the immune sera on a protein A coupled Sepharose 4B column.[12] Obviously, an immunization like this mainly gives rise to antibodies recognizing common portions of rat immunoglobulin. The immunoglobulin fractions from the two immune sera were thus absorbed on affinity columns containing covalently coupled

FIGURE 1. Schematic outline of the reasoning behind the experiments. See text for explanation. H = hormone, R = receptor

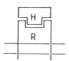 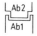

normal rat immunoglobulin.[10] Once all reactivity against the constant portions of rat immunoglobulins had been removed, the antibodies were examined for presence of anti-idiotypic antibodies to anti-RBP antibodies. If the above outlined reasoning is valid, such anti-idiotypic antibodies should encompass reactivity towards PA, since RBP and PA interact with each other.

Highly purified human PA was labeled with ^{125}I and incubated with serial dilutions of the absorbed anti-idiotypic antibodies. As shown in FIGURE 2A the anti-idiotypic antibodies precipitate PA, although the titer is low. Preimmune serum do not bring down any labeled prealbumin. The specificity of the anti-idiotypic antibody preparation is further ascertained by the fact that rat anti-RBP antibodies can abolish the binding of the anti-idiotypic antibodies to PA, whereas nonimmune rat antibodies have no effect (FIGURE 2B). Furthermore, human RBP does also inhibit the interaction between PA and the anti-idiotypic antibodies (FIGURE 2b). This is, of course, to be anticipated, because the anti-idiotypic antibodies should only bind to PA at its site of interaction with retinal-binding protein.

STOICHIOMETRY OF BINDING OF THE ANTI-IDIOTYPIC ANTIBODIES TO PREALBUMIN

Prealbumin is composed of four identical protein subunits.[9] It thus seems reasonable to assume that each subunit or pair of subunits carries one RBP-binding site,

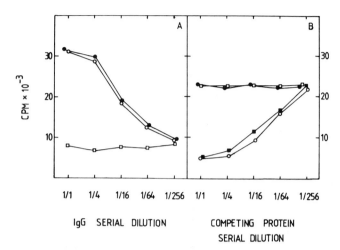

FIGURE 2. A. Reactivity of anti-idiotypic antibodies to anti-RBP antibodies with ^{125}I-labeled prealbumin. Anti-idiotypic IgG fractions from two different rabbits were used (O–O and ●–●), both at initial concentrations of 2 mg ml^{-1}. Serial dilutions of the different sera were mixed with 32,000 cpm of the ^{125}I-labeled prealbumin. The mixtures were incubated for 6 hours at +4° C and immune complexes collected with protein-A-containing *Staphylococcus aureus*.[11] Serial dilutions of preimmune rabbit IgG (□–□; initial concentration 4 mg ml^{-1}) were used as a control. B. Inhibition of the binding between anti-idiotypic antibodies to anti-RBP antibodies and ^{125}I-labelled prealbumin. ^{125}I-labeled PA (32,000 cpm) was mixed with enough IgG from one of the anti-idiotypic IgG fractions used in FIGURE 2A to cause a 70% binding. Serial dilutions of rat anti-RBP antibodies (O–O; initial concentration 0.5 mg ml^{-1}), nonimmune rat serum (●–●; initial concentration 1 mg ml^{-1}), RBP (■–■; initial concentration 0.25 mg ml^{-1}), and soybean trypsin inhibitor (□–□; initial concentration 0.25 mg ml^{-1}) respectively, were included in the reaction mixtures as well. Immune complexes were analyzed as described in FIGURE 2A.

although at physiological conditions, only one of these is occupied by retinol-binding protein. Several investigations have been carried out to study the stoichiometry of the PA-RBP interaction. This has, however, led to some controversy as to whether PA exhibits one, two, or four RBP binding sites.

Raz *et al.*[13] obtained evidence for a single RBP binding site of prealbumin. Peterson and Rask,[14] using fluorescence-quenching techniques, came to the same conclusion. In a study, however, employing fluorescence polarization and sedimentation velocity analyses, van Jaarsveld *et al.*[15] concluded that PA displays four binding sites for retinol-binding protein. Nilsson *et al.*[16] showed that the isolated PA subunit retains binding affinity for retinol-binding protein. In a study carried out by Vahlquist and Peterson,[17] it was demonstrated that out of the twelve anti-PA Fab fragments that could simultaneously be bound to PA, four were displaced by the binding of RBP to prealbumin. We thus reinvestigated this issue using the anti-idiotypic antibodies to anti-RBP antibodies. This was possible because of the exclusive reactivity that these antibodies have with the RBP binding site of prealbumin.

Fab fragments were prepared[1] from the specific anti-idiotypic immunoglobulin fraction and from normal rabbit IgG. ^{125}I-labeled PA was incubated with an excess amount of the anti-idiotypic Fab fragments and the nonimmune Fab fragments respectively. The mixtures were subjected to gel chromatography analyses on Sepharose 6B columns (130 × 1 cm) equilibrated with 0.02 *M* TRIS-HCl pH 8.0, containing

0.15 M NaCl. The complex between ^{125}I-labeled PA and RBP, as well as ^{125}I-labeled PA only, were analyzed similarily (original data not shown).

The Stoke's radii obtained from these analyses (see TABLE 1) were calculated realtive to the elution profile of the ^{131}I-labeled marker proteins, IgM, IgG, and albumin, that were included in each run. The behavior of the same set of mixtures on analytical sucrose density gradient ultracentrifugation was also examined. The gradients were 5 to 20% sucrose in 0.02 M TRIS-HCl buffer pH 8.0, containing 0.15 M NaCl. Centrifugations were carried out at 224000 × g for 16 hours at +4° C. Each run included the ^{131}I-labeled marker proteins, IgG (6.7S) and ovalbumin (3.4S). (Original data not shown.) TABLE 1 gives the sedimentation coefficients obtained for the different ^{125}I-labeled PA incubation mixtures.

As can be deduced from the table, where also the molecular weights calculated for the different complexes are given, the ratio of anti-idiotypic Fab to PA is 2.0. This is calculated on the assumption that the molecular weights of PA and the Fab fragments are 60,000 and 50,000, respectively. Fab fragments derived from nonimmune IgG do not bind to PA as also shown by the table. The tetrameric PA molecule thus exhibits two sites for the anti-idiotypic antibodies. In view of the specificity of the anti-idiotypic antibodies, we would argue that PA displays two RBP-binding sites. One may ask whether two Fab fragments bound to PA may sterically exclude the binding of further Fab fragments. That situation does not, however, seem to be the case, because previously published studies from this laboratory[17] have shown that twelve Fab fragments of antibodies raised directly against PA can bind PA simultaneously. This further indicates that the anti-idiotypic antibodies to the anti-RBP antibodies interact with PA in a more "RBP like manner" than do regular anti-PA antibodies.

PRODUCTION OF ANTI-IDIOTYPIC ANTIBODIES TO ANTI-INSULIN ANTIBODIES

Another system in which we raised anti-idiotypic antibodies was the insulin anti-insulin antibody system. Rat antibodies to crystalline bovine insulin were raised according to the same procedure as the one used for obtaining the rat anti-RBP antibodies (see above). Specific antibodies were purified on an affinity column containing covalently coupled bovine insulin.[10] The antibodies were further purified on gel filtration in propionic acid, and all steps were carried out as described above for the rat anti RBP-antibodies.

The specific rat anti-insulin antibodies were used to immunize two rabbits (see above). The rabbit immune sera were enriched for IgG on a protein A coupled immunosorbent column[12] and thereafter absorbed on normal rat immunoglobulin coupled columns. The remaining immunoglobulin fraction was analyzed for anti-idiotypic activity.

TABLE 1.

PA Complex	Stokes' Radius	Sedimentation Coefficient	Molecular Weight[a]
	Å	S	
PA	31	4.2	60,000
PA-RBP	38	4.7	77,000
Fab-anti-idiotype	53	6.9	160,000
Fab-NRS	31	4.2	60,000

[a]Calculated from Stokes' radii and sedimentation coefficients.

First, however, it was very important to ascertain that the anti-idiotypic IgG fractions did not contain any insulin or antibodies to insulin. The presence of insulin was examined by trying to inhibit the binding between ^{125}I-labeled insulin and rabbit anti-insulin antibodies with the anti-idiotypic IgG fraction. No such inhibition could be detected even at concentrations as high as 25 mg/ml of anti-idiotypic IgG. Neither did the anti-idiotypic IgG fractions react with ^{125}I-labeled bovine insulin, which indicates that they do not contain any anti-insulin antibodies, especially because, in this assay, rat anti-insulin antibodies at high dilutions could bring down all of the labeled insulin.

INTERACTION OF THE ANTI-IDIOTYPIC ANTIBODIES WITH THE INSULIN RECEPTOR

The absorbed anti-idiotypic IgG fraction was shown to react with ^{125}I-labeled rat anti-insulin antibodies, whereas no reactivity towards ^{125}I-labeled nonimmune rat IgG could be demonstrated. Furthermore, the interaction between the ^{125}I-labeled rat

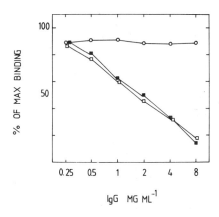

FIGURE 3. Binding of ^{125}I-labeled insulin to epididymal fat cells in the presence of anti-idiotypic antibodies against anti-insulin antibodies. The reaction mixtures contained 6×10^4 epididymal fat cells, ^{125}I-labeled insulin to give 90% of the maximal specific binding, serial dilutions of the anti-idiotypic anti-insulin IgG fractions (□–□ rabbit no 1 ■–■ rabbit no 2), and the anti-idiotypic anti-RBP IgG fraction (O–O).

anti-insulin and the anti-idiotypic IgG could be completely abolished by an excess of cold bovine insulin, thus ascertaining the specificity of the anti-idiotypic antibodies. (data not shown)

To investigate whether some of the anti-idiotypic antibodies were similar enough to the receptor-binding domain of the insulin molecule to interact with the insulin receptor, we performed competition experiments with the anti-idiotypic IgG fractions. Rat epididymal fat cells were used as a source of insulin receptors.[18] Bovine insulin was labeled with ^{125}I, and its binding to the fat cell preparation was measured[19] in the presence and absence of the anti-idiotypic IgG. FIGURE 3 shows that ^{125}I-labeled insulin is displaced from its receptor by the anti-idiotypic antibodies, although the effect is rapidly reversed upon dilution of the antibodies. No such displacement of the ^{125}I-labeled insulin can be detected when an IgG fraction isolated from the anti-idiotypic antiserum raised against antibodies to RBP was used.

One of our reasons for producing anti-idiotypic antibodies was to obtain reagents against cell-surface structures that otherwise might prove difficult to isolate. The anti-idiotypic antibodies were therefore tested for their ability to immunoprecipitate

FIGURE 4. Sodium dodecyl sulfate-polyacrylamide gel electrophoresis of the [³H]leucine-labeled rat liver insulin receptor immunoprecipitated with the anti-idiotypic anti-insulin antibodies (O–O). Pre-immune IgG was used for a control immunoprecipitation (●–●). The arrows from left to right denote the migration positions of the marker proteins phosphorylase B, albumin, ovalbumin, and the tracking dye bromphenol blue.

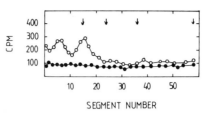

SEGMENT NUMBER

the insulin receptor. Rat liver cells were metabolically labeled with [³H]leucine and the washed cells subsequently solubilized with 1% T-X-100 in 0.02 M TRIS-HCl buffer pH 8.0, containing 0.15 M NaCl. The immunoprecipitation was carried out according to standard methods,[20] and the material brought down by the antibodies was analyzed on SDS-polyacrylamide gel electrophoresis.[20] FIGURE 4 shows the result of one such immunoprecipitation. The anti-idiotypic antibodies specifically precipitate two components of molecular weights 130,000 and 90,000. The reactivity, however, is weak, and a considerable amount of IgG had to be used (50 μg) to get a positive immunoprecipitation.

The insulin receptor has recently been isolated in several laboratories,[21–23] and it has been shown that the receptor is composed of two types of subunits with molecular weights of 135,000 and 90,000, respectively, when analyzed on SDS-polyacrylamide gel electrophoresis. In the light of these data, it seems reasonable to conclude that the material brought down by the anti-idiotypic antibodies is indeed the rat liver insulin receptor.

INSULIN-LIKE EFFECT OF THE ANTI-IDIOTYPIC ANTIBODIES

Because the anti-idiotypic antibodies should bind to the insulin receptor in an insulin-like fashion, it was, of course, of interest to examine whether they could also mediate any of the known biological effects of insulin. This possibility was studied in two different systems. First, we examined the effect of the anti-idiotypic IgG fractions on the uptake of α-amino-isobutyric acid (AIB) by young rat thymocytes, a system that is known to be stimulated by insulin.[24] Two different anti-idiotypic IgG fractions were analyzed corresponding to the two rabbits immunized with the rat anti-insulin antibodies. As can be seen in FIGURE 5, the two anti-idiotypic IgG fractions stimulate

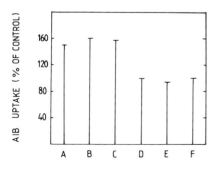

FIGURE 5. Effect of the anti-idiotypic antibodies on the uptake of α-amino-isobutyric acid (AIB) by young rat thymocytes. The thymocytes (6 × 10⁷ cells/ml) were incubated with 5 μg/ml of insulin (A), 5 mg/ml of anti-idiotypic anti-insulin IgG (from two different rabbits B and C), 5 mg/ml of nonimmune rabbit IgG (D) and 5 mg/ml of an IgG fraction against AgB antigen (E). The uptake of AIB in the absence of any additive served as the control (F).

the uptake to a similar extent. Moreover, the effect of the anti-idiotypic antibodies on the uptake is as pronounced as that of insulin, although at a much higher concentration than that needed for insulin. Nonimmune IgG or IgG isolated from a rabbit anti-rat transplantation antigen serum have no effect on the thymocyte uptake of α-amino-isobutyric acid. In the second system the effect of the anti-idiotypic antibodies on the blood glucose level of diabetic mice was examined. The anti-idiotypic IgG fraction from one of the immunized rabbits, nonimmune IgG, insulin, and phosphate-buffered saline, respectively, were injected into four groups of Streptozotocin-induced diabetic mice. Each group comprised 6 to 8 mice, and they all had high blood glucose levels. After injecting the mice with the different substances, blood samples were collected at various times, and the blood glucose concentrations were determined. FIGURE 6 shows the outcome of this *in vivo* study. As can be seen, insulin produced the expected highly significant decrease in the blood glucose level. The effect of insulin reaches its maximum within thirty minutes after its administration. Nonimmune IgG and phosphate-buffered saline had no significant effect. The anti-idiotypic IgG fraction, however, lowered the blood glucose levels considerably. The kinetics of the effect exerted by the anti-idiotypic IgG is quite different from that of insulin. Not until 3

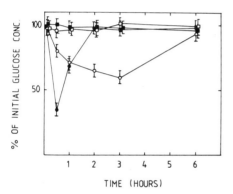

FIGURE 6. Effect of the anti-idiotypic antibodies on the blood glucose level in Streptozotocin-induced diabetic mice. The diabetic mice had an initial glucose level of 616 ± 123 mg percent. Six to eight animals were injected intravenously with 0.25 ml of phosphate-buffered saline pH 7.4 (□–□), 0.1 U of insulin (●–●), 2.5 mg of anti-idiotypic anti-insulin IgG (O–O), and 2.5 mg of nonimmune IgG (■–■), respectively. The values have been calculated as the percentage of the initial blood glucose level for each animal. The mean and the S.E.M. are indicated in the figure.

hours after injection of the antibodies is the full effect obtained. The difference in kinetics, however, between insulin and the antibodies is not unexpected, because the antibodies have a much longer half-life *in vivo* than insulin. In addition, the anti-idiotypic antibodies, at the concentration used (5 mg/ml), did not manage to lower the blood glucose levels to the same extent as did insulin. In this context it is interesting to note that there are cases of insulin resistant diabetes reported in the literature,[25] where it has been shown that the disease is caused by antibodies to the insulin receptor. These antibodies seem to bind to the insulin-binding portion of the receptor rather than to other parts. When using the antibodies from these patients in *in vitro* studies, it turns out that they have insulin-like activity, although a chronic exposure to the anti-receptor antibodies produces insulin resistence. The insulin-resistence *in vivo* is most probably due to the downshift of the insulin receptors.[26]

CONCLUDING REMARKS

The results presented here describe a way to raise antibodies recognizing molecules with which the animals were never challenged. Elegant studies by Schreiber *et al.*[27] and by Wasserman et al.[28] have confirmed the possibility of raising antibodies in this fashion. Whether this will turn out to be a general phenomenon is, of course, too early to conclude. The major drawback of this method has, in our hands, been to produce these antisera with a titer that was high enough. Although not calculated very precisely, an estimate of the amount of anti-idiotypic antibodies with insulin-like activity is in the order of 0.1 to 0.2% of the immunoglobulin fraction. Furthermore, one may have to catch the anti-idiotypic antibodies at a precise time during the immunization period. When samples from early and late bleedings of the same anti-idiotypic antiserum were pooled, the anti-idiotypic activity of the early bleedings was extinguished. The reason for this is unclear, but this data could mean that the rabbit had produced auto-anti-idiotypic antibodies to the anti-idiotypic antibodies. In other experimental systems it has been shown that auto-anti-itiotypic antibodies can indeed arise spontaneously during an immunization.[29]

ACKNOWLEDGMENTS

The experiment described in FIGURE 6 was performed in collaboration with Dr. A. Andersson and Dr. C. Hellerström. Ms. Margareta Moliteus is gratefully acknowledged for expert secreterial help.

REFERENCES

1. NISONOFF, A., J. E. HOPPER & S. B. SPRING. 1975. The antibody molecule. Academic Press. New York.
2. CAZENAVE, P-A. 1977. Proc. Natl. Acad. Sci. USA 74: 5122–5125.
3. URBAIN, J., M. WIKLER, J. D. FRANSSEN & C. COLLIGNON. 1977. Proc. Natl. Acad. Sci. USA. 74: 5125–5130.
4. JERNE, N. K. 1974. Ann. Immunol. Inst. Pasteur (Paris) 125C: 373–389.
5. SEGE K. & P. A. PETERSON. 1978. Nature (London) 271: 167–168.
6. SEGE, K. & P. A. PETERSON. 1978. Proc. Natl. Acad. Sci. USA 75: 2443–2447.
7. SEGE, K. & P. A. PETERSON. 1980. In Immunology of Diabetes. W. J. Irvine, Ed.: 195–204. Teviot.
8. TRÄGÅRDH, L., H. ANUNDI, L. RASK, K. SEGE & P. A. PETERSON. 1980. J. Biol. Chem. 255: 9243–9248.
9. PETERSON, P. A. 1971. J. Biol. Chem. 246: 44–49.
10. CUATRECASAS, P. 1970. J Biol. Chem. 245: 3059.
11. ÖSTBERG, L., K. SEGE, L. RASK & P. A. PETERSON. 1976. Folia Biol. (Prague) 22: 372–373.
12. In Affinity Chromatography—Principles and Methods. Pharmacia Fine Chemicals, Uppsala, Sweden.
13. RAZ, A., T. SHIRATORI & DE W. S. GOODMAN. 1970. J. Biol. Chem. 245: 1903–1912.
14. PETERSON, P. A. & L. RASK. 1971. J. Biol. Chem. 246: 7544–7551.
15. VAN JAARSVELD, P. P., H. EDELHOCK, DE W. S. GOODMAN & J. ROBBINS. 1973. J. Biol. Chem. 248: 4698–4705.
16. NILSSON, S. F., L. RASK & P. A. PETERSON. 1975. J Biol. Chem. 250: 8554–8563.
17. VAHLQUIST, A. & P. A. PETERSON. 1973. J. Biol. Chem. 248: 4040–4046.
18. GLIEMANN, J. 1967. Diabetologia 3: 382–388.
19. CUATRECASAS, P. 1971. Proc. Natl. Acad. Sci. USA 68: 1264–1268.
20. SEGE, K., L. RASK & P. A. PETERSON. 1981. Biochemistry 20: 4523–4530.
21. JACOBS, S., E. HAZUM & P. CUATRECASAS. 1980. J. Biol. Chem. 255: 6937–6940.
22. MASSAGUE, J., P. F. PILCH & M. P. CZECH. 1980. Proc. Natl. Acad. Sci. USA 77: 7137–7141.
23. KASUGA, M., E. VAN OBBERGHEN, S. P. NISSLEY & M. M. RECHLER. 1981. J. Biol. Chem. 256: 5305–5308.

24. GOLDFINE, I., J. D. GARDNER & D. M. NEVILLE JR. 1972. J. Biol. Chem. **247:** 6919–6926.
25. KAHN, C. R., J. S. FLIER, R. S. BAR, J. A. ARCHER, P. GORDEN, M. M. MARTIN & J. ROTH. 1976. N. Engl. J. Med. **294:** 739–845.
26. KAHN, C. R., J. S. FLIER, M. MUGGEO & L. C. HARRISON. 1980. *In* Immunology of Diabetes. W. J. Irvine Ed.: 205–218. Teviot.
27. SCHREIBER, A. B., P. OLIVER COURAND, C. ANDRE, B. VRAY & A. D. STROSBERG. 1980. Proc. Natl. Acad. Sci. USA **77:** 7385–7389.
28. WASSERMAN, N. H., A. S. PENN, P. I. FREIMUTH, N. TREPTOW, S. WENTZEL, W. L. CLEVELAND & B. F. ERLANGER. 1982. Proc. Natl. Acad. Sci. USA **79:** 4810–4814.
29. SHECHTER, Y., R. MARON, D. ELIAS & I. R. COHEN. 1982. Science **216:** 542–545.

DISCUSSION OF THE PAPER

UNIDENTIFIED SPEAKER: I am interested in the biological significance of the anti-idiotypes with respect to insulin resistance. Some patients with insulin resistance spontaneously lose that resistance. My question to you is, Have you studied the sera of some of those patients to see if they have developed anti-idiotype?

K. SEGE: We have never worked with sera from these patients. The work I referred to was carried out by J. Roth and his coworkers, and as far as I know they have only tested the patient sera for anti-receptor activity.

C. A. BONA (*Mt. Sinai School of Medicine, New York*): I would like to ask you two questions. The first is, Do you think that this anti-idiotype antibody in the retinal system can play a role in absorption of vitamins and hormones?

SEGE: I do not know. We have never looked at anything like that.

BONA: My second is, Do you have a clear picture about what kind of insulin functions are mimicked by anti-idiotypes and what function anti-idiotypes fail to mimic?

SEGE: We have only tested the insulin dependent functions that I have been talking about.

Induction of Anti-Arsonate CRI Positive Antibodies in BALB/c Mice[a]

O. LEO, M. MOSER, J. HIERNAUX, AND J. URBAIN

Laboratory of Animal Physiology
Department of Molecular Biology
Free University of Brussels
Brussels, Belgium

INTRODUCTION

When injected with the same antigen, different individuals of the same species generally synthesize specific antibodies bearing different idiotypic specificities. Cross-reactive idiotypes, however, are frequently expressed by all members of an inbred strain of mice immunized with a given antigen. Recurrent idiotypes provide an attractive model system for the study of immune regulation and repertoire expression.

One system involving such a public idiotype is the arsonate system.[1] After immunization with arsonate-coupled keyhole limpet hemocyanin (KLH-Ars), all A/J mice synthesize anti-arsonate antibodies bearing a cross-reactive idiotype (CRI_A^+). Expression of this major idiotype is linked to the IgC_H locus (d or e allotype). Amino acid sequence analysis of monoclonal anti-arsonate antibodies have shown that CRI_A^+ proteins constitute a family of closely related but distinct molecules that appear to be encoded for by one, or a very few germ-line genes.[2,3]

Recent data[4,5] suggest that the CRI_A^+ structural gene is absent in the genome of CRI_A^- strains as BALB/c mice (a allotype).

In this report, we demonstrate that it is possible, by idiotypic manipulation, to induce CRI_A^+ anti-arsonate antibodies in BALB/c mice that never express this idiotype upon antigen stimulation.

RESULTS

We have previously shown that it is possible to induce the expression of silent idiotypes in rabbits by sequential anti-idiotypic immunization[6] (see also J. Urbain *et al.,* this volume). Similar experiments have been performed in this study. Briefly, Ab_1 antibodies (purified A/J anti-arsonate antibodies) are injected into a rabbit to induce Ab_2 antibodies (rabbit anti-CRI_A^+). These purified rabbit anti-idiotypic antibodies are injected into naive BALB/c mice that then synthesize Ab_3 antibodies (or anti-Ab_2). After a rest period, these mice are immunized with KLH-Ars and produce Ab_1, antibodies (anti-arsonate antibodies of BALB/c manipulated mice). When immunized with KLH-Ars, normal BALB/c mice never express the CRI_A^+ idiotype, but synthesize anti-arsonate antibodies carrying another cross-reactive idiotype called CRI_C^+.[7] This CRI_C^+ idiotype is serologically unrelated to the major CRI_A^+ idiotype of A/J mice, but is expressed by a minor subpopulation of anti-arsonate antibodies present in

[a]The Laboratory of Animal Physiology is supported by grants from the Belgian State and Euratom. O. Leo and M. Moser have a fellowship from the National Foundation for Scientific Research.

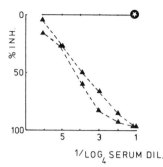

FIGURE 1. Inhibition of binding of labeled, purified A/J anti-Ars antibodies to the rabbit anti-CRI$_A$ antibodies. Unlabeled inhibitors: – BALB/c anti-Ars sera; ▲ A/J anti-Ars sera; ⊘ BALB/c and A/J normal sera.

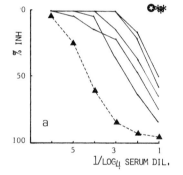

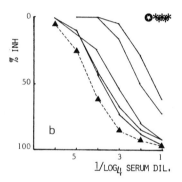

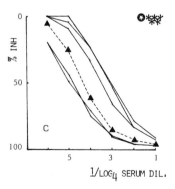

FIGURE 2. Inhibition of the binding of labeled purified A/J anti-Ars antibodies to rabbit anti-CRI$_A$ serum. Unlabeled inhibitors: ▲ A/J anti-Ars sera (secondary response); ⊘ normal A/J sera; (a) —— BALB/c Ab$_3$ sera * BALB/c anti-normal rabbit Ig sera; (b), (c) —— BALB/c Ab$_{1'}$ sera; (b) primary and (c) secondary response; * BALB/c untreated sera; (b) primary and (c) —— secondary response.

all A/J mice immune serum. The rabbit anti-idiotypic serum is therefore rendered specific for the CRI_A^+ idiotype by first adsorbing it on normal A/J globulin conjugated to Sepharose followed by further adsorption on Sepharose, coupled to a pool of anti-arsonate antibodies from BALB/c mice.

FIGURE 1 described the experiments demonstrating the specificity of the rabbit Ab_2 serum for the major A/J idiotype (CRI_A^+). Five BALB/c mice are injected with

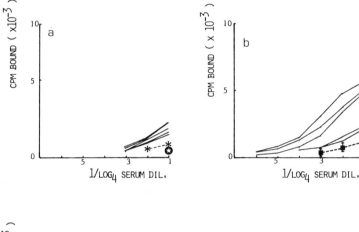

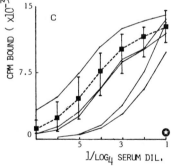

FIGURE 3. Antigen-binding capacity of BALB/c immune sera. Individual mice are assayed for anti-Ars antibodies with a solid phase radioimmunoassay by incubating serum dilutions on polyvinyl microtiter wells coated with bovine serum albumin-arsonate (BSA-Ars). Bound anti-Ars antibodies are detected by the uptake of labeled purified goat anti-mouse Ig. (a) ——— BALB/c Ab_3 sera; * BALB/c anti-normal rabbit Ig (mean); (b), (c) ——— BALB/c Ab_1 sera; (b) primary and (c) secondary response; ■ BALB/c untreated sera; (b) primary and (c) secondary response.

purified rabbit anti-idiotypic antibodies. After five successive immunizations, the serum of these Ab_3 mice are tested for anti-anti-idiotypic activity (Ab_3). As indicated in FIGURE 2a, all Ab_3 serum significantly inhibit the binding of purified and radiolabeled A/J Ab_1 to rabbit Ab_2 antibodies. When tested for specific anti-arsonate activity, these sera specifically bind the antigen [bovine serum albumin-arsonate

TABLE 1. CRI_A^+ Anti-Arsonate Antibodies Assays[a]

	Inhibition of the Binding of Radiolabeled Goat Anti-Mouse Ig by Rabbit Anti-CRI_A^+ (Percent)				
Mice No.	1	2	3	4	5
A/J	36.1	46.3	—	—	—
BALB Untreated	7.9	5.4	1.2	1.6	5.0
BALB AB_1'	19.2	63.1	73.8	45.5	21.1

[a]The binding of unlabeled anti-arsonate antibodies to insolubilized BSA-Ars was inhibited by rabbit anti CRI_A^+ serum. CRI_A^+ antibodies are quantified by measuring the inhibition of the uptake of ^{125}I-labeled goat anti-mouse Ig.

(BSA-Ars)] as compared to the sera of nonimmune BALB/c mice or of mice injected with normal rabbit immunoglobulins. Moreover, the Ab_3 sera contain higher concentrations of anti-arsonate antibodies than the sera of control mice primed only with KLH-Ars (FIGURE 3a).

Two (group I) or three (group II) months after the last injection of Ab_2 antibodies, the Ab_3 mice are injected with KLH-Ars. Analysis of these $Ab_{1'}$ sera can be summarized as follows. The sera of $Ab_{1'}$ mice collected after a single injection of antigen ($Ab_{1'}$ primary response) contains more anti-arsonate antibodies than control mice (see particularly group I mice). After a second challenge with KLH-Ars, manipulated and control mice show similar antigen binding activity (FIGURES 3b and 3c). The sera of $Ab_{1'}$ mice completely inhibit the binding of A/J Ab_1 antibodies to rabbit Ab_2 antibodies : a clear positive correlation is observed between the concentration of anti-arsonate antibodies and the inhibitory activity of a given serum.

The injection of rabbit Ab_2 antibodies probably induced a subpopulation of anti-arsonate antibodies. We can therefore assume that this population carries the CRI_A^+ idiotopes and is expanded after antigenic stimulation.

To assess the presence of CRI_A^+ anti-arsonate antibodies in the serum of manipulated mice, the following experiments were performed. The binding of unfractionated A/J anti-Ars sera on unsolubilized antigen can be inhibited by increasing concentration of rabbit anti-idiotypic antibodies. This system was shown to be specific for the CRI_A^+ idiotype and provides a correct measurement of the percentage of anti-arsonate antibodies bearing the CRI_A^+ idiotype. TABLE 1 shows that the binding of manipulated sera to the antigen is significantly inhibited by the rabbit Ab_2 serum. Similar results have been obtained by using a polyclonal BALB/c anti-CRI_A^+ serum as an inhibitor of the same reaction (TABLE 2). Moreover, anti-arsonate antibodies of $Ab_{1'}$ mice have been isolated on a Sepharose column coupled to BSA-Ars. These

TABLE 2. CRI_A^+ Anti-Arsonate Antibodies Assays[a]

	Inhibition of the Binding of Radiolabeled Goat Anti-Mouse Ig by BALB Anti-CRI_A^+ (Percent)				
Mice No.	1	2	3	4	5
A/J	19.5	27.0	—	—	—
BALB Untreated	0.0	0.0	0.0	0.0	0.0
BALB AB_1'	14.6	57.0	44.0	19.6	4.5

[a]The binding of unlabeled anti-arsonate antibodies to insolubilized BSA-Ars was inhibited by a BALB/c anti-CRI_A^+ serum.

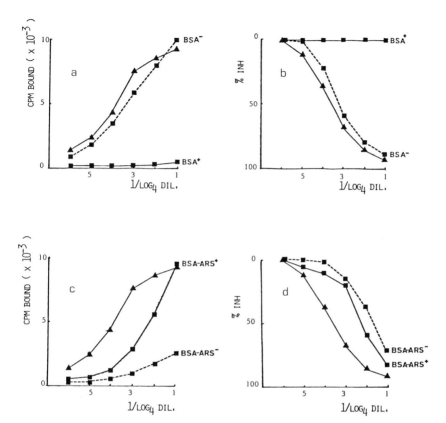

FIGURE 4. Anti-arsonate (a, c) and CRI_A^+ (b, d) assay of a fractionated Ab_1; ▲ Unfractionated serum of hyperimmune Ab_1 mouse no. 3; Serum fractionated on a sepharose-BSA column (a, b) or on a sepharose BSA-Ars column (c, d); ■ unbound fraction (−) ▬■▬ bound fraction (+) (acid elution).

affinity-purified antibodies inhibit the binding of A/J Ab_1 to rabbit anti-CRI_A^+ serum (FIGURE 4).

DISCUSSION

It now seems clear that recurrent idiotypes are encoded by germ-line genes. Indeed, there is a linkage between idiotype expression and the IgC_H locus. Recent DNA studies suggest, for example, that the V_H CRI_A^+ gene is absent in the BALB/c genome.[4,5] This report and others, however, indicate that BALB/c mice can synthesize CRI_A^+ antibodies. Lucas and Henry[8] recently found CRI_A^+ plaque-forming cells in 3 out of 17 BALB/c mice injected with the T-independent antigen Ars-*Brucella abortus*. N. Sigal identified 2 out of 10 naive BALB/c mice able to generate monoclonal CRI_A^+ when tested by the splenic focus assay.[9]

To explain these apparently contradictory results, the following (although not exclusive) hypothesis is proposed. The genes responsible for the expression of $CRI_A{}^+$ molecules are indeed absent in the BALB/c genome, as suggested by DNA studies, but are present in some lymphocyte clones. These $CRI_A{}^+$ genes could arise in $CRI_A{}^-$ strains by a process of somatic modification. $CRI_A{}^+$ clones, very rare in nonmanipulated BALB/c mice, could be specifically expanded, upon idiotypic manipulation in Ab_3 mice. Our data suggest that the putative "somatic event" leading to the generation of $CRI_A{}^+$ molecules in BALB/c occurs in all mice tested. Moreover, preliminary data obtained in our laboratory suggest that these clones are present in the spleen of naive BALB/c mice.

We think, therefore, that a process of genic conversion between two or several genes is responsible for the appearance of such $CRI_A{}^+$ clones. This could represent a one-step phenomenon that could repeatedly generate similar somatic variants in many members of an inbred strain. In order to pursue this study at the structural level, we are now preparing $CRI_A{}^+$ monoclonal antibodies of BALB/c origin. This observation also implies that public idiotypes cannot simply be ascribed to the presence of a particular germ-line gene. The frequency of Ars specific $CRI_A{}^+$ B cells in A/J mice as determined by a splenic focus assay is not very high and does not seem to be responsible for the clonal dominance observed in the serum of immune A/J mice.[9] The frequency of B-cell $CRI_A{}^+$ clones only increased upon immunization in previously $CRI_A{}^+$ scored strains. As proposed by Sigal, these data are more consistent with the notion that T cells are involved in the selection of expressed repertoire. Our experiments show, however, that upon idiotypic manipulation, $CRI_A{}^+$ B-cell products can be synthesized, probably in a T-dependent manner, suggesting the existence in this strain of a functional set of T-helper cells able to collaborate with these clones. In nonmanipulated mice, these T-helper cells could be very rare or possibly under the control of specific T-suppressor cells.

The unraveling of cellular events leading to the expression of $CRI_A{}^+$ in BALB/c mice could be very helpful in the understanding of clonal dominance phenomena.

ACKNOWLEDGMENT

The authors thank Lea Neirinckx for editorial assistance.

[NOTE ADDED IN PROOF: We have recently generated monoclonals $Ab_{1'}$ antibodies from manipulated BALB/c mice. These antibodies bind arsonate and display most of the CRI_A idiotopes on the same molecule.]

REFERENCES

1. GREENE, M. I., M. J. NELLES, M. S. SY & A. NISONOFF. 1982. Regulation of immunity to the azobenzenearsonate hapten. Adv. Immunol. 32: 253.
2. MARSHAK-ROTHSTEIN, A., M. SIEKEVITZ, M. N. MARGOLIES, M. MUDGETT-HUNTER & M. L. GEFTER. 1980. Hybridoma proteins expressing the predominant idiotype of the antiazophyenyl-arsonate response of A/J mice. Proc. Natl. Acad. Sci. USA 77: 1120.
3. ESTESS, P., E. LAMOYI, A. NISONOFF & J. D. CAPRA. 1980. Structural studies on induced antibodies with defined idiotypic specificities IX. Framework differences in the heavy and light chain variable regions of monoclonal anti-p-azophenylarsonate antibodies from A/J mice differing with respect to a cross-reactive idiotype. J. Exp. Med 151: 863.
4. GEFTER M., M. SIEKEVITZ & R. RIBLET. 1982. The genetic basis of expression of the Ars

idiotype. *In* Idiotype, Antigens on the inside. I. Schnurr, Ed.: 27. Editions Roche. Basel, Switzerland.

5. ESTESS P., F. OTANI, E. C. B. MILNER, J. D. CAPRA & P. W. TUCKER. 1982. Gene rearrangements in monoclonals A/J anti-arsonate antibodies. J. Immunol. **129:** 2319.

6. URBAIN J., M. WIKLER, J. D. FRANSSEN & C. COLLIGNON. 1977. Idiotypic regulation of the immune system by the induction of antibodies against anti-idiotypic antibodies. Proc. Natl. Acad. Sci. USA **74:** 5126.

7. BROWN A. R. & A. NISONOFF. 1981. An intrastrain cross-reactive idiotype associated with anti-p-azophenylarsonate antibodies of BALB/c mice. J. Immunol. **126:** 1263.

8. HENRY L. & A. LUCAS. 1982. The relation of idiotype expression to isotype and allotype in the anti-p-azobenzenearsonate response. Eur. J. Immunol. **12:** 175.

9. SIGAL N. H. 1982. Regulation of azophenylarsonate-specific repertoire expression I. Frequency of crossreactive idiotype-positive B cells in A/J and BALB/c mice. J. Exp. Med. **156:** 1352.

DISCUSSION OF THE PAPER

J. CERNY (*University of Texas Medical Branch, Galveston, Tex.*): Would the injection of normal BALB/c spleen cells into rabbit Ab_2-treated mice suppress the expression of $CRI_A{}^+$ antibodies after antigenic challenge?

O. LEO: We have not done the experiment. Data from Dr. Nisonoff's laboratory, however, suggest that idiotype ($CRI_A{}^+$) specific suppressor cells do not occur in naive BALB/c mice.

A. NISONOFF (*Brandeis University, Waltham, Mass.*): I think your experiments with monoclonal antibodies will be very important, because formally, there still exists the possibility that you are inducing a collection of molecules, each of which shares an idiotope with the A/J mice. Collectively they inhibit, but none of them actually bears the idiotype.

C. A. BONA (*Mt. Sinai School of Medicine, New York*): Can you give us any more explanation about how you envisage the gene conversion?

LEO: What could be the genetic origin of $CRI_A{}^+$ antibodies in BALB/c mice? $CRI_A{}^+$ genes could arise in negative strains by a process of somatic diversification such as genic conversion. It has been recently shown that recombination between V-region genes may contribute to the somatic generation of new antibodies molecules. A new serological marker ($CRI_A{}^+$ idiotype) could result at the DNA level from a mechanism of genic conversion between two $CRI_A{}^-$ encoding germ line genes.

H. KOHLER (*Roswell Park Memorial Institute, Buffalo, N.Y.*): Your data indicate that these events are really directed by the injection of Ab_3.

LEO: We believe that it is a matter of selection, because of the experiments showing that the injection of arsonate coupled to a T-cell independent antigen gives (at least with a difference of rates) similar results. We are not creating any new molecules; we are just selecting them.

KOHLER: If you select, then you could also say you select an internal image of Ab_1.

LEO: You are right. $CRI_A{}^+$ antibodies in BALB/c mice could represent an internal image of $CRI_A{}^+$ antibodies of A/J origin. In other words, different amino acid sequences could give rise to similar serological markers. This would represent a new example of molecular mimicry.

J. A. BLUESTONE (*National Cancer Institute, Bethesda, Md.*): Is it not still formally possible that BALB/c mice have the CRI_A germ line gene but that this gene is not turned on after antigen exposure?

LEO: Yes, but this idea is not consistent with recent data obtained at the DNA level, suggesting indeed that BALB/c mice do not possess the A/J CRI_A^+ germ line gene. We hope that the analysis of monoclonal BALB/c CRI_A^+ proteins will help in the understanding of the genetic origin of such antibodies.

W. E. PAUL (*National Institutes of Health, Bethesda, Md.*): I just want to express the same point of view. The idea that it is not a germ line gene really can only be determined after you make a probe from a hybridoma of that type. The fact that the A/J probe does not cross-hybridize does not prove that the reason that the idiotope is not expressed is because the gene does not exist. To develop the recombinational mechanisms would be a little premature. Also, I would imagine that you could do the same, could you not, with recombination rather than gene conversion?

LEO: Yes, although different, the two mechanisms can lead to the same result, especially in inbred strains.

K. RAJEWSKY (*University of Cologne, Cologne, F.R.G.*): First, there is very clear evidence for the work of Gefter in a paper in press that states that there is genetic polymorphism of the gene encoding CRI. The second point is that I think one should be clear that it is always possible to squeeze a system that is locked into any kind of expression. One can get by somatic mutation conversions with any marker that one wishes. On the other hand, it is also clear from very strong evidence, that in many immune responses, the animal will pick a particular germ line gene and will not obscure the repertoire by a somatic mutation that would be there. So somatic mutation is not good enough to disturb this very clear pattern of germ line determination. Finally, I would like to say that whenever one talks about these silent clones (the gene may still be there and there may be T cells present), one has to keep in mind that the control in these cases of the gene expression that you are looking at is always by the IgH locus or by the IgL locus and not by any other locus. So, in fact, when you think about T cells that are doing this job, these must be controlled by something in the structural gene locus for immunoglobulins. Maybe they are anti-idiotypic, for example, but one has to come back again to polymorphism in the structural genes for immunoglobulins.

Idiotypes of Anti-Major Histocompatibility Complex Antibodies

DAVID H. SACHS, JEFFREY A. BLUESTONE,
SUZANNE L. EPSTEIN, AND RUTH RABINOWITZ

Transplantation Biology Section
Immunology Branch
National Cancer Institute
National Institutes of Health
Bethesda, Maryland 20205

Class I and Class II antigens of the major histocompatibility complex (MHC) are of major importance in determining the fate of allografts. In addition, both classes of antigens have been shown to participate in physiologic immune reactions, because nominal antigens are generally seen by T cells in the immune system not alone, but rather in association with either Class I or Class II products.[1–3] Therefore, the MHC antigens and the receptors that specifically recognize these antigens are extremely important to the study of immunologic interactions.

In order to study these antigens and receptors more precisely, we and other laboratories have recently developed a series of monoclonal antibodies recognizing individual murine Class I (H-2) and Class II (Ia) antigens.[4–6] Availability of large quantities of monoclonal antibodies directed against the individual MHC antigens has made it possible to study the nature of antibody receptors for these antigens. To this end we have raised anti-idiotypic reagents specific for several of our panel of monoclonal anti-MHC antibodies, and we have studied the reactivity of these anti-idiotypic reagents with monoclonal antibodies and with conventional alloantisera.[7–9] We have also administered these anti-idiotypic reagents *in vivo* in an attempt to manipulate the immune response to MHC antigens specifically.[10–12] In addition to their potential usefulness in modifying anti-MHC immune responses, these manipulations have provided information on the nature of immune interactions of relevance to idiotype–anti-idiotype networks. In the present paper we shall review a variety of these studies to date.

ANTI-IDIOTYPIC REAGENTS

Approximately 10 anti-H-2 and 5 anti-Ia monoclonal antibodies have been used to produce anti-idiotypic reagents in this laboratory to date. In all cases, it has been relatively easy to produce xenogeneic reagents of reasonable titer and specificity. Miniature swine and rabbits were immunized with each monoclonal antibody purified from the culture supernatant. The antisera obtained were then purified by extensive absorption on immunoabsorbent columns containing myeloma proteins of the same class as the immunizing antigen and, in some cases, normal serum globulins. The resulting serum depleted of antibodies against constant region determinants was then further purified by adsorption to and elution from a Sepharose column bearing the hybridoma protein, this time obtained from ascites fluid in order to minimize the chance of identical contaminants occurring in both the immunizing and affinity column preparations.

TABLE 1. The 14-4-4 Monoclonal Antibody

Immunization:	C3H.SW anti-C3H
Fusion Partner:	SP2/0
Class:	IgG_{2a}, κ
Reactivity:	Cytotoxic to B cells of all strains expressing I-E antigens; corresponds to specificity Ia.7

In addition, in several cases we have produced anti-idiotypic reagents in mice. For this purpose we have used the protocol of Buttin et al.,[13] coupling the hybridoma protein first to keyhole limpet hemocyanin with glutaraldehyde in order to increase immunogenicity. Sera have been produced by this means both in mice allogeneic to the producer of the original hybridoma antibody and in syngeneic animals.

14-4-4 IDIOTYPE SYSTEM

As shown in TABLE 1, 14-4-4 is a monoclonal antibody produced from a C3H.SW anti-C3H immunization. A striking finding with xenogeneic anti-idiotypes to 14-4-4 was that they reacted with conventional alloantisera from virtually all C3H.SW animals immunized against C3H tissues.[8] At least some of the idiotopes detected were

TABLE 2. Penetrance of Induction of Anti-I-E Activity by Treatment with Pig Anti-14-4-4 Antibodies[a]

		Fluorescence Units[c] on		
In Vivo Treatment	Animal Number[b]	2R[d]	4R	Specific Fluorescence
Pig anti-idiotype	1	338	66	272
	2	322	68	254
	3	352	78	274
	4	764	192	572
	5	202	87	115
	6	350	66	284
	7	193	54	139
	8	122	52	70
Normal pig Ig	9	52	57	−5
	10	51	54	−3
	11	51	52	−1
	12	51	51	0
	13	54	53	1
	14	55	56	−1
	15	52	54	−2
	16	52	56	−4
Controls				
C3H.SW normal serum		53	60	−7
Staining reagent alone		52	46	−6

[a]From Reference 12.
[b]Test sera were from C3H.SW mice primed with pig anti-14-4-4 tested at 4 weeks.
[c]Mean fluorescence adjusted to the same gain.
[d]Strains 2R and 4R are genetically different only in the I region, 2R, but not 4R, expressing I-E antigens.

therefore "public" by definition, similar to idiotopes detectable in several other model antigen systems previously reported.[14-19] Such public idiotypes probably represent the expression of germ line genes,[20] which would be represented to a large extent among the B-cell repertoire and might therefore be expected to arise following immunization in a very large percentage of animals. The idiotype expressed in conventionally immunized C3H.SW mice was indeed found on anti-I-E antibodies, as indicated by the fact that absorption of alloantisera in strains expressing Ia.7 removed the idiotype, whereas absorption in strains not expressing Ia.7 did not.[8]

When xenogeneic anti-idiotype to 14-4-4 was injected into virgin mice, 100% of the animals so treated developed high titers of idiotype detectable by either an hemagglutination inhibition assay or an enzyme-linked immunosorbent inhibition assay.[12] In addition, when sera from such animals were examined by flow-microfluorometry (FMF) for specific binding to lipopolysaccharide blasts, a large percentage of the sera showed significantly greater binding to cells from Ia.7$^+$ strains than to cells from Ia.7$^-$ strains (TABLE 2). Induction of specific anti-Ia.7 antibodies was also virtually 100% penetrant; however, whereas absorption of anti-Ia.7 activity from alloantisera with Ia.7$^+$ cells removed all 14-4-4 idiotype, absorption of anti-Ia.7 reactivity from serum of anti-idiotype treated mice removed only a very small fraction of the total induced idiotype. This finding indicates that much of the induced idiotype represents 14-4-4 idiotopes on antibody molecules nonreactive with Ia.7.

ANTI-H-2K^k SYSTEMS

Among the anti-H-2 monoclonal antibodies that have been studied idiotypically, three of the anti-H-2K^k antibodies are indicated in TABLE 3 along with some of the

TABLE 3. Anti-H-2K^k Hybridomas Studied

Hybridoma	11-4.1	3-83	36-7-5
Immunization	BALB/c anti-CKB	BALB/c anti-C3H	A.TL anti-A.AL
Fusion partner	NS-1	P3U1	SP2/0
Class	IgG$_{2a}$, κ	IgG$_{2a}$, κ	IgG$_{2a}$, κ
Reactivity	Cytotoxic to all lymphoid cells	Cytotoxic to all lymphoid cells	Cytotoxic to all lymphoid cells
Specificity	K^k	K^k	K^k
Cross-reactions	K^q, p, r	D^k, K^b, p, q, r, s	—
Reference	24	5	25

properties of these antibodies. Unlike the 14-4-4 system, all of the anti-H-2K^k idiotypes we have examined have appeared to be "private" in nature, in that conventional alloantisera showed only rare reactivity with anti-idiotypic reagents.[7] These results could be interpreted either to indicate that the monoclonal antibodies used to generate the anti-idiotypes did not represent products of germ line genes, and were therefore found only occasionally in conventional antisera, or that there are such a large number of genes devoted to anti-H-2 specificities that any one was just a very small fraction of the antibodies produced.

Treatment of animals with xenogeneic anti-idiotype in these systems led, however, to a result similar to that observed for the 14-4-4 system. One hundred percent of animals so treated developed circulating idiotype detectable by assays such as hemagglutination inhibition or enzyme-linked immunosorbent inhibition assay.[10,11] In the case of 11-4.1 and 3-83 antibodies, approximately 20% of BALB/c animals treated with anti-idiotype developed detectable anti-H-2K^k activity as detected by FMF analysis on the fluorescence-activated cell sorter (FIGURE 1). In order to determine whether or not the induced idiotypes showed structural similarity to the original idiotype, several hybridomas were produced by fusion of spleens from anti-idiotype treated mice.[21] Four hybridoma antibodies bearing 11-4.1 idiotypes were produced, purified, and studied by sequence analysis in collaboration with Dr. Krutzsch, Dr. Cazenave, and Dr. Kindt.[21] None of these idiotype-bearing monoclonal antibodies showed detectable reactivity with H-2K^k. Nevertheless, one of the four antibodies was found to have a heavy chain with identical sequence to 11-4.1 throughout the first 40

ANTIGEN SPECIFICITY OF ANTI-H-2 ANTIBODIES
INDUCED BY ANTI-ID

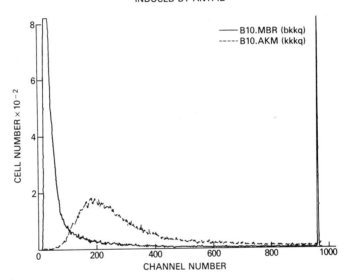

FIGURE 1. Approximately 20% of BALB/c animals treated with pig anti-idiotype to 11-4.1 or 3-83 developed anti-K^k serum antibodies. Shown here is the analysis of serum from one such animal by FMF using H-2 congeneic lymph node cells stained with test sera from an anti-idiotype treated mouse and counter stained with a mixture of fluoresceinated anti-mouse IgG antibodies. Staining of lymph node cells of the inappropriate H-2 haplotype was not significantly greater than the fluorescence of the cells in the absence of sera.[11]

amino acid residues. In addition, when the heavy chain from this monoclonal antibody was recombined with 11-4.1 light chain, a substantial amount of anti-H-2K^k activity was generated. Therefore, it seems likely that anti-idiotype induction of idiotypes stimulates a B-cell repertoire derived at least in part from the same germ line genes that gave rise to the original hybridoma antibody. This experiment has only been performed for the 11-4.1 antibody, so it is not clear that it can be generalized to all induced idiotype systems. These results, however, favor the hypothesis that the 11-4.1 antibody represents the product of either a germ line gene or a very close derivative of such a gene.

INVOLVEMENT OF T CELLS IN EFFECT OF
ANTI-IDIOTYPE TREATMENT

Although the 11-4.1 idiotype was only rarely detectable in conventional alloanti-sera, sera from animals first treated with anti-idiotype and then immunized with C3H skin grafts showed a high percentage of idiotype positive anti-H-2K^k antibody production.[22] In order to determine whether this effect on the expressed repertoire involved only interactions at the B-cell level or also required T cells, adoptive transfer experiments were performed. It was found that T cells from anti-idiotype primed mice were capable of altering the response of recipient mice to alloantigen to the extent that a large percentage of such recipient mice produced the 11-4.1 idiotype following subsequent immunization with a C3H skin graft.[22] These results are therefore consistent with an idiotypic network in which both T cells and B cells are involved in regulating the idiotype expressed.

The next steps in determining which T cells were responsible for this effect and in studying the mechanism of the interaction were to isolate these T cells, characterize them, and possibly clone them. Unfortunately, in more recent studies in our laboratory the 11-4.1 idiotype has become more public, that is, we are now finding that a larger percentage of BALB/c mice immunized with C3H skin grafts produce this idiotype among their anti-H-2K^k antibodies. This difference may represent a change in the mice themselves, because we and others have previously noted marked differences in the idiotypes expressed by closely related but distinct strains.[11,23] Alternatively, this change represents some unintentional difference in our immunization or test systems. It may therefore be necessary to develop similar protocols in one of our other private idiotype systems in order to study further the involvement of the T-cell compartment.

SUMMARY

Our studies to date indicate that treatment with anti-idiotype to monoclonal anti-MHC antibodies can markedly influence the repertoire of anti-MHC antibodies expressed. The antibodies discussed here appear to represent two classes, one of which is public, probably representing expression of a germ line gene, and the second of which probably represents either a somatic variant of a germ line gene or one of a very large number of germ line genes devoted to the same specificity. In either case, this class of idiotype arises only rarely following antigen, but is readily induced by anti-idiotype treatment. There may indeed exist a third class of anti-MHC monoclonal antibodies representing distant somatic diversification from a germ line gene. Our only indication of this so far is that certain idiotypes are only induced after multiple boosts with anti-idiotypes rather than a single treatment. This finding, however, may reflect again the enormous number of different ways in which anti-MHC antibodies to the same nominal specificity can be produced. Finally, our results in adoptive transfer systems indicate that manipulation of idiotype expression by anti-idiotype treatment probably involves a complex pathway of cellular interactions. If, as we expect, these intercellular interactions involve idiotype and/or anti-idiotypic receptors, they should provide a model for mechanistic studies of the *in vivo* immune network.

REFERENCES

1. SHEARER, G. M., T. G. REHN & C. A. GARBARINO. 1975. J. Exp. Med. **141:** 1348.
2. ZINKERNAGEL, R. M. 1978. Immunol. Rev. **42:** 224.

3. HODES, R. J., K. S. HATHCOCK & A. SINGER. 1980. J. Exp. Med. **152:** 1779.
4. LEMKE, H., G. J. HÄMMERLING & U. HÄMMERLING. 1979. Immunol. Rev. **47:** 175.
5. OZATO, K., N. MAYER & D. H. SACHS. 1980. J. Immunol. **124:** 533.
6. PIERRES, M., C. DEVAUX, M. DOSSETO & S. MARCHETTO. 1982. Immunogenetics **14:** 481.
7. SACHS, D. H., J. A. BLUESTONE, S. L. EPSTEIN & K. OZATO. 1981. Transplant. Proc. **13:** 953.
8. EPSTEIN, S. L., K. OZATO, J. A. BLUESTONE & D. H. SACHS. 1981. J. Exp. Med. **154:** 397.
9. BLUESTONE, J. A., J.-J. METZGER, M. C. KNODE, K. OZATO & D. H. SACHS. 1982. Mol. Immunol. **19:** 515.
10. BLUESTONE, J. A., S. O. SHARROW, S. L. EPSTEIN, K. OZATO & D. H. SACHS. 1981. Nature (London) **291:** 233.
11. BLUESTONE, J. A., S. L. EPSTEIN, K. OZATO, S. O. SHARROW & D. H. SACHS. 1981. J. Exp. Med. **154:** 1305.
12. EPSTEIN, S. L., V. R. MASAKOWSKI, J. A. BLUESTONE, S. O. SHARROW, K. OZATO & D. H. SACHS. 1982. J. Immunol. **129:** 1545.
13. BUTTIN, G., G. LEGUERN, L. PHALENTE, E. C. C. LIN, L. MEDRANO & P. A. CAZENAVE. 1978. Curr. Top. Microbiol. Immunol. **81:** 27.
14. PAWLAK, L. L., E. B. MUSHINSKI, A. NISONOFF & M. POTTER. 1973. J. Exp. Med. **137:** 22.
15. EICHMANN, K. 1973. J. Exp. Med. **137:** 603.
16. RIBLET, R., B. BLOMBERG, M. WEIGERT, R. LIEBERMAN, B. A. TAYLOR & M. POTTER. 1975. Eur. J. Immunol. **5:** 775.
17. SACHS, D. H., J. A. BERZOFSKY, D. S. PISETSKY & R. H. SCHWARTZ. 1978. Springer Semin. Immunopathology **1:** 51.
18. KARJALAINEN, K. & O. MÄKELÄ. 1978. Eur. J. Immunol. **8:** 105.
19. COSENZA, H. & H. KÖHLER. 1972. Proc. Natl. Acad. Sci. USA **69:** 2701.
20. SACHS, D. H. 1980. In Immunology 80. M. Fougereau and J. Dausset, Eds.: 478–495. Academic Press. New York.
21. BLUESTONE, J. A., H. C. KRUTZSCH, H. AUCHINCLOSS, JR., P.-A. CAZENAVE, T. H. KINDT & D. H. SACHS. 1982. Proc. Natl. Acad. Sci. USA **79:** 7847.
22. AUCHINCLOSS, H., JR., J. A. BLUESTONE & D. H. SACHS. 1983. J. Exp. Med. **157:** 1273–1286.
23. LEGUERN, C., F. B. AISSA, D. JUY, B. MARIAMÉ, G. BUTTIN & P.-A. CAZENAVE. 1979. Ann. Immunol. Inst. Pasteur (Paris) **130c:** 293.
24. OI, V. T., P. P. JONES, L. A. GODING, L. A. HERZENBERG & L. A. HERZENBERG. 1978. Curr. Top. Microbiol. Immunol. **81:** 115.
25. SACHS, D. H., N. MAYER & K. OZATO. In Monoclonal Antibodies and T Cell Hybridomas. C. Janeway, E. E. Sercarz and J. F. Kearney, Eds.: 95–101. Academic Press. New York.

DISCUSSION OF THE PAPER

H. KOHLER (*Roswell Park Memorial Institute, Buffalo, N.Y.*): Dr. Sachs, I have two questions. Have you tried to induce with your anti-idiotype treatment anti-self Ia antibody? The second question is, Have you looked at T-cell function in your anti-idiotype-treated animals?

D. H. SACHS: The answer to both of those questions is yes, we have tried. With regard to inducing systems, if we treat C3H mice with the anti-14-4-4 anti-idiotype, 100% of the animals will produce 14-4-4 idiotype. None of that antibody appears to bind Ia.7. Whether it is binding to a modified-self receptor is something we have considered, but we have not done the kind of experiments that would rule that hypothesis true or false.

Your second question was whether we examined T cells from such animals, and we have done that quite extensively. Unfortunately, to date, we do not have data that would indicate that we have changed any T-cell phenotype by this treatment, but these studies are still in progress.

Internal Images of Major Histocompatibility Complex Antigens on T-Cell Receptors and Their Role in the Generation of the T-Helper Cell Repertoire[a]

GEK KEE SIM AND ANDREI A. AUGUSTIN

National Jewish Hospital and Research Center
National Asthma Center
and
University of Colorado Medical Center
Denver, Colorado 80206

Soon after the discovery of the major histocompatibility complex (MHC) restriction, it was noted that T cells displayed their restricted repertoire subsequent to adaptive differentiation and independently of their genomic elements.[1] The "learning" of this repertoire in the thymus[2] was interpreted to be a result of a positive recognition of MHC-encoded antigens on thymus epithelial cells. It was implicitly considered that the learning pathway takes place exclusively in this organ and that once the mature T cells exit, the self-restricted T-cell repertoire is frozen by virtue of the clonal distribution of antigen specific receptors. Originally, it has been stated that only self-restricted T cells are mutated progenies of self-reactive T precursors.[3] More recently, however, it appeared that the self-restricted and alloreactive sets are both selected by the thymic MHC environment.[4] One could conclude from this finding that the repertoire of T-cell specificities allows a smooth transition from self-reactive to alloreactive steric conformations. In these terms it will be difficult to accept a) that any mutants generated from a self-reactive pre-T-cell pool will be necessarily self restricted (indeed we would expect the persistence of a significant number of allo-restricted T cells in the adult set), and b) that the self-restricted mutants (which after their emergence cannot be stimulated any more by the self epithelial cells) will be numerous enough to constitute the entire self-restricted repertoire. In the frame of the original Jerne theory,[3] or of its more recent variants, one could only postulate that thymus epithelial cells have the special ability of triggering T cells that bind to them even with low affinity (i.e. precisely those that would react to modified self). Because we do not possess any data supporting this idea, we propose an alternate view of the expansion of the self restricted T-cell population. It emerged from the theoretical necessity of finding a mechanism able to enhance this preferential expansion of T-cell clones and from the evaluation of some recent data obtained in our laboratory.

We shall now expose briefly the sequence of events that lead, according to our view, to a self-restricted repertoire of T-helper cells.

[a]This work was supported by grants AI17263 and AI19760 from the National Institutes of Health.

NETWORK INTERACTIONS IN THE GENERATION OF THE T–HELPER CELL REPERTOIRE

We will start by assuming with Jerne[3] that immature T cells arriving at the thymus will express preferentially clonally distributed MHC receptors. Recognition of I region antigens on the thymus epithelium will result, in the case of helper cells, in a specific proliferation of the clones with anti-self specificity. Subsequently, genomic events such as DNA rearrangement or single base mutations will diversify the progeny of such cells, and those remaining strictly anti-self will be deleted to prevent self-aggression. At this point, we postulate that an important event occurs: T cells that recognize determinants close to self I-region (set T_I) will induce further the proliferation of a second set of T cells (T_{II}) that exhibit internal images of such MHC encoded determinants. The assumption that T-cell receptors could mimic MHC encoded determinants could have a precedent in a series of experiments that prove that "physiological" membrane receptors to a certain ligand can also interact with anti-idiotypic antibodies raised against antibodies that bind this ligand.[5] The T_{II} set will exhibit imperfect images of MHC antigens. It follows that the T_{II} set will present structures that are rather similar to modified self than to self. This is likely to be so because in the case of antibodies as well, internal images are only infidel copies (i.e. topochemical copies) of the antigen, a product of steric resemblance and not of identity in amino-acid sequence. In our case, their divergence from mimicking self would be also due to the fact that they are selected by complementarity by T cells whose receptors also mutated away from strict self-MHC recognition. The interaction between T_I and T_{II} set will allow the expansion and selection of the T-cell repertoire after the first interaction with the thymus epithelium MHC antigens occurred. It would favor the persistence of clones that are restricted to modified self, without the complicated play of high affinity/low affinity interactions with self that is so often involved in theories dealing with the generation of the T-cell repertoire. Indeed, we can assume that channeled by the stimulating signals between the two sets of T cells, there would be a tendency of selecting for the "better fit" for the interacting receptors, and this "better fit" would be best when some T cells mimic modified self (which is close to self) and their counterparts would react to such structures (which would functionally be equivalent to self MHC restriction. We can imagine that such a mechanism of selection of the T-helper cell repertoire can allow the recruitment in the restricted set of T cells of clones that arose independently from the anti-allo-MHC pool and not only from the progenies of the original anti-self set. It also appears that according to this view the conservation of the restricted T-cell repertoire can actively take place in the periphery, after the T cells leave the thymus, in a fashion that is independent of the presence of nonself conventional antigenic determinants.

We limited this view of the expansion and conservation of the T-cell repertoire to T-helper cells. In the case of cytotoxic T cells it is probable that T-T interactions would have to be considered differently. A model in which immune response (Ir) genes function by way of an active mechanism of idiotype-anti-idiotype suppression has been proposed by Mullbacher.[6] In this model "... those anti-idiotype structures that resemble the antigen suppress the response, therefore an anti-idiotype to one clone of a response may theoretically be cross-reactive and suppressive to the total number of clones making up a T_c-cell response to the given antigen X." It is possible indeed that the T-T interactions for helper cells have a different value, because the restriction element that mediates them (bona fide I region determinants or an internal image of such a determinant) is not present on all the cells like the class I determinants that mediate the restriction of cytotoxic T cells. The existence of self I-region specific reactivity, which has been recently proven beyond any doubt with the help of IL-2 secretor hybridomas, suggests that I-region reactive T cells in an immune state, can exhibit reactivities very close to self without acting as dangerous aggressors.[7]

Our tentative model, exposed above, presents, in our opinion, some interesting theoretical arguments in its favor and can explain satisfactorily several experimental findings.

1. The diversification of the T repertoire can continue after the encounter of the pre-T cells with the thymus epithelium.

2. The repertoire of T-cell receptors, as expressed in the relative frequencies of reactive T cells, can be preserved as MHC restricted in adult populations of T lymphocytes in an antigen-independent fashion.

3. There is a high frequency of alloreactive cells. The internal image of the I region is interposed between the set of self I-A or I-E epitopes and the T-cell receptors, encoded very probably in separate genetic regions. In this way, the T_{II} set is the phenetic link between a fixed set of restriction elements (H-2 encoded) and a set of variable receptors recognizing them (with possible fluctuating frequencies within a repertoire that is basically self restricted).

4. This type of selection of the repertoire would predict that the active self-restricted T-cell repertoire can be recruited also from allo-MHC reactive pre-T cells. The active role of internal images of MHC would necessarily lead to changes in the quality of the alloreactive pool as a function of the initial direction of selection given by the thymic epithelium. Such an observation was already made for cytotoxic T cells.[3]

The idea that T cells exhibit internal images of MHC determinants could probably explain the discrepancy between the data of Belgrau and Wilson[8] and Binz and Wigzell[9] concerning the polymorphism of the alloreactive T-cell receptors. Belgrau and Wilson demonstrated that T cells responsible for the suppression of alloreaction in graft versus host reaction (GvH) can exert their function upon alloreactive T cells independent of the genetic background that generated the alloreaction. While demonstrating to the authors that the alloreactive receptor, as detected by anti-idiotypic T cells, has a very limited or no polymorphism in the species, these results suggest to us that the T-suppressor cell could not detect any polymorphism because it exhibits the internal image of the MHC encoded antigen recognized by the GvH effector T cells. It would result that these T cells carrying an internal image of MHC are frequent enough to inhibit GvH in any genetic combination. According to Binz and Wigzell,[9] in a very similar experimental model, the alloreactive T cells, responsive for GvH, share idiotypes with anti-allo MHC antibodies. The idiotypes are polymorphic and probably immunoglobulin (Ig)-heavy chain linked. In these experiments, however, the "probe" detecting polymorphism was an anti-T-receptor (idiotype) antiserum. We could assume that a simple explanation for the controversy would be the fact that anti-idiotypic T receptors express frequently internal images of MHC, whereas antibodies do not.

The "aberrant recognition" of modified non-self observed by Doherty and Bennink[10] would be a case in which T-T interactions could be invoked in order to explain the existence of such a recognition in normal animals and its disappearance in animals neonatally tolerized to the H-2 that should have provided the "aberrant restriction." We consider the model of Mullbacher, based on T-T interactions,[6] a more elegant explanation than the one recently provided by Schwartz and Doherty for their results.[11] This latter explanation assumes that clones reacting to a potential modified self could be eliminated prethymically. It would be, however, very strange for the T-cell system to eliminate such clones and then to replace them, during the thymus-induced generation of diversity, with mutants similar to them, but of a dubious origin.

Several observations originating in our laboratory support the idea that T cells are able to present internal images of conventional antigens or MHC encoded epitopes at the level of their receptors.

ANTI-TEPC 15 T-HELPER CELLS CAN EXHIBIT AN INTERNAL IMAGE OF THE HAPTEN PHOSPHORYLCHOLINE

In this particular experimental system, it has been previously demonstrated that in BALB/c mice, T-helper cells that react to phosphorylcholine (PC) exhibit idiotype-like determinants very similar to those present on the TEPC 15 (T15) myeloma protein.[12,13] It has been also shown that one could raise in BALB/c mice, subsequent to the appropriate priming *in vivo*, T-helper cells that recognize the T15 idiotype.[14] It

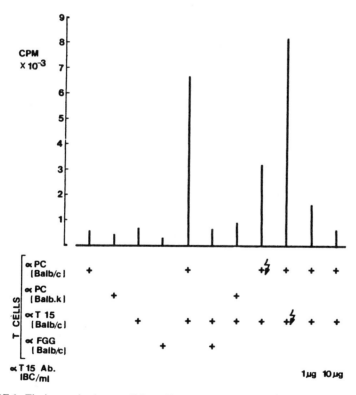

FIGURE 1. The interaction between PC specific and T15 specific T-helper cells enriched *in vitro* results in the enhanced proliferation of both T-cell populations. The interaction is specific, MHC restricted, and can be inhibited by anti-T15 idiotypic antibodies. Whenever two T-cell populations were cocultured, 10^5 cells of each population were mixed in 0.2 ml/culture. The backgrounds were established by culturing each population of T cells at a concentration of 2×10^5 cells in the same volume of culture medium. Proliferation was estimated by [^{3}H]TdR uptake after 3 days of culturing, subsequent to a 16 hour pulse. Columns represent counts per minute (CPM) ($\times 10^{-3}$).

appears that these anti-idiotypic T-helper cells, after *in vitro* enrichment, can recognize anti-PC precursor B cells and induce in the absence of any conventional antigen (PC carrier) a strong anti-PC specific B-cell response. These same anti-idiotype helper cells are able to interact specifically with anti-PC T-helper cells, which by our criteria are T15$^+$. This T-T interaction results in the proliferation of both T-cell populations (FIGURE 1), an event probably due to the secretion of interleukin 2 (IL-2) by the activated T cells. It appeared also that both T-B and T-T idiotype mediated cellular interactions are H-2 restricted. The MHC restriction of anti-idiotypic T cells in a T-B collaboration assay is not a surprising observation because one can consider these T cells as bona fide helper cells with the only distinction being that the nominal antigen they recognize happens to be an idiotypic determinant exhibited by membrane-associated immunoglobulin receptors. The MHC restriction of the T-T collaboration, however, is more intriguing because both reacting T populations do not exhibit I region determinants. This suggested to us the possibility that some T cells could present, at the level of their receptors, structures that would resemble MHC encoded determinants, thus allowing their recognition by the other T cells. Such structures could be described as internal images of H-2 antigens.

Experimentally, however, it would be rather difficult to establish which of the many possible T-cell defined determinants encoded in the I region would be mimicked by our T cells. Therefore, we made a further assumption that led to a feasible experiment: if some of the anti-T15 helper cells exhibit I region-like determinants, these determinants would mimic the modified self (i.e. PC modified). Among the various T clones that fulfull the requirement, some might display the "PC-like" component of their receptor in a fashion that could make it detectable independently of the rest of the receptor. Thus, we tried to investigate the presence of internal images of PC at the level of anti-T15 helper cells. We generated from BALB/c mice a line of T-helper cells specific for the T15 idiotype. Out of this line, 19 individual T-cell clones were isolated by limiting dilution and further expanded in the presence of antigen (T15 protein) and limited amounts of interleukin 2. When the clones reached a size of approximately 10^6 cells, they were tested for their ability to induce B cells to synthesize anti-PC antibodies in the absence of antigen. Seventeen of them were able to provide help to PC-specific B cells. A line of PC-specific cytotoxic T cells (CTL) was also obtained from BALB/c mice. These cells lyse only H-2^d target cells coupled to phosphorylcholine. Of the seventeen anti-T15 helper T-cell clones, however, three were found to be targets of the PC-specific CTL (FIGURE 2). Furthermore, the lysis of these clones was inhibited by competing PC coupled syngeneic cold target cells, and the inhibition could be titrated. These results indicate that epitopes seen by PC-specific CTL on the anti-T15 T-helper clones can represent a PC-like structure and that from a sample of anti-T15 T cells, a good proportion of them (15–20%) can exhibit on their surface an internal image of phosphorylcholine. It appears that such an internal image can be recognized in conjunction with class I MHC determinant(s) by cytotoxic T cells.

T-CELL HYBRIDS BEARING INTERNAL IMAGES OF H-2 I REGION DETERMINANTS ON THEIR RECEPTOR

Our theory on the expansion and maintenance of a restricted T-helper cell repertoire is only valid if the internal image of H-2 exhibited by some T-helper cells can be demonstrated experimentally in a direct fashion. To this end, we took advantage of the T-cell hybridoma technology.

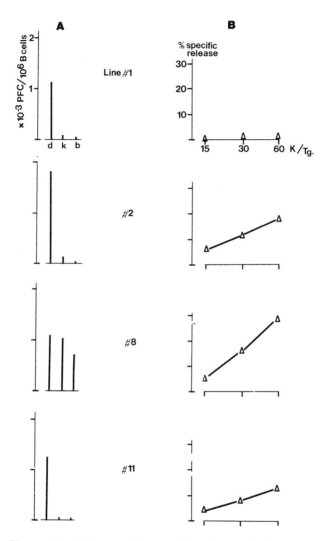

FIGURE 2. Three anti-T15 T-helper cell clones are lysed by cytotoxic T cells specific for PC + H-2^d. In column A, it is shown that such T-helper clones collaborate with PC-specific B cells, in the absence of soluble antigen. 10^5 B cells were cocultured with 2 × 10^4 T cell in 0.2 ml cultures. The immune response was measured on day 5 and expressed as PC-specific plaque forming cells (PFC) per 10^6 input B cells. The responses obtained with B cells from BALB/c, BALB/k, and BALB/b mice are marked respectively as d, k, b, l, according to their H-2 haplotype.

In column B, clones 2, 8, and 11 are lysed by syngeneic PC specific cytotoxic T cells. Results are expressed as specific ^{51}Cr release at various target/killer ratios (Tg/k). Phosphorylcholine-coupled syngeneic lymphocytes inhibit the lysis (data not shown). Clone 1 is one of the 14 T15 specific T-helper cell clones that are not recognized by PC-specific cytotoxic T cells.

BALB/c mice were injected at the base of the tail with BALB/k spleen cells in complete Freund's adjuvant. Five days later, lymphocytes from the regional lymph nodes were restimulated *in vitro* with 3300 rads irradiated BALB/k spleen cells, according to a described procedure.[15] Six days later T-cell blasts were isolated from the preparative cultures and fused with the BW5147 T-cell lymphoma according to the procedure of Kappler *et al.*[16] The anti-I^k region specificity of the resulting hybrids was assayed by an IL-2 secretion assay, according to Kappler *et al.*[16] Out of the several positive hybrids obtained, one was selected and cloned for further experimentation (BdK-4.10). This T hybrid exhibited a high cloning efficiency, high stability, and secreted upon induction large amounts of interleukin 2.

This hybrid was subsequently used as antigen in a second set of immunizations of BALB/c mice, followed by *in vitro* expansion and T-cell hybridization. It appears that

TABLE 1. Specific Interaction between Two T-Cell Hybrids that Do Not Express I-Region Products[a]

	Responder (response measured as units of IL-2 produced)	
Stimulator	BDK.4.10	Ddk455
CBA/J	>160	<10
CBA/N	>160	<10
BALB/k	>160	<10
BALB/b	<10	<10
BALB/c	<10	<10
ATL	>160	<10
ATH	<10	<10
BW5147	<10	<10
BdO540	<10	<10
Ddk455	>160	<10
Bdk4.10	<10	>160
Bdk11.02	<10	<10

[a] The reactivity of various T-cell hybrids to other cells was estimated by measuring the secretion of IL-2 in the culture supernatants. The concentration of IL-2 was established according to the ability of supernatants to support the proliferation of the HT-2 T-cell line. The assay was performed, and results are expressed in IL-2 units according to Kappler *et al.*[16] All T-cell hybridomas are generated by fusing BALB/c T-cell blasts to the BW5147 thymoma line. BdO 540 is specific for ovalbumin when presented by H-2^d cells. DdK455 was obtained in response to BdK4-10 (used as immunogen). BdK4-10 was obtained in response to BALB/k spleen cells. BdK1 1-02 is specific for keyhole limpet hemocyanin when presented by H-2^d cells.

BALB/c mice exhibit a strong reactivity to this hybrid. Subsequent to the hybridization of the *in vitro* expanded T-cell blasts, a large number of viable T hybrids was obtained. None of these hybrids exhibited the pattern of reactivity of Bdk-4.10, indicating that γ-irradiation of the stimulator T-hybrid cells (10,000 rads) completely eliminated them. Four of the tested hybrids, when mixed with BdK-4.10 cloned T cells in the absence of any antigen-presenting cells, led to production of interleukin 2. These hybrids reacted to neither the BW5147 T-cell line, nor to several tested anti-ovalbumin and anti-keyhole limpet hemocyanin T-cell hybrids generated by hybridization with BALB/c blasts (TABLE 1). We consider that such hybrids that react specifically with I-region specific T-cell hybrids, but that do not express conventional I-region products, are likely to exhibit, at the level of their receptor, an internal image of the I-region determinant recognized by the respective alloreactive receptor.

The present attempt to describe network interaction events as a necessary step in the selection of the T-helper cell repertoire is open to experimental investigation. The estimation of the frequency of T-helper cells exhibiting internal images of MHC encoded epitopes in the mature T-cell pool has yet to be performed. Receptor-mediated T-T interactions might be involved in the establishing of T-cell clonal dominance or selection of high responder and low responder phenotypes. The present technology based on the use of functional T-cell clones and hybrids should facilitate experiments testing the value of such interactions.

REFERENCES

1. BEVAN, M. J. 1977. In radiation chimera, host H-2 antigens determine immune responsiveness of donor cytotoxic cells. Nature (London) **269:** 417–419.
2. ZINKERNAGEL, R. M., G. N. CALLAHAN, A. ALTHAGE, S. COOPER, P. A. KLEIN & J. KLEIN. 1978. On the thymus in the differentiation of "H-2 self recognition" by T cells: evidence for dual recognition? J. Exp. Med. 147:882–891.
3. JERNE, N. K. 1971. The somatic generation of immune recognition. Eur. J. Immunol. **1:** 1–7.
4. HÜNIG, T. & M. J. BEVAN. 1980. Self H-2 antigens influence on specificity of alloreactive cells. J. Exp. Med. **151:** 1288–1298.
5. SEGE, K. & P. A. PETERSON. 1978. Use of anti-idiotypic antibodies as cell-surface receptor probes. Proc. Nal. Acad. Sci. USA **75:** 2443–2447.
6. MULLBACHER, A. 1981. Natural tolerance: a model for Ir gene effects in the cytotoxic T cell response to H-Y. Transplantation **32:** 58–67.
7. GLIMCHER, L. H. & E. M. SHEVACH. 1982. Production of autoreactive I region-restricted T cell hybridomas. J. Exp. Med. **156:** 640–645.
8. BELGRAU, D. & D. B. WILSON. 1979. Immunological studies of T cell receptors. II. Limited polymorphism of idiotypic determinants on T-cell receptors specific for major histocompatibility complex alloantigens. J. Exp. Med. **149:** 234–243.
9. BINZ, H. & H. WIGZELL. 1975. Shared idiotypic determinants of B and T lymphocytes reactive against the same antigenic determinants. I. Demonstration of similar or identical idiotypes on IgG molecules and T cell receptors with specificity for the same alloantigens. J. Exp. Med. **142:** 197–207.
10. DOHERTY, P. C. & J. R. BENNINK. 1979. Vaccinia-specific cytotoxic T cell responses in the context of H-2 antigens not encountered in the thymus may reflect aberrant recognition of a virus-H-2 complex. J. Exp. Med. **149:** 150–158.
11. SCHWARTZ, D. H. & DOHERTY, P. C. 1982. Induction of neonatal tolerance to H-2^k in B6 mice does not allow the emergence of T cells specific for H-2^k plus vaccinia virus. J. Exp. Med. **156:** 810–821.
12. JULIUS, M. H., H. COSENZA & A. A. AUGUSTIN. 1977. Parallel expression of new idiotypes on T and B cells. Nature (London) **267:** 437–439.
13. AUGUSTIN, A. A., M. H. JULIUS, H. COSENZA & T. MATSUNAGA. 1980. Expression of idiotype-like determinants on hapten specific, MHC-restricted T helper cells enriched *in vitro* in "Regulatory T lymphocytes." B. Pernis and H. Vogel, Eds. 171–184. Academic Press. New York.
14. JULIUS, M. H., A. A. AUGUSTIN & H. COSENZA. 1977. Recognition of a naturally occurring idiotype by autologous T cells. Nature (London) **265:** 251–253.
15. AUGUSTIN, A. A. & A. COUTINHO. 1980. Specific T helper cells that activate B cells polyclonally. *In vitro* enrichment and cooperative function. J. Exp. Med. **151:** 587–601.
16. KAPPLER, J. W., B. SKIDMORE, J. WHITE & P. MARRACK. 1981. Antigen-inducible, H-2 restricted, interleukin-2-producing T cell hybridomas. Lack of independent antigen and H-2 recognition. J. Exp. Med. **153:** 1198–1214.

DISCUSSION OF THE PAPER

C. A. BONA (*Mt. Sinai School of Medicine, New York*). The research that we have seen in this paper illustrates that immunology has grown from microbiology. A long time ago, it was shown that cardiolipin antigens look like Treponema antigens. You showed that the phosphocholine from *Ascarisis sum* or from *Streptococcus pneumoniae* looks like the receptor of T15 idiotype-specific T cells.

A. A. AUGUSTIN: I think I should actually qualify that. I do not think or believe that there is a T-cell structure that really mimics PC perfectly. It is interesting that whatever that structure is it can be recognized probably in combination with something that we think looks like Ia, by a T-helper cell. It can, however, also modify, probably, appropriately K or D encoded determinants so that it can be killed by T-killer cells. That is all I am saying. I do not know how it is; I am very curious.

UNIDENTIFIED SPEAKER: Can any of your TT or TB interactions with the anti-T15 line and PC-specific B cells, for example, be blocked by antibodies against MHC determinants?

AUGUSTIN: I did not try that. I assume that any restricted interaction can be blocked. In the case of the TB, I am sure that it can be blocked. Any MHC restriction interaction can be blocked. Actually you block more than only one. For instance, John Sprent related to me the fact that you can block MLS specific TB interactions even if you come with an anti-Ia, which can bind to any I region determinant of the stimulator cell.

UNIDENTIFIED SPEAKER: It would be particularly interesting because you said that by fluorescence you cannot detect any Ia determinants from either of the two T-cell lines.

AUGUSTIN: The prediction would be that if you screen enough monoclonal antibodies, for instance, you would find that at a certain point one of them would probably bind something on T cells as Dr. Tada did.

D. E. MOSIER (*Institute for Cancer Research, Philadelphia, Pa.*): In the same vein, have you tried the antiserum that Dr. Swearcont has made against I-J, so-called anti-I-J antiserum on these T-cell lines?

AUGUSTIN: No, I have not.

MOSIER: I presume you have not tried any of Dr. Tada's.

AUGUSTIN: No, we did not try any of them.

D. H. SACHS (*National Institutes of Health, Bethesda, Md.*): Dr. Augustin, I am confused by your experiment. Your hypothesis was that some of your anti-T15 helpers were actually recognizing Ia—being recognized as Ia—because they had on them an internal image, that is, an anti-anti-Ia. So you produced a PC-CTL that recognized a T15 helper.

AUGUSTIN: That is right. That was the second experiment. They are not connected. They are separate.

SACHS: Would not the obvious reason for that, however, be then to see if those cells that you made, which now really are anti-Ia, would also be stimulated by the cells you were proposing had internal images of Ia on them? You did not show that.

AUGUSTIN: Right. When I am talking about internal image of Ia, I do not think that a T-cell receptor can possibly have a lot of the Ia-like determinants.

SACHS: What about the ones that are relevant for stimulating?

AUGUSTIN: I do not know which of them are there, you see. That was exactly the problem. In the case of the PC system, all you need is probably one determinant there, one or two epitopes. Out of the many that are possible, which of them am I going to look for?

SACHS: Then, did you examine the reactivity of the T cell that you made, the anti-anti-Ia T cell that you made, against any of your possible cells that you have internal images on, that is, your T15 helpers?

AUGUSTIN: No, that I did not do.

SACHS. Would not that be the experiment? Why else would you want that anti-Ia T cell? Why did you want the anti-Ia T cell that you made in the last experiment?

AUGUSTIN: Well, the experiment started as an experiment looking at T-T interactions of the PC system. As I tried to point out, however, I think that the important finding during this experiment is that the T-T interactions are possible. They look restricted, but the restriction element is not there. So I deviated completely from my plan from that moment. So what I am interested in now is how these Ia determinants are there. What are they; how do they look? If I turn back to the PC system, I do not know which of them to look for. In experiments that I have done since that time, I refer to an Ia-alloreactive system.

SACHS: You have no proof, however, at this point that there is Ia, or of them recognizing anything like an internal image?

AUGUSTIN: No, there is no formal proof.

Idiotype Connection Between Anti-Arsonate and Anti-Dinitrophenyl Responses in BALB/c Mice[a]

GEORGE K. LEWIS, ZEHRA KAYMAKCALAN,
JOHN YAO, AND JOEL W. GOODMAN

Department of Microbiology and Immunology
University of California
San Francisco, California 94143

Two major conceptual advances in recent years have profoundly altered our perception of the way in which the immune system is regulated. First there was the realization that immune responses were regulated by distinct functional classes of T lymphocytes. Then came the proposal by Niels Jerne of the network theory of the immune system.[1] Jerne postulated that communication between lymphocytes occurs by way of idiotype-anti-idiotype interactions, and that for every antibody (or lymphocyte antigen receptor) combining site, there exists another combining site capable of recognizing a determinant, or idiotype, on the first site. He, therefore, perceived the immune system as a complex network of interacting elements in which the level of expression of each element is regulated by the other members of the network that directly interact with it. Experimental evidence supporting immune regulation by way of idiotype-anti-idiotype interactions has been cascading,[2-4] and the network hypothesis is now widely accepted.

Two ramifications of the network hypothesis hold particular significance. One is the rather obvious deductive conclusion that if every combining site, or paratope, recognizes an idiotope, then the determinants of conventional "foreign" antigens, or epitopes, which are also recognized by the same arsenal of paratopes, must mimic idiotopes. Jerne described this mimicry by referring to idiotypes as "internal images" of the epitopes of nominal antigens.[1]

The second offshoot of the network hypothesis, with which this report is especially concerned, has to do with idiotope sharing by antibodies (or receptors) that recognize non-cross-reactive epitopes, designated "unspecific parallel sets" by Jerne.[1] A number of studies have demonstrated idiotype sharing by antibodies specific for different determinants of the same antigen molecule,[5-9] as well as by antibodies induced against a particular hapten and naturally occurring antibodies that do not bind the hapten.[10,11] Evidence for functional connection, however, between unspecific parallel sets is meager. The strongest functional data come from the hen egg lysozyme system,[5,12] where antibodies directed against different epitopes share idiotypy. Production of these idiotypically connected antibodies is apparently favored by an anti-idiotypic T-helper cell acting in concert with a classical antigen-specific T-helper cell. On the other hand, in several experiments where idiotypy is shared between hapten-binding and nonbinding antibodies, immunization with the hapten selectively called forth only the hapten-binding set,[10,11,13] clouding the physiological relevance of unspecific parallel sets.

[a] This work was supported by United States Public Health Service Grants AI-05664 and AI-17090.

We now report idiotype sharing between arsonate-binding and dinitrophenylated (DNP)-binding antibodies in BALB/c mice. The sharing occurs between members of the CRI[cl4] and 460[11] idiotypic families that represent major idiotypes of anti-arsonate and anti-DNP antibodies, respectively, in the BALB/c strain. This connection is shown to be physiologically relevant inasmuch as the induction of suppression by an arsonate tolerogen also leads to suppression of the shared idiotypic set in the response to dinitrophenylated proteins.

LOCAL SITES OF ABA-SPECIFIC HELP AND SUPPRESSION

We have previously shown that intraperitoneal (i.p.) immunization of mice with bifunctional antigens of the form dinitrophenyl-spacer-L-tyrosine-*p*-azobenzenearson-

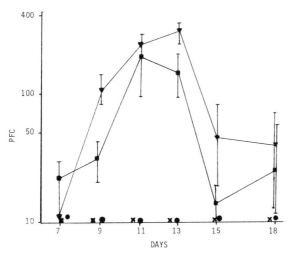

FIGURE 1. BALB/c mice were injected i.p. with CFA alone (■), DNP-lysine (▼), ABA-T (●) or DNP-(Proline)$_{22}$-ABA-T (**X**). Two weeks later, all mice were immunized with DNP-(Proline)$_{22}$-ABA-T in the hind footpads. Anti-DNP IgG PFC from the popliteal and inguinal nodes were assayed on the days indicated. PFC are expressed per 10^6 viable cells.

ate (DNP-spacer-ABA-T) in complete Freund's adjuvant (CFA) induce very weak anti-DNP IgM plaque-forming cell (PFC) responses in the spleen and virtually no IgG responses.[15] The IgM PFC responses peaked at two- to fivefold above controls immunized with CFA alone (10^3–10^4 PFC per spleen). By contrast, the same dose of antigen (0.1 mg of DNP-(Proline)$_{22}$-ABA-T) administered in the footpads in CFA gave rise to 100–400 anti-DNP IgG PFC per 10^6 viable lymph node cells (LNC) in the draining popliteal and inguinal lymph nodes. In order to determine the basis for this marked discrepancy between the IgG antibody responses to the same bifunctional antigen in spleen versus lymph node, BALB/c mice were injected i.p. with CFA alone, DNP-lysine, ABA-T, or DNP-(Proline)$_{22}$-ABA-T. All animals were immunized two weeks later with DNP-(Proline)$_{22}$-ABA-T in the footpads. The anti-DNP IgG PFC responses of the mice are shown in FIGURE 1. Animals preimmunized with CFA or

DNP-lysine gave responses similar in magnitude and kinetics to mice immunized locally with the bifunctional antigen alone, whereas those preimmunized with ABA-T or the bifunctional were profoundly suppressed to subsequent local challenge. The findings demonstrate that splenic immunization induces suppression of a normally strong lymph node response and that the epitope responsible for the induction of suppression is ABA-T. This suppression was transferred to normal syngeneic mice with spleen cells from suppressed donors, and suppression was eliminated by treatment of the spleen cells with anti-Thy-1.2 serum and complement (FIGURE 2). The antigen specificity of suppression was shown by the inability of transferred spleen cells to alter

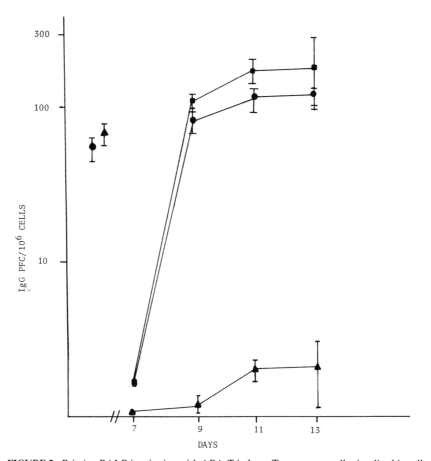

FIGURE 2. Priming BALB/c mice i.p. with ABA-T induces T-suppressor cells visualized in cell transfer experiments. Day (-14): BALB/c mice immunized i.p. with 100 μg DNP-SAC-ABA-T emulsified in CFA (▲) or with CFA alone (■). Day (-1): 5×10^7 cells transferred intravenously into naive recipients. One aliquot was depleted of T cells with anti-Thy-1.2 and C'(●). Day 0: Mice immunized in the footpads with 100 μg of DNP-(Proline)$_{22}$-ABA-T or sheep red blood cells (SRBC) (10^7 cells) emulsified in CFA. IgG PFC responses were determined on days 7–13 in the draining lymph nodes. Anti-DNP responses are shown to the right of the slash; anti-SRBC response was significant only on day 7, and is shown to the left of the slash.

TABLE 1. Preimmunization of BALB/c mice with ABA-T Specifically Suppresses CRI^c (+) Anti-Dinitrophenylated Antibody Responses

Immunization Day − 14^a	Immunization Day 0^b	Anti-DNP-PFC/10^6 LNC	Percent Suppression	Percent CRI^c
Saline/CFA	DNP-OVA	898 ± 101	—	30 range (22–55)
ABA-T/CFA	DNP-OVA	393 ± 21	56	1
Saline/CFA	BSA	321 ± 121	—	
ABA-T/CFA	BSA	265 ± 20	17	

^a100 μg antigen in CFA, i.p. inoculation
^b100 μg antigen in CFA, footpad inoculation
^cDetermined by PFC inhibition with a rabbit anti-CRI^c antiserum. This antiserum was made in rabbits against affinity-purified BALB/c anti-ABA antibodies and was adsorbed on BALB/c myeloma proteins. This antibody had no inhibitory activity on anti-SRBC PFC, anti-BSA PFC, or on CRI^a (+) anti-ABA PFC.

the response to sheep red blood cells (RBC). Thus, ABA-T-specific suppression is mediated by a Thy-1-positive cell.

SUPPRESSION INDUCED BY ABA-T OF ANTI-DINITROPHENYLATED RESPONSES WITH UNRELATED CARRIERS

The suppression observed by splenic immunization with ABA-T followed by lymph node immunization with DNP-spacer-ABA-T bifunctional antigens appeared to be an example of classical carrier-specific suppression. In addition to the sheep RBC specificity control (FIGURE 2), other responses assayed in the suppression protocol included BSA (bovine serum albumin), DNP-BSA, and DNP-OVA (ovalbumin). The anti-BSA PFC response, like the RBC response, was unaffected by preimmunization with ABA-T (TABLE 1), but the anti-DNP PFC responses elicited by either DNP-BSA (not shown) or DNP-OVA (TABLE 1) were diminished by approximately 50 percent. This seemed very curious, but a possible explanation that engaged our attention was that we had happened upon an unspecific parallel set in the idiotypic network. The plausibility of this explanation was strengthened by amino acid sequence data that showed that the ABA-binding strain A/J hybridoma protein 36-60 and the trinitro-phenylated (TNP)-binding BALB/c myeloma protein mouse plasmacytoma cell (MOPC)-460 both belong to the V_H1 subgroup and differ in only 3 of the first 30 residues of the heavy chains.[16,17] Protein 36-60 is a prototype of the cross-reactive idiotypic (CRI^c) family, which constitutes only a minor set of anti-ABA antibodies in A/J mice, but represents a major idiotypic family in the anti-ABA response of BALB/c mice. This sequence homology suggested the possibility of shared idiotypy between anti-ABA and anti-DNP responses in BALB/c mice.

In order to investigate the possibility of idiotype-specific suppression in the anti-DNP responses of BALB/c mice preimmunized with ABA-T, an anti-CRI^c reagent was incorporated into the plaquing medium to detect CRI^c-positive anti-DNP plaque-forming cells. This reagent was prepared by immunizing rabbits with affinity-purified anti-ABA antibodies from BALB/c mice. The rabbit antiserum was absorbed with a series of BALB/c myeloma proteins until it no longer reacted with normal BALB/c immunoglobulin, but reacted strongly with anti-ABA antibodies and with hybridoma 36-60. Plaque inhibition with anti-CRI^c revealed that in mice receiving

CFA/saline prior to immunization with DNP-OVA, approximately 30% of the anti-DNP plaques were inhibited (TABLE 1). On the other hand, hardly any (1%) of the anti-DNP plaques elicited by DNP-OVA in mice preimmunized with ABA-T were inhibited by anti-CRI^c antibody. These results indicate that a fraction of BALB/c anti-DNP antibodies do, indeed, express CRI^c idiotypes, and that the cells secreting these antibodies are selectively suppressed by ABA-T. A likely mechanism is that ABA-T stimulates a population of T-suppressor cells that recognize the common idiotope(s) and turn off that segment of the anti-DNP response. If such is indeed the case, then the population of T-suppressor cells specific for a common idiotope denote functional (regulatory) connection between the two non-cross-reacting systems.

SEROLOGICAL EVIDENCE FOR SHARED IDIOTYPY BETWEEN ANTI-ABA AND ANTI-DINITROPHENYLATED ANTIBODIES IN BALB/c MICE

To garner independent evidence for idiotype sharing between anti-ABA and anti-DNP antibodies in BALB/c mice, an enzyme-linked immunosorbent assay (ELISA) was used with several preparations of anti-CRI^c and anti-MOPC-460 idiotypes. The anti-MOPC-460 preparations were made as described elsewhere,[18] using DNP-glycine to elute rabbit anti-idiotype antibodies from an MOPC-315 immunosorbent. This procedure yielded an anti-"public" idiotype shared by the two DNP-binding myelomas (MOPC-315 and MOPC-460). In the ELISA, the anti-idiotype was incubated with various inhibitors prior to adsorption onto plates coated with hybridoma protein 36-60 or with MOPC-460. After adsorption, unbound antibodies were washed away, and the plates were developed with alkaline phosphatase-conjugated goat anti-rabbit immunoglobulin, followed by the p-nitrophenylphosphate substrate. The plates were incubated at 37° C and then read at 405 mμ. Positive controls (without inhibitor) always had optical density (O.D.$_{405}$) readings of at least 0.2.

Anti-MOPC-460 idiotype bound to plates coated with 36-60. The binding was inhibited by MOPC-460 and 36-60, but not by T15, a BALB/c phosphorylcholine-binding myeloma protein, or hybridoma protein 36-65, an A/J anti-ABA antibody bearing the strain-specific major idiotype (CRI^a) (TABLE 2). This experiment demonstrated cross-idiotypic binding between the anti-DNP-binding myeloma protein and 36-60, the ABA-binding hybridoma protein. Furthermore, only those proteins bearing the appropriate idiotopes inhibited this binding.

TABLE 2. Shared Idiotypy between Anti-Dinitrophenylated and Anti-ABA Antibodies[a]

Inhibitor	Immunoglobulin Class	Strain of Origin	Idiotype	Percent Inhibition
MOPC-460	IgA,κ	BALB/c	CRI^{460}(+)	70%
T15	IgA,κ	BALB/c	T15(+)	0%
36-60	IgG$_{2a}$,κ	A/J	CRI^c(+)	76%
36-65	IgG$_1$,κ	A/J	CRI^a(+)	0%

[a]Inhibitors (10,000 ng/ml) incubated with rabbit anti-MOPC-460 idiotype, prepared according to Rosenstein et al.,[18] prior to adsorption onto plates coated with 36-60. After adsorption, unbound antibodies were washed away, and the reaction developed with an alkaline-phosphatase conjugated goat anti-rabbit immunoglobulin antiserum.

TABLE 3. Shared Idiotypy between Anti-Dinitrophenylated and Anti-ABA Antibodies Experiment 1[a]

Inhibitor	Immunoglobulin Class	Strain of Origin	Idiotype	Percent Inhibition
MOPC-460	IgA,κ	BALB/c	CRI^{460}(+)	75%
T15	IgA,κ	BALB/c	T15(+)	0%
36-60	IgG$_{2a}$,κ	A/J	CRI^c(+)	70%
MKD6	IgG$_{2a}$,κ	(B6xA/J)F$_1$	CRI^a(−), CRI^c(−)	0%

Reaction done as described in TABLE 2.

Experiment 2[b]				
MOPC-460	IgA,κ	BALB/c	CRI^{460}(+)	89%
T15	IgA,κ	BALB/c	T15(+)	0%
36-60	IgG$_{2a}$,κ	A/J	CRI^c(+)	86%
MKD6	IgG$_{2a}$,κ	(B6xA/J)F$_1$	CRI^a(−), CRI^c(−)	0%

[a]Inhibitors (10,000 ng/ml) incubated with rabbit anti-CRI^c prior to adsorption onto plates coated with MOPC-460. Reaction developed with an alkaline-phosphatase conjugated goat anti-rabbit-Ig antiserum. The anti-CRI^c was made in rabbits against affinity-purified BALB/c anti-ABA antibodies and was absorbed until specific, using BALB/c myeloma proteins.
[b]Assay performed as described above except that plates were coated with 36-60 and inhibitors incubated with anti-MOPC-460 idiotype.

Reciprocal experiments in which anti-CRI^c antibodies were reacted with plates coated with MOPC-460 also disclosed cross-idiotypy (TABLE 3). Here, MOPC-460 and 36-60 inhibited binding, whereas T-15 and MKD$_6$, an IgG$_{2a}$, k hybridoma immunoglobulin, like 36-60, but lacking CRI^c idiotypy, did not. Additional data is also given for the anti-460 assay on 36-60 coated plates, confirming the findings in TABLE 2 and showing that MKD$_6$ was negative in this reaction as well as in the reciprocal one.

CONCLUSION

The findings presented in this communication establish the existence of shared idiotypy between anti-ABA and anti-DNP antibodies in BALB/c mice, including, at least in part, the CRI^c and MOPC-460 idiotypic families. In addition, linked regulation of ABA-specific and DNP-specific responses, apparently based on idiotypic connection, has been demonstrated in one direction here, but presumably operates in the other direction as well. Thus, idiotype sharing between immune responses elicited by non-cross-reacting epitopes assumes functional relevance. The results fit well into Jerne's general network hypothesis. Further investigation of linked regulation between these idiotypic systems will include the effect of ABA-induced suppression on the level of endogenous non-DNP binding 460 idiotype in BALB/c mice,[10] and the influence of anti-DNP and anti-ABA responses on the idiotypic profile of the reciprocal responses. It will also be important to confirm the findings reported here using monoclonal anti-idiotype reagents.

ACKNOWLEDGMENT

We wish to thank Dr. Ann Rothstein for supplying hybridoma protein 36-60.

REFERENCES

1. JERNE, N. K. 1974. Ann. Immunol. Inst. Pasteur (Paris) **125C:** 373.
2. BOTOMLY, K., B. J. MATHIESON & D. E. MOSIER. 1978. J. Exp. Med. **148:** 1216–1227.
3. BONA, C. & W. E. PAUL. 1979. J. Exp. Med. **149:** 592–600.
4. SY, M. S., M. H. DIETZ, R. N. GERMAIN, B. BENACERRAF & M. I. GREENE. 1980. J. Exp. Med. **151:** 1183–1195.
5. METZGAR, D. A., A. MILLER & E. SERCARZ. 1980. Nature (London) **287:** 540–542.
6. JU, S. T., B. BENACERRAF, & M. DORF. 1980. J. Exp. Med. **152:** 170–182.
7. KOHONO, Y., I. BERKOWER, J. MINNA & J. A. BERZOFSKY. 1982. J. Immunol. **128:** 1742–1748.
8. OUDIN, J. & P. A. CAZENAVE. 1971. Proc. Natl. Acad. Sci. USA **68:** 2616–2620.
9. URBAIN, J., C. COLLINGNON, J. D. FRANSSEN, B. MARIAME, O. LEU, G. URBAIN-VANSANTEN, P. VAN DE WALLE, M. WIKLER & C. WUILMART. 1979. Ann. Immunol. Inst. Pasteur (Paris) **130C:** 281.
10. DZIERZAK, E. A. & C. A. JANEWAY. 1981. J. Exp. Med. **154:** 1442–1454.
11. WYSOCKI, L. J. & V. L. SATO. 1981. Eur. J. Immunol. **11:** 832–839.
12. ADORINI, L., M. HARVEY & E. SERCARZ. 1979. Eur. J. Immunol. **9:** 906–909.
13. JULIUS, M., C. HEUSSER & J. W. JOHNSON. 1981. J. Supramol. Struct. Supp. **5:** 34.
14. BROWN, A. R. & A. NISONOFF. 1981. J. Immunol. **126:** 1263–1267.
15. CHEN, P., D. E. NITECKI, G. K. LEWIS & J. W. GOODMAN. 1980. J. Exp. Med. **152:** 1670–1683.
16. MARSHAK-ROTHSTEIN, A., M. N. MARGOLIES, J. P. BENEDETTO & M. L. GEFTER. 1981. Eur. J. Immunol. **11:** 565–572.
17. MILNER, E. B. & J. D. CAPRA. 1982. J. Immunol. **129:** 193–199.
18. ROSENSTEIN, R. W., J. B. ZELDIS, W. H. KONIGSBERG & F. F. RICHARDS. 1979. Mol. Immunol. **16:** 361–370.

DISCUSSION OF THE PAPER

J. ARMAND (*Yale University School of Medicine, New Haven, Conn.*): I have a question with regard to the surface of the T cells that are mediating the suppression.

J. W. GOODMAN: I do also.

ARMAND: My question is, Are the T-suppressor cells specific for the idiotype, and what is the idiotype specificity of monoclonal anti-Id antibodies that are directed against CRI of Ars of 36-60 or to the MOPC 460?

GOODMAN: We, of course, predict that it would be directed against an idiotope that would be common to both 460 and 36-60. There must be at least one common idiotope, and the suppressor cells that are used in the suppression of the anti-DNP response, induced by DNP-ovalbumin, must be directed against an idiotope expressed on MOPC 460.

We have performed some experiments to get at this problem, but so far they are inconclusive. What Dr. Kaymakcalan has done is show that she can enrich suppressors by plating on ABA-coated plates, but she can not remove all the suppression by absorption onto ABA-coated plates. We have not yet done the other experiment that would tell us if we can enrich suppressors on idiotype-coated plates—in fact on MOPC 460 as well as 36-60.

ARMAND: My interest is whether you have a heterogeneous population of T-suppressor cells that are somewhat specific for arsonate and dinitrophenyl.

GOODMAN: We are very interested in that possibility too, but I cannot really answer your question.

C. A. BONA (*Mt. Sinai School of Medicine, New York*): I am interested in the inhibition of PFC that you get with monoclonal anti-460 Id antibody.

GOODMAN: The following is the reason that I did not present that material. What we find is that the monoclonal anti-"public" will inhibit anti-ABA secreting cells in the plaque assay. What we have not found is that this antibody will react in the ELISA with 36-60. What I think is that the monoclonal may be directed against an idiotope that is not expressed on 36-60, but is expressed on a fraction of the anti-ABA antibody. Of course we are looking at a much narrower specificity with 36-60.

BONA: This antibody that actually was prepared by Gerard Buttin was obtained by using MOPC 21. A researcher in the Cazeneve Laboratory found that these hybridomas produce a mixture of H and L chains of MOPC 21 and F(5), some of them having anti-460 Id activity.

GOODMAN: Are they all combinations of the two? Maybe that would be a factor.

The Level of Expression and the Molecular Distribution of ABPC 48 Idiotopes in Levan- or Anti-Idiotope- Primed BALB/c Mice

PIERRE LEGRAIN AND GÉRARD BUTTIN

Laboratory of Somatic Genetics
Pasteur Institute
Paris, France

Idiotypic manipulations carried out in several systems strongly suggest that B and T cells are involved in specific idiotypic interactions. The structural basis of such interactions, however, requires further characterization. The serological analysis of idiotopic specificities and the molecular biological approach to the identification of V_H genes are powerful tools for evaluating physiological network theories. Here we present results on the idiotypic repertoire related to the anti-levan response of BALB/c mice and to the ABPC 48 (A 48) idiotype, a levan-binding myeloma protein. Stimulation with the antigen (bacterial levan) or with a monoclonal anti-idiotypic antibody gives rise to different, but structurally related antibodies: their serological pattern reveals common idiotopes, and the molecular analysis of their genetic origin shows that similar or identical V_H genes encode their heavy chains.

A 48-CROSS-REACTIVE IDIOTYPES CONTRIBUTE TO THE IMMUNE RESPONSE AGAINST BACTERIAL LEVAN IN BALB/c MICE

Three syngeneic monoclonal anti-idiotypic antibodies, IDA 10, IDA 16, and IDA 17 define three different idiotopes on ABPC 48: Id 10, Id 16, and Id 17.[1] We quantified the presence of such idiotopes in BALB/c sera by enzyme-linked immunosorbent assay (ELISA) sandwich-binding assays that allow the detection of one idiotope, or of two different idiotopes on one immunoglobulin (Ig) molecule.[2]

TABLE 1 shows that preimmune sera already contain a high titer of anti-levan antibodies and detectable amounts of the three idiotopes. (The Id 17 level is only slightly above the detection threshold.) After immunization of BALB/c mice with 50 μg of bacterial levan, the increase of anti-levan titer is correlated to that of Id 10 and Id 16. In sharp contrast, the Id 17 titer does not change for at least 50 days after immunization. These results demonstrate that the three idiotopes analyzed here are not expressed on the same Ig molecules. By using binding-inhibition assays, as well as sandwich-binding assays designed to detect only Ig molecules with two given idiotopes, we have established that all Ig molecules bearing Id 16 are also Id 10 positive (Id (10–16)). To confirm that Id (10–16) molecules contribute effectively to the anti-levan response, we preincubated sera with bacterial levan before performing the idiotype binding assays. In this case, neither idiotope was detected, showing that Id (10–16) molecules have levan-binding sites. From these results, we conclude that A 48-cross-reactive idiotypes participate in the anti-levan response of normal BALB/c mice.

IDIOTYPIC DIVERSITY OF THE RESPONSE TO IMMUNIZATION WITH MONOCLONAL ANTI-IDIOTYPIC ANTIBODY

Mice were injected intraperitoneally with the different IDA antibodies copolymerized with lipopolysaccharide (LPS). Mice injected with polymerized antibody alone, with LPS alone, or with their mixture served as controls: none of those mice showed an increase in circulating Ig molecules binding the corresponding anti-idiotypic antibody. Results obtained upon immunization with IDA 10-LPS, IDA 16-LPS, or a mixture of IDA 10-LPS and IDA 16-LPS are presented in FIGURE 1. Individual sera were analyzed for the presence of Id 10, Id 16, and Id (10–16) molecules, and for anti-levan titers. The kinetics of these responses disclose two consecutive phases. The first part of the response is characterized by an increase of Id (10–16) molecules that correlates with an increased anti-levan titer, and is observed with all three immunogens (IDA 10, IDA 16, or both). The second phase of the response shows a selective increase of antibodies that are strictly specific for the corresponding immunogen. Mice injected with both anti-idiotypic antibodies respond with a high level of molecules binding either IDA 10 or IDA 16. Very few Id (10–16) molecules, that is, binding both antibodies, are found. To investigate the exact proportion of anti-levan antibodies

TABLE 1. Increase of ABPC 48 Idiotopes during the Immune Response to Bacterial Levan[a]

| | Preimmune Sera | Immune Sera | |
		7 Days	50 Days
Anti-levan	1,000	2,500	1,750
Id 10	17.5	160	130
Id 16	14	294	200
Id 17	2.4	1.4	1.8

[a]Measurements of the ABPC 48 idiotopes were done by sandwich binding assays. Anti-levan activity was measured in ELISA, using levan-coated plates. Results are given in $\mu g/ml$ of equivalent ABPC 48 idiotype (standard binding assay).

among these idiotope-positive molecules, we repeated the same binding assays using sera preincubated with bacterial levan, because levan binding has been previously shown to abolish the interaction between IDA 10 or IDA 16 and the corresponding idiotopes on anti-levan antibodies[1] (and this paper). The results from mice injected with IDA 10 and IDA 16 are given in FIGURE 2. It is clear that anti-levan antibodies constitute an important fraction of the idiotope-bearing molecules during only the first phase of the response. Strikingly, the peak of Id 16 response, repeatedly found at day 7, is no longer detected when anti-levan antibodies are removed. These observations indicate that the response to anti-idiotypic immunization actually comprises two partially overlapping waves of Id 16 bearing antibodies of which only the first carries anti-levan activity.

Similar results were obtained in the Id 10 response. In contrast, however, with Id 16, preimmune sera already contain an important level of Id 10 molecules, 30%–100% of which, depending on the individual donor, do not bind levan. Consequently, the first phase of the response does not exclusively comprise anti-levan antibodies.

In conclusion, the long-lasting response to the injection of anti-idiotypic antibodies is mainly composed of Ig molecules without demonstrable levan-binding activity, whereas anti-levan idiotype-positive molecules constitute the initial and transient response to the injection.

HETEROGENEITY OF ANTIBODIES RAISED AGAINST MONOCLONAL ANTI-IDIOTYPIC ANTIBODIES

Two batteries of monoclonal antibodies had been obtained from mice hyperimmunized with two different IDAs.[3,4] We previously showed, using polyclonal anti-

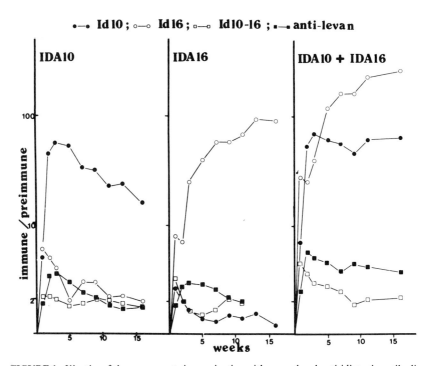

•—• Id 10 ; o—o Id 16 ; □—□ Id 10-16 ; ■—■ anti-levan

FIGURE 1. Kinetics of the responses to immunization with monoclonal anti-idiotypic antibodies. Monoclonal anti-idiotypic antibodies were coupled to LPS and injected separately or together into mice (immunogenic doses: 5 to 50 μg per mouse). Increases of titer of the Id 10, Id 16, and Id (10–16) idiotopes and increase of the anti-levan titer are calculated, and means of values for five animals are given.

anti-idiotypic antisera, that 10 out of 17 IDAs were cross-reactive idiotypes.[1] With a large battery of 23 monoclonal antibodies (Ab₃) raised against IDA 10, it was now possible to analyze the individual idiotope basis of cross-reactive IDAs antibodies. In this analysis, we used the inhibition of a rosette assay between Ab₃ hybridoma cells and IDA 10-coated sheep red blood cells. Each anti-idiotypic (Ab₂) antibody was tested for inhibition of IDA 10 binding to each Ab₃ hybridoma. Results are presented in FIGURE 3. Ten idiotypically cross-reactive anti-idiotypic antibodies (Ab₂) inhibit, with various degrees of efficiency, the different rosette assays. Furthermore, direct

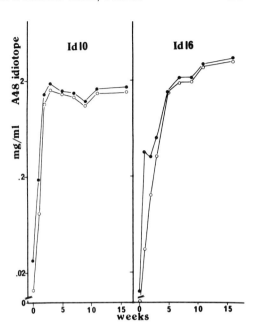

FIGURE 2. Levan binding by a fraction of antibodies induced by anti-idiotypic immunization. Mice were injected with IDA 10 LPS and IDA 16 LPS. Sandwich binding assays for Id 10 and Id 16 were carried out in absence (●——●) or in presence (O——O) of bacterial levan (10 μg/ml). The results, expressed in mg per ml of ABPC 48 idiotype, were calculated from a standard binding curve of ABPC 48.

binding assays between these Ab$_2$ and the battery of Ab$_3$ antibodies show that all but 6 Ab$_3$ do in fact bind these 10 Ab$_2$ antibodies (results not shown, see reference 3). These results are not compatible with the interpretation that Ab$_3$ antibodies define several discrete idiotopes on IDA 10, one or more of which would be shared by the cross-reactive IDAs. On the contrary, these observations strongly suggest that Ab$_3$

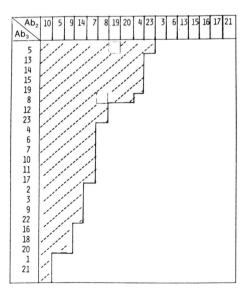

FIGURE 3. Inhibition of the binding of anti-IDA 10 monoclonal anti-idiotypic antibodies (Ab$_3$) to IDA 10 (Ab$_2$) by the different Ab$_2$ raised against ABPC 48. Ab$_2$ antibodies were assayed for the inhibition of the binding of Ab$_3$ hybridoma cells to sheep red blood cells coupled to IDA 10 (more than 95% rosetting cells). Hatched bars represent successful inhibition (<5% rosetting cells).

antibodies define closely related overlapping idiotopes on IDA 10 molecules. Accordingly, Ab_3 antibodies would carry slightly different binding sites to IDA 10, such that Ab_2 antibodies structurally related to IDA 10 bind most Ab_3 antibodies, as they share a similar idiotope with IDA 10. The different affinity patterns in binding to Ab_3 are probably related to the small structural differences between IDA 10 and the other 10 Ab_2. Among the 23 monoclonal Ab_3 antibodies, 6 have been found to bind levan with low avidity. It is possible that most Ab_3 antibodies share idiotope(s) with A 48, and only some of these might have enough structural homology to this molecule to display levan-binding activity. Alternatively, most Ab_3 might be true anti-anti-idiotypic antibodies raised against "dominant" idiotopes of Ab_2, that is, without structural homology to A 48. One approach to answer this question is to compare the V_H genes expressed by A 48 and by Ab_3 hybridomas. To this end, we have obtained from Dr. F. Rougeon (Pasteur Institute, Paris) a V_H probe ($_pV_H$ 441-4) prepared from the M 173 myeloma, that is closely related to A 48.[5] Northern blot analysis of polyA RNA from several hybridoma lines have been carried out under low stringency and high

TABLE 2. Characteristics of Several Ab_3 Monoclonal Antibodies

Ab_3	Raised Against	Binding Specificities IDA 10, IDA 23, Levan			Northern Blot Analysis with V_H 173 Probe
AIDA 10/16	IDA 10	+	+	+	+
AIDA 10/19	IDA 10	+	−	+	+
AIDA 23/1	IDA 23	+	+	−	+
AIDA 23/2	IDA 23	−	+	−	−
AIDA 23/3	IDA 23	+	+	−	+
AIDA 23/8	IDA 23	+	+	−	+
AIDA 23/9	IDA 23	−	+	−	−

The specificity for IDA 10 and IDA 23 was analyzed by direct binding assay, (ELISA and rosette assay). The levan-binding activity was detected in ELISA. Diluted ascitic fluid of Ab_3 hybridomas were adsorbed on plates, then bacterial levan and anti-levan antibodies labeled with β galactosidase were added in sequence. Northern blot analysis was carried out under low stringency (hybridization: 30% Formamide, 36° C; washing: 30% Formamide, 5 × SSC, 25° C) and under high stringency conditions (hybridization: 50% Formamide, 42° C; washing: 0.1 × SSC, 50° C). The different stringency conditions gave identical results.

stringency conditions. RNA extracted from five different Ab_2 hybridomas and from the SP2oAg line did not hybridize with the V_H 173 probe under any conditions. The results obtained with mRNA from seven of the Ab_3 hybridomas are shown in TABLE 2. No hybridization was found with two RNA preparations from Ab_3 hybridomas that define private idiotopes on IDA 23, as previously shown.[4] Five RNA preparations were positive in this analysis and the intensity of hybridization for any of these RNAs was the same under both stringency conditions. These 5 Ab_3 hybridomas whose message is homologous to the probe used, secrete antibodies that recognize a large spectrum of IDA antibodies, and two of them bind levan.

These preliminary results show that a large fraction of antibodies raised against an anti-idiotypic (Ab_2) antibody share idiotope(s) with Ab_1 (A 48) and that this serological property is correlated with the expression of the same (or closely related) V_H gene(s).

Taken together, the results presented here suggest that even if antibodies raised against antigen or anti-idiotypic antibodies are serologically different, they may be generated by a limited set of V_H genes. The absence on these antibodies of idiotopes detected on ABPC 48 can be explained by somatic diversification of V_H sequences, or, more likely, by the association of these V_H sequences to various D region genes, and by the expression of different κ chains. In fact, a correlation between specific D regions and anti-levan activity has already been shown.[6]

REFERENCES

1. LEGRAIN, P., D. VOEGTLE, G. BUTTIN & P. A. CAZENAVE. 1981. Eur. J. Immunol. 11: 678–685.
2. LEGRAIN, P. & G. BUTTIN. 1983. J. Exp Med. 158. In press.
3. LEGRAIN, P., G. BUTTIN & P. A. CAZENAVE. 1982. In Monoclonal Antibodies and T Cell Hybridomas. G. J. Hämmerling, U. Hämmerling and J. K. Kearney, Eds.: 416–422. Elsevier/North-Holland Biomedical Press. Amsterdam, The Netherlands.
4. LEGRAIN, P., D. JUY & G. BUTTIN. 1983. In Methods in Enzymology. S. Colowick and N. Kaplan, Eds.: 92: 175–182. Academic Press. New York.
5. OLLO, R., C. AUFFRAY, J. L. SIKORAV & F. ROUGEON. 1981. Nucleic Acids Res. 9: 4099–4109.
6. AUFFRAY, C., J. L. SIKORAV, R. OLLO & F. ROUGEON. 1981. Ann. Immunol. Inst. Pasteur (Paris). 132 D: 77–88.

Regulation of the Response to α1-3 Dextran in IghC^b Mice^a

JÉRÔME PÈNE, HABIB ZAGHOUANI,
AND MARC STANISLAWSKI

Institute for Scientific Research on Cancer
Villejuif, France

Responsiveness to the α1-3 glucosidic linkage of Dextran B-1355 is dictated by the IghC complex.[1,2] In "responder" IghC^a mice, this thymus-independent antibody response is typified by the IdX Dex VH marker and the almost exclusive use of the λ1 light chain.[1-3] Whereas in "responders" this VH idiotype (Id) marker characterizes a large pauciclonal response ($\sim$50% of anti-α1-3 dextran antibodies[3]), "non-responder" IghC^b mice synthesize small amounts of κ-bearing anti-α1-3 dextran antibodies that lack this VH idiotype. Although the titer of these antibodies can rise to high levels in hyperimmune C57B1/6 (IghC^b) mice with a concomitant switch to λ1 chain synthesis, the antibodies still remain IdX Dex-negative.[4,5] Thus, CH allotype appears to determine both the quality and the magnitude of this response.

This basic response pattern has led Cohn[4] and his associates to propose that the immune status of these mice reflects the absence of a CH allotype-linked VH^{Dex} structural gene coding for the IdX Dex idiotype in opposition to the situation in IghC^a animals.

Whereas the expression of various other idiotype-characterized antibody responses is also under the control of CH allotype,[6] there have been reports that "non-responder" mice do synthesize minute amounts of idiotypic antibodies,[7] or have a low frequency representation of such clones.[8] The serum concentration of these antibodies can be increased to easily detectable levels by pretreatment of these mice with anti-idiotypic antibodies raised against myeloma or hybridoma antibodies or normal serum antibodies of "responder" mice.[9] There are at least three recently published instances where this has been achieved.[10-12] Thus, in spite of the failure to detect idiotypic antibody by standard immunization procedures, the synthesis of gene products of allotype-linked idiotypic responses can be activated in these "non-responders" by pretreatment with anti-idiotype. Mechanisms based on idiotope recognition[13] may be responsible for this activation.

The precursor clones of these idiotypic antibodies may represent "minor"[14] or "silent"[11] clones resulting from homeostatic active suppression, down regulating the product to undetectable levels. For example, 460-idiotype-specific T-suppressor cells were shown to specifically suppress the synthesis of 460-idiotype-bearing anti-dinitrophenyl (DNP) antibodies in BALB/c mice.[15] The available repertoire of antibody specificities thus may exceed in size the expressed repertoire.[16]

Recent work from our laboratory[5] indicated that it was possible to induce the synthesis of λ1-bearing IdX Dex-positive anti-α1-3 dextran antibodies by administration of anti-IdX558 antibodies into the two IghC^b mouse strains, C57B1/6 and CB 20. We have since been able to reproduce these results in four Bailey RI strains, CXBK, CXBD, CXBE, and CXBH.

^{a}This work was supported by a Grant from the National Center for Scientific Researche ATP No. 60-80-846.

The mice synthesize IgM, IgG$_3$, and proportionately large amounts of IgG$_1$ class antibodies. Furthermore, all of the IgG$_1$ antibodies bear the Igh$_{4b}$ allotype determinants, which is not an unexpected finding, because these mice are homozygous at the IghC complex. (It is suspected that the IgM and IgG$_3$ antibodies are likewise products of the b haplotype IghC loci).

This finding is, in effect, paradoxical as the IdX Dex is found associated here with the wrong CH allotype.[2] As IdX Dex, however, in BALB/c mice is structurally determined by only two amino-acid residues in VH CDR2,[17] only this idiotypic determinant, or idiotope, need be expressed on Igh^b VH Dex, which otherwise may differ from the BALB/c VH Dex sequence. According to this view, this short stretch of the VH would encode the structural gene for IdX Dex. VH gene polyporphism, such as is encountered in the (4-hydroxy-3-nitrophenyl) acetyl (NP) system,[18] may account for the occurrence of IdX Dex in other than IghC^a mouse strains. Alternatively, gene "conversion"[12] has been proposed to account for the anti-Id-induced appearance of CRI^a idiotype-positive anti-*p*-azophenylarsonate (Ar) response in the wrong allotype BALB/c mice. The exact structural correlates of IdX Dex expression in IghC^b haplotype mice must, however, await the sequencing of the VH of these antibodies. Here, we report some of the main findings concerning the induction of this idiotype in the CB 20 congeneic mouse strain.

IdX DEX SPECIFICITY OF ANTI-IDIOTYPE REAGENTS

Anti-IdX Dex antibodies were purified from the serum of a single rabbit hyperimmunized with the mouse α1-3 dextran-binding myeloma antibody J558 (IdX Dex$^+$). The serum was preabsorbed on various myeloma protein immunoabsorbents in order to remove anti-α and anti-λ1 class-specific antibodies, and the anti-IdX558 antibodies were purified over a column of another IdX Dex$^+$ myeloma protein, M104E.

For the purpose of these experiments, it was important that the reagent be specific for the product of the structural VH^{Dex} gene of BALB/c, namely, the IdX Dex idiotope, that is, that it be able to discriminate between a λ1, IdX Dex$^+$ from a λ1, IdX Dex$^-$ response. The later type of response is frequently encountered in dextran B-1355-immune C57B1/6[4,5] mice. TABLE 1 summarizes the results of competitive radioimmunoassays showing that this reagent specifically discriminates between IdX Dex$^+$ and IdX Dex$^-$ λ1-positive α1-3 dextran-binding myeloma and hybridoma antibodies. In the panel tested, the first 6 IdX Dex$^+$ antibodies gave an I_{50} in the range of 7 to 200 ng, whereas the two IdX Dex$^-$ antibodies, Hdex14 and Hdex8, gave only around 20% inhibition at a concentration of 10,000 ng. Myeloma and hybridoma antibodies displaying various other antigen-binding specificities were not significantly inhibitory. The reagent was 40% binding-site inhibitable[19] by B-1355 using either J558 or M104E as target antibodies.

Two mouse IdX Dex-specific reagents were also used in this study. One was BALB/c anti-J558, and the other was a BALB/c anti-M104E. Both were made IdX Dex-specific by immunoabsorption, and were 60% binding site inhibitable by B-1355.

RESPONSE TO DEXTRAN B-1355 FOLLOWING ANTI-IdX558 SENSITIZATION OF CB 20 MICE

Two injections of the rabbit anti-IdX558 in complete Freund's adjuvant (CFA) resulted in substantial amounts of IdX Dex$^+$ inhibitory material appearing in the

TABLE 1. IdX Dex Specificity of Rabbit Anti-J558 in Competitive Immunoassay[a]

Competitor	Binding Specificity	NG for 50 Percent Inhibition	Percent Inhibition by Large Amounts
M104E	α1-3 Dex[b]	7	100 (900 ng)
J558	α1-3 Dex	16	100 (900 ng)
Hdex1	α1-3 Dex	25	100 (900 ng)
Hdex3	α1-3 Dex	27	95 (900 ng)
Hdex12	α1-3 Dex	200	75 (900 ng)
Hdex8[d]	α1-3 Dex	>10,000	20 (10,000 ng)
Hdex14	α1-3 Dex	>10,000	20 (10,000 ng)
B1–8	NP[b]	>10,000	10 (10,000 ng)
93G7	Ar[b]	>10,000	5 (10,000 ng)
J606	Inulin	>10,000	
UPC10	Levan	>10,000	10 (10,000 ng)
McPc603	PC[b]	<1/30[c]	2 (1/30)
J539	Galactan	<1/30	2 (1/30)
BALB/c serum		1/65	95 (1/5)
CB 20 serum		<1/5	10 (1/5)

[a]The solid-phase microplate radioimmunoassay was carried out as described by Pene et al.[5] The proband was [^{125}I]M104E (4 ng, ~3,000 cpm).
[b]α1-3 Dex = α1-3 dextran; NP = (4-hydroxy-3-nitrophenyl) acetyl; Ar = p-azophenylarsonate; PC = phosphorylcholine.
[c]Dilutions of ascites or serum.
[d]Hdex 8 was typed by Clevinger et al.[17] to express 20% of IdX Dex.

serum of CB 20 mice. TABLE 2 indicates that as little as 10 IBC of anti-Id still induced significant amounts of IdX Dex in all tested mice. Similar results were obtained thus far in a total of 32 CB 20 mice, 5 C57B1/6 mice, and 14 Bailey RI (Igh[b]) mice. The mice also responded with ~10 μg/ml of λ1-positive anti-α1-3 dextran antibodies whose titer was porportional to the IdX Dex titer. It is possible that these antibodies appear in

TABLE 2. Dose Response for Induction of an IdX Dex$^+$ Response and α1-3 Dex-Binding Antibodies in CB 20 Mice Sensitized with Rabbit Anti-IdX558[a]

IBC Anti-IdX558 Injected in CFA	Day 21 Titer (Av ± SD)		Day 38 Titer (Av ± SD)	
	IdX Dex$^+$ (μg/ml)	anti-α1-3 Dex(μg/ml)	IdX Dex$^+$ (μg/ml)	anti-α1-3 (Dex(μg/ml)
122	262 ± 102	11.7 ± 4.6	570 ± 140	201 ± 98
25	272 ± 56	11.8 ± 3.4	625 ± 140	218 ± 99
5	47 ± 10	4 ± 2.1	231 ± 53	75 ± 62
NRIgG 100μg in CFA	1.3 ± 2.5	0.75 ± 0.4	1.3 ± 2.2	0.58 ± 0.27
B-1355 100 μg in CFA	≤20	1.1 ± 1.7		

[a]Groups of 4 CB 20 mice were given two subcutaneous injections, spaced at 14 days, of the indicated amounts of anti-IdX558 (1.27 IBC/μg), and the serum response was measured 7 days later (day 21). Six days later, they were given three injections, spaced two days apart, of a B-1355-ConA precipitate, intraperitoneally, and the response was measured seven days after the last injection (day 38). IdX Dex was determined as in the legend of TABLE 1, and antibodies in a microplate binding assay using ^{125}I-labeled rabbit anti-λ1 antibodies, as described by Geckeler et al.[37]

response to intestinal flora microorganisms having dextran in their envelope. Alternatively, the antibodies may represent a subpopulation of the IdX Dex$^+$ clones similarly induced by anti-IdX558. As will be discussed below, these antibodies likewise express IdX Dex.

Control mice immunized with B-1355 or injected with an equivalent weight of normal rabbit IgG (NRIgG) in CFA never responded with significant levels of IdX Dex or anti-α1-3 antibodies[5] (TABLE 2). Furthermore, when there animals were now immunized with a B-1355-concanavalin A (ConA) precipitate 13 days after the second anti-IdX558 injection, there was a 2- to 3-fold increase of the IdX Dex response reaching ~600 μg/ml, and a 10- to 20-fold increase in the antibody response in all three groups of animals (TABLE 2). Thus, small amounts of antibodies can be induced by anti-IdX558 treatment alone, and their titer increases significantly when followed by immunization with dextran.

SEROLOGICAL CHARACTERISTICS OF THE RESPONSE

Independent experiments indicated that the inhibitory material in serum was not the residual rabbit anti-IdX558. A rapid clearance follows two injections of 23 μg of ^{125}I-labeled rabbit antibodies spaced 14 days apart, and $\leq$10 ng/ml remain in the serum 7 days later. Second, all the inhibitory activity could be eliminated by a preabsorption with anti-λ1 coupled to Sepharose 4B. This finding strongly suggested that the Id activity is associated with an immunoglobulin (Ig) bearing a λ1 light chain.

The higher levels of this Id-positive Ig compared to antibody seen at all times (TABLE 2) suggested that a part of Id represented nondextran binding immunoglobulin. The two serum components were, therefore, studied separately. Pooled sera, from either anti-IdX558-sensitized mice or followed by immunization with B-1355-ConA (termed Ab$_3$ in FIGURE 1), were preabsorbed sequentially on a column of NRIgG to eliminate the corresponding antibodies. The sera were then preabsorbed on a column of dextran B-512 in order to purify anti-α1-6 antibodies (ā-B512 in FIGURE 1), and finally preabsorbed on a column of dextran B-1355 to purify anti-α1-3 antibodies (Ab$_1'$ in FIGURE 1).

As can be seen in FIGURE 1, the inhibition curve of the purified anti-α1-3 antibodies is indistinguishable from that of the M104E proband in the IdX Dex assay. Independent calculations indicated that most or all of these antibodies expressed this idiotype. The antibodies were also completely inhibitory in the IdX Dex assay using the BALB/c anti-IdX reagents, suggesting a strong idiotypic similarity, or identity with the IdX Dex$^+$ reference BALB/c myeloma antibodies. It does not exclude, however, a sequence heterogeneity in VH CDR2 of a minor portion of the antibodies that would go undetected in this type of assay.

With rare exceptions, anti-α1-6 antibodies purified from the same serum pools and from NRIgG-sensitized control groups, did not type positively in this assay (FIGURE 1). Whenever an inhibition was observed, the sera came from anti-IdX558-sensitized pools and were contaminated by ~6% of anti-α1-3 antibodies. These antibodies may have been coabsorbed on the B-512 column, as this dextran contains 4% of α1-3 linkages.[20]

Finally, FIGURE 1 illustrates that the whole serum depleted of both anti-α1-3 and anti-α1-6 antibodies remains completely inhibitory, albeit with a distinct slope compared to proband, suggesting some idiotope deficiency or a substantial content of idiotope-related immunoglobulin. This dextran nonbinding component represents 90%

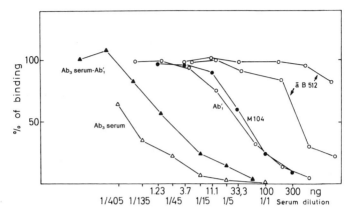

FIGURE 1. Idiotypic properties of specifically purified anti-α1-3 dextran (Ab$_1'$) and anti-α1-6 dextran ($\bar{a}$-B512) antibodies, and whole serum devoid of dextran binding activity (Ab$_3$-Ab$_1'$) from CB 20 mice sensitized with rabbit anti-IdX558. Ab$_3$ serum is the starting serum from which the above three components were obtained. See text for details. The IdX Dex assay was performed as in the legend of TABLE 1. M104E is an Id Dex$^+$ BALB/c myeloma antibody having α1-3 dextran binding activity.

of the total IdX Dex$^+$ response in anti-IdX558-sensitized CB 20 mice and remains at elevated levels throughout the investigated period (50–160 days).[5]

Thus, these Ig represent a major Id-positive component in this system, and their induction has been reported in a number of previous studies in the mouse and in the rabbit.[21-26] They have been defined as Ab$_3$ by Urbain *et al.*[26] to distinguish them from the Id-positive antibodies defined as Ab$_1'$. In the present system these Ig, in addition, bear a λ1 light chain identical to that of BALB/c mice, as the CB 20 strain is CH allotype congeneic with BALB/c. Thus, although devoid of antibody function, the Ab$_3$ Ig bear a strong serological similarity with the Ab$_1'$ component. The present data do not exclude, however, that these Ig, in addition, contain anti-(anti-IdX Dex) antibodies, that is, antibodies recognizing noninternal image related idiotopes[27] expressed on the injected rabbit antibodies.

Margolies[28] reported the first structural study of CRI^a idiotype-bearing Ig devoid of Ar hapten binding activity. A strong homology with a CRI^a-positive anti-Ar hybridoma antibody was apparent by only four substitutions throughout the VH region, whereas JH2 was used by the antibody and JH4 by the Ab$_3$. The VL region sequences were also similar.

An important regulatory role of these Ig was suggested by their capacity to transfer *in utero* responsiveness to offspring rabbits.[29] Also, the injection of small amounts of idiotypic myeloma antibody into neonate mice was reported to induce subsequent responsiveness.[30]

CLASS COMPOSITION

A striking finding in the present study was the prominent IgG$_1$ class anti-α1-3 antibody response in anti-IdX558 sensitized CB 20 mice. A similar situation held with respect to the Ab$_3$ Ig, with the difference that this class was the major heavy chain component. In both cases, and with rare exceptions, the light chain was entirely $\lambda 1$. Typical examples with purified antibodies are shown in TABLE 3.

Following immunization with B-1355, the ratio of IgG_1 to IgM was reversed, with IgM becoming the major class of antibody response. As a result, the response appears to partially revert to its typical thymus-independent form characterized by high levels of IgM. In BALB/c mice, the use of IgG_1 by anti-α1-3 dextran antibodies has not been reported[31] and was not detected by us. Anti-α1-6 dextran antibodies purified from the same serum pools were almost entirely IgM, κ.

The induction of this strongly thymus-dependent class, characteristic of many secondary responses, strongly suggests the aid of T-helper cells in this response. These cells may recognize regulatory idiotopes[10,30] shared by anti-α1-3 dextran antibodies of the two haplotype mice. It has recently been shown, for instance, that T-helper cells appear to recognize a shared idiotope on two idiotypically distinct BALB/c anti-PC myeloma antibodies, T15 and M167.[32] Previous studies have also clearly implicated the participation of specifically anti-Id-induced T-helper cells in such immune responses.[33,34]

CH ALLOTYPE

We took advantage of the presence of these IgG_1 antibodies by attempting to determine their CH allotype. Anti-α1-3 dextran antibodies were purified from CB 20 sera selected for high (35 to 70%) IgG_1 antibody content, and run in parallel in the Igh_4^b and Igh_{4^a} allotype competitive radioimmunoassays.[35]

The specificity of each assay for the respective IgG_1 allelic variant is evident by examining the data shown in TABLE 4. Only the M245 IgG_1 myeloma protein (from C57B1/6 origin) and purified C57B1/6 normal serum IgG_1 were inhibitory in the Igh_4^b assay—not the IgG_{2^a} myeloma protein CBPC101. In addition, enriched prepara-

TABLE 3. Class Representation of CB 20 Anti-α1-3 Dextran Antibodies and IdX Dex$^+$ Immunoglobulin (Ab$_3$).

Source	Percent of Class Response[a]						
	$\lambda 1$	κ	μ	$\gamma 1$	$\gamma 2$	$\gamma 3$	α
CB 20 Anti-α1-3[c]	100	—[d]	44	34	3	18	—
BALB/c Anti-α1-3	100	—	90	—	—	4	7
CB 20 Ab$_3$[b]	100	—	35	55	4	3	3
CB 20 Anti-α1-6[c]	—	100	78	—	—	12	12

[a]Determined in a binding assay according to Geckeler *et al.*[37] using specifically purified ^{125}I-labeled rabbit anti-mouse heavy or light chain antibodies.

[b]Determined in a microplate binding assay using 1.5 μg/ml of anti-IdX558 as coat, and as control 1.5 μg/ml of NRIgG. The whole CB 20 sera were preabsorbed with NRIgG coupled to sepharose 4B.

[c]Anti-α1-3 and anti-α1-6 antibodies were purified from the same serum pool of CB 20 mice sensitized with five injections of anti-IdX558. The anti-α1-6 response pattern of NRIgG-sensitized control mice is basically similar.

[d]Not detectable in the assay.

TABLE 4. Allotype Assignment of CB 20 IgG$_1$ Anti-α1-3 Dextran Antibodies

Competitor[a]	NG required for 50 Percent Inhibition in	
	Igh$_{4b}$ Assay[b]	Igh$_{4a}$ assay[b]
M245 (Igh$_{4b}$)	7.5	ND
C57B1/6 (IgG$_{1c}$)	450	ND
CBPC 101 (Ig$_{1b}$)	>2,700	ND
CB 20 normal serum	1/900	<1/10
CB 20 antibodies	4.5 ; 10 ; 19[d]	>80 ; >750 ; >65
M21 (Igh$_{4a}$)	ND	22
M173 (Igh$_{1a}$)	ND	>2,700
BALB/c normal serum	<1/10	1/2,900

[a]All the myeloma proteins were purified preparations.

[b]The competition radioimmunoassays were performed according to Bosma et al.[35] using a BALB/c anti-C57B1/6 serum for the Igh$_{4b}$ assay, and specifically purified C57B1/6 anti-BALB/c antibodies in the Igh$_{4a}$ assay. The proband in the Igh$_{4b}$ assay was [^{125}I]M245, and for the Igh$_{4a}$ assay [^{125}I]M21.

[c]Purified from normal serum on an ethylchloroformate[36] specific rabbit anti-mouse Fcγ1 immunoabsorbent.

[d]Values obtained from three separate pools of purified anti-α1-3 dextran antibodies from CB 20 mice sensitized with two or five injections of rabbit anti-IdX558.

tions of M352 and CBPC112, respectively IgG$_{2b}$ and IgM of C57B1/6 origin, were likewise not inhibitory (not shown).

It can be seen that 4 to 19 ng of three purified antibody preparations sufficed for 50% inhibition, the values being in the range found with the reference Igh$_{4b}$ immunoglobulins. None of the antibodies were inhibitory in the specific Igh$_{4a}$ assay, suggesting that all, or most of the antibodies were Igh$_{4b}$

In addition, all of the inhibitory activity was abrogated by a preabsorption with rabbit anti-λ1 or anti-IdX558 antibodies coupled to Sepharose 4B, but not with anti-κ absorbent. This experiment ensured that the CH allotype determinants were on the antibody IgG$_1$ and not on possible contaminant normal serum IgG$_1$.

ACKNOWLEDGMENTS

We thank Dr. Brian Clevinger for the generous gift of Hdex hybridoma antibodies, Dr. Klaus Rajewsky for the B1-8 hybridoma, Dr. D. J. Capra for the 93G7 hybridoma, Dr. Melvin Cohn for the J606 myeloma antibody, and Dr. Michael Potter for the McPC603 and J539 ascites fluids. The BALB/c anti-C57B1/6 serum was a gift of Dr. Melvin Bosma, the C57B1/6 anti-BALB/c serum from Dr. Michel Seman, and the BALB/c anti-J558 serum from Dr. P. A. Cazenave.

REFERENCES

1. BLOMBERG, B., W. R. GECKELER & M. WEIGERT. 1972. Genetics of the antibody response to dextran in mice. Science 177: 178.
2. RIBLET, R., B. BLOMBERG, M. WEIGERT, R. LIEBERMAN, B. A. TAYLOR & M. POTTER. 1975. Genetics of mouse antibodies. I. Linkage of the dextran response locus, VH-Dex, to allotype. Eur. J. Immunol. 5: 775.
3. HANSBURG, D., D. E. BRILES & J. M. DAVIE. 1976. Analysis of the diversity of murine antibodies to dextran B1355. I. Generation of a large pauciclonal response by a bacterial vaccine. J. Immunol. 117: 569.

4. GECKELER, W., B. BLOMBERG, C. DE PREVAL & M. COHN. 1977. On the genetic dissection of a specific humoral immune response to $\alpha(1,3)$ dextran. Cold Spring Harbor Symp. Quant. Biol. **41:** 743.

5. PÈNE, J., F. BEKKHOUCHA, C. DESAYMARD, H. ZAGHOUANI & M. STANISLAWSKI. 1983. Induction of an IdX Dextran-positive antibody response in two IghC[b] mouse strains treated with anti-IdX558 idiotype antibodies. J. Exp. Med. **157:** 1573.

6. WEIGERT, M. & R. RIBLET. 1978. The genetic control of antibody variable regions in the mouse. Springer Semin. Immunopathology. **1:** 133.

7. SLACK, J. H., M. SHAPIRO & M. POTTER. 1979. Serum expression of a VK structure, VK-11, associated with inulin antibodies controlled by gene(s) linked to the mouse IghC complex. J. Immunol. **122:** 230.

8. CANCRO, M. P., N. H. SIGAL & N. R. KLINMAN. 1978. Differential expression of an equivalent clonotype among BALB/c and C57B1/6 mice. J. Exp. Med. **147:** 1.

9. EICHMANN, K. & K. RAJEWSKY. 1975. Induction of T and B cell immunity by anti-idiotypic antibody. Eur. J. Immunol. **5:** 661.

10. BONA, C., E. HEBER-KATZ & W. E. PAUL. 1981. Idiotype-anti-idiotype regulation. I. Immunization with a levan-binding myeloma protein leads to the appearance of auto-anti-(anti-idiotype) antibodies and to the activation of silent clones. J. Exp. Med. **153:** 951.

11. LE GUERN, C., F. BEN AÏSSA, D. JUY, B. MARIAMÉ, G. BUTTIN & P. A. CAZENAVE. 1979. Expression and induction of MOPC-460 idiotopes in different strains of mice. Ann. Immunol. Inst. Pasteur (Paris). **130C:** 193.

12. LEO, O. 1983. Induction of anti-arsonate CRI positive antibodies in BALB/c mice. Ann. N.Y. Acad. Sci. **418:** 257–264. This volume.

13. JERNE, N. K. 1974. Towards a network theory of the immune response. Ann. Immunol. Inst. Pasteur (Paris). **125C:** 373.

14. WUILMART, C., M. WIKLER & J. URBAIN. 1979. Induction of autoantiidiotypic antibodies and effects on the subsequent immune response. Mol. Immunol. **16:** 1085.

15. BONA, C., R. HOOGHE, P. A. CAZENAVE, C. LE GUERN & W. E. PAUL. 1979. Cellular basis of regulation of expression of idiotype. II. Immunity to anti-MOPC-460 idiotype antibodies increases the level of anti-trinitrophenyl antibodies bearing 460 idiotypes. J. Exp. Med. **149:** 815.

16. URBAIN, J., C. WUILMART & P. A. CAZENAVE. 1981. Idiotypic regulation in immune networks. Contemp. Top. Mol. Immunol. **8:** 113.

17. CLEVINGER, B., J. SCHILLING, L. HOOD & J. M. DAVIE. 1980. Structural correlates of cross-reactive and individual idiotypic determinants on murine antibodies to $\alpha(1 \rightarrow 3)$ dextran. J. Exp. Med. **151:** 1059.

18. BOTHWELL, A. L., M. PASKIND, M. RETH, T. IMANISHI-KARI, K. RAJEWSKY & D. BALTIMORE. 1981. Heavy chain variable region contribution to the NP[b] family of antibodies: somatic mutation evident in a $\gamma 2a$ variable region. Cell **24:** 625.

19. CARSON, D. & M. WEIGERT. 1973. Immunochemical analysis of the cross-reacting idiotypes of mouse myeloma proteins with anti-dextran activity and normal anti-dextran antibody. Proc. Natl. Acad. Sci. USA **70:** 235.

20. JEANES, A. & F. R. SEYMOUR. 1979. The α-D-glycopyranosidic linkages of dextrans: comparison of percentages from structural analysis by periodate oxidation and by methylation. Carbohydr. Res. **74:** 31.

21. WYSOCKI, L. J. & V. L. SATO. 1981. The strain A anti-p-azophenyl-arsonate major cross-reactive idiotypic family includes members with no reactivity toward p-azophenyl-arsonate. Eur. J. Immunol. **11:** 832.

22. ENGHOFFER, E., C. P. J. GLAUDEMANS & M. J. BOSMA. 1979. Immunoglobulins with different specificities have similar idiotypes. Mol. Immunol. **16:** 1103.

23. EICHMANN, K., A. COUTINHO & F. MELCHERS. 1977. Absolute frequencies of lipopolysaccharide-reactive B cell producing A5A idiotype in unprimed, streptococcal A– carbohydrate-primed, anti-A5A idiotype sensitized and anti-A5A idiotype-suppressed A/J mice. J. Exp. Med. **146:** 1436.

24. OUDIN, J. & P. A. CAZENAVE. 1971. Similar idiotypic specificities in immunoglobulin fractions with different antibody functions or even without detectable antibody function. Proc. Natl. Acad. Sci. USA **68:** 2616.

25. SACHS, D. H., M. EL-GAMIL & G. MILLER. 1981. Genetic control of the immune response to staphylococcal nuclease. XI. Effects of *in vivo* administration of anti-idiotypic antibodies. Eur. J. Immunol. **11:** 509.
26. URBAIN, J., M. WIKLER, J. D. FRANSSEN & C. COLLIGNON. 1977. Idiotypic regulation of the immune system by the induction of antibodies against anti-idiotypic antibodies. Proc. Natl. Acad. Sci. USA **74:** 5126.
27. JERNE, N. K., J. ROLAND & P. A. CAZENAVE. 1982. Recurrent idiotopes and internal images. Eur. Mol. Biol. Org. J. **1:** 247.
28. MARGOLIES, M. N. 1983. Structural correlates of idiotypy in the arsonate system. Ann. N.Y. Acad. Sci. **418:** 48–64. This volume.
29. WICKLER, M., C. DEMEURE, G. DEWASME & J. URBAIN. 1980. Immunoregulatory role of maternal idiotypes. J. Exp. Med. **152:** 1024.
30. RUBINSTEIN, L. J., M. YEH & C. BONA. 1982. Idiotype-anti-idiotype network. II. Activation of silent clones by treatment at birth with idiotypes is associated with the expansion of idiotype-specific helper T-cells. J. Exp. Med. **156:** 506.
31. HANSBURG, D., R. M. PERLMUTTER, D. E. BRILES & J. M. DAVIE. 1978. Analysis of the diversity of murine antibodies to dextran B1355. III. Idiotypic and spectrotypic correlations. Eur. J. Immunol. **8:** 352.
32. GLEASON, K. & H. KÖHLER. 1982. Regulatory idiotypes. T helper cells recognize a shared VH idiotype on phosphorylcholine-specific antibodies. J. Exp. Med. **156:** 539.
33. EICHMANN, K., J. FALK & K. RAJEWSKY. 1978. Recognition of idiotypes in lymphocyte interactions. II. Antigen-dependent cooperation between T- and B-lymphocytes that possess similar and complementary idiotypes. Eur. J. Immunol. **8:** 853.
34. MILLER, G. G. P., P. I. NADLER, R. J. HODES & D. H. SACHS. 1982. Modification of T cell antinuclease idiotype expression by *in vivo* administration of anti-idiotype. J. Exp. Med. **155:** 190.
35. BOSMA, M. J., R. MARKS & C. L. DE WITT. 1975. Quantitation of mouse immunoglobulin allotypes by a modified solid-phase radioimmune assay. J. Immunol. **115:** 1381.
36. AVRAMEAS, S. & T. TERNYNCK. 1967. Biologically active water insoluble protein polymers. Their use for the isolation of antigens and antibodies. J. Biol. Chem. **242:** 1651.
37. GECKELER, W., J. FAVERSHAM & M. COHN. 1978. On a regulatory gene controlling the expression of the murine λ1 light chain. J. Exp. Med. **148:** 1122.

DISCUSSION OF THE PAPER

C. A. BONA (*Mt. Sinai School of Medicine, New York*): I think that these data and the data reported in the arsonate system (and in other systems) show that the family of the idiotypes association with a particular allotype became smaller.

Induction of Multi-Specific Antibodies to Bovine Serum Albumin after Production of Anti-Idiotype Antibodies to an Albumin-Specific Monoclonal Antibody[a]

NANCY J. KRIEGER,[b] AMADEO J. PESCE,[c]
AND J. GABRIEL MICHAEL[b]

[b]Department of Microbiology and Molecular Genetics
and
[c]Department of Pathology
University of Cincinnati College of Medicine
Cincinnati, Ohio 45267

INTRODUCTION

Considerable evidence is now available to suggest that anti-idiotype antibodies have an important function in both regulation and diversification of the immune response.[1-10] Anti-idiotype antibodies are capable of regulating relevant idiotypic responses as demonstrated by antibody production[1] and the induction of T-suppressor cells.[2] Furthermore, anti-idiotypic antibodies stimulate the production of antibodies with distinct paratopes, but while sharing common idiotopes.[3,4] Until recently, the regulatory function of such stimulation appeared questionable, however, with the demonstration of common idiotopes on antibodies directed to different epitopes on the same protein, that is, myoglobin and human serum albumin,[5,6] a regulatory function can be described. Although unproven, such idiotypes may function as determinants for control of responses to complex molecules, a role suggested by Paul and Bona[11] in their description of regulatory idiotopes.

In the present study, using a complex protein, bovine serum albumin (BSA), we investigated the ability of anti-idiotypic antibodies to regulate the poly-specific anti-BSA response. Anti-idiotypic antibodies generated to a monoclonal anti-BSA antibody, induced anti-BSA antibodies in the absence of antigen. Most importantly, the anti-BSA response in these mice was not limited to antibodies of the same paratope as the monoclonal antibody. Anti-BSA antibodies were found to bind epitopes located between amino acids 1-306, 307-505, as well as the amino acids 505-582 bound by the monoclonal antibody. We believe this is the first demonstration of a polyspecific antibody response to multiple determinants of an antigen generated by an anti-idiotypic mechanism.

[a]This investigation was supported by Grant A115520 from the National Institutes of Health.

MATERIALS AND METHODS

Animals

A/J, B6D2F$_1$/J(BDF$_1$), and CAF$_1$/J(CAF$_1$) female mice 6 to 9 weeks old were obtained from the Jackson Laboratory, Bar Harbor, Maine.

Antigens

Bovine serum albumin was purchased from Miles Laboratories, Elkart Indiana. Bovine serum albumin fragments produced by peptic digestion were generous gifts of Dr. Peters, Jr. and Dr. Reed of Cooperstown, N.Y. The preparation, purity, and localization of the three peptic fragments BSA P$_{1-306}$, (P$_{1-306}$), BSA P$_{307-582}$ (P$_{307-582}$), and BSA P$_{505-582}$ (P$_{505-582}$) have been described.[12]

Production of P$_{505-582}$ Specific Hybridomas

Hybridomas were produced by fusion of spleen cells from A/J mice, hyperimmunized with BSA prior to fusion, with a BALB/c myeloma SP2/0, a nonsecreting line. In brief, fusion was performed by mixing the two cell populations with polyethylene glycol[13] and seeding washed cells into 96 well microtiter plates using supplemented RPMI-1640 media containing Garamycin (50 µg/ml), 2-mercaptoethanol ($5 \times 10^{-5}M$), sodium pyruvate (100 mM), and nonessential amino acids (0.6 ml of 100× concentration). After 24 hours 2× HAT media (hypoxanthine, aminopterin, and thymidine) was added.[14] Ten days after fusion, aminopterin was removed from the media, and wells were subsequently screened for visible growth. Hybridomas secreting P$_{505-582}$ specific antibodies were transferred to tissue culture flasks. The hybridoma in this report was prepared as described and was a gift of Dr. D.C. Benjamin of Charlottesville, Virginia. For use in immunizations, the hybridoma was transferred into Pristane primed CAF$_1$ mice for ascites production.

Preparation of the Monoclonal Antibody 17.5.5E

Ascites fluid from mice were precipitated twice with ammonium sulfate (33%) followed by extensive dialysis against phosphate-buffered saline, pH. 7.4. Following dialysis, the monoclonal antibodies were concentrated by ultrafiltration using a Millipore CX-10 ultrafiltration unit. Antibodies were further purified by affinity chromatography using BSA coupled CNBr-activated Sepharose CL-4B. Specific antibodies were eluted with 0.05 M glycine-HCl buffer pH 2.5, pooled and dialyzed against phosphate-buffered saline. Immunoglobulin class was determined by enzyme-linked immunosorbent assay (ELISA) using the MONO-Ab-ID kit (Zymed Laboratories).

Production of Anti-Idiotypic Antibody to 17.5.5E

Anti-idiotypic antibody was prepared by immunizaiton with affinity purified 17.5.5E. Mice received 100 µg of 17.5.5E in complete Freund's adjuvant (CFA) on day 0, and 50 µg of antibody in incomplete Freund's adjuvant (IFA) on days 30 and 45. All immunizations were performed intraperitoneally (i.p.).

Enzyme-Linked Immunosorbent Assay

Enzyme-linked immunosorbent assays were performed as described elsewhere.[15] Briefly, polystyrene, 96 well plates (Immulon II, Dynatech) were coated with 50 μg/ml of antigen in 0.1 M carbonate buffer, pH. 9.5. Before use, excess antigen was removed by washing with 0.1 M phosphate buffer containing 0.1% Tween-20. Antiserum or supernatants were then dispensed in 0.1 ml aliquots and incubated for 1 hour at 37° C. Following incubation, plates were washed and 0.2 ml of a 1/1000 dilution of alkaline phosphatase-conjugated rabbit-anti-mouse immunoglobulin (Zymed Lab, Burlingame, Calif.) were added to each well. Plates were reincubated for an additional hour and washed. Substrate, *p*-nitro-phenylphosphate (Sigma) 1 mg/ml, in 0.5 mM MgCl$_2$ and 1 M ethanolamine-HCl was then added to each well. The reaction was allowed to develop for 20 minutes at which time 1 N NaOH was added to terminate the reaction. Absorbance was determined at 405 nm using a Microelisa Reader (Dynatech). Antibody concentration was determined by comparison of absorbancies between experimental wells and known concentration standards. Values are reported as μg of antibody/ml.

TABLE 1. Characteristics of the Monoclonal Antibody 17.5.5E[a]

Class	BSA (1-582)	Domain I[b] (1-183)	Domain II[b] (184-316)	P307-582[c]	Domain III[b] (377-582)	P505-582[c]
IgG$_1\kappa$	+ +	− −	− −	+ +	+ +	+ +

[a]The monoclonal antibody was produced by fusion of A/J spleen cells hyperimmunized with BSA and a BALB/c myeloma SP2/0. The hybridoma was a generous gift of Dr. D.C. Benjamin (Charlottesville, Va.).
[b]Determined by Benjamin *et al.* (personal communication).
[c]Determined by this lab using the ELISA technique; see MATERIALS AND METHODS.

Determination of Anti-Idiotypic Antibodies to 17.5.5E

The presence of anti-idiotypic antibody was determined by an inhibition assay. The inhibition assays were performed by first diluting affinity purified 17.5.5E monoclonal antibodies to a concentration of 500 ng antibody/ml. Sera to be assayed were serially diluted, beginning at a dilution of 1/5. Five hundred microliters of both monoclonal antibodies and sera were then incubated for 1 hour in glass tubes at 37° C. Following incubation, 200 μl of each mixture were placed in P$_{505-582}$ coated wells for assay in the ELISA system as described above.

RESULTS

Specificity and Characteristics of the Monoclonal Antibody 17.5.5E

The monoclonal antibody, 17.5.5E, produced by fusion of A/J spleen cells from BSA immune mice, has been characterized in this lab[16] and that of Benjamin.[17] The monoclonal antibody, an IgG$_1\kappa$, with a binding specificity to epitopes within Domain III of BSA (aa. 377–582) has further been characterized to bind specifically to an epitope localized within the terminal 78 amino acids on the carboxy end of BSA (TABLE 1). Furthermore, the monoclonal antibody has been shown to be capable of regulating the anti-BSA antibody response when given prior to antigen.[16] This regulation demonstrated by suppression of antibodies to all determinants has been found to be due to nonblocking mechanisms of regulation, operative in both syngeneic and allogeneic mice.

Production of Anti-Idiotypic Antibodies to 17.5.5E

BDF$_1$ mice were given 100 μg of affinity-purified monoclonal antibodies in CFA i.p. on day zero. On days 30 and 45 mice received additional injections of 50 μg of 17.5.5E in incomplete Freund's adjuvant. Prior to the second and third immunizations, on days 29 and 44, mice were bled. Their sera were pooled and tested for the presence of anti-idiotypic antibody. Anti-idiotypic antibody was demonstrated by the ability of the pooled sera to inhibit the monoclonal antibody from binding to P$_{505-582}$ coated plates in an ELISA assay. Serum obtained on day 29 was capable of inhibiting 500 μg of 17.5.5E from binding at a dilution of 1/5, but was negative at all higher dilutions. Serum from day 44 had the ability to inhibit binding of the monoclonal at dilutions up to 1/80 (TABLE 2). Normal pooled BDF$_1$ sera did not inhibit the monoclonal antibody from binding at the lowest dilution used (1/5). Furthermore, anti-idiotypic antibodies had no inhibitory capacity towards affinity-purified human serum albumin antibodies from A/J mice (data not shown). Sera taken five days after the last immunization (day 50) failed to demonstrate inhibition of 17.5.5E from binding to P$_{505-582}$. In fact,

TABLE 2. Demonstration of Anti-Idiotypic Antibodies to 17.5.5E Monoclonal Antibodies

Serum Dilution[a]	Amount of 17.5.5E Bound to Fragment P$_{505-582}$[b] (ng/ml)	Percent Inhibition[c]
1/5	34.1	86
1/10	46.5	81
1/20	57.3	77
1/40	175.0	30
1/80	225.0	10
1/160	249.0	0.4
1/320	251.0	0
Control[d]	250.1	0
Buffer	251.8	—

[a]Pooled sera from eight mice receiving two injections of 17.5.5E monoclonal antibody; 100 μg in CFA on day 0 and 50 μg in IFA on day 30. Sera were obtained 44 days after the initial injection.

[b]Affinity-purified monoclonal antibody, 17.5.5E, was diluted to a concentration of 500 ng/ml. The assay was performed by mixing equal volumes of monoclonal antibody with various dilutions of anti-idiotypic serum or buffer and pre-incubating the mixture for 1 hour at 37° C. These mixtures were then incubated in BSA fragment P505–582-coated wells for 1 hour. Binding of the monoclonal antibody to P505–582 was detected using alkaline-phosphatase conjugated rabbit anti-mouse Ig as described in MATERIALS AND METHODS.

[c]The percent of inhibition of binding of the monoclonal antibody to P505–582 was calculated according to the equation:

$$\% \text{ Inhibition} = \left(1 - \frac{\text{ng of 17.5.5E bound in the presence of serum}}{\text{ng of 17.5.5E bound in buffer}}\right) \times 100$$

[d]Control consisted of a 1/5 dilution of pooled normal B6D2F$_1$/J serum.

TABLE 3. Anti-Borine Serum Albumin Antibodies Produced in the Absence of Antigen Following Demonstration of Anti-Idiotypic Antibodies[a]

Day[c]	1-306	Binding of Anti-BSA Antibodies to BSA and Fragments (μg/ml)[b] 307-582	505-582	1-582
29	0[d]	0	0	0
44	0	0	10 ng[e]	10 ng
50	322.8	127.4	33.9	569.1

[a]BDF$_1$ mice that received the monoclonal antibody 17.5.5E were tested for the presence of anti-BSA antibodies in their sera after a third immunization failed to elicit anti-idiotypic antibodies as demonstrated by inhibition.

[b]Antisera binding specificities were determined by screening the sera on polystyrene plates coated with BSA, P1-306, P307-582, or P505-582.

[c]Days refers to days after the initial immunization with 17.5.5E. Immunization schedule is listed in MATERIALS AND METHODS. Briefly, mice received antibody on days 0, 30, and 45.

[d]Sensitivity of the assay as used was 1.0 ng/ml.

[e]Some antibodies detected below the quantitation limits of 10 ng/ml of antibody.

dilutions of 50 day sera up to 1/320 demonstrated enhancement of the 17.5.5E binding of P$_{505-582}$.

Demonstration of Anti-Bovine Serum Albumin Antibodies in the Sera of 17.5.5E Primed Mice

Demonstration of the enhancing capacity of the 50 day sera with 17.5.5E to bind P$_{505-582}$ suggested that anti-P$_{505-582}$ antibodies may have been produced in the absence of antigen by the anti-idiotypic response. Screening of 29, 44, and 50 day sera on P$_{505-582}$ coated plates revealed no such antibody at day 29, trace quantities at day 44 (10 ng/ml), and a clear response (33.9 μg/ml) on day 50 (TABLE 3). Additional screening of the 50 day sera on BSA-coated plates revealed that a substantial anti-BSA response (569.1 μg/ml) was produced. These antibodies could not be accounted for entirely by antibodies to P$_{505-582}$, therefore the sera was screened on other BSA fragments for binding specificity. Analysis of the sera (TABLE 3) determined the presence of antibodies directed toward epitopes in the region of amino acids 1-306 and 307-505.

Effect of Anti-Idiotypic Antibodies on the Anti-Bovine Serum Albumin Response

To determine what effect immunization with the monoclonal antibodies and the resulting responses (anti-idiotype antibody and anti-BSA antibodies) had on the ability to respond to BSA, the same mice were immunized with bovine serum albumin. Mice were rested for seventeen days after the third immunization with 17.5.5E and then given 100 μg of BSA in alum (1 mg). Mice from the same shipment as the monoclonal antibody treated mice, were also immunized with 100 μg of BSA for comparison. Eight days after immunization, both groups were bled and the anti-BSA titers determined (TABLE 4). The typical primary anti-BSA response was demonstrated by the control mice[18] as indicated by a predominance of antibodies to the carboxy terminal (307-582) amino acids. Later bleedings on days 16 and 23 also demonstrated this trend. Antibody titers of the control animals peaked on day 16, typical of primary responses when BSA was administered in alum. Mice immunized with 17.5.5E antibodies also demonstrated peak anti-BSA response on day 16, however, unlike control mice, the percentage of antibodies towards 1-306 epitopes was 50% or greater of the total anti-BSA antibodies. Furthermore, the quantity of antibodies (3–10 mg) was reminiscent of secondary antibody responses produced after multiple injections of BSA in complete Freund's adjuvant. The proportion of antibodies binding $P_{505-582}$ determinants also increased in idiotype (17.5.5E) treated mice; $P_{505-582}$ specific antibodies represented 20 to 30% of the carboxy terminal antibody response compared to 5 to 10% in mice receiving only bovine serum albumin. Increase in antibodies to $P_{505-582}$ determinants also increased in idiotype (17.5.5E) treated mice; $P_{505-582}$ specific antibodies represented 20 to 30% of the carboxy terminal antibody response compared to 5 to 10% in mice receiving only bovine serum albumin. Increase in antibodies to $P_{505-582}$ determinants over those to $P_{307-505}$ determinants also occurred in secondary anti-BSA responses.[18]

TABLE 4. Effect of Anti-Idiotypic Antibodies on the Anti-Bovine Serum Albumin Antibody Response

Group	Day[a]	Binding Profile of Anti-BSA Antibodies			
		1-306	307-582	505-582	1-582
Control	(8)[b]	1.8	39.0	2.0	32.3
ID-Treated[c]	70 (8)	1341.0	1617.0	318.5	3292.8
Control	(16)	12.0	360.8	28.3	376.4
ID-Treated	78 (16)	4407.0	4290.0	1365.0	10920.0
Control	(23)	16.2	85.5	9.2	195.1
ID-Treated	85 (23)	3332.0	4380.0	931.8	7291.0

[a]Day refers to days after the initial injection of monoclonal antibody in CFA.
[b]Numbers in parentheses refer to days after immunization with BSA.
[c]Sixty-two days after immunization with the first dose of 17.5.5E and following two further injections on days 30 and 45, mice received 100 μg of BSA in 1 mg of alum. Control mice received the same dose of antigen in alum.

DISCUSSION

In this study we have described the production of antibody in the absence of antigen following administration of a monoclonal antibody 17.5.5E (Ab$_1$) specific for an epitope localized in the amino acid sequences $N_{505-582}$ of bovine serum albumin. Anti-idiotype antibodies (Ab$_2$) to 17.5.5E were identified after a primary immunization and were identified similarly following a second injection of the monoclonal antibody. After subsequent immunizations with 17.5.5E, the ability of the sera to inhibit binding of the monoclonal antibody to $P_{505-582}$ disappeared; instead enhancement of the binding to the fragment was noted. This enhancement was determined to be the result of antibodies specific for BSA (Ab$_3$). Therefore, we interpreted the results to indicate that the Ab$_2$ (anti-17.5.5E) was the internal image[19] of the epitope recognized by the monoclonal antibody. Surprisingly, a majority of the Ab$_3$ antibodies detected demonstrated binding specificities to epitopes located within the region of a.a. 1-504, serologically unrelated to the region of a.a.505-582 for which Ab$_1$ was specific. Therefore, additional explanations were entertained to describe the anti-BSA response. The initial concern was that the antigen (BSA) may have inadvertently been given as an Ag/Ab complex arising from affinity purification. This possibility, however, was excluded by additional experiments. Rabbits given the same preparation of 17.5.5E failed to elicit anti-BSA antibodies. Furthermore, mice immunized with the immunoglobulin fraction of the 17.5.5E ascites, without affinity purification, also demonstrated anti-idiotope and anti-BSA antibodies in their sera.

It has been demonstrated that anti-idiotype antibody can expand B-cell clones, prime for secondary antibody responses,[20] and protect against parasitic infections.[9] It has generally been assumed, as postulated by Jerne,[19] that these were the result of the anti-idiotype mimicking of the antigen and as a result, the stimulating of the immune response (i.e. internal image). As reported by Rajewsky, Bona, and others, however, a likely result of anti-idiotype production is the increase in idiotope-bearing antibodies without similar increases in epitope-specific antibodies. Paul and Bona[11] have suggested that such a phenomenon is the result of a specialized idiotope located on the antibodies used for immunization. These idiotopes, designated regulatory idiotopes, are thought to interconnect regulatory interactions between idiotopes and paratopes to allow expansion and increased affinity of cells in the absence of antigen. Several investigators using complex molecules as antigens such as myoglobin,[5] lysozyme,[21] and human serum albumin[6] have discovered shared idiotopes among antibodies binding unrelated epitopes on the antigen molecule. It is interesting to speculate that these idiotopes may represent the regulatory idiotopes postulated above. In these cases such idiotopes could effectively control the expansion or downward regluation of the majority of B-cells to the antigen, regardless of specificity, by way of an idiotope-specific T cell. These conclusions have implications for the increase in affinity and dominance of particular clones in secondary antibody responses to protein antigens and may in fact describe how memory-cell selection occurs. Our data suggests that such regulatory idiotopes do occur in the response generated to BSA, and we are currently involved in identifying such idiotopes on anti-BSA antibodies and monoclonals.

REFERENCES

1. LEE, W., H. COSENZA & H. KOHLER. 1974. Clonal restriction of the immune response to phosphocholine. Nature (London) **247:** 55.
2. EICHMANN, K. 1975. Idiotype suppression. II. Amplification of a suppressor T-cell with anti-idiotypic activity. Eur. J. Immunol. **5:** 11.
3. CAPRA, J. D. & J. M. KEHOE. 1975. Hypervariable regions, idiotypy, and the antibody combining site. Adv. Immunol. **20:** 1.
4. NISONOFF, A., J. E. HOPPER & S. B. SPRING. 1975. Idiotypic specificities of immunoglobulins. *In* The Antibody Molecule. 444. F. J. Dixon Jr. and H. Kunkel, Eds. Academic Press. New York.
5. KOHNO, Y., I. BERKOWER, J. MINNA & J. A. BERZOFSKY. 1982. Idiotypes of antimyoglobin antibodies: shared idiotypes among monoclonal antibodies to distinct determinants of sperm whale myoglobin. J. Immunol. **128:** 1742.
6. CAZENAVE, P. A. 1973. Comparison of the idiotypy of antibodies synthesized by rabbits immunized firstly with a fragment of human serum albumin and secondly with whale serum albumin. Biochem. Biophysics Res. Commun. **53:** 452.
7. MILLER, G. G., P. I. NADLER, Y. ASANO, R. J. HODES & D. H. SACHS. 1981. Induction of idiotype-bearing, nuclease-specific helper T-cells by *in vivo* treatment with antiidiotype. J. Exp. Med. **154:** 24.
8. BLUESTONE, J. A., S. O. SHARROW, S. L. EPSTEIN, K. OZATO & D. H. SACHS. 1981. Induction of anti-H-2 antibodies in the absence of alloantigen exposure by *in vivo* administration of anti-idiotype. Nature (London) **291:** 231.
9. SACKS, D. L., K. M. ESSEN & A. SHER. 1982. Immunization of mice against african trypanosomiasis using anti-idiotypic antibodies. J. Exp. Med. **155:** 1108.
10. EICHMANN, K. & K. RAJEWSKY. 1975. Induction of T and B-cell immunity by antiidiotype antibodies. Eur. J. Immunol. **5:** 661.

11.   PAUL, W. E. & C. BONA. 1982. Regulatory idiotypes and immune networks: a hypothesis. Immunology Today. **3:** 230.
12.   JOHANSON, K. O., D. B. WETLAUFER, R. G. REED & T. PETERS, Jr. 1981. Refolding of bovine serum albumin and its proteolytic fragments. Regain of disulfide bonds, secondary structure and ligand binding ability. J. Biol. Chem. **256:** 445.
13.   WAHN, V., T. PETERS, Jr. & R. P. SIRAGANIAN. 1981. Allergenic and antigenic properties of bovine serum albumin. Mol. Immunol. **18:** 19.
14.   BENJAMIN, D. C. 1981. Personal communication.
15.   FERGUSON, T. A., N. J. KRIEGER, A. J. PESCE & J. G. MICHAEL. 1982. Enhancement of antigen specific suppression by muramyl dipeptide (MDP). Infection Immun. **39:** 800.
16.   KRIEGER, N. J., A. J. PESCE & J. G. MICHAEL. 1983. Immunoregulation of the antibovine serum albumin response by polyclonal and monoclonal antibodies. Cell. Immunol. **80:** 279.
17.   BENJAMIN, D. C. 1982. Personal communication.
18.   RILEY, R. L., L. D. WILSON, R. N. GERMAIN & D. C. BENJAMIN. 1982. Immune responses to complex protein antigens. I. MHC control of immune responses to bovine albumin. J. Immunol. **129:** 1553.
19.   N. K. JERNE. 1974. Towards a network theory of the immune system. Ann. Immunol. Inst. Pasteur (Paris) **125C:** 373.
20.   SACHS, D. H., M. E-GAMIL & G. MILLER. 1981. Genetic control of the immune response to staphylococcal nuclease. XI. Effects of *in vivo* administration of anti-idiotypic antibodies. Eur. J. Immunol. **11:** 509.
21.   METZGER, D. W., A. MILLER & E. E. SERCARZ. 1980. Sharing of an idiotypic marker by monoclonal antibodies specific for distinct regions of hen lysozyme. Nature (London) **287:** 549.

DISCUSSION OF THE PAPER

C. A. BONA (*Mt. Sinai School of Medicine, New York*): Did you use, as a probe, an antibody with a very, very high affinity? Eleven mg of anti-BSA per ml is a huge response, and probably is due to the fact that you used a probe in ELISA, an antibody with a very, very high affinity. Did you use such a probe?

N. J. KRIEGER: It could be, yes. I do not think that is the only reason. Even if we immunize with BSA in CFA over a period of three immunizations, we do not get the quantity of antibody that we are seeing here.

R. KALISH (*Downstate Medical Center, Brooklyn, N.Y.*): Do any of these anti-BSA antibodies to other determinants, other than the one you expressed, react with mouse albumin? Have we created an autoimmune phenomenon?

KRIEGER: As yet, we do not think so. We screened the antibodies. They do not appear to bind to mouse albumin, but I cannot specifically say at this point. I do not think so, no. I think that maybe what we have done is eliminated a regulatory mechanism by the induction of these antibodies that would control the amount we are producing. At this point we really cannot say.

Shared and Nonshared Idiotypes on Rabbit Anti-Allotype Antibodies[a]

DENNIS W. METZGER

Division of Immunology
St. Jude Children's Research Hospital
Memphis, Tennessee 38101

The sharing of cross-reactive idiotype IdX markers by rabbit,[1-6] mouse,[7] and human[8,9] anti-allotype antibodies has been described by several laboratories. This report summarizes our studies of idiotypic determinants on rabbit anti-allotype antibodies and discusses the implications of our results with regard to the general nature and biological significance of IdX structures.

We[4] as well as others[5] have previously demonstrated that in every rabbit examined, almost all antibody directed to the rabbit V_H allotype, a1, bears a predominant idiotype (IdX-a1), in addition to unique (IdI) determinants. The presence of IdX-a1 in unrelated animals, initially observed by radioimmunoassay, has also been visualized using anti-idiotype absorption of antibody isoelectrofocusing (IEF) patterns. In this assay, formation of idiotype-anti-idiotype complexes prior to focusing results in the elimination of IdX-positive bands.[10] The IEF patterns of four anti-a1 preparations that had been preincubated with a two-fold excess of either normal rabbit immunoglobulin as a control or with anti-idiotype antibody are shown in FIGURE 1. It can be seen that, in agreement with our earlier results, most of the heterogeneous anti-a1 activity in each case was removed by the anti-idiotype absorption.

Further experiments showed that the IdX-a1 determinant(s) is within, or close to, the antigen-combining site and expressed primarily on isolated H chains, but not L chains, of anti-a1 antibody.[4] In addition, IdX-a1 was found in rabbits that had been completely suppressed for V_H *a* subgroup expression and then autoimmunized to induce anti-a1 antibody. This latter finding demonstrates that a1 rabbits contain IdX-a1 within their genetic repertoire and that IdX-a1 can be associated with both the major (a^+) and minor (a^-) V_H subgroups as well as with various H and L chain allotypes.

At this point, one must ask why heterogeneous anti-a1 antibodies would share an IdX marker. Two explanations can be offered. 1.) IdX-a1 plays an integral role in regulating allotype expression. The highly conserved gene segment encoding IdX-a1 would most likely be carried within the J or D region, thereby allowing rearrangement with various V_H genes. 2.) Injection of anti-a1, rather than inducing classical anti-idiotype, actually stimulates the production of molecules expressing "a1-like" determinants in the antigen-combining site, that is, internal images of the a1 antigen. Reaction of anti-allotype antibody with internal image epitopes would thus give the appearance of IdX sharing. This concept has been advanced by Jerne *et al.*[6] to explain the sharing of idiotypes by rabbit anti-b6 antibodies.

In order to distinguish between these two possibilities, anti-a1 antibody was isolated from a goat and tested for the ability to inhibit rabbit IdX-a1 binding to anti-idiotype. As seen in FIGURE 2, goat anti-a1 inhibits binding nearly as well as

[a]This work was supported by Grant IN-99H from the American Cancer Society and by ALSAC.

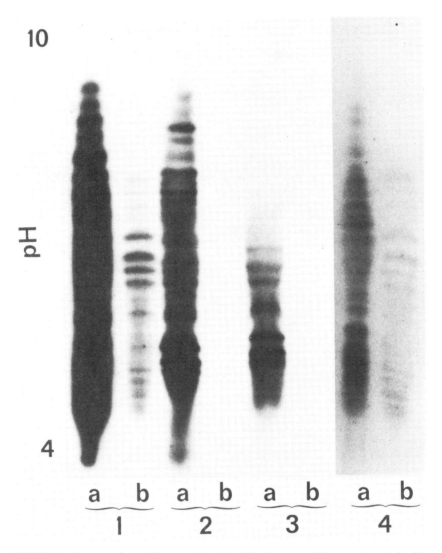

FIGURE 1. Reaction of anti-idiotype with rabbit (#1–3) or goat (#4) anti-a1 antibody. The anti-allotype preparations were incubated with a two-fold excess of normal rabbit Ig (a) or anti-idiotype (b) before focusing. The gels were overlaid with ^{125}I-labeled a1 Fab.

rabbit antibody and therefore must express an idiotype very similar to IdX-a1. In addition, anti-idiotype absorption of IEF bands showed that the bulk of goat anti-a1 bears IdX-a1-like determinants (antibody 4, in FIGURE 1). This finding would tend to rule out a regulatory role for IdX-a1 (because goats have no obvious need to control rabbit allotype expression) and support the idea that our anti-IdX-a1 reagent is indeed an internal image of a1 allotype. Nevertheless, it is clear that the internal image within

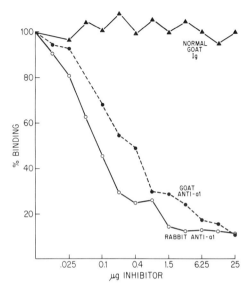

FIGURE 2. Ability of goat (●--●) or rabbit (○——○) anti-al antibody to inhibit binding of ^{125}I-labeled rabbit anti-al to anti-idiotype-coated wells. (▲——▲)-normal goat Ig.

TABLE 1. Lack of Cross-Reactive Idiotype Expression by Anti-b4 Antibodies

Inhibitor[a]	Percent Binding of ^{125}I-Labeled Immunogen Anti-b4 to Anti-Idiotype No.		
	161	191	193
None	100	100	100
Anti-b4 (Immunogen)	11	3	4
Anti-b9 (Control)	92	113	101
Anti-b4			
Rabbit No. 1	88	71	76
Rabbit No. 2	76	68	68
Rabbit No. 3	96	74	77
Rabbit No. 4	90	83	76
Rabbit No. 5	100	76	81
Rabbit No. 6	93	110	85
Rabbit No. 7	97	104	96
Rabbit No. 8	93	118	97
Rabbit No. 9	85	89	85
Rabbit No. 10	86	99	92
Rabbit No. 11	78	94	78

[a]Inhibitors were added at a 1:2 dilution. Anti-b4 numbers 1–7 were derived from a1/b5 rabbits, numbers 8–9 from a1/b9 rabbits, number 10 from an a2/b9 rabbit, and number 11 from an a2/b6 rabbit.

anti-IdX-a1 does not contain the entire set of a1 epitopes, because nonreactive antibody can easily be visualized using the IEF absorption technique.

Our studies have also indicated the presence of IdX markers on anti-a2 and anti-a3 antibodies, in agreement with the findings of others.[3,5] However, we have thus far been unable to detect shared idiotypes on antibodies directed to b4 or b5 κ light-chain allotypes. As shown in TABLE 1, eleven anti-b4 antisera obtained from unrelated rabbits of various H and L chain allotypic phenotypes failed to inhibit the binding of immunogen anti-b4 to its anti-idiotypes. These results again are consistent with reports of others[5] that anti-b locus antibodies do not express IdX markers, yet conflict with the findings of Roland and Cazenave[1,2] who demonstrated shared idiotypes on anti-b4 and anti-b6 antibodies, respectively. The reasons for these discrepant results are unknown, but could be related to the use in the latter study of only rabbits of selected genotypes. For example, anti-b6 prepared in b5 rabbits would show greater epitope restriction and, therefore, idiotype restriction, than antibody obtained from b4 or b6 animals. This possibility is currently under investigation in our laboratory.

In summary, we have found that IdX-a1 is present not only on most anti-a1 antibody in every rabbit, but also on goat antibody. We have failed, however, to detect IdX markers on anti-b locus antibodies. Future studies will allow a better understanding of the molecular basis for shared idiotypes on anti-allotype antibodies and the conditions needed for demonstrating this sharing.

REFERENCES

1. ROLAND J. & P.-A. CAZENAVE. 1979. Mise en évidence d'idiotypes anti-b4 apparentés chez les lapins de phénotype a3+ immunisés contre l'allotype b4. C.R. Acad. Sci. **288:** 571–574.
2. ROLAND, J. & P.-A. CAZENAVE. 1981. Rabbits immunized against b6 allotype express similar anti-b6 idiotopes. Eur. J. Immunol. **11:** 469–474.
3. GILMAN-SACHS, A., S. DRAY & W. J. HORNG. 1980. A *common* idiotypic specificity of rabbit antibodies to the a2 allotype of the immunoglobulin heavy chain variable region. J. Immunol. **125:** 96–101.
4. METZGER, D. W. & K. H. ROUX. 1982. A predominant idiotype on rabbit anti-V_H a1 allotype antibodies: sharing by both major and minor V_H subgroups. J. Immunol. **129:** 1138–1142.
5. GILMAN-SACHS, A., S. DRAY & W. J. HORNG. 1982. Idiotypic specificities of rabbit antibodies to immunoglobulin allotypes. J. Immunol. **129:** 1194–1199.
6. JERNE, N. K., J. ROLAND & P.-A. CAZENAVE. 1982. Recurrent idiotypes and internal images. Eur. Mol. Biol. Org. J. **1:** 243–248.
7. BONA, C., P. K. A. MONGINI, K. E. STEIN & W. E. PAUL. 1980. Anti-immunoglobulin antibodies. I. Expression of crossreactive idiotypes and *Ir* gene control of the response to IgG2a of the b allotype. J. Exp. Med. **151:** 1334–1348.
8. FEIZI, T., H. G. KUNKEL & D. ROELCKE. 1974. Cross idiotypic specificity among cold agglutinins in relation to combining activity for blood group-related antigens. Clin. Exp. Immunol. **18:** 283–293.
9. FØRRE, Ø, J. B. NATVIG & T. E. MICHAELSEN. 1977. Cross-idiotypic reactions among anti-Rh(D) antibodies. Scand. J. Immunol. **6:** 997–1003.
10. METZGER, D. W., A. FURMAN, A. MILLER & E. E. SERCARZ. 1981. Idiotypic repertoire of anti-hen eggwhite lysozyme antibodies probed with hybridomas. Selection after immunization of an IdX marker common to antibodies of distinct epitope specificity. J. Exp. Med. **154:** 701–712.

Bi-Directional Immune Responses within an Idiotype Network[a]

WAYNE J. HORNG[b] AND DORI S. KAZDIN[c]

Department of Pathology and Laboratory Medicine
The University of Texas Health Science Center at Houston
Houston, Texas 77025

Recently, common or cross-reacting idiotypic specificities among rabbit anti-allotype antibodies to a $V_H a$ or κb locus allotype have been found and described.[1-4] In our laboratory, we identified a common idiotypic specificity (IdC) among rabbit anti-a2 antibodies.[2] The anti-IdC antibody (Ab) not only reacted with its immunogen anti-a2 Ab, but also reacted with all of the allo- and auto-anti-a2 antibodies tested.[2,3] When an $a^1 a^1$ homozygous rabbit was immunized with an anti-IdC Ab (bearing the a1 allotype) population, two distinct Ab populations were induced.[5] One of these Ab populations is the anti-a2 Ab that reacts with a2 immunoglobulin (Ig) and inhibits the reaction between the a2 allotype and anti-a2 Ab (FIGURE 1). The other Ab population is anti-anti-IdC Ab, which is specific for the immunogen anti-IdC antibody. In another experiment, when an $a^1 a^2$ heterozygous rabbit was immunized with the anti-IdC Ab, only anti-anti-IdC Ab was induced (FIGURE 1), which appears to be identical to the anti-anti-IdC Ab induced in the $a^1 a^1$ rabbit. When the expression of the a2 allotype in an $a^1 a^2$ heterozygous rabbit, however, was suppressed neonatally and then immunized with the anti-IdC Ab, both anti-a2 Ab and anti-anti-IdC Ab were induced.[5] We concluded from these observations that a bi-directional immune response occurred within this immune network. According to Jerne's network theory,[6] the anti-anti-IdC Ab appears to be induced through a stimulation by the idiotope of the immunogen anti-IdC Ab, whereas the anti-a2 Ab appears to be induced through a reverse stimulation by the paratope of the immunogen anti-IdC antibody.

Because this bi-directional immune response mechanism affects the reverse induction of an idiotype population through anti-idiotype immunization, one must be certain that the immunogen anti-idiotype contains molecules, such as the antigen, that could themselves induce this idiotype population. Accordingly, the specificity of the anti-IdC Ab, used as immunogen in our experiments, was carefully considered. This immunogen anti-IdC Ab was isolated from sera of an $a^1 a^1 x^{32} x^{32} y^{33} y^{33}$ homozygous rabbit (S246-4). Thus, the majority, if not all, of these anti-IdC Ab molecules should have either the a1, x32, or y33 V_H-region allotypic markers. We could account for only a total of 57% of these molecules, however, having the a1, x32, or y33 allotypic specificity, whereas 80% of these molecules reacted with anti-a2 antibody.[2] Thus, we could not determine the Ig V_H-region allotypic marker for 23% of the immunogen anti-IdC Ab population. It is possible that this 23% of immunogen anti-IdC Ab has an Ig V_H-region allotypic specificity that has yet to be identified. It is also possible, however, that the immunogen anti-IdC Ab not only contains an anti-idiotype Ab

[a]This work was supported in part by research grants PHS AI-15228 and PHS AI-07043 from the National Institutes of Health.

[b]Present address: Abbott Laboratories, 14th and Sheridan Rd. N. Chicago, Ill. 60064.
[c]In partial fulfillment of the Doctor of Philosophy degree in the Graduate College of the University of Illinois at Chicago Health Science Center, Chicago, Illinois 60612.

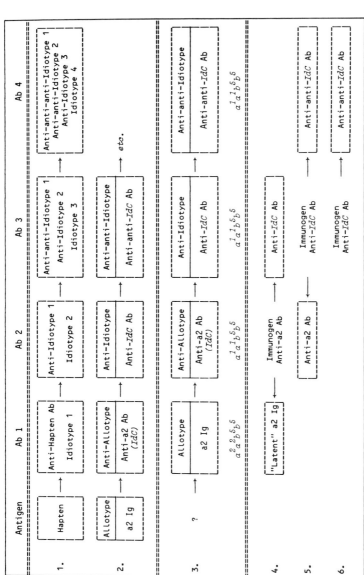

FIGURE 1. The relationship of each antibody involved in an immune network. The arrows indicate the direction of stimulation. Line 1: the nonallotypic idiotypic network system; line 2: the allotypic idiotype network system that is generally understood; line 3: the position of an allotype in the allotypic idiotype system should be considered; line 4: the result of a bi-directional immune response in rabbit S246-4 when immunized with anti-a2 Ab; line 5: the result of a bi-directional immune response in rabbit T117-4 (an a^1a^1 homozygote) and rabbit S218-4 (an a2-suppressed a^1a^2 heterozygote); line 6: the result of immunizing an a^1a^2 heterozygous rabbit (S8-5) with anti-IdC Ab; the absence of a reverse immune response was probably due to the presence of a2 . . .

population (i.e., the "true" anti-IdC Ab), but also contains a population of molecules having a "latent" a2 allotypic specificity. In this instance, the bi-directional immune response would have also occurred when the anti-IdC was induced (FIGURE 1). To examine this possibility, the following experiments using an H-L chain recombination were performed.

Through an anti-a1-Ab-containing immunosorbent column, we separated an anti-IdC Ab population (from an $a^1a^1b^5b^5$ homozygous rabbit) into two populations, the a1 anti-IdC Ab and the non-a1 anti-IdC antibody. When the H-chains of these a1 and non-a1 anti-IdC antibodies were recombined with the L-chains of non-anti-IdC Ig molecules (from a virgin $a^3a^3b^4b^4$ homozygous rabbit), 43% of the recombined Ig molecules having the H-chain of the a1 anti-IdC Ab reacted with anti-a2 Ab, whereas 69% of the recombined Ig molecules having the H-chain of the non-a1 anti-IdC Ab reacted with anti-a2 antibody. This result suggests that approximately 26% of the non-a1 anti-IdC Ab molecules may be bearing the "latent" a2 allotypic specificity. Thus, we suggest that the bi-directional immune response has also occurred when the rabbit (S246-4) was immunized with anti-a2 Ab to induce anti-IdC antibody. This 26% of the non-a1 anti-IdC Ab molecules, however, represents approximately 6% (23% × 26%) of total immunogen anti-IdC Ab population (used to immunize rabbits that produce both anti-a2 Ab and anti-anti-IdC Ab). Although it is possible that these "latent" a2 Ig molecules induce the production of anti-a2 Ab, it is unlikely that, in rabbits immunized with anti-IdC Ab, the production of anti-a2 Ab is solely due to the presence of these "latent" a2 Ig molecules. Because the production of anti-a2 Ab represents a predominant immune response (80%) in rabbits immunized with anti-IdC Ab, we suggest that it is resulted from both the stimulation by "latent" a2 allotype and the reverse stimulation by the anti-IdC antibody. In other words, the bi-directional immune responses have occurred at each step of the immunization cascade employing idiotype and anti-idiotype. These bi-directional immune response phenomena may also represent the function of an idiotype network.

In 1977, Cazenave,[7] using anti-ribonuclease as the idiotype (Ab 1), and Urbain *et al.*,[8] using anti-*Micrococcus lysodeikticus* as the idiotype (Ab 1), induced anti-idiotype Ab (Ab 2) and anti-anti-idiotype Ab (Ab 3) through a series of immunization of outbred but allotype-matched rabbits. Although Ab 3 did not react with the antigen (as did the Ab 1), it was found to modulate the expression of Ab 1.[7,8] Wikler *et al.*[9] carried these experiments further by inducing anti-anti-anti-idiotype Ab (Ab 4) in both the anti-*Micrococcus lysodeikticus* and anti-tobacco mosaic virus idiotype systems. These Ab 4 reacted with their respective Ab 3 as well as their respective Ab 1. They concluded that Ab 1 and Ab 3 share a cross-reacting idiotypic specificity and that Ab 2 and Ab 4 are also similar idiotypically. Recently, a similar finding was reported by Bona *et al.*[10] with their A48 (i.e., ABPC48, a BALB/c levan-binding myeloma protein) idiotype system; again, the Ab 4 was found to react with the Ab 1. Paul and Bona[11] suggested that this phenomenon is due to the presence of a regulatory idiotope (in addition to nonregulatory idiotopes) on the Ab 1 molecules.

More recently, similar to our observations in the a2 allotype system, Jerne *et al.*[12] immunized a rabbit with antibodies (Ab2β) to a public idiotypic specificity of anti-κb6-allotype antibodies, which resulted in the induction of an Ab 3 population (Ab3α) that reacted wtih both Ab 2 and the b6 allotype (the antigen). They observed that, whereas this Ab 3 reacted with the b6 allotype, it could not precipitate the b6 allotype as strongly as normal anti-b6 antibody. In addition, this Ab 3 could not induce b6-allotype suppression and did not cross-react with the b95 allotype as did the normal anti-b6 antibody. Thus, it appears that, whereas this Ab 3 was similar to Ab 1, it was not identical to Ab 1. Based on these observations, these authors concluded that their Ab2β was an "internal image" of the b6 allotype and, thereby, could induce an Ab 3 population that reacted with both Ab 2 and the antigen (the b6 allotype). Our findings, however, of "latent" allotype in the Ab 2 population argue against the occurrence of an "internal image" in our system. In our opinion, the "latent" a2 allotype was induced through a reverse stimulation by the paratope of the immunogen anti-a2 Ab, in addition to the idiotope-induced anti-IdC antibody. With the following considerations, this bi-directional immune response phenomenon can be interpreted within the content of the idiotype network theory proposed by Jerne.[6]

Our observations and the observations of Jerne et al.[12] in an allotypic idiotype network system are strikingly similar to the observations of Urbain and his associates,[9] and of Paul and Bona[10,11] in the nonallotypic idiotype network systems. In an allotypic system, Ab 3 reacted with the antigen (the allotype), whereas, in a nonallotypic system, Ab 4 reacted with the Ab 1 (the idiotype). Because both the antigens (the a2 and b6 allotypes) used in the allotypic systems are the Ig molecules, their antigenic specificities (epitopes) can be found on the lymphocyte surface. Therefore, both a2 and b6 allotypic markers may have been involved in cell-cell interactions and the regulation of immune responses. In other words, like idiotypes, allotypes can be considered as integral parts of an immune network. In a functional immune network, one should consider the allotype as Ab 1, anti-allotype as Ab 2, and anti-idiotype to an anti-allotype (e.g., anti-IdC Ab) as Ab 3. Thus, the observations among the allotypic and nonallotypic idiotype network systems would be essentially identical, and the bi-directional immune responses may represent a general phenomenon occurring in immune networks. As illustrated in the lower portion of FIGURE 2, the major immune regulatory pathway is and remains to be as follows: the foreign stimulus stimulates the synthesis of Ab 1 (p_1, i_1) through the interaction of its epitope (e) with the p_1, the idiotope (i_1) of Ab 1 stimulates the synthesis of Ab 2 (p_2, i_2) through the i_1-p_2 interaction, and the idiotope (i_2) of Ab 2 stimulates the synthesis of Ab 3 (p_3, i_3) through the interaction of i_2 and p_3, etcetera. Concomitantly at each step, however, the paratope (e.g., p_n) of each stimulating molecule can also stimulate the synthesis of molecules bearing the complementary idiotope (i.e., i_{n-1}) in a reverse direction. For example, when Ab 2 (i.e., anti-allotype in an allotypic system and anti-idiotype in a nonallotypic system) is used as the immunogen, i_2 stimulates the lymphocytes bearing the complementary p_3 to synthesize the Ab 3 (p_3, i_3) molecules. At the same time, p_2 stimulates the lymphocytes bearing its complementary i_1 to synthesize the Ab 1 (p_1, i_1) in a direct reverse direction and/or the "latent" Ab 1 (p_x, i_1) molecules (i.e., the unspecific parallel set as suggested by Jerne) in an alternate reverse direction. In a random interaction of p_2 with lymphocytes bearing the complementary i_1, the lymphocytic clones synthesizing the "latent" (or the unspecific parallel set) Ab 1 become the predominant responding lymphocytes that are stimulated. This indicates that the number of lymphocytes bearing the "latent" Ab 1 (p_x, i_1) must be larger than the number of lymphocytes bearing the Ab 1 (p_1, i_1). Thus, the "latent" Ab 1, concomitantly induced with Ab 3 by Ab 2, does not react with the epitope (of the antigen), although it bears a similar or identical idiotope (i_1). Similarly, when Ab 3 is used as the immunogen, i_3 stimulates the synthesis of Ab 4 (p_4, i_4) molecules and, concomitantly, p_3 stimulates the synthesis of i_2-bearing molecules, that is, the Ab 2 (p_2, i_2) molecules are stimulated in a direct reverse direction and the "latent" Ab 2 (p_y, i_2) molecules are stimulated in an alternate reverse direction. Due to the presence of the latent" Ab 1 population in the Ab 3 immunogen, however, the direct reverse stimulation of the Ab 2-bearing clone increases significantly; this may be due to the modulating or priming effect of the i_1-p_2 interaction (or, conversely, of the p_3-i_2 interaction) on the stimulation of i_2 by p_3 (or p_2 by i_1). Therefore, the Ab 4 populations, consisting of Ab 4 (p_4, i_4), Ab 2 (p_2, i_2), and possibly the "latent" Ab 2 (p_y, i_2) molecules, were found to react with the Ab 1.[5,9,10,12] This same line of reasoning can be

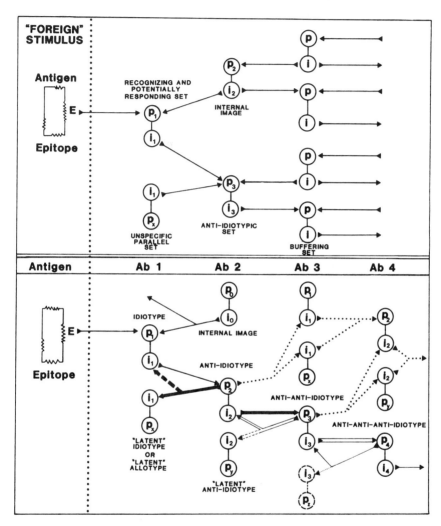

FIGURE 2. The upper portion of this figure represents the original network concept proposed by Jerne in 1974. (N.K. Jerne.[6] With permission from *Annales d'Immunologie de L'Institut Pasteur (Paris)*.) The lower portion of this figure represents the incorporation of the bi-directional immune response into Jerne's network theory. See text for detailed explanations. The arrows indicate the direction of stimulation. The two heavy arrows show the bi-directional stimulation when Ab 2 is the immunogen, and the double-lined arrows indicate the bi-directional stimulation when Ab 3 is the immunogen.

continued with the Ab 4, Ab 5, etcetera, as immunogen. In each successive step, however, the direct reverse stimulation would gradually become more significant due to the increased number of idiotope-bearing "latent" and native molecules in the immunogen. For example, when Ab 4 is used as the immunogen, because the presence of a large number of Ab 2 (p_2, i_2) and possibly of "latent" Ab 2 (p_y, i_2) molecules, the major immune response would, predictably, be the Ab 3 (p_3, i_3) molecules. Furthermore, the idiotope of a given responding Ab set (e.g., the i_1 of Ab 1 population) is relatively heterogeneous as compared to its paratope (p_1), because the paratope is a complementary site for an epitope that is generally rather restricted in heterogeneity. Therefore, the stimulation of an Ab (e.g., Ab 4) by an idiotope (i_3) would become less significant than the reverse stimulation of the idiotope (i_2) by its paratope (p_3). This may also account for the reason that the majority of immune responses (80%) in our rabbits immunized with anti-IdC Ab (an Ab 3 in allotypic network) were anti-a2 Ab (Ab 2) rather than the anti-anti-IdC Ab (Ab 4).

Similar consideration may also apply to the immunization of an animal with Ab 1 (p_1, i_1); i_1 stimulates the synthesis of Ab 2 (p_2, i_2) through the i_1-p_2 interaction and, at the same time, p_1 stimulates the synthesis of a "latent" Ig population (p_0, i_0) that has the "internal image" (i_0) of the epitope. Unfortunately, judging from the data obtained by Urbain and associates[9] and by Bona et al.,[10] the presence of an "internal image" in the Ab 2 population appears to be insignificant, because the immunization of animal 3 with Ab 2 did not induce the production of a detectable amount of Ab 1 (p_1, i_1). In order to demonstrate the presence of an "internal image," we suggest that the interaction of i_1-p_2 must be inhibited, which will in turn allow the i_0-bearing clones to be stimulated by the p_1. Furthermore, when the molecules bearing the "internal image" of an epitope are used as immunogen, the major response to the stimulation by the i_0 may be the parallel set of molecules (p_1, i_x) rather than the Ab 1 molecules (p_1, i_1) for the same reason discussed earlier. Therefore, the responding set of molecules, resulting from the immunization with the molecules having the "internal image" of an epitope, will react with the epitope, but will probably not react with the Ab 2 (p_2, i_2). Also, in order not to confuse between the "latent" (or unspecific parallel set) population and the "internal image," the system chosen to demonstrate the "internal image" should have a nonlymphocyte surface market as the epitope.

ACKNOWLEDGMENTS

We would like to thank Dr. Sheldon Dray, Dr. Katherine L. Knight, Dr. Constantin A. Bona, and Dr. L. Scott Rodkey as well as Ms. Alice Gilman-Sachs for their valuable suggestions and criticisms during the development of this bi-directional immune network concept.

REFERENCES

1. ROLAND, J. & P.-A. CAZENAVE. 1979. Mise en evidence d'idiotypes anti-b4 apparentes cex les lapins de phenotype a3$^+$ immunises centre l'allotype b4. C. R. Acad. Sci. **288:** 571.
2. GILMAN-SACHS, A., S. DRAY & W. J. HORNG. 1980. A common idiotypic specificity of rabbit antibodies to the a2 allotype of the immunoglobulin heavy chain variable region. J. Immunol. **125:** 96.
3. GILMAN-SACHS, A., S. DRAY & W. J. HORNG. 1982. Idiotypic specificities of rabbit antibodies to immunoglobulin allotypes. J. Immunol. **129:** 1194.

4. METZGER, D. W. & K. H. ROUX. 1982. A predominant idiotype on rabbit anti-VHa1 allotype antibodies: sharing by both major and minor VH subgroups. J. Immunol. **129:** 1138.

5. KAZDIN, D. S. & W. J. HORNG. 1983. A bi-directional immune network mechanism: Simultaneous induction of idiotype and anti-anti-idiotype in rabbit immunized with antibody to a common idiotypic specificity of anti-VHa2-allotype antibodies. Mol. Immunol. **20:** 819.

6. JERNE, N. K. 1974. Towards a network theory of the immune system. Ann. Immunol. Inst. Pasteur (Paris) **125C:** 373.

7. CAZENAVE, P.-A. 1977. Idiotype-anti-idiotype regulation of antibody synthesis in rabbits. Proc. Natl. Acad. Sci. USA **74:** 5122.

8. URBAIN, J., M. WIKLER, J.-D. FRANSSEN & C. COLLIGNON. 1977. Idiotypic regulation of the immune system by the induction of antibodies against anti-idiotype antibodies. Proc. Natl. Acad. Sci. USA **74:**5126.

9. WIKLER, M., J.-D. FRANSSEN, O. LEO, B. MARIME, P. VAN DE WALLE, D. DEGROOTE & J. URBAIN. 1979. Idiotypic regulation of the immune system. Common idiotypic specificities between idiotypes and antibodies raised against anti-idiotypic antibodies in rabbits. J. Exp. Med. **150:** 184.

10. BONA, C., E. HEBER-KATZ & W. E. PAUL. 1981. Idiotype-anti-idiotype regulation. I. Immunization with a levan-binding myeloma protein leads to the appearance of auto-anti-(anti-idiotype) antibody and to the activation of silent clones. J. Exp. Med. **153:** 951.

11. PAUL, W. E. & C. BONA. 1982. Regulatory idiotopes and immune networks: a hypothesis. Immunology Today **3:** 230.

12. JERNE, N. K., J. ROLAND & P.-A. CAZENAVE. 1982. Recurrent idiotypes and internal image. Eur. Mol. Biol. Org. J. **1:** 243.

Anti-Immunoglobulins and Their Idiotypes: Are They Part of the Immune Network?

HENRY G. KUNKEL,[a] DAVID N. POSNETT,[a] AND
BENVENUTO PERNIS[b]

[a]The Rockefeller University
New York, New York 10021
and
[b]Department of Microbiology
College of Physicians and Surgeons
Comprehensive Cancer Center
Columbia University
New York, New York 10032

The human anti-immunoglobulins, (Ig), frequently termed rheumatoid factors, represent a very diverse group of antibodies that also might be considered part of the immune network. Most of these are directed against the Fc portion of IgG, but others react with the Fab fragment, apparently against antigens in the C1 area that are revealed by enzymatic splitting.[1] The latter have presented special problems when Fab fragments are used for the isolation of anti-idiotypic antibodies. Anti-light chain antibodies also occur in rheumatoid arthritis as well as other sera that may react with the Fab fragments.[2] Anti-γ globulins directed against the C regions of IgD and IgE also have been described.[3]

Special attention has been directed to the IgM anti-γ globulins because of their dominant reaction in various agglutination systems used for assay. The IgG and IgA anti-γ globulins, however, are widely prevalent. Most of the anti-γ globulins show isotype specificity. In the human they are primarily directed to IgG_1, IgG_2, and IgG_4 and show little reaction with IgG_3.[4] A wide assortment of isotype specificities have been observed recently in the mouse.[5] Both in the human and in the mouse an increase in anti-γ globulins is observed after polyclonal activation of lymphocytes in vitro; this is especially striking with lipopolysaccharide stimulation of mouse spleen cells.[6] As much as half of the indirect plaque forming cells that develop with lipopolysaccharide have anti-γ globulin activity.[7] They clearly represent the most widely occurring autoantibodies and are present at low levels in all normal sera.[8] They reach very high levels in many pathological states and can circulate in the blood despite the presence of the antigen, IgG, primarily because of their low binding affinity for monomeric IgG. The 22S complex of IgM anti-γ globulin and IgG apparent by analytical ultracentrifuge analysis is readily dissociable, does not fix complement, and therefore remains in the circulation. The IgG anti-γ globulins are of special interest because of their self-associating character.[9]

In the past, primary attention has been directed to the possible pathological role of the anti-γ globulins, primarily because of their special occurrence in rheumatoid arthritis sera. The possibility, however, that they play an immunoregulatory role requires consideration. Naturally occurring anti-idiotypes may be present that are directed against these anti-γ globulins, and thus they would clearly be part of a network. Such natural anti-idiotypes have not thus far been described. They should be looked for carefully. Possibly some of these might behave like anti-receptor antibodies and be directed toward the Fc receptors that are widely present on lymphocytes and

324

certain other cells. This might be another mechanism by which the anti-γ globulins could play a regulatory role. Still a further potential relationship concerns the possibility that anti-γ globulin binding activity is a secondary property of a number of different antibodies.

GENERAL PROPERTIES OF MONOCLONAL IgM ANTI-γ GLOBULINS

These proteins probably represent the most common types of monoclonal protein with combining activity found in human sera. They bind IgG through the Fc portion and frequently precipitate as cryoglobulins in the form of immune complexes. Many of the patients with these proteins develop severe kidney disease, and these immune complexes can be identified in the glomerular deposits with anti-idiotypic sera.[10] These IgM proteins almost invariably possess κ light chains, and these very commonly are of the VKIIIb type.[11] Anti-idiotypic sera are readily produced in rabbits to these proteins, and these invariably show specificity for private idiotypes. In addition, however, a number of cross-idiotypic specificities have been demonstrated.[12] The most striking is the Wa specificity that separates approximately 65% of the IgM anti-γ globulins from the others. Very few IgM proteins without anti-IgG activity were positive in this initial study.[12] In addition, there is a Po group that has a striking cross-reactive idiotype (CRI), totally different from the Wa group. Sequence analyses of two of the latter group proteins have shown great similarity in the heavy chains.[13] The sequence studies on the major Wa group are not as complete, but two typical Wa group proteins differ strikingly in heavy chain sequence from the two proteins of the Po group.[14] Several additional CRI reactions also have been observed among the anti-γ globulins that do not relate to the two types described above.

OCCURRENCE OF THE Wa CROSS-REACTIVE IDIOTYPE IN RHEUMATOID ARTHRITIS PATIENTS

Evidence was obtained by Natvig and associates[15] that certain of the monoclonal IgM anti-γ globulins related in cross-idiotypic specificities to the IgM and IgG anti-γ globulins formed in rheumatoid arthritis (RA) sera. More recently the Wa CRI has been shown to be widely prevalent in rheumatoid arthritis.[16] This was most strikingly demonstrated in studies of the plasma cells from these patients formed in response to stimulation with pokeweed mitogen. TABLE 1 shows such results with one rabbit antiserum that was made specific for the Wa CRI. Careful absorption with large amounts of polyclonal IgM deprived of anti-IgM activity was required in these cellular studies. The lymphocytes of RA patients gave approximately 10% plasma cells after mitogen stimulation, which was not significantly different from normal lymphocytes. The percentage, however, of plasma cells showing the CRI was markedly increased for the RA cells; up to 20% of the plasma cells showed fluorescence with the specific antiserum as compared to levels below 3% in the controls. Double labeling experiments indicated that all the cells showing the CRI were IgM-forming cells. In some cases as much as 50% of the IgM-plasma cells expressed the cross-reactive idiotype.

The studies at the cellular level using the CRI antisera provided quantitative data on the expression of the CRI in plasma cells. It was evident that the Wa CRI was widely present among polyclonal anti-Ig in rheumatoid arthritis. In fact, the anti-CRI proved to be a valuable reagent for the detection of anti-γ globulins; the direct cellular

TABLE 1. Cytoplasmic Immunoglobulins and Cross-Reactive Idiotype Detected in Rheumatoid Arthritis and Control Cells after a Six-Day Culture of PBL with Pokeweed Mitogen

RA	Percentage Plasma Cells of All Cells	Percentage RCRI Cells of All Plasma Cells
E.F.	8.0 (5.4–10.4)	11.2 (7.7–13.9)
M.S.	5.5 (5.0–5.9)	12.0 (11.3–13.3)
E.C.	12.0 (10.0–14.0)	13.9 (13.8–14.0)
M.J.	8.3 (7.0–9.6)	10.8 (9.4–12.2)
J.J.	10.4 (8.6–12.2)	18.0 (16.0–20.0)
H.L.	12.0	17.1
B.B.	10.6	7.9
Normal		
N.A.	13.3 (9.7–18.7)	1.5 (0.0–3.0)
V.B.	11.1 (6.8–14.4)	2.8 (2.1–3.5)
D.E.	18.0 (17.0–19.0)	1.9 (1.6–2.2)
L.K.	11.3 (8.5–14.0)	2.0 (1.8–2.2)
P.R.	9.0 (8.5–9.5)	2.5 (2.0–3.0)

demonstration of anti-γ globulin activity is very difficult primarily because of the low affinity of the IgG-IgM reaction.

MONOCLONAL ANTI-IDIOTYPIC ANTIBODIES WITH CROSS-REACTIVE IDIOTYPE SIMILAR TO THE Wa CROSS-REACTIVE IDIOTYPE

Monoclonal antibodies were made against a number of the IgM anti-γ globulins, and cloned lines were obtained that showed varying specificities for anti-γ globulins. FIGURE 1 illustrates the results obtained with three of these hybridoma antibodies.

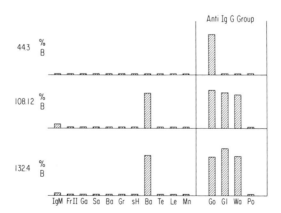

FIGURE 1. Radioimmune assay showing the binding of three monoclonal antibodies with anti-γ globulins on the right side of the figure. Control monoclonal IgM proteins were all negative except for protein Ba. The anti-γ globulin protein Po that did not belong in the Wa CRI group is negative. The bars show the percent binding as compared to the binding of a monoclonal anti-IgM protein. Polyclonal IgM is represented by the bars at the extreme left side.

Clone P44.3 showed only private idiotype reactivity. P108.12 and P132.4 showed specificity for the anti-γ globulins, however, reacting with three of the four anti-γ globulins. The one that did not react belonged to the Po group; the three Wa proteins reacted strongly. There was, however, one protein, Ba, that lacked anti-Ig activity but still reacted with both monoclonal antibodies. In addition, there was slight but definite reactivity with the polyclonal IgM. Additional Wa CRI proteins were positive and most other control proteins were negative. Thus similarity in reactivity of the monoclonal hybridoma antibodies and the rabbit antisera to the Wa CRI group was evident, although the specificity for the anti-γ globulins appeared lower.

Analyses of the plasma cells produced by pokeweed mitogen stimulation also gave results somewhat similar to the rabbit antisera. TABLE 2 shows some of these results. It is apparent that some plasma cells from normals were stained with the monoclonal antibodies in the indirect fluorescent assay, but more were stained in the preparations from RA patients. Again, approximately 50% of the IgM-producing cells reacted as compared to a lower percentage in the controls. Thus, at least two hybridomas have become available that appear to reflect at least some of the CRI previously described with rabbit antisera; certain differences, however, have been noted that remain to be

TABLE 2. Percent Plasma Cells Positive with Two Hybridomas (P14 and P108) after Pokeweed Mitogen Stimulation of Cells from Four Rheumatoid Arthritis Patients and Five Normal Patients

	P.G.[a]	R A				Normal				
		J	DC	EF	LO	N_1	N_2	N_3	N_4	N_5
P14	42	18	16	21	18	0	5	4	12	0
P108	20	18	10	20	16	2	0	1	10	2

[a]P.G. is the patient with the monoclonal protein used for immunization.

clarified. The details of these studies will be published separately by Posnett and associates.[17]

QUESTIONS CONCERNING THE ANTI-γ GLOBULINS AND THEIR CROSS-REACTIVE IDIOTYPE

There remain a number of special questions concerning the anti-γ globulins that require consideration. Perhaps foremost of these is the possibility that reactivity for γ globulin is a secondary property of a group of different antibodies, possibly of naturally developing anti-idiotypic antibodies. This would go along with their characteristic of low binding affinity. Such a hypothesis also might explain the large number of such anti-γ globulin reactive molecules that appear after polyclonal activation of mouse spleen cells with lipopolysaccharide. It might also fit in well with a role in a network system. Low binding affinity for other γ globulin molecules might be an advantageous property of specific antibodies and also aid their polymerization around a foreign antigen.

Considerable work has been carried out on the sequence of different anti-γ globulins particularly by Capra and associates.[13,14] The minor Po group defined by one type of CRI showed a remarkable similarity in the complementary determining residues of the heavy chains. These might be considered truly related antibodies. The major Wa group, however, proved much less definable by sequence analysis.[14] The two proteins analyzed showed marked similarity in the light chains, but this was not greatly different from random proteins of the VKIIIb type. It had previously been shown that all of the Wa proteins had L chains of the VKIIIb type and that this appeared to be their common feature;[11] their heavy chains appeared very different antigenically. The heavy chain sequences also proved to be very different except for the J segment, where similarities were discernible. There are clearly IgM as well as other proteins that have VKIIIb light chains, but that lack anti-γ globulin binding properties. It is possible that VKIIIb light chains, together with the appropriate J segment of the heavy chain, convey anti-γ globulin reactivity to these molecules without involvement of the primary complementary determining residues of the heavy chains.

Also in the Wa CRI system, it is clear that the VKIIIb light chains are involved in the CRI antigen or antigens. In both the rabbit antisera, however, and in the monoclonal hybridoma antibodies, some additional specificities appeared to be influential. Absorption with VKIIIb light chains does not take out the reactivity. A number of the specific antisera and monoclonal antibodies also reacted only with IgM proteins. This was manifest in a variety of ways. Pooled polyclonal IgM removed the reactions when added in large amounts, whereas pooled IgG had no effect. In the fluorescent antibody work with plasma cells, only cells with IgM were stained; IgG-bearing cells were entirely negative. IgG anti-γ globulins also were never reactive with these antibodies. It would appear that the Wa CRI antigenic site as detected with certain of the monoclonal antibodies involved the VKIIIb light chains plus a part of the C region of IgM and perhaps a specific J segment of the heavy chains. These interpretations may explain the difficulty in a previous study of relating the Wa CRI to specificity for IgG from different species.[12]

Further work with additional monoclonals is required. Absorbed rabbit antisera present special problems in this system. Solid absorptions are essential because of the strong reactivity of the anti-γ globulin with immune complexes. Even with solid absorptions, however, some antigen frequently comes off the column to form complexes; the individual anti-γ globulins then react differently with these complexes. These reactions have lead to false interpretations in some past studies. Even with the monoclonal antibodies, spurious results may be obtained because of reactivity of certain anti-γ globulins with mouse IgG. Numerous controls are essential.

SUMMARY

The anti-γ globulins represent a very heterogeneous group of proteins with widely different specificities that might be considered a portion of the immune network. The hypothesis is presented that at least some of these proteins have other specificities, with the anti-γ globulin reactivity being a secondary property. Anti-idiotypic antibodies are possible candidates. This is based on the low binding affinity for γ globulin of many of these proteins and the results of CRI and sequence studies. All the proteins of the major CRI group have VKIIIb light chains, and these have a dominant but not total influence on this CRI. This has been evident from studies with rabbit antibodies and recently also with monoclonal hybridoma antibodies. Sequence studies have also demonstrated the similarity in light chains that, however, are not greater than with other VKIIIb chains; the heavy chains show little similarity except possibly in the J segment. The possibility is discussed that antibodies with secondary anti-γ globulin binding properties might have selective advantages.

REFERENCES

1. OSTERLAND C. K., M. HARBOE & H. G. KUNKEL. 1963. Anti-γ globulin factors in human sera revealed by enzymatic splitting of anti-Rh antibodies. Vox Sang. **8:** 133.
2. WILLIAMS, R. C. 1964. Heterogeneity of L-chain sites on Bence-Jones proteins reacting with anti-γ globulin factors. Proc. Natl Acad. Sci. USA **52:** 60.
3. WILLIAMS, R. C., R. W. GRIFFITHS, J. D. EMMONS & R. C. FIELD. 1972. Naturally occurring human antiglobulins with specificity for γE. J. Clin. Invest. **51:** 955.
4. ALLEN, J. C. & H. C. KUNKEL. 1966. Hidden rheumatoid factor with specificity for native gammaglobulins. Arthritis Rheum. **9:** 758.
5. VAN SNICK, J. L. & P. COULIE. 1982. Monoclonal anti-IgG autoantibodies derived from lipopolysaccharide-activated spleen cells of 129/Sv mice. J. Exp. Med. **155:** 219.
6. DZIARSKI, D. 1982. Preferential induction of autoantibody secretion of polyclonal activation by peptidoglycan and lipopolysaccharide. 1. *In vitro* studies. J. Immunol. **128:** 1018.
7. DRESSER, D. W. 1978. Most IgM-producing cells in the mouse secrete autoantibodies (rheumatoid factor). Nature (London) **274:** 480.
8. MÜLLER-EBERHARD, H. J. & H. G. KUNKEL. 1961. Isolation of a thermolabile serum protein which precipitates γ-globulin aggregates and participates in immune hemolysis. Proc. Soc. Exp. Biol. Med. **106:** 291.
9. POPE, R. M., D. C. TELLER & M. MANNIK. 1974. The molecular basis of self-association of antibodies to IgG (rheumatoid factors) in rheumatoid arthritis. Proc. Natl. Acad. Sci. USA **71:** 517.
10. AGNELLO, V., D. KOFFLER, J. W. EISENBERG, R. J. WINCHESTER & H. G. KUNKEL. 1971. C1q precipitins in the sera of patients with systemic lupus erythematosus and other hypocomplementemic states: characterization of high and low molecular weight types. J. Exp. Med. **134:** 228s.
11. KUNKEL, H. G., R. J. WINCHESTER, F. G. JOSLIN & J. D. CAPRA. 1974. Similarities in the light chains of anti-γ globulins showing cross-idiotypic specificities. J. Exp. Med. **139:** 128.
12. KUNKEL, H. G., V. AGNELLO, F. G. JOSLIN, R. J. WINCHESTER & J. D. CAPRA. 1973. Cross-idiotypic specificity among monoclonal IgM proteins with anti-γ globulin activity. J. Exp. Med. **137:** 331.
13. KLAPPER, D. G. & J. D. CAPRA. 1976. The amino acid sequence of the variable regions of the light chains from two idiotypically cross reactive IgM anti-gamma globulins. Ann. Immunol. Inst. Pasteur (Paris) **127C:** 261.
14. ANDREWS, D. W. & J. D. CAPRA. 1981. Complete amino acid sequence of variable domains from two monoclonal human anti-gamma globulins of the Wa cross-idiotypic group: Suggestion that the J segments are involved in the structural correlate of the idiotype. Proc. Natl. Acad. Sci. USA **78:** 3799.
15. FORRE, O., J. H. DUBLONG, T. E. MICHAELSEN & J. B. NATVIG. 1979. Evidence of similar idiotypic determinants on different rheumatoid factor populations. Scan. J. Immunol. **9:** 281.
16. BONAGURA, V. R., H. G. KUNKEL & B. PERNIS. 1982. Cellular localization of rheumatoid factor idiotypes. J. Clin. Invest. **69:** 1356.
17. POSNETT, D. N., H. G. KUNKEL & B. PERNIS. Manuscript in preparation.

Immune Networks in Immediate Type Allergic Diseases[a]

K. BLASER,[bc] A. WETTERWALD,[b] E. WEBER,[b]
V. E. GERBER,[b] AND A. L. DE WECK[d]

[b]Institute of Clinical Protein Research
[d]Institute of Clinical Immunology
University of Bern
Bern, Switzerland

INTRODUCTION

Idiotypes (Id) are antigenic structures expressed on receptor molecules that are displayed by immunocompetent cells and their secreted products, such as antibodies and regulatory T-cell factors.[1,2] A number of experimental findings suggest that some immune responses are regulated at least in the early stages by a network of complementary Id that recognize each other. It has been demonstrated in several systems that the production of antibodies expressing the respective Id or cross-reactive Id can be suppressed or enhanced by active or passive immunization with anti-idiotypes.

Moreover, Id or anti-idiotypes are expressed on different functional subsets of regulatory T lymphocytes, such as T-helper (T_H) and T-suppressor (T_S) cells.[3-5] Accordingly, Id and anti-idiotypes, together with antigen, provide three specific elements of immunoregulation that bring about functional regulatory circuit(s) by acting through a cellular network.[2-5] These cells express one or the other of these elements. Accordingly, an immune response, being in a highly equilibrated steady state, can be modulated by the interaction of one of the elements of immunoregulation with the regulatory circuit(s).

The genes encoding the heavy chain isotype classes of immunoglobulins (Ig), including C_ϵ, are all located on the same chromosome, together with the V, D, and J genes coding for the variable region.[6] Accordingly, it is possible that the same Id can be expressed on different Ig classes,[7] that is, IgE was found to express similar or identical Id to IgG, IgM, and IgA antibodies.[2,8-10]

An excessive formation of IgE antibodies against an antigen (allergen) leads to allergic reactions of the immediate type upon reexposure to the same antigen. In this report we describe our attempts to regulate the IgE response in mice in an antigen-specific way by external interactions with the regulatory network of complementary Id by way of antigen, Id, or anti-idiotype. These studies are performed in BALB/c mice in two antigenic systems, the IgE response against the phosphorylcholine (PC) hapten and the benzylpenicilloyl (BPO) group. The anti-PC response was chosen because a large fraction of antibodies in mice bear the T15 Id that is represented by the BALB/c myeloma TEPC 15, HOPC-8, and S 107. On the other hand, the BPO group represents

[a]This work was supported by the Swiss National Foundation for Scientific Research, grant number 3.537.074 and in part by the Stanley Thomas Johnson Foundation.
[c]Address correspondence to: K. Blaser, PhD, Institute of Biochemistry, University of Bern, CH-3012 Bern, Switzerland.

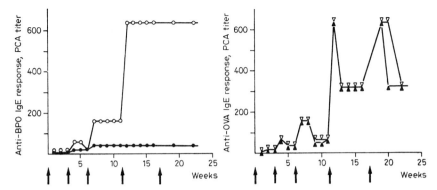

FIGURE 1. Formation of anti-BPO IgE antibodies in BALB/c mice upon immunization with BPO₄-OVA in alum (↑). Mice actively producing anti-BPO anti-idiotype (●) suppressed the formation of anti-BPO IgE antibodies, compared to age-matched control mice (O). Both groups showed the same titers for IgE antibodies against the carrier protein (OVA) (▲, ▽).

one of a few chemically defined haptens that play a role in human allergic diseases. We have shown in these models that an IgE antibody response is regulated by network interactions similar to antibodies of other isotype classes. Attempts were undertaken to suppress specific IgE responses by interactions with the cellular network of idiotypes.

REGULATION OF THE PRIMARY IgE RESPONSE BY ANTI-IDIOTYPES

In order to study the role of Id-anti-idiotype network in the regulation of IgE synthesis at the initial phase of the response, we made attempts to suppress a primary IgE formation by active or passive immunization with anti-idiotype. BALB/c mice that produced anti-idiotype directed against purified anti-BPO antibodies of syngeneic mice (anti-BPO anti-idiotype) upon repeated immunization with antibodies were sensitized several months later with BPO₄-ovalbumin (OVA) in alum. As is shown in

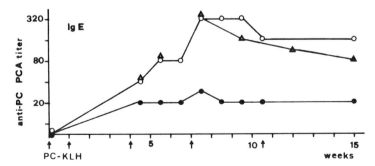

FIGURE 2. Formation of anti-PC IgE antibodies in BALB/c mice upon immunization with PC-KLH in alum (↑). The mice (five per group) that produced anti-T15 anti-idiotype (●) suppressed the formation of anti-PC IgE antibodies compared to a group of control mice (O), and to a group that produced anti-M 167 anti-idiotype (△).

FIGURE 1 mice that produced anti-BPO anti-idiotype selectively suppressed the formation of anti-BPO IgE antibodies for a long period of time. The production of anti-OVA IgE, on the other hand, was not impaired. The production of anti-BPO IgG[10] was also suppressed, but to a lesser extent.

We made similar observations in BALB/c mice that produced isologous anti-T15 anti-idiotype. In this case, as demonstrated in FIGURE 2, the formation of anti-PC IgE was suppressed for a prolonged period of time. The titers of anti-PC IgG_1, IgG_2, IgG_3, and IgM also remained in an enzyme-linked immunosorbent assay (ELISA) with isotype-specific antibodies at 4 to > 5 serial dilution steps lower than controls. These titers increased to almost control levels after four months, including five injections of PC keyhole limpet hemocyanin (KLH) in alum.[2] The IgA-antibody synthesis was not significantly affected throughout. From this we conclude that a considerable proportion of anti-PC IgE antibodies express Id that react with anti-T15 anti-idiotype at the beginning of the response, similar to other isotypes. That anti-PC IgA is not affected indicates that the T15 Id is not expressed on this isotype if induced in a immunization procedure that leads to IgE production. Indeed, it was found by Gearhart and Cebra[11] that only a minority of IgA antibodies in Peyer's patches express the T15 idiotype.

Furthermore, suppression of primary IgE responses was achieved in mice that were two to three times preinjected with 5×10^7 syngeneic spleen cells chemically coupled with Id-expressing antibodies or with cells naturally bearing the relevant Id on the cell surface. FIGURE 3 shows the effect that resulted from five injections of spleen cells or ascitic leucocytes from BPO_{42}-bovine-γ-globulin (BGG) primed BALB/c mice into syngeneic animals. These were sensitized three months later with BPO_4-OVA in alum. Mice that were shown to produce anti-idiotypes were suppressed for IgE production against the BPO hapten, whereas no effect was observed for the response against ovalbumin. Matched control groups produced comparable normal levels of IgE antibodies. The suppression of anti-BPO IgE could be transferred by whole spleen cells to 650 R irradiated mice, but not with T T_S cell-depleted spleen cells. T-suppressor

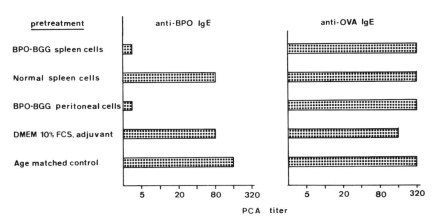

FIGURE 3. Anti-BPO and anti-OVA IgE antibodies produced after four immunizations with 10 μg BPO_4-OVA in alum in BALB/c mice. Levels of IgE antibodies are estimated by PCA titration in rats. BALB/c mice injected with spleen cells or peritoneal cells from BPO_{42}-BGG immunized syngeneic animals show suppressed anti-BPO IgE and normal anti-OVA IgE-antibody content compared to age matched control and animals injected with culture medium.

TABLE 1. Production of IgE Antibodies in 650 R Irradiated BALB/c Mice After Adoptive Transfer of Spleen Cells of Suppressed (I) and Control Mice (II)

Treatment of Mice	Treatment of Transferred Cells	PCA-Titer of Recipients
I BPO-BGG primed spleen cells	anti-Lyt-2.2 + C'	160
	normal Ig + C'	<10
II normal syngeneic spleen cells	anti-Lyt-2.2 + C'	640
	normal Ig + C'	320

cells were lysed in these fractions with monoclonal anti-Lyt-2.2 antibodies plus complement (TABLE 1).

Whereas in these mice, however, the anti-BPO IgE response was suppressed, stimulation of the IgG response against this determinant was observed. Again, as for IgE, the IgG response against OVA was not affected (FIGURE 4). Similar results were achieved in BALB/c mice injected with syngeneic spleen cells (SC) chemically modified with anti-BPO antibodies.

We have also injected BALB/c mice with SC-T15, whereas the T15 protein was mildly reduced and alkylated. As shown in FIGURE 5, two injections of 5×10^7 SC-T15 suppressed the anti-PC IgE formation to a titer of 20, compared to 320 of controls. SC-M 167 injected mice reached one dilution step less than controls. M 167 is another IgA/κ anti-PC myeloma protein of BALB/c mice, but not expressing the T15 idiotype. After 14 weeks, including five immunizations with PC-KLH, the passive cutaneous anaphylaxis (PCA) titers reached 40 for SC-T15, 80 for SC-M 167, and 640 for SC treated mice. As expected, the IgE response towards the KLH carrier remained equal for all three groups, namely 20–40.

It was found by Chang *et al.*[12] that PC-KLH elicits two different species of anti-PC antibodies: group I antibodies are directed exclusively against the PC moiety of the PC hapten and express the T15 idiotype. This group consists mainly of IgM, IgA, and IgG$_3$ antibodies. By contrast, group II anti-PC antibodies are mainly of the IgG$_{2a}$, IgG$_{2b}$, and IgG$_1$ class, do not express the T15 Id, and recognize structures of the antigenic carrier, in addition to phosphorylcholine. We have adsorbed anti-PC IgE containing serum from PC-KLH immunized BALB/c mice onto PC-tyrosyl-Sepharose 4 B and eluted the antibodies with carbobenzoxy-glycin, phosphoryl-choline-chloride and *p*-nitrophenyl-phosphorylcholine. After extensive dialysis, PCA titers of effluents were estimated. Elicitation was performed with 2 mg (PC)$_{25}$-HSA/1% Evan's Blue in 1 ml saline. After four weeks, including two immunizations with 2 μg PC-KLH in alum, > 90% anti-PC IgE antibodies belonged to group I. After seven weeks, including three immunizations, 6–10% of group I and 90–95% of group II anti-PC IgE antibodies were observed.

REGULATION OF A PRIMARY IgE RESPONSE BY (ANTI-CARRIER) ANTI-IDIOTYPES

It was established by several investigators that the participation of an immunogenic carrier molecule is of crucial importance in the initial phase of an IgE-antibody response against a hapten. This so called carrier effect, also required for the establishment of an IgE response, is the result of cooperation between different populations of immunologically competent cells with distinct specificities for hapten or

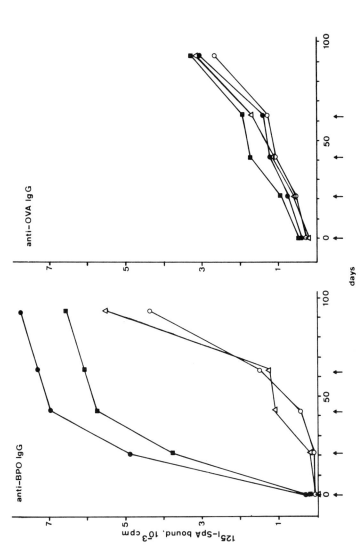

FIGURE 4. Formation of anti-BPO and anti-OVA IgG antibodies in BALB/c mice in the course of immunization with 10 µg (BPO)$_4$-OVA in alum. The arrows indicate the days of antigen administration. IgG antibodies are estimated by radioimmunoassay with Staphylococcus protein A. Mice injected with spleen cells (●) or peritoneal cells (■) from BPO$_{42}$-BGG immunized syngeneic animals show enhanced induction of anti-BPO IgG, but not anti-OVA IgG antibodies, compared to controls. (○) age matched control group. (△) age matched control group.

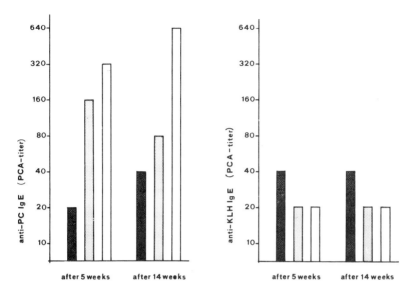

FIGURE 5. Levels of anti-PC IgE antibodies (PCA titers) of BALB/c mice injected twice with 5×10^7 syngeneic spleen cells chemically coupled with purified T15 (▩) or M167 (▨) protein and in a control group (□). Sera were taken after 5 weeks (two injections of 2 μg PC-KLH/alum) and 14 weeks (four injections of 2 μg PC-KLH/alum).

carrier antigenic determinants. Recognition and regulation in a carrier-dependent response acts through receptor molecules expressing anti-hapten Id or anti-carrier idiotypes. Accordingly, we immunized BALB/c mice with purified syngeneic anti-carrier antibodies, in this case anti-OVA IgG. The mice produced anti-OVA anti-idiotype as demonstrated by a radioimmunoassay.[13] These mice, sensitized three months later with BPO$_4$- or DNP$_4$-OVA were suppressed for the production of IgE

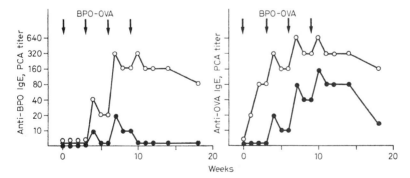

FIGURE 6a. Primary IgE antibody responses upon repeated immunizations with 10 μg BPO$_4$-OVA in alum (↓) in BALB/c mice producing isologous (anti-OVA) anti-idiotype (●), compared with control groups (○). The left figure represents the anti-BPO IgE, the right figure the anti-OVA IgE antibody titers estimated by PCA in rats.

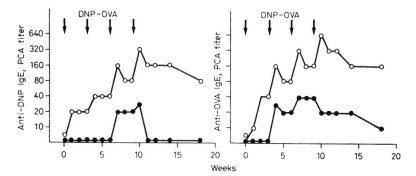

FIGURE 6b. Primary IgE antibody responses upon repeated immunizations with 10 μg DNP$_3$-OVA in alum ($\downarrow$) in BALB/c mice producing isologous anti-OVA anti-idiotype ($\bullet$), compared with control groups (O). The left figure represents the anti-DNP, the right figure the anti-OVA IgE antibody titers estimated by PCA in rats.

against both haptens (FIGURE 6a, 6b). If, however, they were sensitized with an antigen consisting of the same haptens, but bound to an OVA unrelated carrier, such as ascaris protein extract (ASC), they showed normal levels of anti-hapten and anti-carrier IgE (FIGURE 6c). In anti-OVA anti-idiotype-producing mice, anti-OVA IgE was depressed, but to a lesser extent. The lesser degree of anti-OVA suppression could be due to new antigenic determinants developing on the carrier upon hapten conjugation and raising antibodies cross-reacting with the native carrier protein. In addition, the anti-OVA anti-idiotype was obtained from antibodies raised against the native protein. It may therefore not include all anti-idiotypes required for total suppression of the anti-carrier response evoked with hapten conjugates. Another possibility is that antibodies against a total protein with many antigenic determinants are more diverse than anti-hapten antibodies, and only a small part of anti-protein antibodies may be recognized with anti-idiotypes produced against antibodies of another individual.

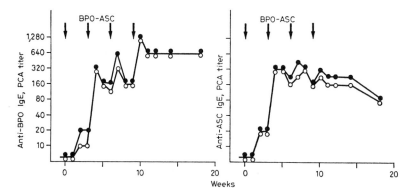

FIGURE 6c. Primary IgE antibody responses upon repeated immunizations with 10 μg BPO$_5$-ASC in alum ($\downarrow$) in BALB/c mice producing isologous anti-OVA anti-idiotype ($\bullet$) compared with control groups (O). The left figure represents the anti-BPO, the right figure the anti-ASC IgE antibody titers estimated by PCA in rats.

REGULATION OF A PRIMARY RESPONSE BY ANTIGEN COUPLED TO SYNGENEIC SPLEEN CELLS

As mentioned before, an immune response is regulated by three specific elements: antigen, Id, and anti-idiotype. These may reach optimal functional efficacy if processed by immunoregulatory cells expressing major histocompatibility complex (MHC)-encoded structures. Moreover, antigen and anti-idiotype may possess similar immunological properties, as both can bind to idiotypes. With this finding in mind, we coupled BPO or PC antigens onto spleen lymphocytes of BALB/c mice. Syngeneic mice were injected four times intravenously (i.v.) with 5×10^7 SC-PC. After 13 weeks, they received the first PC-KLH antigen administration for IgE sensitization. In FIGURE 7, it is shown that the anti-PC IgE response remained suppressed for a long time despite four additional administrations of PC-OVA in alum. A slight suppressive effect was also observed on the anti-OVA IgE response.

The time that is required to establish a suppressive state by SC-antigen may be several weeks. We learned this from an experiment in which BALB/c mice were injected twice in two weeks with syngeneic 5×10^7 benzylpenicilloyl spleen cells. The animals received the first dose of BPO_4-OVA antigen in alum after five weeks, followed by booster injections at week 7, 9, and 11. As shown in FIGURE 8, mice that were treated twice with SC-BPO produced normal levels of anti-BPO IgE at the beginning, but showed decreased IgE synthesis after 10 weeks. The anti-OVA IgE response, again, was not affected throughout, indicating antigen-specific suppressive effects.

ATTEMPTS TO REGULATE AN ESTABLISHED IgE RESPONSE BY ANTI-IDIOTYPES

Considering the practical problems in allergic diseases, it would be of the greatest relevance to be able to suppress IgE responses that are already established in sensitized patients. We have shown that an established IgE response against the BPO hapten can be suppressed specifically in BALB/c mice for two to three weeks by a single intravenous injection of isologous anti-BPO anti-idiotype (FIGURE 9). At the moment, the exact mechanism of anti-idiotype administration in an ongoing IgE response, however, is not fully established.

One could argue that the suppressive effect is the result of the formation of complexes between free Id and anti-idiotype rather than of real suppression of IgE synthesis. The amount of injected anti-idiotype, however, was small and would not suffice to complex all anti-BPO antibodies in a mouse. Furthermore, PCA titration of anti-BPO antiserum, preincubated with anti-idiotype, showed no reduction of the titer. From the experiment shown in FIGURE 9, which includes one single injection of anti-idiotype, we suggest that the first suppressive effect is due to direct inactivation or depletion of B cells expressing idiotype. Later, specific T_S cells may be generated and act at a later stage of the response.

Similar experiments were performed in guinea pigs. Animals of strain 13 were first sensitized with BPO-BGG and OVA and then injected four times every following day with isologous anti-BPO anti-idiotype. As shown in FIGURE 10, the anti-BPO IgE levels remained low, with titers of 200 in anti-idiotype-treated animals, compared to controls that showed titers of 800–1600. The IgE response against the BGG carrier and the unrelated OVA antigen was slightly depressed for two weeks, but reached control levels after a further booster injection with antigen. This newly injected antigen at

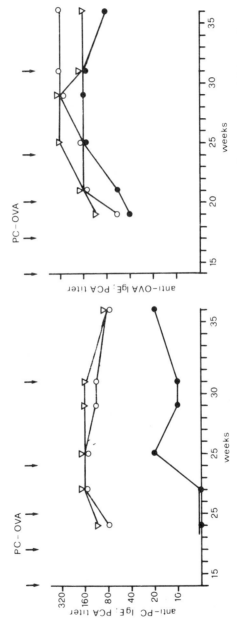

FIGURE 7. Formation of anti-PC IgE antibodies in BALB/c mice four times injected with 5 × 10⁷ syngeneic SC-PC (●) at week 0, 2, 6, and 8. Mice were sensitized with 2 μg PC-OVA in alum at days indicated by arrows. Control groups received normal spleen cells (○) or were not pretreated (▽). The left figure shows the PCA titers of anti-PC IgE, the right figure the titers of anti-OVA.

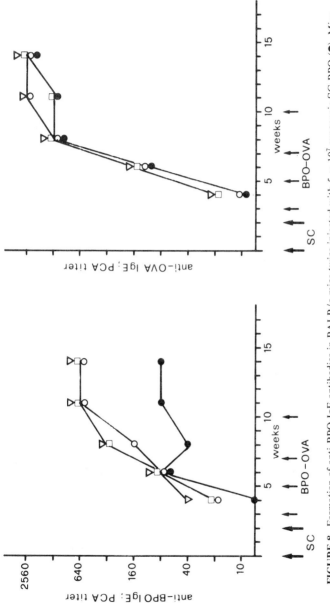

FIGURE 8. Formation of anti-BPO IgE antibodies in BALB/c mice twice injected with 5×10^7 syngeneic SC-BPO (●). Mice were sensitized with 2 μg BPO-OVA in alum at the days indicated by arrows. Control groups received normal spleen cells (○), 50 μg BPO$_{20}$-HSA (□) or were not pretreated (▽). The left figure shows the PCA titers of anti-BPO IgE, the left figure the titers of anti-OVA IgE.

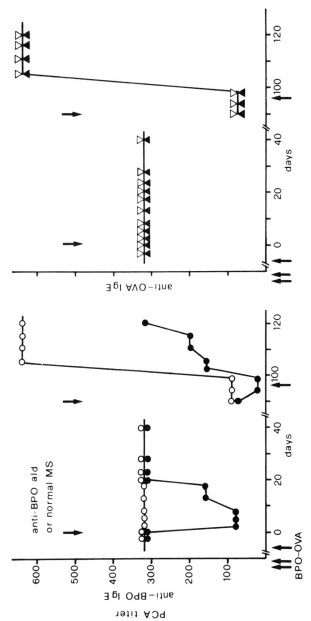

FIGURE 9. Effect of passively administered isologous anti-BPO anti-idiotype on the ongoing IgE response induced with three injections of BPO₄-OVA in two-week intervals (↓). BALB/c mice administered with anti-idiotype (●) showed depressed anti-BPO IgE formation for two to three weeks, compared with BALB/c mice that were given normal serum (○). No effect was observed on the anti-OVA IgE response (▲ ▽).

week 6, on the other hand, did not increase anti-BPO IgE levels in anti-BPO anti-idiotype-injected guinea pigs.

These two experiments, however, dealt with IgE responses that were established for only a few months. It remains to be established whether an IgE response established for a long time can also be suppressed.

CONCLUSIONS

Our results demonstrate that IgE synthesis is regulated by Id-anti-idiotype network interactions, similar to that of other isotypes. The IgE response, however, is

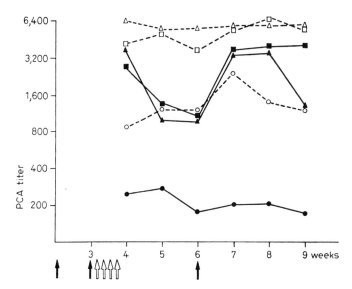

FIGURE 10. Effect of administration of isologous anti-BPO anti-idiotype on the response of homocytotropic antibodies to BPO (●), BGG (▲), and OVA (■) in guinea pigs of strain 13, compared with animals injected with normal immunoglobulins (○, △, □). Closed arrows indicate day of injection of BPO-BGG and OVA, open arrows the day of anti-BPO anti-idiotype administration.

more accessible to network regulation at early stages than in later phases. Particularly, initial elicitation of IgE antibodies could be suppressed in an antigen-specific way with actively produced or passively administered anti-idiotype. It was shown that anti-idiotypes, produced in the same mouse strain against Id from a pool of antibodies from many donors, possess enough cross-reactivity to affect a major part of the total IgE response against a hapten (BPO). On the other hand, polyclonal anti-idiotype raised against monoclonal anti-PC antibody of the TEPC 15 myeloma (T-15 Id) could cause suppression also of antibodies that do not express the T-15 Id, but possess single cross-reactive epitopes in the variable region. As shown in FIGURE 11, mildly reduced and alkylated T15 protein elicits isologous anti-idiotypes that probably recognize most anti-PC antibodies, in contrast to M 167. A substantial number of anti-PC IgE antibodies in a later stage of the response are group II anti-PC antibodies and do not express T15 idiotype. This finding is reflected by the fact that four hybridomas from BALB/c mice were obtained that produced group II anti-PC IgE antibodies (Heusser and Blaser, unpublished). At the beginning of the anti-PC IgE response, however, most IgE antibodies are of group I. The amounts of group I antibodies remain at the same level throughout, and group II IgE is formed after five weeks. This is evidence for different clonal origin of group I and group II IgE antibodies. It also explains that the primary response is more accessible to regulation by anti-T15 anti-idiotype.

Another finding is that syngeneic immunization with purified anti-OVA antibodies to raise antibodies against Id specific for carrier epitopes, suppressed both anti-hapten and anti-carrier (OVA) IgE production. These results are summarized in TABLE 2. It shows that the regulation of IgE at its initial phase dissociates into two distinct compartments. One operates by way of carrier recognition and processing antigen, the other regulating specifically the anti-hapten response. In this context one has to keep in mind that antibodies against the carrier, in fact, recognize "haptenic epitopes" of the protein itself. Benzylpenicilloyl and phosphorylcholine are just additional artificially grafted haptens on the carrier protein. The exact way of regulation by anti-carrier anti-idiotype is not yet fully understood. We suggest that anti-carrier anti-idiotypes either induce carrier-specific T_S cells or that it blocks carrier-specific T_H cells, or cells

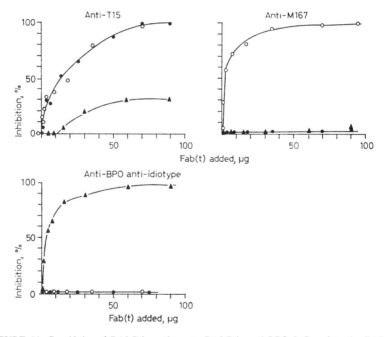

FIGURE 11. Specificity of BALB/c antisera to BALB/c anti-BPO IgG and to the BALB/c myeloma proteins T15 and M 167. Each quadrant shows the inhibitory activity of three different Fab(t) in radioimmunoassays of antisera and the corresponding ^{125}I-labeled Fab(t) fragment. The reaction of anti-T15 antiserum with ^{125}I-labeled T15-Fab(t) can be inhibited with unlabeled Fab(t) of T15 (●) and M 167 (○) and to 30% with anti-BPO Fab(t) (▲). Anti-M 167 and (anti-BPO) anti-idiotype reactions with their ^{125}I-labeled Fab(t) can be inhibited with their own unlabeled Fab(t) but not with any of the other unlabeled Fab(t).

TABLE 2. Formation of Anti-Hapten and Anti-Carrier IgE Antibodies in Mice Actively Producing Isologous Anti-Idiotype of Different Specificities

Antigen	T15-Anti-Idiotype		Anti-BPO-Anti-Idiotype		Anti-OVA-Anti-Idiotype	
	Anti-hapten Response	Anti-carrier Response	Anti-hapten Response	Anti-carrier Response	Anti-hapten Response	Anti-carrier Response
BPO-OVA	+	+	−	+	−	−
DNP-OVA[a]	n.d.	n.d.	+	+	−	−
BPO-ASC/KLH	+	+	−	+	+	+
PC-KLH	−	+	+	+	n.d.	n.d.

[a]DNP-OVA = dinitrophenylated ovalbumin.

processing antigen at initiation of the response. It is not an isotype-specific mechanism, because IgG antibodies are also suppressed.

T-dependent immune responses, such as IgE elicitation, are regulated by a cellular network among antigen, Id, and anti-idiotype together with MHC encoded products. Therefore syngeneic lymphocytes coupled with antigen or Id may interact with the regulatory circuits of cells. We observed prolonged suppression of the primary IgE antibody response against PC and BPO to see if these groups were coupled to syngeneic SC and repeatedly injected into BALB/c mice before sensitization with antigen. The suppression is specific for the respective antigens, because little or no effects were observed on the anti-OVA IgE response. We suggest that antigen-modified syngeneic spleen cells directly interact with the cellular circuits of complementary idiotypes. Some evidence for this appears from preliminary results demonstrating that injection of SC-PC induce $T15^+$ T_S cells.

Several authors demonstrated in different experimental systems that SC coupled with Id induces Id^+ and/or anti-idiotype$^+$ T_S cells.[3-5] We injected SC-T15 and SC-M 167 into BALB/c and observed suppression of the anti-PC IgE response measured at the fifth week after injection of cells in SC-T15 injected animals. Mice injected with SC-M 167 were only slightly depressed. After 14 weeks both groups showed suppressed IgE compared to the controls.

These results that demonstrate network regulation of IgE at initiation of the response are of basic interest for further understanding of regulation of this Ig class. Of clinical relevance would be antigen-specific suppression of a long-established response and the understanding of isotype-switch mechanisms.

We were successful in suppressing ongoing anti-BPO and anti-PC IgE responses in BALB/c mice and in guinea pigs. Although these animals produced high titers of specific antibodies at the moment of anti-idiotype administration, the response was not established longer than two months. We do not know at the moment whether a long-established IgE response can be regulated and whether "late" B_ϵ cells can escape network regulation. This does not necessarily mean that once committed, B_ϵ cells are not accessible to regulation by some T_S and T_SF.

No conscious effort to administer anti-idiotype in man has yet been made, although the therapeutic administration of Ig (gamma-globulin therapy) for a variety of medical indications may sometimes represent anti-idiotype therapy. It must be assumed that parts of normal human Ig preparations possess anti-idiotype specificity and that Id-expressing antibodies can interact with the immunoregulatory network.

In order to study network regulation in a human system, we produced anti-idiotype antibodies in rabbits against human anti-bee-phospholipase A_2 (anti-PLA) anti-idiotype antibodies. This protein is the major allergen of beevenom, and high amounts of anti-PLA IgG antibodies are produced in bee keepers. We produced heterologous anti-PLA anti-idiotype in rabbits that were made tolerant at birth with normal human γ-globulin. After additional adsorption of anti-PLA anti-idiotype onto a Sepharose-γ-globulin column, anti-idiotype reacted strongly with anti-PLA of the respective donor, and to some extent with anti-PLA of other individuals, but not with Ig of normal individuals. Further studies of network regulation and network therapy in the bee-venom system are in progress.

ACKNOWLEDGMENTS

We thank Dr. C. H. Heusser, Ciba-Geigy Ltd., for substantial discussions and support of our work. Laboratory facilities were generously provided by Professor P. Zahler at the Institute of Biochemistry, University of Bern.

REFERENCES

1. BONA, C. A. 1981. Idiotypes and Lymphocytes. Academic Press. New York.
2. BLASER, K. & A. L. DE WECK. 1982. Regulation of IgE antibody response by idiotype-anti-idiotype network. *In* Progress in Allergy 32: 203. S. Karger. Basel.
3. TADA, T., K. OKUMURA, K. HAYAKAWA, G. SUZUKI, R. ABE & Y. KUMAGAI. 1981. Immunological circuitry governed by MHC and V_H gene products. *In* Immunoglobulin Idiotypes. ICN-UCLA Symp. Mol. Cell. Biol. C. JANEWAY, E. E. SERCARZ and H. WIGZELL, Eds.: XX: 563.
4. GERMAN, R. N., M.-S. SY, K. ROCK, M. H. DIETZ, M. I. GREENE, A. NISONOFF, J. Z. WEINBERGER, S.-T. JU, M. E. DORF & B. BENACERRAF. 1981. The role of idiotype and the MHC in suppressor T cell pathways. *In* Immunoglobulin Idiotypes. ICN-UCLA Symp. Mol. Cell. Biol. C. JANEWAY, E. E. SERCARZ and H. WIGZELL, Eds.: XX: 709.
5. GREENE, M. I., J. S. BROMBERG, J. NEPOM, R. FINBERG, K. ROCK, B. WHITAKER, R. N. GERMAIN, I. FOX, L. PERRY, R. WETZIG, M. TAKAOKI, A. NISONOFF, B. BENACERRAF & M.-S. SY. 1981. The role of idiotype in guiding cellular responses. *In* Immunoglobulin Idiotypes. ICN-UCLA Symp. Mol. Cell. Biol. C. JANEWAY, E. E. SERCARZ and H. WIGZELL, Eds.: XX: 725.
6. NISHIDA, Y., T. KATAOKA, N. ISHIDA, S. NAKAI, T. KISHIMOTO, I. BOTTCHER & T. HONJO. 1981. Cloning of mouse immunoglobulin-epsilon gene and its location within the heavy chain cluster. Proc. Natl. Acad. Sci. USA 78: 1581.
7. RETH, M., T. IMANISHI-KARI & K. RAJEWSKY. 1979. Analysis of the repertoire of anti-NP antibodies in C 57 B1/6 mice by cell fusion. II. Characterization of idiotypes by monoclonal anti-idiotype antibodies. Eur. J. Immunol. 9: 1004.
8. DESSEIN, A., S.-T. JU, M. E. DORF, B. BENACERRAF & R. N. GERMAIN. 1980. IgE response to synthetic polypeptide antigens. II. Idiotypic analysis of the IgE response to L-Glutamic acid^{60}-L-Alanine^{30}-L-Tyrosine^{10} (GAT). J. Immunol. 124: 71.
9. BLASER, K., M. GEISER & A. L. DE WECK. 1974. Suppression of phosphorylcholine-specific IgE antibody formation in BALB/c mice by isologous anti-T 15 antiserum. Eur. J. Immunol. 9: 1017.
10. BLASER, K., T. NAKAGAWA & A. L. DE WECK. 1980. Suppression of the benzylpenicilloyl (BPO)-specific IgE formation by isologous anti-idiotypic antibodies in BALB/c mice. J. Immunol. 125: 24.
11. GEARHART, P. J. & J. J. CEBRA. 1979. Differentiated B Lymphocytes. Potential to express particular antibody variable and constant regions depends on site of lymphoid tissue and antigen load. J. Exp. Med. 149: 216.
12. CHANG, S. A., M. BROWN & M. B. RITTENBERG. 1982. Immunologic memory to

phosphorylcholine. II. PC-KLH induces two antibody populations that dominate different isotypes. J. Immunol. **128:** 702.
13.   BLASER, K., T. NAKAGAWA & A. L. DE WECK. 1981. Suppression of anti-hapten IgE and IgG antibody responses by isologous anti-idiotypic antibodies against purified anti-carrier (Ovalbumin) antibodies in BALB/c mice. J. Immunol. **126:** 1180.

DISCUSSION OF THE PAPER

N. ABDOU (*University of Kansas Medical Center, Kansas City, Kans.*): It is very nice that you have shown that the anti-idiotype will decrease the IgE in levels in the serum. What happens to the IgE that is already bound to the basophils? Do you have any information showing that the anti-idiotype binds to the IgE on those cells, and if so, does it enhance or suppress mediator release?

K. BLASER: We have shown that isologous anti-idiotypic antibodies from mice can elicit Prausnitz-Küster type reactions in rat skin, but we have not observed systemic reactions, either in mice or in guinea pigs. In contrast to elicitation of skin reactions, anti-idiotypic manipulations require very little amounts of anti-idiotype, probably too little to be dangerous.

A. R. PACKNER (*Yale University, New Haven, Conn.*): I just want to get something straight with regard to your experimental protocol. Did you give idiotype and spleen cell with idiotype on the surface before immunization?

BLASER: Yes.

PACKNER: Did you ever try to give the spleen cells with idiotype during an ongoing response?

BLASER: That is what we are trying now, and that would be the real experiment with respect to allergic diseases.

PACKNER: I would like to let you know that we have been doing similar experiments using spleen cells from animals immunized with a different antigen, acetyl-choline receptor, injecting those intravenously both before and during the course of the response. We got the same results that you did, in that when given to four mice, the immunization resulted in a marked suppression of the response. The suppression was much less marked when it was given during the course of the immune response, but it was still there.

UNIDENTIFIED SPEAKER: Did you ever have any experiments where the IgE level went up rather than down?

BLASER: In IgE, no. It seems to me that the IgE is particularly susceptible to suppression, maybe more so than other isotypes. Mainly we have observed in some cases a stimulation of IgG synthesis at the beginning of the response.

Cellular and Molecular Mechanisms that Regulate Idiotype Expression in Myeloma Cells

RICHARD G. LYNCH AND GARY L. MILBURN

Department of Pathology
College of Medicine
The University of Iowa
Iowa City, Iowa 52242

INTRODUCTION

Myeloma is an example of idiotype expression carried to an extreme. Whereas neither the extent of dominance of the single clone in myeloma nor the extraordinary serum levels of the single idiotype in myeloma have obvious counterparts in normal immune responses, the analyses of myeloma cells and myeloma proteins have continued to provide important information that has improved our understanding of immune responses.

This laboratory has employed antigen-binding murine myelomas as monoclonal B-cell models and has established that these myelomas differentiate during *in vivo* growth, are responsive to antigen-specific and idiotype-specific immunoregulatory signals, and induce an extraordinary expansion of immunoregulatory T-suppressor cells. Those studies have recently been reviewed.[1,2] The present report reviews our studies on the regulation of idiotype expression in myeloma cells by idiotype-specific immunoregulators.

Previous studies identified three idiotype (Id^{315})-specific events that followed immunization of BALB/c mice with the IgA anti-trinitrophenyl (TNP) antibody (M315) produced by MOPC-315: a) induction of anti-idiotypic (anti-Id^{315}) antibodies, predominantly of the IgG_1 subclass,[3] b) development of anti-Id^{315} T-suppressor cells,[4] and c) establishment of Id^{315}-specific protection from challenge with lethal numbers of MOPC-315 cells.[5]

Subsequent studies of MOPC-315 cells enclosed in peritoneal diffusion chambers[4] suggested that anti-Id^{315} antibodies inhibited surface membrane expression of M315, and anti-Id^{315} T-suppressor cells inhibited secretion of M315. More recently an extensive *in vitro* study of the role of anti-Id^{315} antibodies in the regulation of Id^{315} expression was completed.[6] This established that anti-Id^{315} antibodies inhibited surface membrane expression of M315 by a process in which the antibody-aggregated surface M315 was shed attached to membranous vesicles. The anti-Id^{315} antibodies did not influence M315 secretion or the growth and viability of MOPC-315 cells.[6] This was true for syngeneic, polyclonal anti-Id^{315} antibodies in the presence or absence of guinea pig complement, as well as for a syngeneic, γ_1 monoclonal anti-Id^{315} antibody. In the *in vitro* studies, as well as the *in vivo* studies that employed MOPC-315 cells enclosed in diffusion chambers, the anti-Id^{315} antibodies were able to interact with the MOPC-315 cells, but were not able to interact with MOPC-315 cells in the presence of host cells. Thus our finding that anti-Id^{315} antibodies simply modulate surface idiotype on MOPC-315 cells does not rule out the possibility that under appropriate conditions *in vivo*, the anti-Id[315] antibodies might work in concert with another host element to achieve additional target-cell effects.

INHIBITION OF M315 SECRETION BY ANTI-IDIOTYPIC[315] T-SUPPRESSOR CELLS *IN VITRO*

Idiotype-specific T cells were induced in BALB/c mice by hyperimmunization with a mildly reduced and alkylated form of M315. Each mouse received a total of six weekly injections of 200 μg each. The primary injection was in complete Freund's adjuvant, the second in incomplete Freund's adjuvant, and all subsequent injections were in phosphate buffered saline. The first and second injections were distributed over the hind footpads and four dorsal subcutaneous sites. The subsequent injections were in the hind footpads and the peritoneal cavity. For optimal generation of idiotype-specific

TABLE 1. Effect of Anti-Id[315]T Cells on MOPC-315 Cells *In Vitro*

Effector:MOPC-315 Cell Ratio[a]	Effector Cells	Viability	Percent MOPC-315 with Surface M315	Percent MOPC-315 Cells that Secrete M315
MOPC-315 cells alone	None	93 ± [b]	89 ± 2	44 ± 3
50:1	Normal spleen T cells	86 ± 3	89 ± 2	41 ± 5
100:1	Normal spleen T cells	85 ± 5	84 ± 3	40 ± 4
200:1	Normal spleen T cells	83 ± 5	82 ± 3	38 ± 3
50:1	RA315 immune spleen T cells	78 ± 3	82 ± 4	36 ± 4
100:1	RA315 immune spleen T cells	78 ± 5	79 ± 5	8 ± 2
200:1	RA315 immune spleen T cells	76 ± 2	77 ± 5	3 ± 2

[a]MOPC-315 cell number was typically 10^5 viable cells per ml, and the effector cell number was adjusted according to the ratio indicated.
[b]Mean ± standard error of the mean for three experiments.

T-suppressor cells, each mouse received a 50 μg boost of M315 intravenously in phosphate buffered saline (PBS) three days prior to sacrifice. Splenic T cells were prepared by nylon wool column passage and were mixed directly with, or separated by a 0.2μ pore membrane from an *in vitro*-adapted line of MOPC-315.[7] The usual T cell: MOPC-315 cell ratio was 100:1. The cells were harvested after 24 to 48 hours of culture, and MOPC-315 viability and M315-secreting frequency were determined.

As shown in TABLE 1, splenic T cells from M315-immunized mice had little or no effect on MOPC-315 viability or surface M315 expression, but inhibited the secretion of M315 by as much as 90% when compared to control cultures containing myeloma cells and normal spleen cells. The secretory inhibition is spleen cell dose-dependent. At a T cell:MOPC-315 cell ratio of 800:1, complete (98%) suppression occurred, whereas an 800-fold excess of normal T cells had little effect on secretion of M315.

Previous experiments both *in vivo* and *in vitro* had established that the suppressive activity was totally abrogated after treatment of the immune cells with anti-θ and complement. Monoclonal anti-Lyt-1 and anti-Lyt-2 antibodies were coupled to

Sepharose-6MB beads, and columns were constructed for specific cell-depletion studies. We observed that only cells that passed through the anti-Lyt-1 column were effective as secretory inhibitors, thus defining the phenotype of the regulatory T cell as Lyt1⁻2⁺. Furthermore, when equal numbers of Lyt1⁺ and Lyt2⁺ cells were mixed together, the Lyt1⁺ cells did not enhance or interfere with the suppressive activity of the Lyt2⁺ cells.

To determine whether adherent accessory cells (macrophages) played any role in the inhibition of M315 secretion, depletion studies were performed. Nylon wool-passed immune spleen cells were further depleted by two consecutive adherence steps on plastic petri dishes at 37° C for 60 minutes. Using the nonadherent cells as effectors, identical suppression was observed. This finding suggests that macrophages are not required at the effector stage of secretory inhibition.

To investigate the idiotype specificity of secretory inhibition, affinity columns were prepared using M315 or M460 idiotypes conjugated to Sepharose 6MB beads. M460 is the murine IgA anti-TNP myeloma protein produced by MOPC-460, and serves as an excellent control, because even though both M315 and M460 are IgA anti-TNP antibodies, they have dissimilar idiotypes. The data in TABLE 2 show that the regulatory T cells responsible for secretory inhibition were removed by the M315-Sepharose, but not by the M460-Sepharose column. In addition, the T cells eluted from the M315-Sepharose column with soluble M315 (2mg/ml) were enriched for the specific regulatory cells. A cell ratio of only 12:1 was now effective in mediating secretory inhibition, and M315 secretion was virtually nil at higher ratios. These observations indicate that the regulatory T cells have surface recognition structures specific for M315 idiotypes.

All of the data presented thus far reflect measurement of M315 secretion after 24 hours of coculture of MOPC-315 cells and regulatory T cells. To determine the kinetics of inhibition, we measured M315 secretion at 2-hour intervals following the

TABLE 2. Depletion and Enrichment of Anti-Id³¹⁵ T Cells on Idiotype Columns

Effector:MOPC-315 Cell Ratio	Treatment of Added RA315 Immune T cells	Percent MOPC-315 Cells that Secrete M315
MOPC-315 cells alone	No treatment	43 ± 3[a]
50:1	No treatment	12 ± 3
100:1	No treatment	8 ± 3
200:1	No treatment	3 ± 1
50:1	Id⁴⁶⁰ Absorption[b]	16 ± 4
100:1	Id⁴⁶⁰ Absorption	10 ± 5
200:1	Id⁴⁶⁰ Absorption	7 ± 2
50:1	Id³¹⁵ Absorption[c]	35 ± 3
100:1	Id³¹⁵ Absorption	36 ± 5
200:1	Id³¹⁵ Absorption	34 ± 6
12:1	Eluted from Id³¹⁵ absorbant[d]	11 ± 5
25:1	Eluted from Id³¹⁵ absorbant	4 ± 4
50:1	Eluted from Id³¹⁵ absorbant	1 ± 1

[a]Mean ± standard error for three experiments.
[b]RA315 Immune Spleen T Cells were passed over an Id⁴⁶⁰-Sepharose-6MB column, and the nonadherent cells were used as effectors.
[c]RA315 Immune Spleen T Cells were passed over an Id³¹⁵-Sepharose-6MB column, and the nonadherent cells were used as effectors.
[d]Cells that adhered to the Id³¹⁵-Sepharose-6MB column were eluted with soluble RA315 in PBS at a concentration of 2 mg/ml.

TABLE 3. Effect of Pronase on Suppressed MOPC-315 Cells

Effector:MOPC-315 Cell Ratio	Effector Cells	Pronase Treatment[a] Prior to Plaque Assay	Percent MOPC-315 Cells That Secrete M315
MOPC-315 cells alone	None	–	41 ± 1[b]
MOPC-315 cells alone	None	+	43 ± 1
100:1	Normal spleen T cells	–	37 ± 1
100:1	Normal spleen T cells	+	39 ± 1
100:1	RA315 immune spleen T cells	–	7 ± 1
100:1	RA315 immune spleen T cells	+	27 ± 1

[a]Cells were subjected to a 30 minute treatment with 0.5% pronase at room temperature immediately prior to plaquing.
[b]Mean ± standard error for three experiments.

addition of Id[315]-immune splenic T cells to MOPC-315 cells. Inhibition of M315 secretion was first detected after only 6 hours of coculture and progressed until an inhibition of 80 to 90% of the control value was observed at 24 hours.[7] This result suggests that the regulatory T cells are already programmed for the suppressive activity when added to the culture and probably require little further proliferation or differentiation. Furthermore, because MOPC-315 cells were secreting M315 at the time that the suppressor cells were added to the culture, the T-suppressor cells acted directly on the actual antibody-secreting cell rather than on a precursor to the antibody-secreting cells.

Because the *in vivo* findings implied that secretory blockade was effected by a diffusible T-cell product, *in vitro* experiments were undertaken in which the T cells were separated from the MOPC-315 cells by a 0.2μ pore membrane. Idiotype[315]-specific inhibition of secretion was observed even though the target cells and regulatory T cells were prevented from any direct contact. Interestingly, the inhibition of M315 secretion was gradually reversed when the immune T cells were removed from the system. These observations suggest that the secretory inhibition is mediated by a diffusible product and that for the inhibition to persist, the T-cell environment must be maintained.

In the *in vivo* studies, MOPC-315 cells were released from secretory inhibition after a brief treatment *in vitro* with 0.5% pronase. To determine whether the *in vitro* induced secretory inhibition could also be reversed by pronase, we treated suppressed MOPC-315 cells with 0.5% pronase for 30 minutes at room temperature prior to washing and plaquing. The data in TABLE 3 show that secretory inhibition was to a large degree reversed by pronase treatment, whereas pronase treatment had little effect on MOPC-315 cells cultured either alone or with normal splenic T cells. These findings imply that 1) the suppressive factor is retained at the surface of the myeloma cell and is susceptible to proteolytic digestion, or 2) an activation signal generated by pronase can override the T-suppressor cell signal.

Because the Id[315]-specific T cells were retained on M315-Sepharose, we investigated whether excess soluble M315 could block the T-suppressor cells. The data in TABLE 4 show that soluble M315, added at the start of the coculture, abrogated secretory inhibition. This interference was modest at an M315 concentration of 20 μg/ml, but was almost complete at 100 μg/ml. M460 at 100 μg/ml had no effect on the secretory inhibition. These results suggest that soluble M315 may have bound to the suppressive component and neutralized its effect. In similar experiments, using the constitutive polypeptide chains and enzymatically prepared fragments of M315, we have found that the Id[315]-specific T-suppressor cells recognize determinants located in the V_H region of the M315 molecule.

Collectively, these studies have established that M315 secretion can be inhibited by Id[315]-specific T-suppressor cells. Inhibition of M315 secretion could have resulted from inhibition of M315 release without inhibition of M315 synthesis, inhibition of transcription or translation of M315 mRNA, or an increased rate of intracellular degradation of M315. The first possibility was considered highly unlikely because continued M315 synthesis in the presence of a block in release would be expected to result in the intracellular accumulation of large masses of cytoplasmic M315. In a previous study, tunicamycin was shown to inhibit secretion but not synthesis of M315,[8] and this was accompanied by striking dilatation of endoplasmic cisternae filled with

TABLE 4. Inhibition of Anti-Id[315] T-Suppressor Cells by Soluble Idiotype

Effector:MOPC-315 Cell Ratio	Effector Cells	Inhibitor Added[a]	Percent MOPC-315 Cells that Secrete M315
MOPC-315 cells alone	None	None	39 ± 2[b]
100:1	RA315 immune spleen T cells	None	6 ± 3
100:1	RA315 immune spleen T cells	RA460 (100 µg/ml)	8 ± 2
100:1	RA315 immune spleen T cells	RA315 (20 µg/ml)	20 ± 3
100:1	RA315 immune spleen T cells	RA315 (100 µg/ml)	34 ± 4

[a]The inhibitor was added to cultures of the effector T cells just prior to the addition of the MOPC-315 cells.
[b]Mean ± standard error for three experiments.

M315. In the present studies, inhibition of M315 secretion by T-suppressor cells was not accompanied by ultrastructural changes in the MOPC-315 cells.

To evaluate changes in M315 synthesis, we measured incorporation of [³H]leucine into secreted and intracellular M315. We observed (TABLE 5) a marked decrease of incorporation into both intracellular and secreted M315 in the presence of Id[315]-specific T-suppressor cells. Incorporation of [³H]leucine into cellular and secreted M315 was decreased by greater than 95% when cells were pulsed from 24 to 48 hours after the start of coculture.

To determine whether inhibition of M315 synthesis was selective, studies were performed in an apparatus that allows the total protein synthesis by MOPC-315 cells to be measured. [³H]leucine incorporation into intracellular M315 and into the trichloroacetic acid (TCA)-precipitable fraction of MOPC-315 cells showed that the inhibition of protein synthesis was selective for M315 (TABLE 6). When T-suppressor cells and MOPC-315 cells were incubated in separate compartments of the diffusion apparatus for 48 hours and then pulsed with [³H]leucine for 24 hours, we observed a

TABLE 5. Inhibition of M315 Synthesis and Secretion by Anti-Id[315] T-Suppressor Cells

| | [³H]Leucine Incorporated Into M315[a] | |
Effector Cells	Supernatants[b]	Intracellular[c]
None	34,119 ± 2,539[d]	144,868 ± 2,319
100× normal spleen T cells	31,919 ± 3,630	108,329 ± 1,705
100× RA315 immune spleen T cells	1,285 ± 245	2,932 ± 1,212

[a]Effector and tumor cells were cocultured for 24 hours prior to a 24 hour pulse of [³H]leucine. Specific immunoprecipitation of M315 was then employed.
[b]One ml supernatant from the 48 hour coculture was immunoprecipitated for [³H]leucine incorporation into secreted M315.
[c]The cocultured cells were lysed with 0.5% NP40, the subcellular organelles were removed by centrifugation, and the supernatant was immunoprecipitated.
[d]Mean CPM ± standard error for three experiments.

50% decrease in total protein synthesis in MOPC-315 cells, and the entire decrement could be accounted for by the decrease in M315 synthesis. These findings strongly suggested that inhibition of M315 secretion by the T-suppressor cell product was achieved by a selective down regulation of M315 synthesis. Although the inhibition of secretion could have been accounted for by increased intracellular degradation of M315, this possibility was unlikely for two reasons: because non-M315 protein synthesis was not influenced by the T-suppressor cells, intracellular catabolism of M315 was highly selective; and when secretion but not synthesis of M315 was blocked by tunicamycin,[25] no evidence for intracellular degradation of M315 was detected.

The selective inhibition of M315 synthesis in MOPC-315 cells, and the finding that the time-course of onset of M315 inhibition[7] paralleled the known half-life of mRNA for both heavy and light immunoglobulin chains,[9] both suggested that suppression of M315 synthesis was mediated at the level of transcription or translation.

In recent studies[10] Northern blot analysis of suppressed MOPC-315 cells has shown normal levels of heavy chain mRNA, but markedly diminished or nondetected levels of light chain mRNA. It is still unclear whether the alteration in light chain mRNA results from decreased synthesis or increased inactivation.

There are several interesting aspects of these results. Although the anti-Id[315] T-suppressor cell is specific for a V_H^{315} idiotype, the inhibition of M315 synthesis is achieved by regulation of light chain mRNA expression. Although heavy chain

TABLE 6. Diffusable Product Mediates Selective Suppression of M315 Synthesis

| MOPC-315 Cells Added to Upper Chamber with Lower Chamber Containing: | MOPC-315 [³H]Leucine Incorporation Into: | |
	M315[b]	TCA-ppt Protein[c]
Media	124,936 ± 5,158[d]	236,639 ± 6,041
200× normal spleen T cells	107,254 ± 2,593	210,733 ± 6,338
200× RA315 immune spleen T cells	9,092 ± 1,510	112,213 ± 4,481

[a]Effector and tumor cells were cocultured in double chamber culture system for 48 hours prior to a 24 hour pulse of [³H]leucine.
[b]Specific immunoprecipitation of M315 was used.
[c]5% cold TCA precipitation
[d]Mean CPM ± standard error for three experiments.

mRNA is not decreased in suppressed MOPC-315 cells, heavy chain synthesis is suppressed.[7] Although suppressed MOPC-315 cells do not synthesize heavy chains, the mRNA isolated from suppressed MOPC-315 cells is translated *in vitro* in a cell-free translation system.[10]

Collectively, these findings indicate that suppression of light chain mRNA expression in MOPC-315 cells results in the failure of these cells to express the entire immunoglobulin molecule. This situation has features in common with pre-B cells where heavy chains are synthesized but light chains are not. When light chain genes are activated to expression in pre-B cells, the cell becomes an antigen-sensitive B cell that expresses complete immunoglobulin molecules on the surface membrane. Thus, in pre-B cells and suppressed MOPC-315 cells, control of light chain expression controls expression of the complete immunoglobulin molecule.

One could account for this regulatory sequence if light chains had to bind to polysome-associated heavy chains in order for the completed heavy chain to be released from the polysome. Heavy chains are known to be poorly soluble unless glycoslyated or paired with a light chain. If light chain association was required for completed heavy chains to be released from their polysomes, then in the absence of free light chains in suppressed MOPC-315 cells, heavy chains and heavy chains mRNA would remain polysome bound. Further heavy chain synthesis would be blocked. Studies are in progress to test the validity of this hypothesis.

In summary, these data demonstrate that Id^{315}-specific T cells can quickly and specifically down regulate the synthesis and secretion of M315 by MOPC-315 cells. The regulatory T cell acts independently of macrophages; is $Lyt1^- 23^+$; recognizes and binds M315, specifically V_H^{315}; acts by way of a diffusible product; and is an example of a T-suppressor cell that acts directly on the antibody-secreting cell. The mechanism of suppression affects regulation of expression of light chain mRNA.

There are two major unresolved issues that come from these observations. 1) In the absence of light chain synthesis, how does one account for the persistent expression of idiotype and TNP-binding sites on the surface membrane of suppressed MOPC-315? 2) What is it that the anti-Id^{315} T-suppressor cell does that results in the selective regulation of light chain mRNA expression? It is highly unlikely that engagement per se of surface membrane Id^{315} by an anti-Id^{315} product of the T cell could account for the suppression. The engagement of surface membrane Id^{315} on MOPC-315 cells by anti-Id^{315} antibodies results in the clearance of surface Id^{315} without any effect on M315 secretion.[6] Furthermore, engagement of surface Id^{315} by TNP-carrier in the presence of carrier-specific T-helper cells results in an increase of M315 secretion.[11] These findings (and others reviewed in reference 12) support the view that surface membrane Id^{315} functions as a focusing device for a multiplicity of immunoregulatory effectors and that the quality and intensity of the regulatory effect observed is probably dictated by the effector that is focused and not simply by engagement of the membrane Id^{315} as such.

Finally, these studies continue to show that malignant immunoglobulin-producing cells can provide useful tools with which to examine the molecular basis of immunoregulation. Although the objection could be raised that malignant B cells are poor models because they are malignant cells, similar arguments could have been raised against the use of myeloma proteins as antibody models, or the use of mutants in metabolic pathways as biochemical models. Yet, such tools have provided much useful information.

It seems reasonable to anticipate that just as careful studies of aberrant immune systems in individuals with primary immunological deficiency diseases provided great insight into the structural and functional organization of the normal immune system, careful study of the dysfunctional B-cell clones in myeloma and lymphoma will contribute to a more complete understanding of normal B cells.

REFERENCES

1. MILBURN, G. L., R. G. HOOVER & R. G. LYNCH. 1982. The use of myeloma cells to analyze immunoregulatory mechanisms and visualize immunoregulatory circuits. *In* Regulation of Immune Response Dynamics. C. De Lisi and J. R. J. Hiernaux, Eds.: **2**: 141–155. CRC Press. Boca Raton, Florida.
2. MILBURN, G. L., R. G. HOOVER & R. G. LYNCH. 1982. Immunoregulatory cell interactions that govern the growth and differentiation of murine myeloma cells. B and T Cell Tumors: Biological and Clinical Asepcts. *In* UCLA Symposium on Molecular and Cellular Biology. E. Vitetta and C. F. Fox, Eds.: **24**: 335–347. Academic Press. New York.
3. FRIKKE, M. J., S. H. BRIDGES & R. G. LYNCH. 1977. Myeloma-specific antibodies: studies of their properties and their relationship to tumor immunity. J. Immunol. **118**: 2206.
4. ROHRER, J. W., B. ODERMATT & R. G. LYNCH. 1979. Immunoregulation of murine myeloma: isologous immunization with M315 induces idiotype-specific T cells that suppress IgA secretion by MOPC-315 cells *in vivo*. J. Immunol. **122**: 2011.
5. LYNCH, R. G., R. J. GRAFF, S. SIRISINHA, E. SIMMS & H. N. EISEN. 1972. Myeloma proteins as tumor-specific transplantation antigens. Proc. Natl. Acad. Sci. USA **69**: 1540.
6. MILBURN, G. L. & R. G. LYNCH. 1983. Anti-idiotypic regulation of IgA expression in myeloma cells. Mol. Immunol. **20**: 931–940.
7. MILBURN, G. L. & R. G. LYNCH. 1982. Immunoregulation of murine myeloma *in vitro*. J. Exp. Med. **155**: 852–861.
8. HICKMAN, S., A. KULCZYCKI, R. G. LYNCH & S. KORNFELD. 1977. Studies of the mechanism of tunicamycin inhibition of IgA and IgE secretion by plasma cells. J. Biol. Chem. **252**: 4402.
9. COWAN, N. J. & C. MILSTEIN. 1974. Stability of cytoplasmic ribonucleic acid in a mouse myeloma: estimation of the half-life of the messenger RNA coding for an immunoglobulin light chain. J. Mol. Biol. **82**: 469.
10. PARSLOW, T. G., G. L. MILBURN, R. G. LYNCH & D. K. GRANNER. 1983. Suppressor T cell action inhibits the expression of an excluded immunoglobulin gene. Science. **220**: 1389.
11. ROHRER, J. W. & R. G. LYNCH. 1977. Specific immunologic regulation of differentiation of immunoglobulin expression in MOPC-315 cells during *in vivo* growth in diffusion chambers. J. Immunol. **119**: 2045.
12. LYNCH, R. G., J. W. ROHRER, B. ODERMATT, H. GEBEL, J. R. AUTRY & R. G. HOOVER. 1979. Immunoregulation of murine myeloma cell growth and differentiation: a monoclonal model of B cell differentiation. Immunol. Rev. **48**: 45.

DISCUSSION OF THE PAPER

UNIDENTIFIED SPEAKER: Will anti-idiotypic antibody to 315 added to your system of T cells plus MOPC 315 cells inhibit the effect of T cells?

R. G. LYNCH: Do you mean in the presence of the T-suppressor cells?

UNIDENTIFIED SPEAKER: That is right.

LYNCH: That is a very interesting question and has a very interesting result. We can interfere with the T-suppressor cell, finding the myeloma cell by putting in dinitrophenylated (DNP) proteins and binding up the immunoglobulin on the surface, but so far in very preliminary experiments, putting in anti-idiotypic antibody does not interfere with the T cell. We may not be doing it optimally, and if we play with it a little more, we are going to find that anti-idiotype, which we know clears surface idiotype, will in fact inhibit the T cell. The alternative possibility is that there is some free heavy chain on the surface of these cells, and because the T cells see a V_H idiotope, it can find its molecule even though we modulate off the intact immunoglobulin. So we do not know. The prediction was that modulating off the surface immunoglobulin would prevent the suppressor cell, but in fact it did not.

UNIDENTIFIED SPEAKER: Have you done any experiments with other anti-DNP myelomas that would inhibit the anti-idiotypic factor from T cells? What is the specificity of this T-cell factor?

LYNCH: The T-cell factor appears to be specific for an idiotope on the V_H 315 molecule. These T-suppressor cells do nothing to the secretion and synthesis of MOPC 460, for instance, which in fact does have a cross-reacting structure. The target molecule, however, or the region on the target molecule seen by these T-suppressor cells is not that region that is shared between 315 and 460. If one immunizes with 460, however, one can suppress the secretion of 460 with a similar kind of suppressor cell, the difference being that it is specific for the 460 idiotype.

J. CERNY (*University of Texas Medical Branch, Galveston, Tex.*): In the double Millipore Chamber system where you get the suppression across the membrane, what is the stimulus for the T cells? Is it soluble myeloma protein released from MOPC-315 cells?

LYNCH: I believe it is and the reason for saying that is, if we take the idiotype immune spleen cells and put them in with the myeloma cells, we see suppression. If we put the immune T cells in by themselves to try to condition a media, if we just grow the T-suppressor cells by themselves and then take the supernatants, they do not suppress. If we add, however, to the cells cultured alone a 315 signal, then we get a supernatant that works.

CERNY: By signal, do you mean small amounts of 315 protein?

LYNCH: That is right.

CERNY: Thank you.

Z. OVARY (*New York University, New York*): Does the T cell in question have any relationship to the FcR$^+$ T cells you have identified in mice with plasmacytomas?

LYNCH: Dr. Ovary, these cells do not have IgA receptors, so they are not the T-α cells that we have studied in these mice. We really do not know whether they have a γ receptor or another isotype specific receptor, but they do not have an α receptor. One of the predictions of the concept of a light chain specific regulation is that if one had a myeloma-myeloma hybrid that made two different immunoglobulin molecules of different light chain classes, for example, a κ light chain and a λ-2 light chain and then one presented to that cell the idiotype-specific T-suppressor cell that sees the V_H, then one would predict that one would down regulate the expression of the myeloma protein that has a light chain of the λ class, but not the light chain of the κ class. In fact, that is the observation that Abul Abbas and his colleagues in Boston reported earlier in a system where MOPC 315 and MPC11 are fused together, where MPC-11 is a γ-2b-κ, and where 315 is an α-λ-2. They showed that there was independent regulation of the expression of those immunoglobulin molecules in the same cell.

A. K. ABBAS (*Brigham and Woman's Hospital, Boston, Mass.*): In answer to Dr. Cerny's question, we have been doing some similar experiments. We have a fundamentally different way of generating anti-idiotypic suppressors against the same and other myeloma idiotypes. In Millipore systems, however, it looks like soluble myeloma protein is a lot less effective at giving the suppressor cells a final signal than the intact myeloma cells themselves. It might just mean that suppressor cells are at different stages of maturation and/or activation, depending on how you generate them.

LYNCH: In fact, Dr. Abbas, just to simplify the issue, to refer to the point that Dr. Cerny asked about, I said that the soluble idiotype would provide the signal to the T cell. The studies, however, did not distinguish between whether it was secreted idiotype and/or another secreted product that provided the signal. This is an important point and will be addressed in future studies. Presumably what it is secreting across that Marbrook chamber may include more than just the immunoglobulin.

CERNY: What will happen if you use as a source of xenogeneic immune T cells, rat T cells, for example, rat immunized with a MOPC 315 myeloma protein, and add them to the system?

LYNCH: We have never done that. All the studies that we have done have been in the syngeneic system with the idea that we are trying to look at autoregulatory circuitry. So I do not know what the answer is.

Idiotypy of Clonal Responses of Mice to Influenza B Virus Hemagglutinin[a]

Y.-N. LIU, J. L. SCHULMAN, AND C. A. BONA

Department of Microbiology
Mount Sinai School of Medicine
City University of New York
New York, New York 10029

Antigenic variation among influenza viruses in nature constitutes one of the major obstacles to control of pandemic and epidemic influenza. As antigenically novel strains appear in nature, the protective effects of antibody directed to earlier strains are circumvented, and the new strains are freely transmitted. Two forms of antigenic variation among influenza A viruses, antigenic shift and antigenic drift have been described.[1] The former has been attributed to genetic recombination among human influenza A viruses and influenza viruses present in nonhuman populations, resulting in new viruses possessing novel surface antigens derived from the animal influenza virus.[2-4] Antigenic drift on the other hand, which has been observed both in influenza A and influenza B viruses can be defined as stepwise mutations that result in gradual changes in antigenic structure. Subsequent selection of variants in the presence of antibody to previous strains favors the emergence of antigenic variants.[1]

In the past few years, monoclonal antibodies to viral hemagglutinin have been used to select for antigenic variants of influenza viruses in the laboratory. These variants then were compared to wild type virus hemagglutinin (HA) with respect to nucleotide sequences and amino acid sequences determined by peptide mapping to determine the specific amino acid substitutions associated with changes in antigenic sites.[5,6] Information obtained from such analyses, in conjunction with data obtained from x-ray crystallography permitted Wiley, *et al.*[7] to construct a three-dimensional model of the H3 hemagglutinin on which four antigenically important regions could be identified.

We have been interested in the clonal responses of mice to influenza virus hemagglutinin. In particular, we have been concerned with the question of whether antibodies specific for different regions of the HA molecule and antibodies specific for different antigenic variants are derived from distinct germ line genes or from B cells generated from common precursor clones.

In these studies we have relied on idiotypes as phenotypic markers of V-region genes to investigate the diversity of clonal responses to influenza virus hemagglutinin. In our initial studies, we demonstrated extensive cross-reactive idiotypy among monoclonal antibodies to distinct antigenic determinants on the hemagglutinin of influenza A/PR/8/34 (H1N1) virus. Analyses of idiotypes on monoclonal antibodies to the HA of B/Lee virus revealed individual idiotypes not shared by any other monoclonal antibody, idiotypic determinants shared by a few monoclonal antibodies, and cross-reactive idiotypes that could be detected on all of the monoclonal antibodies tested. In addition, we examined the idiotypes expressed during primary and secondary responses of BALB/c mice immunized with influenza B/Lee virus and found that

[a]This work was supported by Research Grants AI14053, AI103304, and AI18316 from the U.S. Public Health Service.

356

some cross-reactive idiotypes were expressed during both primary and secondary responses, whereas others were detected only in the primary or secondary response.[8]

In the present communication, we have extended these observations to examine the ontogeny of the cross-reactive idiotype response and to determine whether its expression is under major histocompatibility complex (MHC) or IghC control. In addition, we have studied the idiotypes expressed by BALB/c mice in response to immunization with natural variants of B/Lee virus.

RESULTS

Shared Idiotypes among Monoclonal Antibodies to B/Lee Virus Hemagglutinin

TABLE 1 summarizes data obtained by competition radioimmunoassay and demonstrates shared idiotypic determinants among different monoclonal antibodies to B/Lee virus hemagglutinin. Although much lower concentrations of B142 and B123 were required to inhibit binding of ^{125}I-labeled B142 to purified anti-B123 coated plates, at higher concentrations, other monoclonal antibodies also were capable of inhibiting

TABLE 1. Sharing of Idiotypic Determinants among Different Monoclonal Antibodies Specific for Influenza B/Lee Virus Hemagglutinin

Monoclonal antibody	Concentration (μg/ml) required for 50% inhibition of binding of ^{125}I-labeled B142 to anti-B123
BY104	70
B109	30
B118	30
B123	0.27
B142	0.23

binding. It should be noted that BY104 is a monoclonal antibody obtained from a different fusion from that from which the other monoclonal antibodies were obtained, indicating that sharing of idiotypes is not restricted to monoclonal antibodies obtained from a single fusion. Similar evidence of cross-reactive idiotypes was obtained in a hemagglutination inhibition assay (data not shown).

Ontogeny of the Cross-Reactive Idiotype Response

BALB/c mice of different ages were immunized with purified B/Lee virus (10 μg protein), and then serum anti-viral and cross-reactive idiotype (IdX) responses were determined 7 days later by assays of anti-viral hemagglutination inhibition (HI) titers and competition radioimmunoassay, respectively. It can be seen in TABLE 2 that newborn mice failed to generate a detectable anti-viral response and that their pooled sera did not contain significant levels of antibody capable of inhibiting the binding of ^{125}I-labeled B142 to plates coated with purified anti-B123. By contrast, immunization of mice 7 days of age or older resulted in the production of both virus-specific antibody and of antibody capable of low but significant levels of inhibition in the B142 anti-B123 system.

TABLE 2. Ontogeny of Cross-Reactive Idiotype Detected by Competitive Radioimmunoassay

Age of Mice (days)	Number of Mice Studied	Anti-viral HI Titer ($\log_2$)	Percent Inhibition of Binding
0	5	0	8.7
7	6	2.7 ± .5	19.3 ± 10.2
14	5	4.0 ± .7	18.3 ± 6.5
21	5	3.2 ± .8	21.6 ± 14.0
28	5	4.2 ± .9	27.3 ± 5.2

Similarly, pools of the same sera were tested by hemagglutination inhibition assay using sheep red blood cells coated with B142 and anti-B123. Again, only the sera obtained from mice 7 days of age or older inhibited agglutination. These results indicate that clones bearing the B142 IdX appear shortly after birth and persist in adult mice.

Genetics of the IdX Response

Various strains of mice of different MHC and IghC haplotypes were immunized with 10 μg of B/Lee virus and 4 weeks later were reimmunized with the same antigen. Sera obtained before immunization and after primary and secondary immunization were tested for anti-viral antibody and expression of cross-reactive idiotype. All of the strains studied showed significant primary and secondary anti-viral responses, and in all strains, anti-viral HI titers were higher after secondary immunization than after primary immunization. No significant differences in titers were detected (data not shown).

The same sera were individually tested by hemagglutination-inhibition assay using sheep erythrocytes (SRBC) coated with B123 and anti-B118. As seen in TABLE 3, all of the strains showed significant increases in the titers of the cross-reactive idiotype in either the primary or secondary response to immunization, or in both. Thus, whereas

TABLE 3. Expression of Cross-Reactive Idiotype in Sera of Different Strains of Mice Immunized with Influenza B Virus

Strain	MHC	Igh-C	Hemagglutinating Inhibiting Titer[a] day		
			0	10 Primary	7 Secondary
BALB/c	d	a	0	6.0	6.4
C.B 20	d	d	0	5.3	6.3
DBA/2J	d	c	1.0	4.2	8.0
CE/J	k	f	0	1.5	8.0
AKR/J	k	d	0	0	7.8
CBA/J	k	j	0	5.0	7.2
DBA/1J	q	c	0	7.3	1.0
A/J	a	e	0	6.0	6.4
RIII S/J	r	g	0	4.8	5.2
PL/J	μ	j	0	8.0	2.3

[a]$\log_2$ serum dilution inhibiting agglutination of SRB2-B123 by anti-B118.

CE/J and AKR/J mice showed significant increases in titer only in the secondary response, titers of IdX in DBA/J and PL/J mice were higher after primary immunization than after secondary immunization. Similar results were obtained using pools of these sera in HI assays with SRBC-B142 and anti-B123 and SRBC-B118 and anti-B142 (data not shown). In addition, the same sera were tested by radioimmunoassay used to measure inhibition binding of ^{125}I-labeled B142 to wells coated with purified anti-B123. Again, increases in the level of inhibition were detected in the sera of all strains following primary and secondary immunization (data not shown). These results demonstrate that the expression of IdX following immunization with B/Lee virus is not under MHC or IghC gene control.

Attempts were also made to detect the expression of IdX in sera of other species (rat, chicken, rabbit, and guinea pig) following immunization with B/Lee virus. The preimmune sera, however, of these species contained varying levels of nonspecific inhibitor so that assessment of the effects of virus immunization could not be readily interpreted.

TABLE 4. Anti-Viral Hemagglutinating Inhibiting Antibody Titers in Mice Immunized with Different Natural Variants of Influenza B Virus

Virus Used in Immunization	HI Titer[a] (log$_2$) Against Immunizing Virus			HI Titer[a] (log$_2$) Against B/Lee/40 Virus		
	Day 0	Primary Day 10	Secondary Day 7	Day 0	Primary Day 10	Secondary Day 7
B/GL/54	0	3.4 ± .7	5.4 ± 2.1	0	0	.8 ± 1.1
B/Md/59	0	3.4 ± .3	5.8 ± 1.1	0	1.0 ± 0	2.8 ± .8
B/Vict/70	0	2.0 ± .7	3.4 ± .3	0	.2 ± .4	1.2 ± .7
B/HK/8/72	0	3.0 ± .7	6.2 ± .8	0	0	1.8 ± .4

[a]Values represent mean ± S.D. for five mice.

Expression of IdX in Mice Immunized with Natural Variants of Influenza B/Lee Virus

In this section of our study we were interested in determining whether antibodies made to naturally occurring variants of B/Lee virus also expressed the same minor cross-reactive idiotype detected in the B142 anti-B123 system. The viruses selected for this study were isolated between 1954 and 1972 and have been shown in conventional serologic assays to be clearly distinguishable antigenically from B/Lee virus. None of the monoclonal antibodies employed in the present study had detectable hemagglutinating inhibiting activity against any of the variants, and neither B142 and B118 showed significant binding to any of the variants in radioimmunoassay (data not shown).

As shown in TABLE 4, all of the mice had significant primary and secondary responses to the immunizing virus when assayed by conventional anti-viral HI titration. Sera obtained after primary immunization had either no detectable activity or very low levels of activity against B/Lee virus, but secondary sera had low levels of cross-reactivity with B/Lee virus.

The same sera were individually employed in competition radioimmunoassay to measure the levels of inhibition in the B142 anti-B123 system. As shown in TABLE 5, significant increases in the expression of the B142 IdX were detected in all cases, although the level of inhibiton was not great.

TABLE 5. Expression of Cross-Reactive Idiotype in Sera of Mice Immunized with Different Natural Variants of Influenza B Virus

Virus Used in Immunization	Idiotype response (percent inhibition of binding)[a]		
	Day 0	Primary Day 10	Secondary Day 7
B/GL/54	−2.3 ± 5.0	14.2 ± 4.7	21.4 ± 6.1
B/Md/59	9.7 ± 12.5	26.4 ± 7.2	40.1 ± 8.9
B/Vict/70	−3.8 ± 10.0	23.1 ± 10.2	20.6 ± 6.9
B/HK/8/72	−7 ± 9.5	15.1 ± 7.8	30.7 ± 6.4

[a]Values represent percent inhibition ± S.D. for five mice in each group. Purified BALB/c αB123Id (30μg/ml) was used to coat the wells. 25λ of undiluted sera along with 25λ of 50,000 cpm of radiolabeled B142 were added to each well.

To confirm these findings, pools were made of the same sera that were then tested in a hemagglutination inhibiton assay, using SRBC coated with B118 and purified anti-B142. As shown in TABLE 6, increases in the expression of IdX were observed following immunization with all of the variants in either the primary or secondary response or in both.

DISCUSSION

In the present studies we have confirmed and extended our earlier observation of cross-reactive idiotypy among monoclonal antibodies to influenza virus hemmagglutinin.[8] This cross-reactivity is not restricted to monoclonal antibodies directed to the same or overlapping epitopes, as evidenced by our earlier observation that monoclonal antibodies to distinct antigenic determinants on the hemagglutinin of PR8 virus also show cross-reactive idiotypy. Similar cross-reactive idiotypy has been observed previously in other systems among monoclonal antibodies to different determinants on the same molecule,[9,10] antibodies to different antigenic molecules,[11–13] and antibodies of unknown specificity.[11,14] It is tempting to speculate that such evidence of shared idiotypy among monoclonal antibodies to different determinants on the same molecule may reflect idiotype regulation mediated by idiotype specific T-helper cells. Other possibilities, however, are equally plausible, and the limited data obtained thus far in the influenza virus system do not provide an adequate basis to distinguish among these possibilities.

TABLE 6. Expression of a Cross-Reactive Idiotype in Sera of Mice Immunized with Natural Variants of Influenza B Virus

Virus Used in Immunization	Hemagglutinating-inhibiting titer[a]		
	Day 0	Primary Day 10	Secondary Day 7
B/GL/54	NA[b]	4	4
B/Md/59	0	4	4
B/Vict/70	0	3	0
B/HK/72	0	3	NA

[a]SRBC coated with B118 plus anti-B142; titers expressed as $\log_2$
[b]Serum pool not available.

The expression of IdX in the immune responses of different strains of mice immunized with B/Lee virus are in accord with those previously observed in BALB/c mice.[8] Although relatively low levels of inhibition were observed in the competition radioimmunoassay system employed, increases in the level of inhibition were observed in all strains of mice irrespective of H_2 or IghC haplotype, and confirmation of the results was obtained in a hemagglutinating inhibiting assay. Taken together, these results suggest that the IdX detected in this system is probably only a minor component of the B/Lee HA repertoire, but that the V-region genes affected are probably of germ line origin and are probably present in all strains of mice.

Similarly, detection of the IdX in the response of BALB/c mice to natural variants of B/Lee virus suggest that the same germ line genes are employed in the response to variants. Although mutations affecting antibody specificity occur during clonal expansion following antigenic stimulation, idiotypic specificities remain unaltered. Thus, although it is possible that the low level of expression of IdX seen following immunization with the variants is restricted to that component of the response that is reactive with B/Lee virus, it is more likely that in part it reflects antibody molecules reactive only with the variants.

REFERENCES

1. WEBSTER, R. G. & W. G. LAVER. 1975. Antigen variation of influenza viruses. *In* The Influenza Viruses and Influenza. E. D. Kilbourne, Ed.: 269–314. Academic Press. New York.
2. SCHOLTISSEK, C., W. ROHODE, V. VON HOYNIGEN & R. ROTT. 1978. On the origin of the human influenza virus subtypes H2N2 and H3N2. Virology 87: 13–20.
3. HINSHAW, V. S., W. J. BEAN, R. G. WEBSTER & G. SPIRAM. 1980. Genetic reassortment of influenza viruses in the intestinal tract of ducks. Virology 102: 412–419.
4. LAVER, W. G. & R. G. WEBSTER. 1973. Studies on the origin of pandemic influenza. Evidence implicating duck and equine influenza viruses as possible progenitors of the Hong Kong strain of human influenza. Virology 51: 383–391.
5. LAVER, W. G., G. M. AIR, R. G. WEBSTER, W. GERHARD, C. W. WARD & T. A. A. DOPHEIDE. 1979. Antigenic drift in type A influenza viruses. Sequence differences in the hemagglutinin of Hong Kong (H3N2) variants selected with monoclonal antibodies. Virology 98: 226–237.
6. SLEIGH, M. J., G. W. BOTH, P. A. UNDERWOOD & J. BENDER. 1981. Antigenic drift in the hemagglutinin of Hong Kong influenza subtype: Correlation of amino acid changes with alterations in viral antigenicity. J. Virol. 37: 845–853.
7. WILEY, D. C., I. A. WILSON & J. J. SKEHEL. 1981. Structural identification of the antibody binding sites of Hong Kong influenza hemagglutinin and their involvement in antigenic variation. Nature (London) 283: 373–378.
8. LIU, Y. N., C. A. BONA & J. L. SCHULMAN. 1981. Idiotypy of clonal responses to influenza virus hemagglutinin. J. Exp. Med. 154: 1524–1538.
9. KAROL, R., M. REICHLIN & R. W. NOBLE. 1978. Idiotypic crossreactivity between antibodies of different specificity. J. Exp. Med. 148: 1488–1497.
10. JU, S-T, B. BENACEROFF & M. E. DORF. 1980. Genetic control of a shared idiotype among antibodies directed to distinct specificities. J. Exp. Med. 152: 170–182.
11. OUDIN, J. & P. A. CAZENAVE. 1974. Similar idiotypic specificities in immunoglobulin fractions with different antibody functions or even without detectable antibody function. Proc. Natl. Acad. Sci. USA 168: 2616–2620.
12. KOHNO, Y., I. BERKOWER, J. MINNA & J. A. BERZOFSKY. 1982. Idiotype of anti-myoglobulin antibodies: shared idiotypes among monoclonal antibodies to distinct determinants of sperm whale myoglobulin. J. Immunol. 128: 1742–1748.
13. HIERNAUX, J. & C. BONA. 1978. Shared idiotypes among monoclonal antibodies specific for

different immunodocument sugars of lipopolysaccharide of different gram negative bacteria. Proc. Natl. Acad. Sci. USA **79:** 1616–1620.

14. EICHMANN, K., A. COUTINHO & F. MELCHERS. 1977. Absolute frequencies of lipopolysaccharide-reactive B cells producing A5A idiotype in unprimed anti-A5A-idiotype serialized and anti A5A idiotype suppressed A/J mice. J. Exp. Med. **146:** 1436–1449.

DISCUSSION OF THE PAPER

H. G. KUNKEL (*The Rockefeller University, New York*): Do you have any evidence that a given cross-reactive idiotype among your monoclonal antibodies reacts with a similar site in the model that you showed in one of your early slides. Is there any evidence that the anti-idiotype selects those monoclonals that react with a certain site?

J. L. SCHULMAN: We do not have sufficient mapping data with regard to our population of monoclonal antibodies to be able to determine the specific sites to which they are directed, so we cannot answer that question. It obviously would be very interesting to address.

D. A. HAFLER (*Harvard Medical School, Boston, Mass.*): Have you had the opportunity to study the binding of the anti-idiotype to the viral receptors themselves?

SCHULMAN: I am familiar with the fact that in the reovirus system, of course, it has been shown that the anti-idiotype antibody binds directly to receptors for HA of virus. This is not the case in influenza. As I pointed out with the model, it is very clear from the structural studies that have been obtained that the binding site or the proposed binding site on the hemagglutinin is not identical with any of those epitopes, or any of those determinants, but is probably in a pocket surrounded by these antigenic determinants. Therefore one would not expect that anti-idiotype reagents would bind to receptors. We have looked at it, and they do not.

J. M. KEHOE (*Northeast Ohio Universities College of Medicine, Rootstown, Ohio*): This may be premature, but have you had any chance to look at the in *vivo* systems? If you prime with any of the monoclonals, do the mice show a differential response to vaccine in any of these systems?

SCHULMAN: Those studies are underway right now. The sera have been obtained and we should have some information shortly.

Anti-Idiotypic Antibodies and Autoantibodies[a]

MAURIZIO ZANETTI

Department of Immunology
Medical Biology Institute
La Jolla, California 92037

INTRODUCTION

To date, Jerne's hypothesis[1] that idiotype (id) and anti-idiotypes, both as soluble products in the serum and as lymphocyte receptors, are involved in a complex network of interactions that regulate immune responsiveness has been supported by many observations. Much of the available information, however, stems from experiments in which anti-idiotypic responses were generated by intentional and often unphysiological immunization with antigen or idiotype. More importantly, in the majority of the cases, the antigens used were foreign to the animal's own internal milieu. Thus, whether, and to what extent, idiotypic network rules apply to regulation of responsiveness to antigens of internal origin (self or autoantigens), in particular those involved in the pathogenesis of autoimmune diseases, is still largely unverified. In the strictest sense, every idiotype within the repertoire of possible idiotypes is in turn a self antigen for complementary anti-idiotype. In this respect, the rules established for regulation of autologous idiotype should be applicable to any autoantigen. Nevertheless, we would like to concentrate on those nonpolymorphic organ-specific self antigens that normally do not stimulate an immune response, and when they do so, autoimmune diseases are often initiated.

As shown in a variety of systems, anti-idiotypic immunity can be a potent and very specific way of inducing immunosuppression[2] and generating tolerance.[3] Because the natural occurrence of anti-idiotypic antibodies to idiotypes associated with autoantibodies has already been suggested in a few instances,[4,5] the possibility that regulation of autoreactivity may be under idiotypic control is not unlikely. Thus, it is not unreasonable to speculate that the production of autoantibodies may be favored by lack of down-regulation of autoreactive clones at their emergence by quantitatively insufficient or functionally inefficient anti-idiotypes or anti-idiotype-driven regulatory mechanisms. Conversely, one should bear in mind that it might also be possible that anti-idiotypes cause direct potentiation of responsiveness to self and/or autoimmune processes.

Elucidating the role of network regulation in the reactivity to autoantigens is important not only for clarifying the physiological role of idiotype-anti-idiotype interactions in the maintenance of immunological tolerance vis-a-vis the components of the body constituents, but also for designing new strategies of treatment for autoimmune diseases. In this paper, we will analyze some of these aspects by using anti-idiotypes as probes for the analysis of the complexity of autoantibodies and as putative candidates for *in vivo* regulation of autoimmune disorders.

[a]This is publication Number 20 from the Medical Biology Institute, La Jolla, California. This work was supported by a research grant from QUIDEL, La Jolla, California.

MATERIALS AND METHODS

All materials and methods are described in detail in the following references (see references 6, 7, 9, 10, and 13).

RESULTS

Anti-Idiotypic Antibodies as Probes for Dissecting the Complexity of Autoantibodies

Autoantibodies are often polyclonal and possibly directed against different regions and epitopes on autoantigens. As a consequence, the relative pathogenicity of the various populations of autoantibodies in the serum is difficult to assess. Because similar idiotypic determinants may be distributed on antibody molecules that have in common their specificity for the same antigen, if not the same epitope, anti-idiotypes can be conveniently used to dissect autoimmune responses.

We have tried to address this question using an experimental model of organ-specific autoimmune disease, the tubulointerstitial nephritis (TIN) in the Brown-Norway (BN) rat. This disease is mediated by deposition, along the tubular basement membrane (TBM) of the kidney, of antibodies whose production is triggered by immunization with heterologous, bovine, crude TBM emulsified in complete Freund's adjuvant. The resulting antibody response is highly heterogeneous, ranging from antibodies reacting with antigenic determinants unique to the species of the immunogen, to others specific for autologous TBM antigens, that is, autoantibodies. Using TBM preparations of different chemical nature, it has been possible to establish that serum antibodies react with collagenous moieties present in the particulate (P) form of TBM and with glycoproteins that remain after collagenase solubilization (CS) of the tubular basement membrane. By contrast, the majority of anti-TBM IgG eluted from kidneys with TIN are primarily reactive with a molecular weight of 42,000 CS TBM antigen. From this, and other criteria, we have suggested that autoantibodies to CS TBM are of pathogenetic importance in this model of disease.[6]

To see whether anti-idiotypic antibodies could be of any advantage in assessing the relative pathogenicity of serum TBM autoantibodies, we prepared anti-idiotypic sera

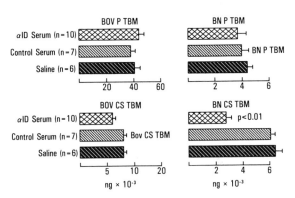

FIGURE 1. Levels of circulating anti-TBM antibodies reacting with P or CS TBM at day 15. Values, ng/ml as detected by solid phase radioimmunoassays, are expressed as mean ± SEM.

TABLE 1. Effects of Anti-Idiotypic Serum on Histological Lesions of Tubulointerstitual Nephritis

Group	Pretreatment	Number of Rats	Cortical Involvement (Percent)			
			0	<25	25–50	50–100
I	Anti-Idiotypic Serum	10	4	3	1	2
II	Normal Rabbit Serum	7	0	2	2	3
III	Saline	6	0	3	0	3

by immunizing rabbits with IgG eluted from TIN kidneys.[7] The obtained antisera were made idiotype specific by extensive adsorption with nonimmune BN gamma globulins and autologous tubular basement membanes. One of the antisera was able to precipitate, albeit only 14%, ^{125}I-labeled anti-TBM IgG eluted from TIN kidneys and partially block the binding of anti-TBM antibodies to TBM in an indirect immuno-fluorescence test. Therefore, this particular serum was retained for this study.

The question we asked was whether this anti-idiotypic serum could affect the *in vivo* production of autoantibodies to CS TBM, and as a consequence of this, the appearance or the severity of tubulointerstitial nephritis. To this end, one ml of anti-idiotypic serum was injected intraperitoneally into rats (group I) 48 hours prior to immunization with bovine tubular basement membrane. Control animals concurrently received normal rabbit serum (group II) or saline (group III). Two weeks after immunization, the levels of circulating antibodies to TBM antigens were determined for each group and compared. As shown in FIGURE 1, anti-idiotype treatment did not induce any noticeable effect on the production of antibodies to heterologous P or CS TBM as compared to control groups. Similarly, the amount of autoantibodies to P TBM was substantially the same in all three groups. Antibodies to autologous CS TBM, however, were significantly lower ($p < 0.01$) in the group that received anti-idiotype. Whereas the difference remained significant through the third week, at the moment of sacrifice, on week four, similar values were found in all three groups (3515 ± 427, 4530 ± 502, and 5361 ± 724 ng/ml, respectively) suggesting the transient nature of the suppressive effect of anti-idiotype treatment. By light micros-copy (TABLE 1), histological lesions of TIN, that is, lymphomonocytic infiltration of cortical interstitium, were clearly less severe in the 10 rats receiving anti-idiotype than in the 13 control rats. By direct immunofluorescence of the kidneys, the majority (6/10) of the anti-idiotype treated rats showed a weaker staining for IgG than control rats. In conclusion, we have verified the premise that anti-idiotypic antibodies against a selected population of autoantibodies, that is, those primarily involved in the pathogen-esis of the disease, could partially suppress both autoantibody production and development of the disease.

Antibodies to Autoantigens Show Large Idiotypic Cross-Reactivity: the Thyroglobulin System

The results obtained in the aforementioned experiment carry a major implication, that is, autoantibodies reacting with the same antigen may have a high degree of idiotypic cross-reactivity. A better analysis of this point can be derived from the studies carried out on the idiotype of autoantibodies to a relatively well-characterized autoantigen, thyroglobulin (Tg). This glycoprotein, which constitutes more than half of the proteins present in the thyroid gland, has been implicated in the pathogenesis of chronic spontaneous thyroiditis in humans and animals and has also been successfully used in experimental animal models to closely duplicate the immunopathological features of the spontaneous disease.[8]

The model we used is the spontaneous autoimmune thyroiditis (SAT) in the inbred strain of Buffalo (BUF) rats. In this strain, spontaneously occurring autoantibodies to thyroglobulin are found in 15% of rats after six months of age and are always associated with the finding of lymphomonocytic infiltration of the thyroid. Interestingly, their incidence is greatly increased by neonatal thymectomy (NTx) suggesting the participation of lymphocytes of thymic origin in the regulation of autoreactivity to autologous thyroglobulin. Thus, because autoantibodies arise from an endogenous stimulation, the conditions of autosensitization, expansion of autoreactive clones, and production of autoantibodies are the product of a very natural event. Similarly, the

TABLE 2. Specificity of Anti-Idiotypic Serum 276

Serum Number	Immunogen Used	Adsorbed With	^{125}I-labeled ART Binding (Percent)	Inhibition (Percent)[a] ^{125}I-labeled RT Binding
274	ART Negative BUF IgG	ART Neg. BUF IgG	1	4
277	BUF IgG Depleted ART	BUF IgG Depleted ART	2	0
276	ART	(a) BUF IgG Depleted ART	31	51
		(b) Effluent of (a) through ART$^+$ IgG column	10	18
		(c) Eluate from column used in b.	24	40
Preimmune			2	0

[a]Percent inhibition calculated through the formula:

$$\frac{\begin{array}{c}\% \text{ binding after preincubation} \\ \text{with preimmune serum}\end{array} - \begin{array}{c}\% \text{ binding after preincubation} \\ \text{with anti-idiotype 276}\end{array}}{\% \text{ binding after preincubation with preimmune serum}} \times 100$$

expression of idiotype on autoantibodies must also be determined through a physiological process within the limits of the natural available repertoire.

Pooled BUF affinity-purified antibodies (IgG$_{2b}$ and IgG$_1$) to rat thyroglobulin (ART) were used to immunize a rabbit whose serum was made specific for ART-idiotype by extensive adsorption on pooled BUF IgG lacking autoantibodies to rat thyroglobulin.[9] The resulting antiserum (#276) was able to directly bind ^{125}I-labeled ART and conversely inhibit the binding of ART to ^{125}I-labeled rat thyroglobulin. As shown in TABLE 2, adsorption of the anti-idiotype through an ART column removed the anti-idiotypic activity. This activity was recovered in the eluate.

Because the binding of ART to ^{125}I-labeled rat thyroglobulin (RT) was only partially inhibited, 51%, we investigated whether this phenomenon was due to a restriction in the recognition of ART by anti-idiotype. To this end, the inhibition assay was repeated on various ART populations as obtained by preparative isoelectrofocusing. As shown in FIGURE 2, all but one fraction were inhibited, with a percentage of

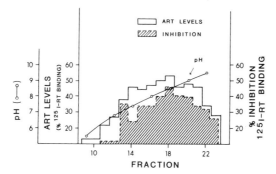

FIGURE 2. Preparative isoelectrofocusing of pooled serum ART IgG from BUF rats with SAT. Presence of a cross-reacting ART-idiotype on ART populations migrating at different isoelectric points as detected by inhibition of the binding of ART to ^{125}I-labeled RT in a fluid phase assay. Percent inhibition calculated as indicated in footnote of TABLE 2.

inhibition ranging from 24% to 45%, hence suggesting that ART migrating at different isoelectric points share idiotype. Using this assay, we then searched for the existence and the distribution of this common idiotype (ART-idiotype) in the serum of individual BUF rats. The results are shown in FIGURE 3. The majority, 67%, of sera tested were inhibited, the percent of inhibition ranging from 11% to 47% of the original ^{125}I-labeled RT binding. No relationship was found between the degree of inhibition and the level of circulating ART, nor did it make any difference whether the sera were from NTx rats. Because the rats used for this study were unrelated to those used to prepare ART idiotype, one must conclude that spontaneous autoantibodies to Tg in BUF rats share idiotype. Because the assay employed, however, was discriminatory only for idiotype located within or close to the antigen-combining site, the likelihood that the same common idiotype may be present in all rats, albeit not always in association with the antigen-combining site, could not be ruled out.

Because a great majority of BUF rats do not usually develop SAT nor have detectable serum ART, it has been possible to search for the existence of ART-idiotype

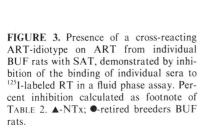

FIGURE 3. Presence of a cross-reacting ART-idiotype on ART from individual BUF rats with SAT, demonstrated by inhibition of the binding of individual sera to ^{125}I-labeled RT in a fluid phase assay. Percent inhibition calculated as footnote of TABLE 2. ▲-NTx; ●-retired breeders BUF rats.

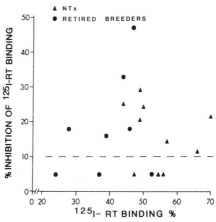

TABLE 3. Presence of Buffalo Autoantibodies to Rat Thyroglobulin Idiotype among Antibodies to Rat Thyroglobulin from Various Species

Species	Type of Antibodies	Individual Sera Inhibited	Percent Inhibition[a]	
			Anti-id	Control
Rat (BUF)	Spontaneous	12/18	23 ± 9	2 ± 2
	Induced	7/9	25 ± 8	1 ± 2
Human	Spontaneous	2/2	58 ± 6	19 ± 8
Guinea Pig	Induced	2/2	66 ± 4	12 ± 4
Rabbit	Induced	2/2	71 ± 1	10 ± 1

[a]Inhibition test and percent inhibition as indicated in footnote of TABLE 2.

on antibodies induced by means of active immunization with RT in adjuvant.[10] Interestingly, seven out of nine rats studied appeared to bear ART-id (TABLE 3). In the course of this investigation, we decided to test antibodies reacting with RT from other species, namely human sera from patients with Hashimoto's thyroiditis and sera from guinea pigs and rabbits immunized with rat thyroglobulin. The results are summarized in TABLE 3 and show that ART-idiotype previously identified on spontaneous rat autoantibodies are also present on spontaneous or induced antibodies to RT from various species.

We made a similar finding recently while studying the degree of idiotypic cross-reactivity among a group of murine monoclonal antibodies reacting with an epitope on the thyroglobulin molecule that is common to human, mouse, and rat antigen.[11] No inhibition was found using a thousand-fold excess of monoclonal antibodies against 2,4-dinitrophenyl. As shown in TABLE 4, not only did a high proportion of the monoclonal antibodies against Tg bear one idiotype (#62), but more surprisingly this was also present on spontaneous antibodies to RT in human and rat sera of the BUF and BB (spontaneously diabetic rat) (TABLE 5). To conclude this section, there is sufficient evidence to support the concept that autoantibodies to Tg are idiotypically cross-reactive. As shown in some instances, this idiotype may rather be conserved.

TABLE 4. Sharing of Idiotype 62 among Murine Monoclonal Antibodies

Antibody	Isotype	Antigen Specificity	Inhibition of the Binding of 62 to Anti-id 4115	Inhibition by Anti-id 4115 of the Binding to Antigen[a]
62[b]	IgG$_1$κ	Tg	+ + + +	+ + + +
60	IgG$_1$κ	Tg	+ + + +	+ + + +
1'15	IgG$_1$κ	Tg	+ + + +	+ + + +
8'2	IgMκ	Tg	0	+
9'1	IgG$_1$κ	Tg	0	+
109'3[c]	IgG$_1$κ	DNP	0	0
10'12	IgG$_{2b}$λ	DNP	0	0
MGG			0	

[a]Binding to RT performed using a solid phase ELISA assay.
[b]Monoclonal antibody used to prepare anti-id 4115.
[c]Courteously obtained from Dr. F.-T. Liu.[12]

TABLE 5. Presence of Idiotype 62 on Spontaneous Autoantibodies to Rat Thyroglobulin

Species	Strain	Individual Sera Inhibited	Percent Specific Inhibition by Anti-id 4115[a]	Range
Human		2/5	30 ± 5	26–34
Rat	BUF	9/20	24 ± 6	18–37
	BB	2/3	29 ± 5	26–33

[a]Inhibition test and percent inhibition as indicated in footnote of TABLE 2. Binding to RT performed using a solid phase ELISA assay.

In Vivo *Effects of Anti-Idiotype on the Ongoing Production of Spontaneous Autoantibodies*

As shown in the first section, the *in vivo* administration of anti-idiotype before induction of autoimmunity resulted in significant suppression of autoantibody formation and partial prevention of the disease. One may argue, however, that this approach is not relevant for already established autoimmunity, as is the case in human autoimmune diseases. In order to explore the possible regulation by anti-idiotype on ongoing production of autoantibodies, the effect of passive anti-idiotypic immunity was investigated in BUF rats with overt spontaneous autoimmune thyroiditis.[10] We had previously estimated that a relatively large number (0.6–1.2%) of spleen lymphocytes from BUF rats with SAT bear ART-idiotype positive receptors.[11] Therefore, to favor any eventual effect by anti-idiotype, we attempted to eliminate most lymphocytes already sensitized to RT by sublethal x-irradiation (675 rads). By doing this, anti-idiotype would only compete with newly emerging autoreactive clones. An initial intraperitoneal injection of anti-idiotype (2 ml) was given 24 hours after x-irradiation followed by five similar injections at weekly intervals.

As shown in FIGURE 4, circulating ART decreased in all rats with SAT (Group I) given anti-idiotype when compared to their pretreatment value. The negative change observed was statistically significant ($p < 0.05–0.01$) throughout the experiment when compared to the percent of change obtained in the control group (II) receiving control

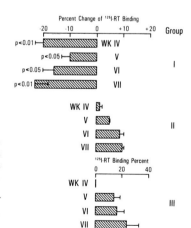

FIGURE 4. *In vivo* effects of treatment with anti-idiotype on the ongoing production of spontaneous ART in BUF rats. Results of group I and II are expressed as mean ± SD of the change of ^{125}I-labeled RT binding percent from the pretreatment value. Results of group III are expressed as mean ± SD of direct ^{125}I-labeled RT binding as determined by a fluid phase assay.

serum (serum from a rabbit immunized with ART negative IgG adsorbed with insolubilized normal rat gamma globulins). In this latter group, serum ART levels showed a modest but continuous increase over pretreatment values. Most likely, this effect resulted from the initial x-irradiation as suggested by the results obtained in group III. Starting from week 5, 4 out of 5 rats that did not have detectable autoantibodies at the beginning of the experiment, became ART positive after x-irradiation. To compensate for such a change, that might have also occurred in the anti-idiotype-treated rats, masking to a certain extent the effects of the treatment, we calculated the *in vivo* inhibition of ART in each rat treated with anti-idiotypic antibodies. This was obtained by adding to the absolute value of the percent change, from the pretreatment levels of serum ART in an individual rat, the mean value of the percent change in rats injected with control serum (Group II). In this fashion, we noticed that the maximum *in vivo* inhibition of ART reached 53%, whereas the minimum was 18 percent. As shown in FIGURE 5, anti-idiotype-treated rats (Group I of FIGURE 4) could be divided into two groups. One group (left panel on FIGURE 5) of four rats showed levels of *in vivo* inhibition between 46% and 53%; another (right panel on FIGURE 5) four rats had much lower inhibition levels, between 18% and 26 percent.

To conclude this section, we would like to summarize. Although in this experiment, treatment by anti-idiotype was only partially effective in reducing autoantibody production, a significant degree of suppression was nevertheless obtained. Thus, sequential passive anti-idiotypic immunity may be usefully adopted in controlling the ongoing production of autoantibodies. It remains to be defined, however, how long this type of immunosuppression may last, and more importantly, by which mechanism it is realized.

Participation of Auto-Anti-Idiotype to Immunopathologic Processes

Because of their integral role during the immune respone, anti-idiotypes represent a potential candidate for participation in immune response that can be harmful to the

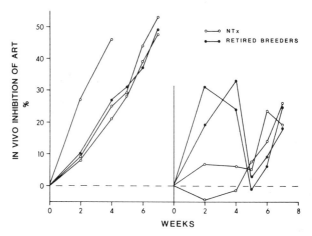

FIGURE 5. *In vivo* inhibition of ART production in individual BUF rats with ongoing SAT by anti-idiotype treatment. Open circles (O—O) refer to NTx and closed circles (●—●) refer to retired breeders BUF rats with SAT.

TABLE 6. Direct ELISA Binding Assay of Serum Fab$'_2$ Idiotype Bovine Serum Albumin[a] to Autologous Anti-Idiotype in the Immune Complexes Eluted from the Kidneys

Wells Coating	Blocking[b]	A$_{492}$
BSA (1 μg/ml)	−	0.341
	+	0.012
Kidney eluted IgG (5 μg/ml)	+	0.218
Autologous serum preimmune IgG	−	0.008
Syngeneic anti-idiotype (1/2000)	−	0.263
Preimmune serum	−	0.018

[a]Idiotype bovine serum albumin directly conjugated to horseradish peroxidase was incubated for 6 hours at +4° C. Bound peroxidase activity was revealed by addition of o-phenylenediamine and H$_2$O$_2$ for 15 minutes in the dark.
[b]Blocking obtained by overnight incubation with undiluted rat serum containing high affinity anti-BSA antibodies.

host. To approach this question, we looked for the presence of auto-anti-idiotype in the glomerular immune deposits of rabbits with chronic serum sickness, induced by daily intravenous injection of bovine serum albumin (BSA).[13]

The Fab$'_2$ fragments of serum anti-BSA antibodies of an early bleeding from one rabbit (#3262) were used as an idiotype probe (id-BSA). Following the daily BSA injections, rabbit #3262 subsequently developed immune-complex glomerulonephritis, as detected by immunofluorescence. The antibodies eluted from its kidneys were studied for the presence of auto-anti-idiotypes. To avoid contamination by BSA, the eluted material was initially adsorbed on a Blue-Sepharose CL-6B column and subsequently fractionated on sucrose gradient centrifugation under acidic conditions, in order to dissociate immune complexes. The 7S fraction (IgG) was collected, tested for anti-BSA activity and used to coat (5 μg/ml) polyvinyl microtiter wells. This material was employed as a source of putative anti-idiotypes in an enzyme-linked immunosorbent (ELISA) binding assay employing horseradish peroxidase-conjugated id-BSA as a probe. Anti-idiotypic antibodies to id-BSA produced in a syngeneic rabbit were used as a positive control.

To rule out the possibility that fragments of BSA could still contaminate the 7S fraction, the microtiter wells were blocked overnight with high affinity rat anti-BSA serum, which in pilot experiments had shown to cause complete abrogation at the binding of id-BSA and other affinity-purified anti-BSA antibodies to BSA-coated wells. The results of the binding experiment are shown in TABLE 6.

As expected, id-BSA bound to wells coated with unblocked BSA and syngeneic anti-idiotype. On the other hand, preventive blocking with rat anti-BSA serum completely abrogated the binding of id-BSA to bovine serum albumin. Finally, binding occurred also in the wells coated with autologous IgG eluted from the kidney similarly blocked with rat anti-BSA serum. Thus, since binding through antigen (BSA) or by rheumatoid factor autoantibodies in the kidney eluate (Fab$'_2$ fragments were used as a probe) can be ruled out, the most likely possibility is that binding occurred because of Fab$'_2$ anti-BSA bound to anti-idiotypes. Whether the idiotype-anti-idiotype complex is formed in the bloodstream or in the tissue is not known. In view of the fact that the dynamics of immune-complex formation and their tissue deposition are subject to continuous variations dependent upon the relative serum concentration of each component, it is possible that the two mechanisms are mutually integrating. Nevertheless, the eventual *in situ* apposition of anti-idiotype to idiotype already bound to glomeruli may constitute a new mechanism of local augmentation and/or perpetuation of immune deposits.

DISCUSSION

It has been our aim to focus on the idiotypic relationship between autoantibodies, the possible use *in vivo* of anti-idiotypic immunity as a means for controlling autoantibodies production, and the eventual participation of auto-anti-idiotypes to diseases of immunological origin.

Antibodies to idiotypic markers on the variable region of the antibody molecules have been instrumental in discovering the existence of relatedness among molecules that have specificity for the same antigen.[14-16] In animals, following immunization with exogenous antigens, idiotypic cross-reactivity has been found among antibodies within the same individual,[17] the same strain,[18] and across strain[19,20] and species[21,22] barriers. Similarly, spontaneously occurring antibodies associated with certain autoimmune conditions have also been found to bear public idiotypes. Thus, in humans, shared idiotypy has been documented among cold agglutinin,[14] monoclonal[23] and polyclonal[24] rheumatoid factors, anti-Rhesus[25] and anti-acetylcholine receptor[26] antibodies, and IgG of the cerebrospinal fluid of individuals with multiple sclerosis.[27] Here, evidence was provided that a cross-reacting idiotype present on spontaneously occurring autoantibodies to thyroglobulin of BUF rats is shared by the majority of individuals in this strain. It was of interest to find that spontaneously occurring human antibodies from patients with Hashimoto's thyroiditis and induced antibodies to RT from various species also possessed the idiotype of BUF autoantibodies. Similarly, a high degree of idiotypic cross-reactivity was found among mouse monoclonal antibodies directed against a highly conserved epitope on mammalian thyroglobulin. This last observation does not substantially differ from what other groups have documented on monoclonal autoantibodies to DNA originated from spontaneously autoimmune mice.[28-31]

The ensemble of these results may have several explanations. It has been known for a long time that in most instances autoantibodies are heterogeneous populations of molecules. Where available, isoelectrofocusing analysis has shown[32,33] patterns with large number of bands, suggesting that the repertoire of autoimmune clones is not limited. On the other hand, idiotype analysis seems to suggest that the idiotypic repertoire used for the V regions of autoantibodies is a rather restricted one. From the few available studies, it has been possible to identify the structural correlate of idiotype to a sequence of very few amino acids.[34] Thus, to explain the observed cross-reactivity among autoantibodies, one would only require very limited structural homology between the various autoantibody molecules. Whether this phenomenon occurs because of the existence of germ line genes or as a consequence of a fortuitous effect of somatic mutation during the response to autoantigens is not known. Alternatively, one may envisage that phylogenetically highly conserved antigens such as autoantigens are immunogenic to the host immune system through an immunodominant domain on the molecule. This will in turn induce the production of antibodies idiotypically cross-reacting. Such an explanation could account for the finding of mouse idiotope 62 on spontaneous human and rat autoantibodies. Finally, one may consider that the immune response to autoantigens may use a limited number of idiotopes, regulatory idiotopes.[35] Compatible with this last possibility could be the hypothesis that the preferential expression of given idiotopes on autoantibodies V regions are associated with a particular, and yet unknown, immunological function as it has been recently shown for the T-15 idiotype in mice.[36]

Manipulation of the immune response in animals by way of idiotype-anti-idiotype interactions has been obtained in a number of antigen systems. There is no doubt that the importance of such an approach lies in its demonstrated usefulness as a specific way for selectively down-regulating biologically relevant phenomena such as alloreactivity in organ transplantation,[37] IgE response in allergic responses,[38] and secretion by myeloma cells.[39] Few attempts have also been made in animal models of autoimmune diseases. In the autoimmune TIN in rodents, passive[40] or active[41] anti-idiotypic immunity have both been able to markedly suppress the production of autoantibodies and diminish the intensity of histological signs of disease. In our hands, passively transferred anti-idiotypic antibodies were capable of selectively suppressing the production of one set of autoantibodies, that is, those specific for that portion of the autoantigen primarily responsible for initiation of the disease.

Considering the practical problems in clinical immunology, the more interesting finding is that sequential anti-idiotype treatment could regulate the formation of autoantibodies produced during an already established spontaneous autoimmune response. As shown in the BUF rats with overt ongoing SAT, a regimen of anti-idiotype given at regular intervals could partially, but significantly, suppress the total amount of circulating autoantibodies to thyroglobulin. We are presently unable to provide an explanation for the possible mechanism through which immunosuppression was obtained. Although the formation of immune complexes idiotype-rabbit anti-idiotype cannot be formally ruled out, we believe it is unlikely because the removal of rabbit immunoglobulin by immunoadsorption did not change the levels of autoantibodies to rat thyroglobulin in the sera of anti-idiotype-treated rats. Furthermore, no evidence of immune complex deposition could be found in any of the various organs examined at sacrifice by immunofluorescence. Suppression of an ongoing antibody production is not an unprecedented observation in the rapidly developing field of idiotypic manipulation of the immune response. In mice, a single treatment with anti-idiotype has been shown to induce a transient but marked depression of ongoing IgE response to benzylpenicilloyl[42] or phosphorylcholine.[38] In humans, it has been recently reported that repeated injections of a monoclonal antibody specific for the idiotype of a B-cell lymphoma were highly effective in inducing biological and clinical improvement.[43] In other systems, however, anti-idiotypic immunity has failed to suppress an already established antibody production.[3] Thus, it is possible that the variability in the results so far observed may reflect different requirements for an efficient immunosuppression, that is, direct action on B-cell clones[44,45] or activation of T-suppressor circuits.[46]

Studies on idiotypic suppression have shown that treatment by anti-idiotype may[45,47] or may not[3] affect the total antibody response to the antigen. Thus, considering the fact that in the few experiments on autoimmune systems, the total amount of autoantibodies affected by anti-idiotype treatment, a possible explanation could be found in the relative idiotypic restriction of autoantibodies.

The presence of circulating idiotype-anti-idiotype complexes has already been shown in the serum of humans[48] and mice.[49] Although their biological significance has not yet been elucidated, they may in fact be involved in regulation of the immune response itself.[50] As auto-anti-idiotypic antibodies are an integral part of the immune response,[51,52] it is evident that they may also be involved in immunological phenomena harmful for the host, such as certain immunopathological conditions. Here, evidence has been provided that glomerular immune deposits from a rabbit with serum sickness induced by means of chronic intravenous injections of BSA, contained autoantibodies that bound the Fab$_2'$ fragments of autologous anti-BSA antibodies. A similar finding has been recently described in mice where immune deposits induced by injection of bacterial lipopolysaccharides contained idiotypic as well as anti-idiotypic immunoglobulin molecules.[53] Whether these observations in animals are pertinent to human immune-complex mediated diseases and in particular glomerular diseases, it is still difficult to assess at the present time. Potentiation and/or perpetuation of immune complex mediated lesions by way of anti-idiotypic antibodies, however, could provisionally explain the lack of satisfactory mechanisms for the chronicity of many immunopathological lesions in autoimmunity.

In conclusion, there is today sufficient evidence to encourage new studies aimed at exploring the mechanisms of responsiveness to self antigens in light of the fine specificity of an idiotype-based regulatory network. Advances in this area will provide essential information not only on the possible use of anti-idiotypic immunity in the treatment of autoimmune diseases in man, but also on the eventual role of natural anti-idiotypic responses in determining the chronicity of autoimmune processes.

SUMMARY

In this paper, we have provided experimental evidence that antibodies to autoantigens bear common idiotypes and that this property makes them susceptible to anti-idiotypic regulation. Spontaneously occurring autoantibodies to Tg in rats have been extensively investigated as a model of immune response responsible for the appearance of autoimmune disease. Large idiotypic cross-reactivity was found among autoantibodies of various individual animals. Similarly, a high degree of idiotypic relatedness was found among mouse monoclonal antibodies reacting with a highly conserved antigenic domain of thyroglobulin. Both rat and mice idiotype were found to be present on spontaneous and induced antibodies to rat thyroglobulin from individuals of other species. In vivo experiments showed that anti-idiotypic antibodies can be effective in suppressing autoantibodies formation. In the induced TIN in BN rats, a single injection of anti-idiotypic serum prior to the induction of autoimmune disease was sufficient to generate a significant selective suppression of autoantibodies produced against a pathogenetic chemical form of the autoantigen, that is, the one against which the autoantibodies used to prepare the anti-idiotypic reagent as mostly reactive. Similarly, it was found that repeated injections of anti-idiotype into rats with ongoing spontaneous production of autoantibodies to thyroglobulin were able to significantly decrease the amount of circulating autoantibodies from the pretreatment values. Thus, although the beneficial effect of anti-idiotype observed in these experiments was only partial, indications were obtained that a specific anti-idiotypic immunity can be used to regulate autoantibody production. Finally, evidence has been provided to support the hypothesis that auto-anti-idiotype, as a normal constituent of the immune response, can be responsible for the potentiation of immune complex-mediated tissue injury that is often the hallmark of autoimmune diseases.

ACKNOWLEDGMENTS

I want to thank Dr. P. E. Bigazzi and Dr. C. B. Wilson for their helpful discussions, Dr. M. De Baets for providing the mouse monoclonal antibodies, Dr. D.H. Katz for a critical reading of the manuscript, Joy Rogers for excellent technical assistance, and Beverly Burgess for typing the manuscript.

REFERENCES

1. JERNE, N. K. 1974. Towards a network theory of the immune system. Ann. Immunol. Inst. Pasteur (Paris) 125: 373.

2. NISONOFF, A. & M. I. GREENE. 1980. Regulation through idiotypic determinants of the immune response to the p-azophenylarsonate hapten in strain A mice. *In* Immunology 80. M. Fougereau and J. Dausset, Eds.: 57. Academic Press. London.

3. BINZ, H. & H. WIGZELL. 1976. Successful induction of specific tolerance to transplantation antigens using autoimmunization against the recipient's own, natural antibodies. Nature (London) **262:** 294.

4. ABDOU, N. I., H. WALL, H. B. LINDSLEY, J. F. HALSEY & T. SUZUKI. 1981. Network theory in autoimmunity. *In vitro* suppression of serum anti-DNA antibody binding to DNA by antiidiotypic antibody in systemic lupus erythematosus. J. Clin. Invest. **67:** 1297.

5. COHEN, P. L. & R. A. EISENBERG. 1982. Anti-idiotypic antibodies to the Coombs antibody in NZB F_1 mice. J. Exp. Med. **156:** 173.

6. ZANETTI, M. & C. B. WILSON. 1983. Characterization of anti-tubular basement membrane antibodies in rats. J. Immunol. **130:** 2173.

7. ZANETTI, M., F. MAMPASO & C. B. WILSON. 1983. Anti-idiotype as a probe in the analysis of autoimmune tubulointerstitial nephritis in the Brown Norway rat. J. Immunol. **131:** 1268.

8. BIGAZZI, P. E. 1979. Thyroiditis as a model of autoimmune disorders in man. *In* Mechanisms of Immunopathology. S. Cohen, P.A. Ward & R.T. McCluskey, Eds.: 157. John Wiley & Sons. New York.

9. ZANETTI, M. & P. E. BIGAZZI. 1981. Anti-idiotypic immunity and autoimmunity. I. *In vitro* and *in vivo* effects of anti-idiotypic antibodies to spontaneously occurring autoantibodies to rat thyroglobulin. Eur. J. Immunol. **11:** 187.

10. ZANETTI, M., R. W. BARTON & P. E. BIGAZZI. 1983. Anti-idiotypic immunity and autoimmunity. II. Idiotypic determinants of autoantibodies and lymphocytes in spontaneous and experimentally induced autoimmune thyroiditis. Cell Immunol. **75:** 292.

11. ZANETTI, M., M. DE BAETS & J. ROGERS. 1983. High degree of idiotypic cross-reactivity among murine monoclonal antibodies to thyroglobulin. J. Immunol. In press.

12. LIU, F.-T., J. W. BOHN, E. L. FERRY, H. YAMAMOTO, C. A. MOLINARO, L. A. SHERMAN, N. R. KLINMAN & D. H. KATZ. 1980. Monoclonal dinitrophenyl-specific murine IgE antibody: Preparation, isolation, and characterization. J. Immunol. **124:** 2728.

13. ZANETTI, M. & C. B. WILSON. 1983. Participation of auto-anti-idiotypes to immune complex glomerulonephritis in rabbits. J. Immunol. In press.

14. WILLIAMS, R. C., H. G. KUNKEL & J. D. CAPRA. 1968. Antigenic specificities related to the cold agglutinin activity of gamma M globulins. Science **161:** 379.

15. CARSON, D. & M. WEIGERT. 1973. Immunochemical analysis of the cross-reacting idiotypes of mouse myeloma proteins with anti-dextran activity and normal anti-dextran antibody. Proc. Natl. Acad. Sci. USA **70:** 235.

16. LIEBERMAN, R., M. POTTER, W. HUMPHREY, E. B. MUSHINSKI & M. VRANA. 1975. Multiple individual cross-specific idiotypes on 13 levan-binding myeloma proteins of BALB/c mice. J. Exp. Med. **142:** 106.

17. URBAIN, J., N. TASIAUX, R. LEUWENKROON, A. VAN ACKER & B. MARIAME. 1975. Sharing of idiotypic specificities between different antibody subpopulations from an individual rabbit. Eur. J. Immunol. **5:** 570.

18. TUNG, A. S. & A. NISONOFF. 1975. Isolation from individual A/J mice of anti-p-azophenylarsonate antibodies bearing a cross reactive idiotype. J. Exp. Med. **141:** 112.

19. PINCUS, S. H., D. H. SACHS & H. B. DICKLER. 1978. Production of antisera specific for idiotype(s) of murine anti-(T,G)-A-L antibodies. J. Immunol. **121:** 1422.

20. JU, S.-T., M. PIERRES, R. N. GERMAIN, B. BENACERRAF & M. E. DORF. 1979. Idiotypic analysis of anti-GAT antibodies. VI. Identification and strain distribution of the GA-1 idiotype. J. Immunol. **123:** 2505.

21. RIESEN, W. F. 1979. Idiotypic cross-reactivity of human and murine phosphorylcholine-binding immunoglobulins. Eur. J. Immunol. **9:** 421.

22. SCHWARTZ, M., D. NOVICK, D. GIVOL & S. FUCHS. 1978. Induction of anti-idiotypic antibodies by immunization with syngeneic spleen cells educated with acetylcholine receptor. Nature (London) **273:** 543.

23. KUNKEL, H. G., V. AGNELLO, F. G. JOSLIN, R. J. WINCHESTER & J. D. CAPRA. 1973. Cross idiotypic specificity among monoclonal IgM proteins with anti-γ-globulin activity. J. Exp. Med. **137:** 331.

24. FØRRE, Ø., J. H. DOBLOUG, T. E. MICHAELSEN & J. B. NATVIG. 1979. Evidence of similar

idiotypic determinants on different rheumatoid factor populations. Scand. J. Immunol. **9:** 281.
25. NATVIG. J. B., H. G. KUNKEL, R. E. ROSENFIELD, J. F. DALTON & S. KOCHWA. 1976. Idiotypic specificities of anti-Rh antibodies. J. Immunol. **116:** 1536.
26. LEFVERT, A.-K., R. W. JAMES, C. ALLIOD & B. W. FULPIUS. 1982. A monoclonal anti-idiotypic antibody against anti-receptor antibodies from myasthenic sera. Eur. J. Immunol. **12:** 790.
27. TACHOVSKY, T. G., M. SANDBERG-WOLLHEIM & L. G. BAIRD. 1982. Rabbit anti-human CSF IgG. I. Characterization of anti-idiotype antibodies produced against MS CSF and detection of cross-reactive idiotypes in several MS CSF. J. Immunol. **129:** 764.
28. ANDRZEJEWSKI, JR., C., J. RAUCH, E. LAFER, B. D. STOLLAR & R. S. SCHWARTZ. 1981. Antigen-binding diversity and idiotypic cross-reactions among hybridoma autoantibodies to DNA. J. Immunol. **126:** 226.
29. RAUCH, J., E. MURPHY, J. B. ROTHS, B. D. STOLLAR & R. S. SCHWARTZ. 1982. A high frequency idiotypic marker of anti-DNA autoantibodies in MRL-Ipr/Ipr mice. J. Immunol. **129:** 236.
30. MARION, T. N., A. R. LAWTON, III, J. F. KEARNEY & D. E. BRILES. 1982. Anti-DNA autoantibodies in (NZB × NZW)F₁ mice are clonally heterogeneous, but the majority share a common idiotype. J. Immunol. **128:** 668.
31. TRON, F., C. LE GUERN, P.-A. CAZENAVE & J.-F. BACH. 1982. Intrastrain recurrent idiotypes among anti-DNA antibodies of (NZB × NZW)F₁ hybrid mice. Eur. J. Immunol. **12:** 761.
32. NYE, L. & I. M. ROITT. 1980. Isoelectric focusing of human antibodies directed against a high molecular weight antigen. J. Immunol. Methods **35:** 97.
33. MATTSON, D. H., R. P. ROOS & B. G. W. ARNASON. 1980. Isoelectric focusing of IgG eluted from multiple sclerosis and subacute sclerosing panencephalitis brains. Nature (London) **287:** 335.
34. CLEVINGER, B., J. SCHILLING, L. HOOD & J. M. DAVIE. 1980. Structural correlates of cross-reactive and individual idiotypic determinants on murine antibodies to α(1-3) dextran. J. Exp. Med. **151:** 1059.
35. BONA, C. A., E. HERBER-KATZ & W. E. PAUL. 1981. Idiotype-anti-idiotype regulation. I. Immunization with a levan-binding myeloma protein leads to the appearance of auto-anti-(anti-idiotype) antibodies and to the activation of silent clones. J. Exp. Med. **153:** 951.
36. BRILES, D. E., C. FORMAN, S. HUDAK & J. L. CLAFLIN. 1982. Anti-phosphorylcholine antibodies of the T15 idiotype are optimally protective against *Streptococcus pneumoniae.* J. Exp. Med. **156:** 1177.
37. BINZ, H. & H. WIGZELL. 1977. Antigen-binding idiotypic T lymphocyte receptors. *In* Contemporary Topics in Immunobiology. O. Stutman, Ed. **7:** 113. Plenum Press. New York.
38. BLASER, K. & A. L. DE WECK. 1982. Regulation of the IgE antibody response by idiotype-anti-idiotype network. Prog. Allergy **32:** 203.
39. LYNCH, R. G., J. W. ROHRER, B. ODERMATT, H. M. GEBEL, J. R. AUTRY & R. G. HOOVER. 1979. Immunoregulation of murine myeloma cell growth and differentiation: A monoclonal model of B cell differentiation. Immunol. Rev. **48:** 45.
40. BROWN, C. A., K. CAREY & R. B. COLVIN. 1979. Inhibition of auto-immune tubulointerstitial nephritis in guinea pigs by heterologous antisera containing anti-idiotype antibodies. J. Immunol. **123:** 2102.
41. NEILSON, E. G. & M. S. PHILLIPS. 1982. Suppression of interstitial nephritis by auto-anti-idiotypic immunity. J. Exp. Med. **155:** 179.
42. BLASER, K., T. NAKAGAWA & A. L. DE WECK. 1980. Suppression of the benzylpenicilloyl-(BPO) specific IgE formation with isologous anti-idiotypic antibodies in BALB/c mice. J. Immunol. **125:** 24.
43. MILLER, R. A., D. G. MALONEY, R. WARNKE & R. LEVY. 1982. Treatment of B-cell lymphoma with monoclonal anti-idiotype antibody. N. Engl. J. Med. **306:** 517.
44. COSENZA, H. & H. KOHLER. 1972. Specific suppression of the antibody response by antibodies to receptors. Proc. Natl. Acad. Sci. USA **69:** 2701.
45. KLUSKENS, L. & H. KOHLER. 1974. Regulation of immune response by autogeneous antibody against receptor. Proc. Natl. Acad. Sci. USA **71:** 5083.

46. GERMAIN, R. N. & B. BENACERRAF. 1981. A single major pathway of T-lymphocyte interactions in antigen-specific immune suppression. Scand. J. Immunol. 13: 1.
47. EICHMANN, K. 1974. Idiotype suppression. I. Influence of the dose and of the effector functions of anti-idiotypic antibody on the production of an idiotype. Eur. J. Immunol. 4: 296.
48. MORGAN, A. C., JR., R. D. ROSSEN & J. J. TWOMEY. 1979. Naturally occurring circulating immune complexes: Normal human serum contains idiotype-anti-idiotype complexes dissociable by certain IgG antiglobulins. J. Immunol. 122: 1672.
49. ROSE, L. M. & P. H. LAMBERT. 1980. The natural occurrence of circulating idiotype—anti-idiotype complexes during a secondary immune response to phosphorylcholine. Clin. Immunol. Immunopathol. 15: 481.
50. KLAUS, G. G. B. 1978. Antigen-antibody complexes elicit anti-idiotypic antibodies to self-idiotopes. Nature (London) 272: 265.
51. SCHRATER, A. F., E. A. GOIDL, G. J. THORBECKE & G. W. SISKIND. 1979. Production of auto-anti-idiotypic antibody during the normal immune response to TNP-Ficoll. I. Occurrence in AKR/J and BALB/c mice of hapten-augmentable, anti-TNP plaque-forming cells and their accelerated appearance in recipients of immune spleen cells. J. Exp. Med. 150: 138.
52. GEHA, R. S. 1982. Presence of auto-anti-idiotypic antibody during the normal human immune response to tetanus toxoid antigen. J. Immunol. 129: 139.
53. GOLDMAN, M., L. M. ROSE, A. HOCHMANN & P. H. LAMBERT. 1982. Deposition of idiotype-anti-idiotype immune complexes in renal glomeruli after polyclonal B-cell activation. J. Exp. Med. 155: 1385.

DISCUSSION OF THE PAPER

I. M. ROITT (*Middlesex Hospital Medical School, London, England*): I have some experimental information that bears on the last point you suggested about the perpetuation of an autoimmune response by anti-idiotype. Studies carried out with Lane DeCavallo and George Wick in the B-strain chicken show that if you thymectomize the B-strain chicken, the level of antibody, once the antibodies are established, goes down in most cases to zero. That suggests that when you remove the antigen there is not the wherewithal within the idiotypic network to maintain that response.

In the light of the results that you have obtained with the Buffalo rat, would you conclude that an approach to trying to abrogate autoimmunity in an established autoimmunity disease by conventionally applying anti-idiotypic serum, even if it is against a major cross-reactive idiotype, is not likely to be as successful? Possibly, other mechanisms using suppression of T helpers may be important, and if so, have you any information in your system as to whether you depressed the response of the T-helper cells as examined by a proliferative response *in vitro* to thyroglobulin?

M. ZANETTI: We have not done any *in vitro* experiments to check for the point that you have made. It is true that it is premature to recommend anti-idiotypic treatment for the treatment of autoimmune diseases. There is an indication, however, that this way, unless disproved from a series of evidence and experiments, should be continued until we find the right approach to down-regulate autoimmune responses.

L. S. RODKEY (*Kansas State University, Manhattan, Kans.*): In your cross-reactive idiotypes that you found between species, have you measured these carefully on a mole to mole basis for inhibitions to see if these are really the same idiotypes? Perhaps they are just structurally similar?

ZANETTI: I have not done that. The experiment was performed, inhibiting by anti-idiotype, limiting dilution of serum reacting with thyroglobulin.

RODKEY: I understand that they inhibit. Are they the same or just similar?

ZANETTI: I cannot answer that question.

H. G. KUNKEL (*The Rockefeller University, New York*): Did you get any inhibition from any serum other than thyroglobulin?

ZANETTI: Do you mean inhibition in other systems?

KUNKEL: I mean other sera than thyroiditis sera. Did you just test the thyroiditis?

ZANETTI: I just tested thyroiditis. There is specific control, however, for that reaction, because I simultaneously used another anti-idiotype made against one of the other five monoclonals. It did not inhibit at all.

N. ABDOU (*University of Kansas Medical Center, Kansas City, Kans.*): I am interested first of all in your thoughts on the *in vivo* model of thyroiditis, the modulation of that by anti-idiotype. What is the mechanism by which suppression was induced? Did you dissect that? My second question is, Was there any lethal effect of that in these same animals, that is, nephritis?

ZANETTI: To answer the second question first, I looked very carefully in various organs to see if there was any deposition of immunoglobulins after treatment with foreign immunoglobulin in the rat. I could see none in the kidney, in the thyroid, or in other tissues.

To answer the first question, I do not have any conclusive evidence. We are in the process of repeating these experiments using anti-idiotype against monoclonal antibodies to thyroglobulin derived from these autoimmune rats. We hope to obtain better insights.

A Monoclonal Antibody That Recognizes Anti-DNA Antibodies in Patients with Systemic Lupus

B. DIAMOND[a] AND G. SOLOMON[b]

Department of Microbiology and Immunology[a]
Department of Medicine
Albert Einstein College of Medicine
Bronx, New York 10461
and
Hospital for Joint Diseases[b]
New York, New York 10003

Patients with systemic lupus erythematosus (SLE) make antibodies to double stranded DNA (dsDNA). The extent of the heterogeneity of these antibodies is not known. In order to examine the heterogeneity of anti-dsDNA, the antibodies from a single patient with SLE, and the similarity of anti-dsDNA antibodies among unrelated patients with SLE, we have produced murine monoclonal anti-idiotypic antibodies to anti-dsDNA antibodies isolated from the serum of a patient with active systemic lupus erythematosus.

MATERIALS AND METHODS

Isolation of Anti-Double Stranded DNA Antibodies

Ten ml of serum from patient AW with active SLE and high titer anti-dsDNA activity were dialyzed against 0.01 M Na phosphate buffer, pH6.6, with 0.01 M NaCl. This was mixed with 10 ml of 0.01 M Na phosphate buffer, pH6.6, with 0.01 M NaCl containing calf thymus DNA (Type 1, Sigma Chemical Co., St. Louis, Mo.) at a concentration of 0.5 mg/ml. The mixture was incubated for 1 hour at room temperature, then overnight at 4° C, and then was chromatographed on a 300 ml DE-52 column equilibrated in 0.01 M Na phosphate, pH 6.6, with 0.01 M NaCl. The column was washed with starting buffer followed by 0.01 M Na phosphate buffer, pH 6.6, with 0.5 M NaCl. Fractions eluted with 0.5 M NaCl were pooled, dialyzed against 8 M urea, and rechromatographed on a DE-52 column equilibrated in 8 M urea with 0.05 M NaCl. The column was washed with solutions of increasing salt concentration, 8 M urea with 0.05 M NaCl, 0.2 M NaCl, and 0.5 M NaCl. The fractions eluted with 0.2 M NaCl were dialyzed against decreasing concentrations of urea, and finally against 0.02 M phosphate-buffered saline (PBS) pH 7.4.

Assay for Anti-ds DNA Activity

Patients' sera and column eluates were tested for anti-dsDNA activity using a Millipore filter assay with ^{125}I-labeled calf thymus DNA.[1,2]

Generation of Hybrid Cells

Three hundred μg of AW-enriched anti-dsDNA antibodies in complete Freund's adjuvant were injected intraperitoneally (i.p.) into BALB/c mice (Jackson Laboratory, Bar Harbor, Maine). Two weeks later, the mice were boosted with an i.p. injection of 100 μg of immunogen without adjuvant. Mice subsequently received weekly i.p. injections of immunogen for 6 to 10 weeks. Three days following the final boost, spleen cells from the immunized mice were fused with polyethylene glycol to the drug marked nonproducing mouse myeloma cell line, P3NP.[3]

Radioimmunoassay for Anti-Idiotypic Activity

A solid phase radioimmunoassay was used to screen both mouse serum and hybridoma supernatants for anti-idiotypic activity. Thirty μg of AW-enriched anti-dsDNA antibodies or an equivalent amount of IgG from control human serum (using an estimated value of 12 mg/ml of IgG) were incubated overnight at 4° C in polystyrene wells (Immulon-2, Dynatech, Alexandria, Va.). Plates were washed with PBS-5% bovine serum albumin (BSA) and incubated for 1 hour at room temperature with PBS-5% bovine serum albumin. This was followed by a 90 minute incubation with mouse serum at a 1:100 dilution or undiluted hybridoma supernatant. After washing with EIA solution (0.5% Tween 20, 0.15 M NaCl, pH 8.3) with 2% BSA, plates were incubated for ninety minutes with ^{35}S methionine-labeled anti-mouse κ chain provided by Dr. M. Scharff. Plates were washed and counted for radioactivity.

In competition studies either 3 mg of pooled human IgG from 5 normal donors or 5 μg of calf thymus DNA were added to the hybridoma supernatant. Human serum was again assumed to contain 12 mg/ml of IgG.

Isolation of Fab'$_2$ Fragments of AW Anti-dsDNA Antibodies

Pepsin digestion for 24 hours at 37° C was used to generate Fab'$_2$ fragments that were then isolated by Sephadex gel chromatography.[4]

Cloning of Hybrid Cells and Production of Ascites

Hybrids with presumed anti-idiotypic activity were cloned in soft agar.[5] Clones were picked, retested, grown to mass culture, and injected into pristane-primed BALB/c mice intraperitoneally.[6] Ascites was harvested 10 to 14 days later.

Screen for Idiotype in Serum Samples

Serum from patients with SLE as defined by the American Rheumatism Association were diluted 1:10 or 1:100 in PBS and incubated in polystyrene wells overnight at 4° C.[7] Wells were washed and incubated for ninety minutes with anti-idiotypic antibodies as undiluted culture supernatant or ascites diluted 1:100 in phosphate-buffered saline. The assay proceeded as previously described.

Coprecipitation Assay

[125]I-labeled calf thymus DNA was incubated with serum from a patient with SLE or a normal control for 15 minutes at 37° C. This was followed by the addition of 100 ml of anti-idiotype supernatant or supernatant from a mouse myeloma cell line, 4T001, for 1 hour. Fifty μl rabbit anti-mouse IgG was added, and the mixture was allowed to precipitate overnight at 4° C. The precipitates were washed in PBS and measured for radioactivity.

Modified Crithidia Assay

A modified crithidia assay was employed in which human serum was diluted 1:10 in PBS and incubated on crithidia slides (Zeus Scientific, Inc., Raritan, N.J.), followed by incubation with anti-idiotype and fluoresceinated goat anti-mouse IgG (Cappel, Cochranville, Pa). Fluorescence of the kinetoplast was scored positive or negative.

Subclass Analysis of 3I Reactive and 3I Nonreactive Antibodies

AW serum was dialyzed against 0.02 M PBS pH 7.4 and applied to a 3I-sepharose column. The column was washed with PBS followed by 2 M KSCN. Fractions eluted with KSCN were dialyzed against phosphate-buffered saline. Protein obtained from the PBS wash and the KSCN elution was incubated overnight on polystyrene wells, and an enzyme-linked immunosorbent assay (ELISA) was performed using polyvalent swine anti-IgG$_1$, IgG$_2$, IgG$_3$, or IgG$_4$ (Nordic Immunological Laboratory, Tilburg, The Netherlands) followed by peroxidase-labeled rabbit anti-swine immunoglobulin (Dako-immunoglobulins, Denmark) and then o-phenylene diamine (Bionetics Laboratory Products, Kensington, Md.). Wells were read on an Artek ELISA reader.

RESULTS

Preparation of Enriched Anti-dsDNA Antibodies

Serum from patient AW was incubated with calf thymus DNA to form DNA-anti-DNA complexes. The complexes were isolated by DE-52 chromatography. Monomeric immunoglobulin eluted in 0.1 M NaCl had no anti-dsDNA activity by Millipore filter assay. Complexes eluted in 0.5 M NaCl possessed anti-dsDNA activity. The complexes were dissociated in 8 M urea, and the antibody was isolated by DE-52 chromatography. IgG with anti-dsDNA antivity was present in the fractions eluted with 0.2 M NaCl. Free DNA was eluted with 0.5 M NaCl. The antibodies recovered by this procedure were enriched 50- to 100-fold over serum for anti-dsDNA activity. As much as 15 mg of IgG in the enriched fraction was obtained from 10 ml of serum, but yields were variable.

Production of Hybridoma Lines

AW enriched anti-dsDNA antibodies were used to immunize BALB/c mice. Mice were presumed to have anti-idiotypic antibodies when their serum had greater reactivity with enriched anti-dsDNA antibodies than with normal human IgG. Three

TABLE 1. Hybrids with Reactivity for Anti-Double Stranded DNA Antibodies

	AW-anti-dsDNA	Normal Human Serum
3I	1996 cpm	146 cpm
9F	2098	134
17A	919	176
3H	207	113
9E	156	99
Control myeloma supernatant	123	114

fusions were performed, using spleen cells from three individual mice. Over one hundred hybrids were screened, and 5 wells were identified as containing cells making presumptive anti-idiotypic antibodies (TABLE 1). The supernatants from these wells bound to AW anti-dsDNA antibodies, but not to pooled normal serum. One of these with high reactivity to AW anti-dsDNA antibodies, 3I, was selected for further study.

Characterization of the 3I Antibody

3I is an IgG_1, κ immunoglobulin. To prove that 3I recognized idiotypic determinants on the enriched AW anti-dsDNA antibodies, we performed several experiments. We reacted 3I with the enriched pool of AW anti-dsDNA antibodies in the presence of a large excess of pooled normal human serum. There was no inhibition by normal serum. We also showed that 3I reacts with Fab'_2 fragments of AW anti-dsDNA antibodies. Furthermore, 3I reactive antibodies were shown to be of all four IgG subclasses. These experiments suggest that 3I does not react with heavy chain constant region determinants as it reacts with Fab'_2 fragments and is not inhibited by normal immunoglobulin. Evidence that it does not react with allotypic determinants comes from the fact that it reacts with antibodies of all IgG subclasses.

3I reactivity with anti-dsDNA antibodies is not inhibited by calf thymus DNA. 3I, therefore, is not anti-"binding site" and does not bind to the variable region in such a way as to sterically inhibit DNA binding. Although 3I does not inhibit the binding of anti-dsDNA antibodies to dsDNA, it does bind to anti-dsDNA antibodies and not solely to contaminating antibodies that may be present in the AW-enriched anti-dsDNA preparation. In the coprecipitation assay, AW serum containing anti-dsDNA antibodies was incubated with radiolabeled DNA, 3I antibody and rabbit anti-serum to mouse IgG. 3I bound to anti-dsDNA antibodies as the rabbit anti-serum precipitated DNA-anti-DNA complexes in the presence of 3I antibody. When a mouse myeloma protein was used in place of 3I, or when normal human serum was used rather than AW serum, the precipitate contained no DNA. Moreover, in a modified crithidia assay, 3I antibody, and not an irrelevant myeloma protein, bound to anti-dsDNA antibodies from the serum of patients with SLE, and gave positive staining of the kinetoplast after incubation with fluoresceinated anti-mouse immunoglobulin antiserum.

Analysis of Serum Samples from Patients with Systemic Lupus Erythematosus

Serum from nine patients with SLE with high titer anti-dsDNA activity in the Millipore filter assay were examined for 3I reactivity. Eight of 9 patients with anti-dsDNA activity had 3I reactivity in their serum (FIGURE 1).

DISCUSSION

The 3I antibody recognizes an idiotypic determinant on anti-dsDNA antibodies from patient AW. That it does not recognize nonpolymorphic constant region determinants is shown by the fact that its reactivity with anti-dsDNA antibodies is not absorbed by normal human serum. That it does not recognize a known heavy chain constant region allotypic determinant is indicated by its reactivity with all IgG subclasses. Although it is possible that 3I recognizes a nonmarker allotypic determinant shared by all IgG subclasses and preferentially expressed in patients with SLE, we feel this is not likely.

Using a radioimmunoassay, we have tested for 3I reactivity sera from nine patients with SLE with anti-dsDNA activity by the Millipore filter assay. Eight showed 3I reactivity. To insure that immune complexes were not preferentially binding to polystyrene wells in the radioimmunoassay, we repeated these experiments, coating the wells first with goat anti-human IgG. The results were unchanged. We have currently found 3I reactivity in serum from 20 of 23 patients with anti-dsDNA activity.

3I, therefore, recognizes a cross-reactive idiotype on anti-dsDNA antibodies from unrelated patients with systemic lupus erythematosus. It is present in the serum of most SLE patients with anti-dsDNA activity. Furthermore, it appears to be present on

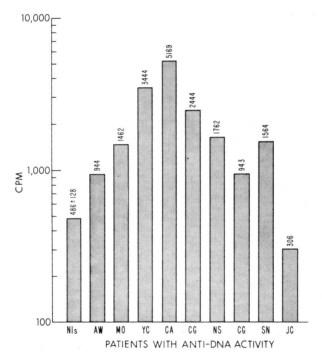

FIGURE 1. Nine patients with SLE and anti-dsDNA activity by Millipore filter assay (nl 1) were tested for 3I reactivity. Five normal controls were also tested. The value for 3I reactivity for these controls was 486 ± 128. All but one SLE patient showed 3I reactivity at least 3 standard deviations greater than the mean of the normal controls.

a significant portion (40% and 70% data not shown) of the anti-dsDNA antibodies from two patients studied.

The extent of the heterogeneity of 3I reactive anti-dsDNA antibodies both in the serum of a single patient and among patients has not yet been determined. We do, however, know that there is some heterogeneity among the antibodies sharing the cross-reactive idiotype recognized by 3I. 17A, a different monclonal anti-idiotypic antibody reacts with only a portion of 3I reactive antibodies (data not shown). This suggests that 3I recognizes a family of structurally related but nonidentical anti-dsDNA antibodies. This family of antibodies comprises a significant portion of anti-dsDNA antibodies in many patients with systemic lupus erythematosus.

REFERENCES

1. GINSBERG, B. & H. KEISER. 1973. Arthritis Rheum. **16:** 199–207.
2. KEISER, H. 1973. Arthritis Rheum. **16:** 468–470.
3. GEFTER, M. L., D. A. MARGULIES & M. D. SCHARFF. 1977. Somatic Cell Genet. **3:** 231–236.
4. STANWORTH, D. R. & N. W. TURNER. 1978. *In* Handbook of Experimental Immunology. D. M. Weir, Ed: Chapter 6. Blackwell. Oxford.
5. COFFINO, P., R. BAUMAL & M. D. SCHARFF. 1972. J. Cell Physiol. **79:** 429–440.
6. POTTER, M., J. G. PUMPHREY & J. L. WALTERS. 1972. J. Natl. Cancer Inst. **49:** 305–308.
7. COHEN, A. S., W. E. REYNOLDS, E. C. FRANKLIN, J. P. KULKA, M. W. ROPES, L. E. SHULMAN & S. L. WALLACE. 1971. Preliminary Criteria for the Classification of SLE. Bull. Rheum. Dis. **21:** 643–648.

DISCUSSION OF THE PAPER

J. CERNY (*University of Texas Medical Branch, Galveston, Tx.*): I would like to know if your 3I antibodies reacted substantially better to complex of antibody to DNA, as opposed to antibody alone.

B. DIAMOND: We have done that experiment and it does not react any better. I did not mention it, but we have added DNA back to the original immunizing preparation to see if we would then get greater reactivity. It does not look like it is reacting to the complexes any better.

N. ABDOU (*University of Kansas Medical Center, Kansas City, Kans.*): The more we look at lupus patients, the way everybody feels, they are heterogeneous individuals, and with monoclonals, we have the proper tools to test that. When you say that your anti-idiotype bound to all anti-DNA from the majority of patients, can you qualify that statement to say what kind of clinical correlates we have? For example, does the anti-idiotype bind to anti-DNA antibodies in serum of a patient whose only clinical symptom is hemolytic anemia the same as it binds to anti-DNA antibodies in a patient with lupus nephritis?

DIAMOND: I do not know that kind of clinical subdivision at this point. We started looking for the presence of the 3I idiotypes and several other of the anti-idiotypes, the 9F and 17A, and another one, C10, in skin and kidneys. We can find some differences there, but I think it is far too preliminary to start talking about it. I think, however, that you are right. The fact that the 3I antibody is present in such a large percentage of patients with lupus and anti-DNA activity means that it is not going to give significant clinical subsets. We have looked in patients without anti-DNA activity and it is much smaller a percentage of them who have the 3I antibody present. We have looked at 71 lupus patients without anti-DNA activity. There are a few there that have 3I reactivity; if we do the modified crithidia assay, they have 3I on anti-DNA antibodies. So even though they were not detected initially as having anti-DNA antibodies, they in fact have them.

UNIDENTIFIED SPEAKER: Have you tested whether any of your patients might be naturally making a 3I-like anti-idiotype antibody?

DIAMOND: We started to look for that. We have looked at 13 patients in remission. In 7 of them, they lose their 3I reactivity; 6 of them still have it. We are trying to look at those 6, where we are hoping we might be able to find an autologous anti-idiotype that is preventing the anti-DNA activity of the antibody. I do not know yet, however.

R. KALISH (*Downstate Medical Center, Brooklyn, N.Y.*): A sizable percentage of these patients will be negative for anti-double-stranded DNA and positive for anti-single-stranded DNA. They may or may not have lupus. Do these antisera react with your anti-idiotype?

DIAMOND: We are just looking at anti-double-stranded DNA. We are using an assay that selects the anti-double-stranded DNA. In answer to your question, these patients all have antibodies to double-stranded DNA, and the 3I antibody sees anti-double-stranded DNA antibodies. Whether the 3I antibody sees anti-single-stranded DNA antibody cannot be completely answered. 3I does not see most lupus patients who do not have anti-double-stranded DNA activity. Many of those will have anti-single-stranded DNA, but that is completely indirect.

N. CHIOROZZI (*Tenafly, N.J.*): Are there significant numbers of B cells circulating that can be bound by the antibody?

DIAMOND: We have attempted the experiment, and we really have not separated B cells and T cells well. We also have not eliminated FcR on the cells very well. If you incubate peripheral blood mononuclear cells overnight, presumably to get rid of 3I positive antibody that might be bound to FcR, and if you then introduce the 3I antibody and a fluoresceinated anti-mouse antibody in maybe 6 or 7 patients, there can be up to 5 to 10% positive peripheral blood mononuclear cells. They are only positive in those patients that have serum that is positive, but we really have not rigorously excluded FcR binding of the serum antibody. We have not separated T and B cells.

Index of Contributors

(Italic page numbers refer to comments made in discussion.)

Abbas, A. K., *354*
Abdou, N., *345, 378, 384*
Adler, F. L., 16–25
Araneo, B., 198–205
Armand, J., *288*
Augustin, A.A., *150, 187–188, 195–196, 272–281*

Bellone, C. J., 74–83
Benjamin, C. D., 140–150, 198–205
Beyreuther, K., 121–129
Bhogal, B. S., 26–30
Binion, S. B., 16–25
Blaser, K., 330–345
Bluestone, J. A., *264*, 265–271
Bona, C., ix, *8, 15, 30, 64, 97*–108, *129, 139, 196,* 220–229, *247, 256, 263, 280, 289, 304, 312,* 356–362
Bottomly, K., 230–239
Bovens, J., 121–129
Brodeur, P., 140–150
Brown, J. C., 16–25
Brüggemann, M., 121–129
Buttin, G., 290–295

Cerny, J., 31–39, *73, 175, 187, 228–229, 238–239, 246, 263, 354–355, 384*
Ch'ng, L. K., 140–150
Couraud, P.-O., 240–247
Cronkhite, R., 31–39

deWeck, A. L., 330–345
Deleo, A. B., 206–219
Diamond, B., 379–385
Dildrop, R., 121–129
Dray, S., 84–96
Dreher, K. L., 109–120
Dunn, E., 230–239

Emorine, L. J., 109–120
Epstein, S. L., *94–95,* 265–271

Flood, P. M., 206–219
Francotte, M., 1–8
Franssen, J. D., 1–8, 9–15

Gearhart, P. J., 171–176
Gefter, M. L., 48–64
Gerber, V. E., 330–345
Gershon, R. K., 206–219
Gibbons, J. J., 26–30

Gilman-Sachs, A., *25,* 84–96
Gleason, K., 65–73
Goidl, E. A., 26–30
Goodman, J. W., 282–289
Gurish, M. F., 40–47

Hafler, D. A., *362*
Harvey, M., 198–205
Hiernaux, J., 1–8, 9–15, 257–264
Horng, W. J., 84–96, 317–323

Jackson, S., 109–120
Jayaraman, S., 74–83
Juszczak, E. C., 48–64

Kalish, R., *170, 312, 385*
Karasuyama, H., 189–197
Kaymakcalan, Z., 282–289
Kazdin, D. S., 317–323
Kearney, J. F., 151–170
Kehoe, J. M., *362*
Kelsoe, G., 121–129
Kenny, J., *237–239*
Kindt, T. J., 109–120
Klinman, N. R., *129,* 130–139
Kohler, H., *25, 39,* 65–73, *108, 229, 263, 270*
Krawinkel, U., 121–129
Kresina, T. F., 40–47
Krieger, N. J., 305–312
Kunkel, H. G., 324–329, *362, 378*

Legrain, P., 290–295
Leo, O., 1–8, 9–15, 257–264
Lewis, G. K., 282–289
Liu, Y.-N., 356–362
Lü, B.-Z., 240–247
Lynch, R. G., 346–355

Mage, R., *96, 120*
Margolies, M. N., 48–64
Marion, T., *15, 108*
Marks, A., *174–175*
Marshak-Rothstein, A., 48–64
Max, E. E., 109–120
McNamara, M., 65–73
Mestecky, J., *227*
Metzger, D. W., 198–205, 313–316
Michael, J. G., 305–312
Milburn, G. L., 346–355
Miller, A., *64,* 140–150, *169,* 198–205
Miyatani, S., 189–197

Moser, M., 1–8, 9–15, 257–264
Mosier, D. E., *73, 169, 176, 228, 280*
Müller, C., 121–129

Nakauchi, H., 189–197
Near, R., 48–64
Nishikawa, S., 121–129
Nisonoff, A., 40–47, *263*

Ochi, A., 189–197
Okumura, K., 189–197
Old, L. J., 206–219
Ovary, Z., *354*

Packner, A. R., *247, 345*
Paul, W. E., *107, 138, 195, 227, 229, 237–239,
     264*
Pène, J., 296–304
Pernis, B., *150,* 220–229, 324–329
Pesce, A. J., 305–312
Pierce, S. K., 177–188
Pollok, B. A., 151–170
Posnett, D. N., 324–329

Rabinowitz, R., 265–271
Radbruch, A., 121–129
Rajewsky, K., *107–108,* 121–129, *175,
     196–197, 264*
Reth, M., 121–129
Riblet, R., 140–150
Riley, R. L., 130–139
Rodkey, L. S., 16–25, *107, 377*
Roitt, I. M., *377*
Rothstein, T. L., 48–64
Rowley, D. A., *170*
Rubinstein, L. J., 97–108

Sachs, D. H., *170, 176,* 265–271, 280–281
Sato, V. L., 48–64
Schmutz, A., 240–247
Schulman, J. L., 356–362
Scott, D. W., *24, 227–228*

Sege, K., 248–256
Sercarz, E. E., 140–150, 198–205
Siekevitz, M., 48–64, 121–129
Sim, G. K., 272–281
Siskind, G. W., 26–30, *150, 169–170, 175–176*
Slaoui, M., 1–8, 9–15
Smith, J. A., 48–64
Sogn, J. A., 109–120
Solomon, G., 379–385
Speck, N. A., 177–188
Stanislawski, M., 296–304
Stohrer, R., 151–170
Stone, M. R., 130–139
Strosberg, A. D., *120,* 240–247

Tada, T., *73,* 189–197
Takemori, T., 121–129
Tesch, H., 121–129
Thorbecke, G. I., 26–30

Urbain, J., 1–8, 9–15, 257–264
Urbain-Vansanten, G., 1–8

Van Acker, A., 1–8
Victor, C., 220–229

Weber, E., 330–345
Weksler, M. E., 26–30
Wetterwald, A., 330–345
Wicker, L., 198–205
Wikler, M., 1–8
Wildner, G., 121–129
Wylie, D., 130–139
Wysocki, L. J., 48–64

Yao, J., 282–289
Yowell, R., 198–205

Zaghouani, H., 296–304
Zaiss, S., 121–129
Zanetti, M., 363–378
Zharhary, D., 130–139

Subject Index

ABPC 48 idiotypes, in anti-levan response of BALB/c mice, 290–295
Adenylate cyclase activity, affected by Ab_2 antibodies, 242–243
Adoptive transfer, and suppression of B-cell responses by T cells, 179–180
β-Adrenergic receptors, DHA binding to, inhibited by Ab_2 antibodies, 242
Affinity of antibodies, somatic mutation affecting, 171–176
Age, and auto-anti-idiotypic antibody production, 27–29
Albumin, bovine serum, antibodies to
  and immune-complex glomerulonephritis, 371
  multi-specific, 305–312
Allergic diseases, immediate type, 330–345
Allotypes
  antibodies to a1, shared and nonshared idiotypes on, 313–316
  latent, in rabbits, 109–120
  suppression induction, 84–96
    allo-anti-allotype antibodies in, 85–86
    auto-anti-allotype antibodies in, 86–93
Antigenic drift, in influenza viruses, 356
Antigenic shift, in influenza viruses, 356
Anti-idiotypic antibodies (Ab_2), 2
  antibodies to (Ab_3), 2, 243–244
    antibodies to (Ab_4), 2, 319
    in arsonate system, 259–261
    to bovine serum albumin, 310
    in CB 20 mice, 300
    heterogeneity of, 292–295
    in lysozyme response system, 198–199
  to anti-BSA monoclonal antibody, 305–312
  anti-IdX558 affecting responses to dextran in IghC^b mice, 296–301
  and anti-levan response of BALB/c mice, 290–295
  and autoantibody production, 363–377. *See also* Autoantibodies, anti-idiotypic
  circulating complexes with idiotypes, 373–374
  cross-reactivity of, 248–256
  to hormones and receptors, 240–247
  and IgE responses in BALB/c mice, 330–344, 373
  to immunoglobulins, 327
  to insulin, 245, 251–254
  interactions with hormone receptors, 241–242
  interactions with idiotypic antibodies, 245

  mimicking actions of hormones, 245, 253–254
  to retinol-binding protein antibodies, 248–249
  to 17.5.5E, 307, 308–309
  3I reactivity with anti-dsDNA antibodies, 382–384
Arsonate system
  antibodies with cross-reactive idiotype, in BALB/c mice, 257–264
  idiotype suppression in, maternal-fetal transfer of, 40–47
  shared idiotypy with DNP-binding antibodies in BALB/c mice, 282–289
  silent idiotypes induced in, 4
  structural studies of idiotypy in, 48–64
  studies with monoclonal antibodies, 9–15
Autoantibodies
  anti-allotype, in allotype-suppressed rabbits, 84–93
  anti-idiotypic, 363–377
    age affecting, 27–29
    artifically induced, 16–18
    characterization of, 165–166
    compared to isologous anti-idiotypic reagents, 17
    cycling of responses in, 21–22, 25
    naturally occurring, 18–25, 255
    and reversible suppression of responses, 22, 26
    and sensitivity of idiotopes to reducing agents, 19, 23
  to renal tubular basement membrane, 364–365
  to thyroglobulin, 365–368

B cells
  antibody-specific regulation of responses in, 177–188
    and generation of refractory B cells, 180–186
  bearing IdXL, 201–202
  developmental stages in, 130–131
  expanded precursor-cell clones, 135, 136
  expansion of, and role of regulatory idiotopes, 311
  Ia antigens of, 230–239
  idiotype recognition by, 65, 70
  inducing idiotype suppression, 41, 43
  interaction with T cells, 81, 126, 129, 149
    MHC restriction of, 180
    MM60-defined, 166, 167

389

B cells *(continued)*
  prereceptor, 131–137
  regulation by anti-idiotypic T-suppressor
    systems, 81
  responses to 2,4-DNP, 132
  responses to 4-hydroxy-3-nitrophenyl-
    acetyl, 134–135
  responses to influenza virus hemagglutin-
    in, 132–133
    inhibition of, 179
  responses to phosphorylcholine, 133–134
  specificity repertoire of, 130–139
  tolerance susceptibility of, 131, 136
Bacterial levan, antibody response to, 97–108,
  290–295
Bee-venom protein, antibodies to, 344
Benzylpenicilloyl, IgE response to, 330–344,
  373
Bi-directional immune responses, 317–323
BisQ antibodies, anti-idiotypic antibodies
  against, 245

Carrier effect, and regulation of IgE
  response, 333–336
Cascade, immunization, 3–4, 11, 13
Catecholamines, internal image of, 240–247
Cellular interaction molecules, 206
  and immunologic tolerance, 215
Clonal selection theory, 1
Contrasuppression, blocked by antisera to
  tumors, 215–216
Contrasuppressor cells, 201
Cross-reactive idiotypes (IdX), 3, 6, 9
  of anti-arsonate antibodies induced in
    BALB/c mice, 257–264
  of antibodies to influenza virus hemagglu-
    tinin, 356–361
  in anti-dextran system, 220
  heterogeneity of, 151–170
  in IghC^b mice, 296–301
  of anti-dsDNA antibodies from lupus
    patients, 383–384
  of anti-immunoglobulins, 324–328
  major idiotype CRI$_A$
    hybridoma products of, 9, 40
    structural studies of, 49–53
    suppression in mothers and offspring, 40–
      47
  minor idiotype CRI$_C$ in BALB/c mice, 40,
    57
  sharing of markers
    by anti-allotype antibodies, 198, 313–316
    by arsonate- and DNP-binding antibod-
      ies, 285–287
    by influenza virus hemagglutinin anti-
      bodies, 357

α1–3 Dextran
  monoclonal antibodies to, 151–170
  response induction in IghC^b mice, 296–304
  response induction in maternally suppressed
    mice, 220–229
Diabetes, antibodies to insulin receptors in,
  254
Diazophenylphosphorylcholine, affinity of
  variant antibodies for, 173
Dihydroalprenolol, binding to β-adrenergic
  receptors, inhibited by Ab$_2$ antibodies, 242
2,4-Dinitrophenyl
  antibodies sharing idiotypy with arsonate-
    binding antibodies in BALB/c mice,
    282–289
  B-cell responses to, 132
    inhibition of, 177–179
DNA, double-stranded, antibodies to, in lupus
  erythematosus, 379–385

Egg-white lysozyme, antibodies to
  epitope specificities of, 148–149
  heavy chain variable regions of, 144–147
  overlap patterns of, 142
  public idiotype of, 140–150
  secondary response, 140
    as Ab$_3$ stage, 198–199
Epitopes
  I region-controlled, associated with T-cell
    factors, 192–193
  specificities of antibodies to egg-white lyso-
    zyme, 148–149
Expansion
  of B cells
    in precursor-cell clones, 135, 136
    and role of regulatory idiotopes, 311
  of self-restricted T-cell population, 272

Gene complements, immunoglobulin, and
  latent allotypes, 114
Genic conversion, 6
  and anti-arsonate response in wrong
    allotype mice, 297
Germ-line encoded antibodies, 3, 6, 104
  affinities of, 171–176
  bearing predominant cross-reactive idio-
    type, 49, 53
  in Id$^{36-60}$ idiotype families, 59
  lacking predominant cross-reactive idiotype,
    54
  nonbinding to arsonate, 60
  recognition by T cells, 183–184
  variable regions in, 48, 121, 124–125

Glomerulonephritis, immune-complex, 371
Graves' disease, anti-idiotypic antibodies in, 245

H-2 antigen
internal image exhibited by T-helper cells, 276–279
monoclonal antibodies to, 267–268
Heavy-chain variable regions
gene products inhibiting interactions between T-cells, identified by antisera to tumors, 206–219
in germ-line encoded antibodies. See Germ-line encoded antibodies
of monoclonal antibodies to egg-white lysozyme, 144–147
as restricting elements, 193–194
Hen's egg lysozyme. See Egg-white lysozyme, antibodies to
Heteroclicity, in murine responses to nitrophenylacetyl, 121, 135
Heterogeneity
of Ab₂ antibodies, 8
of anti-al antibodies, 313
of antibodies to Ab₃ monoclonal antibodies, 292–295
of arsonate-binding antibodies with cross-reactive idiotypes, 49–53
of autoantibodies, 372
of I-region antigens on T cells, 192
idiotopic, of T15-positive lymphocytes, 31–33
idiotypic, analysis of, 151–170
of T15 antibodies to phosphorylcholine, 37
of 3I reactive anti-dsDNA antibodies in lupus patients, 384
Histocompatibility complex
antibodies to, idiotypes of, 265–271
and interactions between T cells and B cells, 180
internal images of antigens, 272–281
products as cellular interaction molecules, 206
restriction
and B-cell activation, 238
and predominance in IdX systems, 200, 203
and T-cell recognition of antigen, 194
Hormones
action mimicked by anti-idiotypic antibodies, 245, 253–254
interaction with receptors, 240–245
Hybridoma proteins
of cross-reactive idiotypes (CRI_A), 9, 40
rabbit-mouse, 114–116
structural studies of, in arsonate system, 48–64

T cell, 190
2D3, 9–15
expression of idiotope in BALB/c mice, 11–12
recognition of HP 36.65 and R 16.7, 10, 15
suppression of idiotope expression in A/J mice, 10–11
36–60
and antibody responses to arsonate and DNP, 285–287
antiserum to, 57
unrecognized by 2D3, 10
4-Hydroxy-3-nitrophenylacetyl
B-cell responses to, 134–135
inhibition of, 179
murine responses to, 121, 125–126, 135
Hypercycle, immune, 1–2
Hyperimmunization
and antibody response to bacterial levan, 99
and maternal-fetal transfer of idiotypic suppression, 40–47
Hypersensitivity
delayed-type, suppression by T-suppressor cells, 74–82
immediate-type allergic diseases, 330–345

I region-controlled determinants, 189–197
Ia antigens, B-cell, 230–239
Idiotopes, 2
expression regulated by anti-idiotope antibodies, 121–127
heterogeneity in splenic foci, 160–165
regulatory, 2, 198–204
and reaction of Ab₄ with Ab₁, 319
and response to autoantigens, 372
and response to bovine serum albumin, 311
Idiotypes
antibodies to. See Anti-idiotypic antibodies
of antibodies to MHC, 265–271
of anti-immunoglobulins, 324–328
circulating complexes with anti-idiotype antibodies, 373–374
cross-reactive, 3, 6, 9. See also Cross-reactive idiotypes
enhancement of expression, 127
expression in myeloma cells, 346–355
heterogeneity of, 151–170
IdXL, 140, 198
in network hypothesis, 2, 6
polymorphism of, 104
predominant, 140, 198
regulatory, 104
repertoires of, 3
in different species, 5
restricted specificities of, 9

Idiotypes *(continued)*
  shared
    in anti-allotype antibodies, 198, 313–316
    in antibodies to influenza virus hemagglu-
      tinin, 357
    between arsonate-binding and DNP-
      binding antibodies in BALB/c mice,
      282–289
  silent, induction of, 1–8, 11–13
    in arsonate system, 4
    in irradiated rabbits, 5
    rabbit idiotypes induced in mice, 4–5
  suppression of, 3
    maternal-fetal transfer of, 40–47
Idiotypic antibodies, interacting with anti-idiotypic antibodies, 245
Immune-complex glomerulonephritis, 371
Immunization cascade, 3–4, 11, 13
Immunoglobulins
  affinities affected by somatic mutation,
    171–176
  allotypes in rabbits, 109–120
  antibodies to, 324–328
    Po proteins of, 325, 327
    Wa proteins of, 325–327, 328
  gene complement of, and latent allotypes,
    114
  idiotype heterogeneity in splenic foci, 160–
    165
  idiotypes expressed on, 330
  IgE antibody responses, 330–345, 373
  immunoregulation of synthesis, 84–96
Influenza virus
  anti-influenza hybridomas, 176
  B-cell responses to, 132–133
    inhibition of, 179
  clonal responses to hemagglutinin, 356–361
Insulin antibodies, and synthesis of anti-idiotype antibodies, 245, 251–254
Interleukin 2, secretion by activated T cells,
  276
Internal images in immune system, 5, 8, 93, 94,
  150, 282
  and Ab$_2$ antibodies, 198
  of anti-17.5.5E, 310
  of catecholamines, 240–247
  in I region, T cells as, 196
  of MHC antigens, 272–281
  responses to, 322

J558 idiotype
  expression by maternally suppressed mice,
    220–229
  monoclonal antibodies to, 153, 156
  IdX Dex specificity of, 297

Kidney tubular basement membrane, antibodies to, 364–365

Latent allotypes, 109–114
  and bi-directional immune responses, 319–
    320
  control of expression of, 110–114
  and immunoglobulin gene complement, 114
  induction by anti-allotype injection, 112,
    113
  structural studies of, 110
Levan, bacterial, antibody response to, 97–
  108, 290–295
Lupus erythematosus, antibodies to double-
  stranded DNA in, 379–385
Lymphocyte activation, in immune response,
  2. *See also* B cells; T cells
Lysozyme system. *See* Egg-white lysozyme,
  antibodies to

M167 idiotype, recognition by T-helper
  cells, 68
M316 secretion, inhibition of, 348–352
Maternal-fetal transfer
  of allotype suppression, 88–93
  and genetic control of activation of A48Id
    silent clones, 102, 104–105
  of idiotypes, 23
  of idiotypic suppression state, 40–47
    and expression of J558 idiotype on lym-
      phocytes, 220–229
Memory B-cell responses, and antibody-specific regulatory function, 177, 186
Methylcholanthrene-induced sarcoma antigens, related to Igh-V-linked T-cell
  interaction molecules, 206–219
Micrococcus antigen, anti-idiotypic antibodies
  to, 5
Minigene hypothesis, 6
Monoclonal antibodies. *See also* Hybridoma
  proteins
  anti-idiotype
    in analysis of idiotypic heterogeneity,
      151–170
    biological activities of, 159–160
    epitope specificity of, 155–156
  arsonate-binding, structural studies of, 49–
    58
  characteristics of 17.5.5E, 307–308
  to double-stranded DNA, in lupus erythe-
    matosus, 379–385
  to egg-white lysozyme, 140
  14-4-4 system, 266–267
  GB4–10 compared to MM60, 166
  to H-2 antigens, 267–268

to I region products on T cells, 190–191
to idiotopes
    regulatory influence of, 121–123, 125–127
    of T15 idiotype, 31–33
to immunoglobulins, 325
to influenza virus hemagglutinin, 356
nonbinding of arsonate by, 59–63
MOPC-104E, monoclonal antibodies to, 153, 156
MOPC-315 cells, 346–355
MOPC-460 idiotype system, 4, 15
    and antibody responses to arsonate and DNP, 285–287
Multi-specific antibodies to bovine serum albumin, 305–312
Mutations, somatic
    and antibody affinity, 171–176
    in B-cell differentiation, 165
Myasthenia gravis, anti-idiotypic antibodies in, 245
Myeloma cells, idiotype expression in, 346–355

Neonatal suppression
    and activation of autologous T cells, 34–36
    and anti-dextran antibody responses, 160
    and factors transmitted in milk, 45–46, 227
    idiotype expression in, 45
    and regulatory influence of anti-idiotope monoclonal antibodies, 125–126
Neonatal treatment with A48Id, and activation of silent clones, 102, 105
Nephritis, tubulointerstitial, autoantibodies in, 364–365
Networks, immune, 2, 6, 13
    and allotype suppression, 84–96
    and auto-anti-idiotypic responses, 18
    and B-cell repertoire expression, 136
    bi-directional concept of, 317–323
    idiotype-specific T-helper cells in, 65–73
    relationship of antibodies in, 318
    and structural studies of idiotypy in arsonate system, 48–64

Ovalbumin
    IgE response to, 332, 336
    IgG response to, 333, 335
    and T-helper cells recognizing Ia on B-cell surface, 231–233

Phosphorylcholine
    affinity of variant antibodies for, 173
    B-cell responses to, 133–134
        Ia antigens affecting, 230–239
        inhibition of, 179

and idiotype-specific T-helper cells, 67–71
IgE response to, 330–344, 373
internal image exhibited by anti-T15 T-helper cells, 275–276
monoclonal antibodies to, 151–170
Prealbumin, binding sites for retinol-binding protein, 249–251
Predominant idiotypes
    IdXL, 140, 198
    and regulatory idiotypes, 198–204
    single or multiple, 199–200

Rabbit idiotypes induced in mice, 4–5
Rabbit-mouse hybridomas, 114–116
Receptors
    hormone interactions with, 240–245
    insulin, anti-idiotypic antibodies interacting with, 252–253
Regulatory idiotopes. See Idiotopes, regulatory
Regulatory idiotypes, 104
Regulatory T cells
    induction by anti-idiotope antibodies, 126
    and secretion of M315, 352
Restriction
    MHC
        and B-cell activation, 238
        and predominance in IdX systems, 200, 203
        and T-cell interactions with B cells, 180
        and T-cell recognition of antigen, 194
        self-restricted repertoire of T-helper cells, 272–281
Retinol-binding protein antibodies
    anti-idiotypic antibodies to, 248–249
    reactivity with prealbumin binding sites, 250–251
Rheumatoid factor idiotypes, 324–328

Self recognition, 6
Self-restricted repertoire of T-helper cells, 272–281
Shared idiotypes
    in anti-allotype antibodies, 198, 313–316
    in antibodies to influenza virus hemagglutinin, 357
    between arsonate- and DNP-binding antibodies in BALB/c mice, 285–287
Silent idiotypes
    activation of A48Id, genetic control of, 97–108
    induction of, 1–8, 11–13
Somatic mutation
    and antibody affinity, 171–176
    in B-cell differentiation, 165

Specificity
  in antibody-specific regulation of B-cell responses, 177–188
  of B-cell repertoire, 130–139
Splenic foci, idiotope heterogeneity of immunoglobulins in, 160–165
Structural studies of idiotypy, in arsonate system, 48–64
  in antibodies bearing predominant cross-reactive idiotype, 49–53
  in antibodies failing to bind arsonate, 59–63
  in antibodies lacking predominant cross-reactive idiotype, 54–56
  in antibodies of second idiotype family, 57–59
Suppression
  of allotypes, induction of, 84–96
  antigen-specific T-suppressor systems, 74–82
  of autoantibody production, by anti-idiotype treatment, 373
  of auto-anti-idiotypic antibody responses, 22, 26
  of B-cell responses, by T cells, 177–188
  of dextran responsiveness in maternally suppressed mice, 220–229
  of idiotypes, 3
  maternal-fetal transfer of, 40–47
  by Ly-1 TsiF, blocked by antisera to tumors, 206–219
Synthetic antigen, inducing T-suppressor systems, 74–82

T cells
  augmenting AgT$_H$ activity, 201
  augmenting factor in, 189–197
  autologous, regulating idiotope expression in T15 complex, 33–39
  bearing IdI, in maternally suppressed mice, 223–226
  helper
    antigen-specific, in lysozyme system, 200–201
    idiotype-specific, 65–73
    ovalbumin-specific, 231–233
    recognition of B-cell Ia antigens, 231
    recognition of IdXL, 199
    recognition of T15 idiotype, 67–71, 275–276
    and response to dextran in CB 20 mice, 301
    self-restricted repertoire of, 272–281
  helper-inducer cells in lysozyme system, 201
  hybridomas, 190
  I region-controlled determinants on, 189–197

inducing idiotype suppression, 41–43
interaction with B cells, 81, 126, 129, 149
  MHC restriction of, 180
modulatory cells, 77–79, 81–82
regulatory
  induction by anti-idiotope antibodies, 126
  and secretion of M315, 352
replacing factor, in reconstitution of idiotype clones, 238
suppressing B-cell responses, 177–188
  and generation of refractory B cells, 180–186
suppressor
  antigen-specific, 74–82, 189–197
  bearing IdXL, relation to B cells with similar idiotype, 201–202
  and predominance in IdX systems, 203–204
suppressor inducer factor
  blocked by antisera to tumors, 206–219
  two chains of, 213, 214
T15 system
  antibodies to
    and function of antibody-recognizing T cells, 184
    and IgE production, 332
  antigenic complexity of, 31–33, 37
  and B-cell clonal antibody product, 134
  expanded anti-T15 B cells, 167
  and Ia antigen expression in B cells, 230–239
  monoclonal anti-idiotypic antibodies reacting to, 156
  recognition by T-helper cells, 67–71, 275–276
Thyroglobulin, autoantibodies to, 365–368
Thyroid disease, Graves, anti-idiotypic antibodies in, 245
TMV, anti-idiotypic antibodies to, 5
Tolerance
  induction in B cells, 131, 136
  and tumor antigen activity, 215
Translocations, and tumor cell activity, 216
Transplantation antigens, 206–219
  gene products on chromosome 12, 211–212, 215, 216, 218
Trimethylammonium
  inducing auto-anti-idiotypic antibodies, 17
  inducing regulatory T-cell populations, 74–82
  inducing T-suppressor systems, 74–82
Trinitrophenyl injections
  in aged mice, 27
  and B-cell response to antigens, 67, 68, 184
Tumor-associated transplantation antigens, 206–219

gene products on chromsome 12, 211–212,
215, 216, 218
Tunicamycin, inhibiting M316 secretion, 350,
351
L-Tyrosine-*p*-azophenyltrimethylammonium,
including regulatory T-cell populations, 74–82

Variant antibodies
affinities affected by somatic mutation,
171–176
and differences in Id expression, 165
recognition by T cells, 183–184
Viruses, influenza. *See* Influenza virus